Y0-EKA-282

Color Atlas and Text of Forefoot Surgery

Edited by

Roger Butterworth, BA, FPodA, MChS, SRCh
*Formerly Head of Northern Ireland
School of Chiropody,
Belfast, Northern Ireland*

Gary L. Dockery, DPM, FACFS
*Seattle Foot and Ankle Clinic,
Seattle, Washington, USA*

Mosby
Year Book

St. Louis   Baltimore   Boston   Chicago   London   Philadelphia   Sydney   Toronto

M Mosby
Year Book

Dedicated to Publishing Excellence

Mosby–Year Book, Inc.
11830 Westline Drive
St. Louis, MO 63146

Copyright © Wolfe Publishing Ltd
All rights reserved.
Published with rights in the USA, Canada and Puerto Rico by Mosby–Year Book, Inc.

ISBN 0-8151-1387-0

English edition first published in 1992 by Wolfe Publishing Ltd,
2–16 Torrington Place, London WC1E 7LT, UK.

All rights reserved. No part of this publication may be reproduced, stored in a retrieval system, or transmitted, in any form or by any means, electronic, mechanical, photocopying, recording, or otherwise, without written permission from the publisher.

Permission to photocopy or reproduce solely for internal or personal use is permitted for libraries or other users registered with the Copyright Clearance Center, provided that the base fee of $4.00 per chapter plus $.10 per page is paid directly to the Copyright Clearance Center, 21 Congress Street, Salem, MA 01970. This consent does not extend to other kinds of copying, such as copying for general distribution, for advertising or promotional purposes, for creating new collected works, or for resale.

Library of Congress Cataloging-in-Publication Data

Butterworth, Roger.
   A colour atlas of forefoot surgery / Roger Butterworth, Gary Dockery.
      p. cm.
   ISBN 0-8151-1387-0
   1. Foot—Surgery—Atlases.   I. Dockery, Gary L. II. Title.
   [DNLM: 1. Forefoot, Human—surgery—atlases.   WE 17 B988c]
RD563.B87 1991
617.5^{1}85059—dc20
DNLM/DLC
for Library of Congress   91-19680
                                                                                                    CIP

Contents

Introduction — 5
Contributors — 6

1 **Principles of Forefoot Plastic Surgery** — 7
   Gary L. Dockery

2 **Local Anaesthetics** — 35
   Roger Butterworth

3 **Nail Surgery** — 65
   Roger Butterworth

4 **Subungual (Periungual) Exostectomy** — 85
   Roger Butterworth

5 **Sesamoidectomy** — 93
   Roger Butterworth

6 **Lesser Metatarsal Surgery** — 111
   Byron L. Hutchinson

7 **Surgery of the Lesser Digits** — 137
   Gerald T. Kuwada

8 **Intermetatarsal Neuromas and Associated Nerve Problems** — 159
   Stephen J. Miller

9 **Soft Tissue Tumours: Diagnosis and Treatment** — 183
   Jeffrey C. Page

10 **Surgical Procedures of the First Ray** — 195
   John M. Schuberth

11 **Surgical Complications of the Forefoot** — 237
   Jeffrey C. Christensen

Index — 259

Introduction

Forefoot surgery, in common with foot care in general, has been a little regarded and, with some notable exceptions, a rather neglected area of medical practice amongst English-speaking peoples. The reasons for this neglect probably relate to the historical disregard of the foot (as with the mouth) by the wider medical profession. The consequence of this lack of interest was an empirical approach to many of the surgical procedures that were used and an outcome that left much to be desired, so that it has only been in the latter half of the twentieth century that forefoot problems have been afforded the attention they deserve.

This still developing interest, together with technological advances, now affords a basis from which to derive a successful surgical treatment for the many previously intractable problems of the forefoot. Many of these procedures remain essentially palliative in nature, but not exclusively so, and perhaps the greatest contribution of the foot surgeon in the latter half of the century will be seen to have been the developments of techniques to restore foot function in the real sense of the word.

This atlas is written primarily for chiropodists and podiatrists, but it is hoped that the wider medical community will also find it useful. It does not attempt to be a definitive text but to provide an introduction to successful surgical practice, using plain solutions of local anaesthetics in an outpatient clinic. The procedures described are all widely practised and have proved reliable and effective in resolving particular conditions.

It is implicit in much of the book that the practitioner will have assessed the underlying pathomechanics of the deformity to be treated at the time of their systemic evaluation of the patient, and that where necessary the orthotic control of the patient's foot, so essential to the post-operative success, will have been achieved.

Originally this atlas was planned as an introduction to surgical techniques for chiropodists and podiatrists in the United Kingdom. Only at a later stage was the proposal made to expand its contents to include some of the techniques being practised in North America, and I am greatly indebted to Gary Dockery and his colleagues for their major contributions to this text. The authority of their contributions evidences to their pre-eminence. I would also wish to thank Dr Kate McClelland for her contribution to the pharmacology of local anaesthetics; my colleagues Steven Urry and Bryan Nelson for their assistance in the production of the illustrations; and Geoff Hannam for much of the photography.

ROGER BUTTERWORTH

The idea for this book came from my friend, colleague, and co-editor, Roger Butterworth. It was originally planned to be a primer for students of the lower extremities and eventually was scheduled for an expanded version. When Mr Butterworth invited me to join in the project, it was an even bigger idea of making the book an atlas of forefoot surgery. As the US editor, I was given the opportunity to invite contributors to write about selected topics in forefoot surgery. From the list of US authors, it can be seen that this task was accomplished by having well-known and outstanding members of the Northwest Podiatric Foundation for Education and Research contribute chapters on their favourite topics. This created a combination of UK and US contributors discussing topics related to the foot in a manner that is enjoyable, as well as enlightening.

This is not a major reference textbook and the references chosen for each of the chapters were done so accordingly. This text is, however, written for students, house officers, teachers, and clinicians who find that foot care must be learned by caring for patients and sharing with colleagues. It is designed to be carried to the clinical setting and used to instruct patients and students: share with peers and review the concepts contained within.

I would like to thank Mr Butterworth for asking me to assist him in this endeavour. I would also like to acknowledge all of the contributors to this text. I respect you all for sharing your time and knowledge with others.

GARY L. DOCKERY

Contributors

Roger F. Butterworth, BA, FPodA, MChS, SRCh
Formerly Head of Northern Ireland School of Chiropody, Belfast, Northern Ireland; Chairman, Faculty of Surgery, Society of Chiropodists, London; Consultant Podiatrist, School of Surgical Chiropody, Cork, Republic of Ireland; Private practice, Belfast, Northern Ireland, Dundalk and Galway, Republic of Ireland.

Jeffrey C. Christensen, DPM, FACFS
Fellow, American College of Foot Surgeons; Diplomate, American Board of Podiatric Surgery; Director of Research, Northwest Podiatric Foundation for Education and Research; Assistant Residency Director, Waldo Podiatric Residency Training Program, Fifth Avenue Hospital, Seattle, Washington, USA; Private practice, Ankle and Foot Clinic of Everett, Washington, USA.

Gary L. Dockery, DPM, FACFS
Fellow, American College of Foot Surgeons; Diplomate, American Board of Podiatric Surgery; Diplomate, American Board of Podiatric Orthopedics; Distinguished Practitioner, National Academies of Practice, Podiatric Medicine and Surgery; Chairman and Founder, Northwest Podiatric Foundation for Education and Research; Former Director of Podiatric Education and Residency Training, Waldo Podiatric Residency Program, Fifth Avenue Hospital, Seattle, Washington, USA; Private practice, Seattle Foot and Ankle Clinic, Seattle, Washington, USA.

Byron L. Hutchinson, DPM, FACFS
Fellow, American College of Foot Surgeons; Diplomate, American Board of Podiatric Surgery; Podiatric Advisor, Northwest Podiatric Foundation for Education and Research, Seattle, Washington, USA; Director of Podiatric Education and Residency Training, Waldo Podiatric Residency Training Program, Fifth Avenue Hospital, Seattle, Washington, USA; Private practice, Highline Foot and Ankle Clinic, Burien, Washington, USA.

Gerald T. Kuwada, DPM, FACFS
Fellow, American College of Foot Surgeons; Fellow, American College of Foot Orthopedics; Diplomate, American Board of Podiatric Surgery; Diplomate, American Board of Podiatric Orthopedics; Distinguished Practitioner, National Academies of Practice, Podiatric Medicine and Surgery; Board of Directors and Co-Founder, Northwest Podiatric Foundation for Education and Research, Seattle, Washington, USA; Private practice, Valley Podiatric Clinic, Renton, Washington, USA.

Steven J. Miller, DPM, FACFS
Fellow, American College of Foot Surgeons; Diplomate, American Board of Podiatric Surgery; Board of Trustees, Northwest Podiatric Foundation for Education and Research; President, Washington State Podiatric Medical Association (1989–91), Seattle, Washington, USA; Private practice, Anacortes, Washington, USA.

Jeffrey C. Page, DPM, FACFS
Fellow, American College of Foot Surgeons; Diplomate, American Board of Podiatric Surgery; Podiatric Advisor, Northwest Podiatric Foundation for Education and Research, Seattle, Washington, USA; Associate Professor, Podiatric Surgery, and Associate Dean for Clinical Affairs, California College of Podiatric Medicine, San Francisco, California, USA.

John M. Schuberth, DPM, FACFS
Fellow, American College of Foot Surgeons; Diplomate, American Board of Podiatric Surgery; Podiatric Advisor, Northwest Podiatric Foundation for Education and Research, Seattle, Washington, USA; Department of Orthopedics/Podiatric Surgery, Kaiser Foundation Hospital, San Francisco, California, USA.

1 Principles of forefoot plastic surgery

GARY L. DOCKERY

Introduction

Until recently, the importance of plastic surgery techniques had been underemphasized in the teaching of surgery of the lower extremity. In the past, most attention was spent on the design of the osseous procedures, the overall correction of the deformity, and the utilization of specialized equipment. Frequently, the planning and design of the incisional approach and the final skin closure was poorly thought-out.

Planning of the surgical incision is the first step necessary to achieve a favourable outcome. This planning must include a complete knowledge of the skin and the principles of wound healing. Understanding how to manipulate the skin incision to obtain better surgical exposure, cover larger defects, and correct excessive scarring, is essential to improve results. Even if the incision is well conceived, the suture closure must also be carried out with some purpose. Regulating this task to unskilled trainees or using improper closure techniques are both to be avoided whenever possible.

Because of poor initial planning of the approach and conclusion of the surgical procedure, the final result may be an unsightly, contracted, or painful surgical scar. It is well known that the final scar is the only thing that the patient can really see, except for obvious positional changes, and it is frequently used as an everlasting testimonial to the surgeon's skill.

In this chapter we focus on multiple aspects of plastic surgery principles, ranging from planning of the skin incision to advanced reconstructive techniques of manipulating skin with flaps and grafts.

Basic considerations

The primary physical properties of skin include the viscoelastic components, skin tension, and skin extensibility. The first viscoelastic property is that of creep, which allows the skin to stretch over a period of time as it is being pulled. This principle is important in delayed primary closure techniques. The second viscoelastic principle deals with stress relaxation. This property of skin allows the force required to maintain stretch to gradually decrease over a period of time.[1] Miller points out that this phenomenon may explain why skin that appears to be sutured too tightly at the conclusion of a surgery will usually become relaxed and viable after a few hours.[2]

Skin tension lines are very important in the process of wound healing. If an incision is placed parallel to the skin tension lines, it will heal with minimal scarring. If, however, the incision is perpendicular to the skin tension line, it will be thicker or tend to hypertrophy. The relaxed skin tension lines (RSTL) are found on the lower extremity by simply placing the part in a relaxed attitude by passive positioning or by active manipulation.[3] The RSTL will then appear as a fold or crease in the skin. In areas where the skin is somewhat more taut, the RSTL may be identified simply by gently pinching the skin between the thumb and finger. Pinching the skin in parallel with the RSTL causes even creases to form (**1.1**) and pinching the skin perpendicularly to the RSTL gives rise to limited skin mobility (**1.2**).

Skin extensibility refers to the adaptability of the skin, which allows it to move and be manipulated to an extended or stretched attitude and then return to a fully relaxed state. This elasticity effect tends to decrease with age and other conditions that deplete the overall elastic fibre network of skin. Older patients tend to show decreased extensibility and increased laxity, and this inability to rebound or adapt to surrounding stresses gives rise to increased wrinkles and sagging of the skin. The end result is that this decrease in normal skin elasticity and extensibility allows for decreased wound tension and therefore fine, subtle, and thin scars.

1.1 Pinching the skin in parallel with the RSTL causes furrows or creases to form.

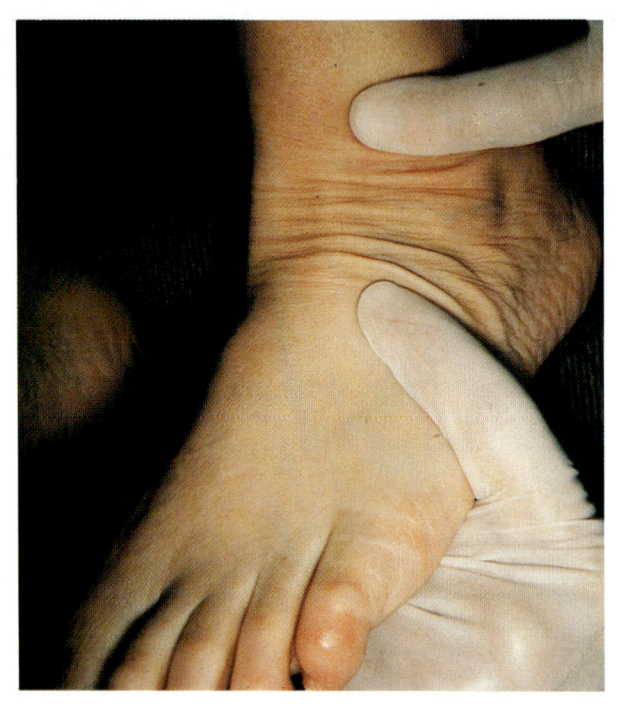

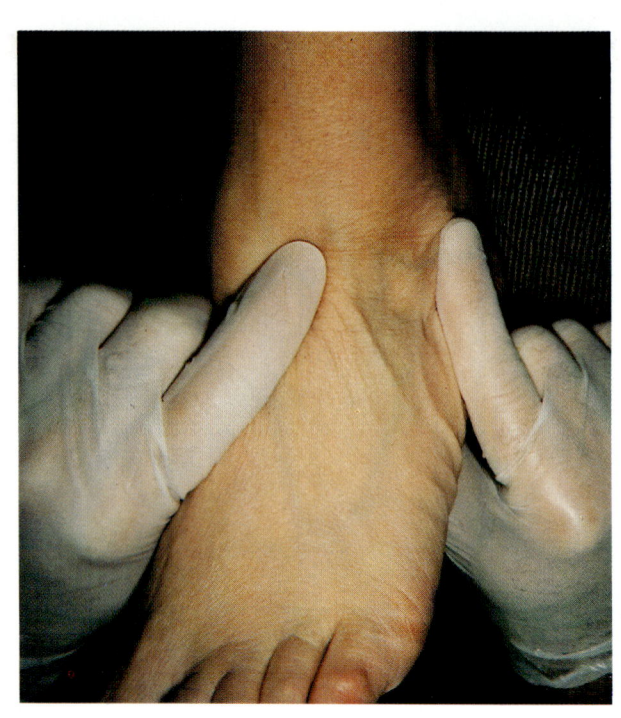

1.2 Pinching the skin perpendicularly to the direction of the RSTL gives rise to limited skin mobility.

Handling of tissues

The general principle of tissue handling is very simple: be gentle. This includes the initial approach of injecting the area, marking the skin, making the incision, and the careful use of instrumentation. Generally, the less the tissue is handled, the better. The use of gauze sponges should be limited and, when used, the mechanism should be one of dabbing the wound rather than wiping or rubbing.

Keeping the tissue layers moist is very important, and the use of cool sterile flush and suction should replace frequent swabbing of the wound. When sterile flush is used, it should be gently applied since forceful sprays of solution may spread tissue layers and cause tissue emphysema. This forceful flushing technique is reserved for wound irrigation in the presence of debris or infection.

The use of skin retractors is recommended in place of handling the tissues with forceps or pick-ups. Tissue forceps should gently retract the tissue layers rather than grabbing or squeezing them. Other instruments, such as clamps and retractors, should be used sparingly, as should the use of electrocautery and sutures. When retractors are used, we recommend manual hand-held instruments rather than self-retaining retractors (**1.3**). Blunt or sharp skin hooks and retractors may be utilized gently for adequate opening of incisions (**1.4**). These instruments should be relocated on slightly different areas of the incision during the procedure to prevent pressure damage to the skin, which is a serious problem with the self-retaining type of retractors. The techniques of incision closure will be discussed later on.

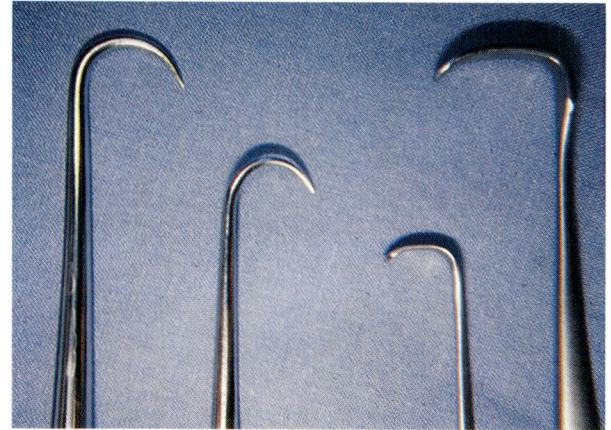

1.3 Blunt and sharp skin hooks and retractors.

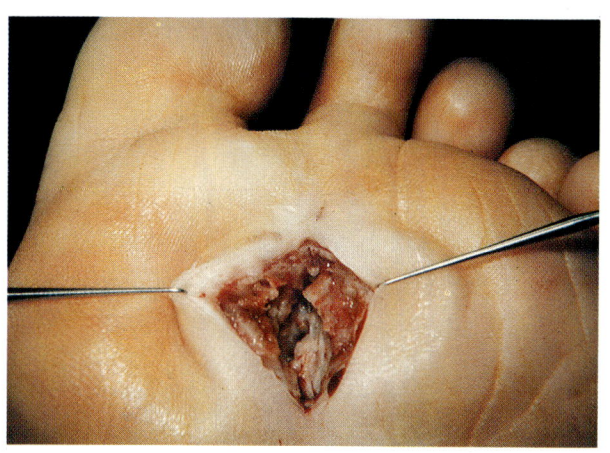

1.4 Retraction on the skin should be gentle. The correct technique (left retractor) lifts the skin edge up and allows better visualization and undermining. The right retractor is depressing the skin edge and placing undue tension on the skin.

Planning the incision

Before the actual skin incision is made, consideration must be given to the underlying anatomical structures. This is usually termed 'surgical anatomy', which refers to the vital structures that will be encountered during the surgical exposure time. The utilization of the skin scribe marker is very important in planning accurate incisions. First, the areas to be avoided may be mapped out with adjacent vital structures outlined. Secondly, the incision itself may be drawn in, which gives the surgeon an opportunity to evaluate its placement before proceeding (**1.5**). Additionally, at our institution, incisions are also frequently marked with crosshatch lines to facilitate accurate final skin closure (**1.6**). This is much more important in planning nonlinear incisions. Using the back of a scalpel blade to 'scratch' the skin to mark out the incision is not recommended because of the damaged done to the epidermal layer. Ideally, the best locations for elective incisions are within the natural flexion and extension creases (parallel to the RSTL) or at right angles to the direction of muscle pull. In the foot and ankle, it is sometimes difficult to gain full exposure to the surgical site by strictly following these guidelines and, at times, it may be necessary to create better exposure and risk a heavier scar. When this is

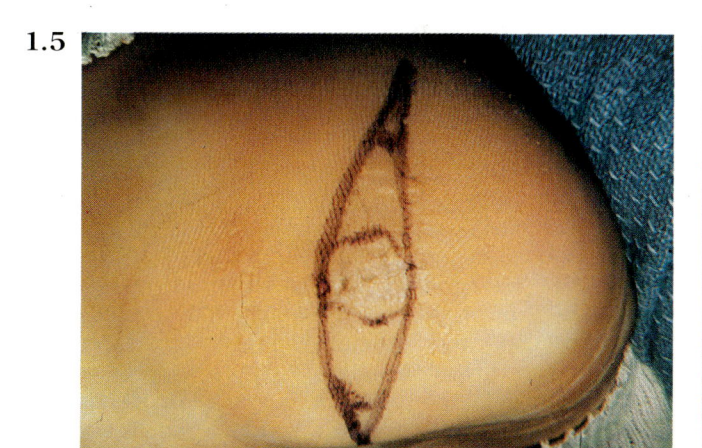

1.5 Skin marker lines drawn out to plan the surgical approach.

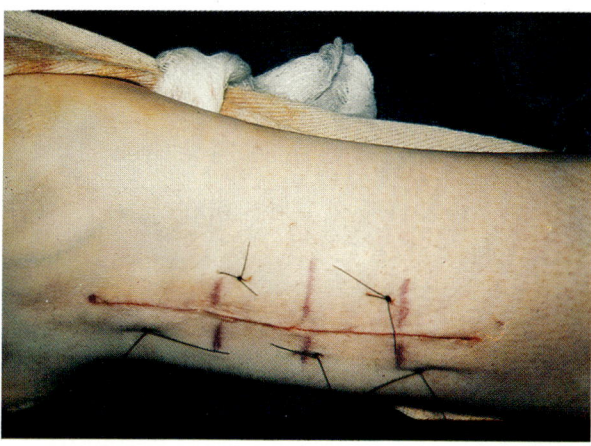

1.6 Skin incision showing crosshatch skin marker lines to help reapproximate the edges.

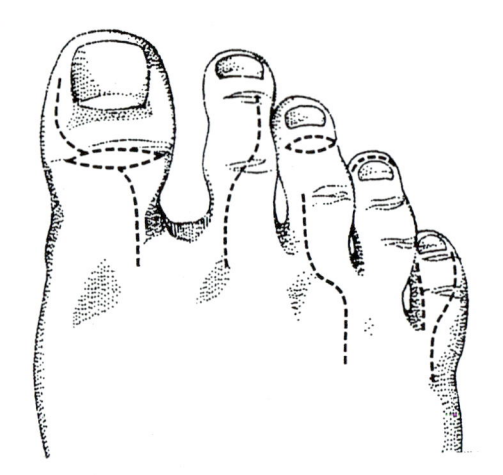

1.7 The utilization of curvilinear or S-shaped incisions on the foot help to gain better exposure and decrease scar contracture. (Redrawn from Miller[2], with permission.)

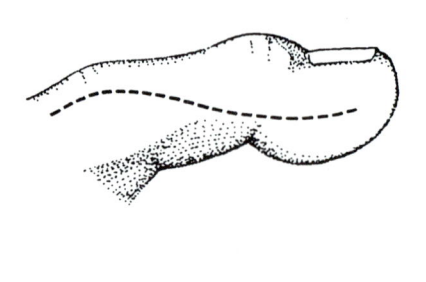

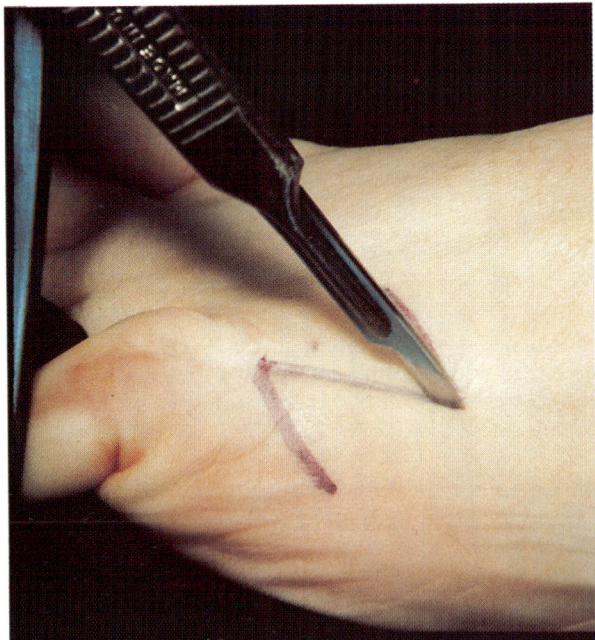

1.8 Starting and finishing the incision with the tip or point of the scalpel blade adds precision and control.

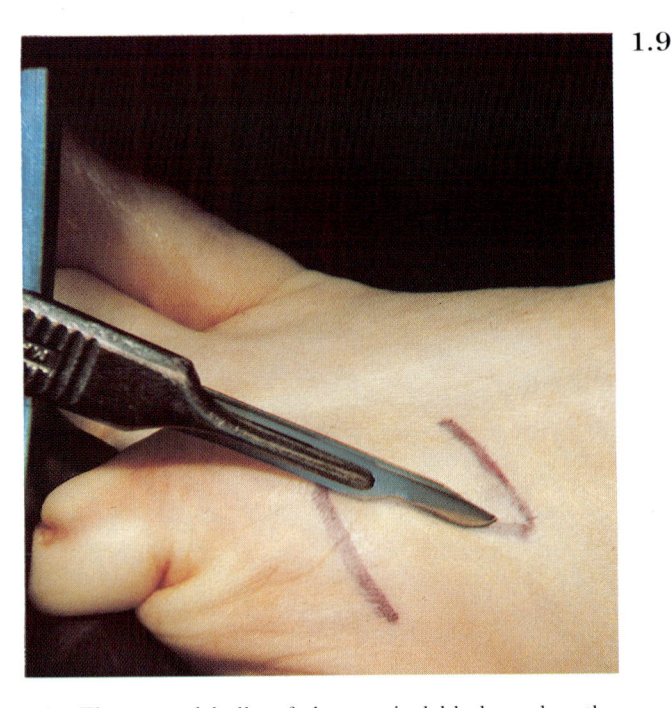

1.9 The curved belly of the surgical blade makes the most efficient skin incision.

done, it is advisable to utilize a curvilinear or S-shaped incision (**1.7**).

The initial skin incision is made with either a No. 15 or No. 10 surgical blade: the No. 15 blade being preferred around the forefoot region and the No. 10 blade around the hindfoot area. The incision is initiated with the tip or point of the blade (**1.8**), and then the surgical scalpel is held in such a manner as to allow the cutting edge of the blade (the belly curve) to contact the skin. The incision is finished again with the tip of the blade (**1.9**). Performing the entire incision with the tip or point of the blade is very inefficient and allows for variability in the depth of the incision.

There is a tradition that the skin blade should be replaced with a new 'deep blade', so that there is no cross-contamination of the deep tissue layer with potential bacteria from the skin blade. However, this is not necessary.[4,5] The primary reason for changing the surgical blade is when it becomes slightly dull: frequent changing of surgical blades during a procedure assures smoother cuts and increases the surgeon's control of the incisions during the case. A dull surgical blade tends to cause the surgeon to press harder on the scalpel and increases the risk of slipping or cutting adjacent tissues.

Once the incision is initiated, it should be completed

through the epidermis and a portion of the dermis in one smooth deliberate stroke, with the blade perpendicular to the skin. A scived or bevelled incision should be avoided at all times since this type of incision is more difficult to close, the skin edge is more likely to necrose, and there is a greater chance for unsightly scarring to occur (**1.10**). The first incision should not completely penetrate the deep dermis (except in those areas where there are no underlying neurovascular structures of any concern). A second incision is then made through the dermal layer to expose the underlying dermal and subdermal vessels. The small skin-edge vessels are not ligated or coagulated, but are simply controlled by local pressure. At this level, it is also very important that no undermining or undercutting of the skin is performed.

A long, smooth continuous stroke of the surgical blade is essential to obtain the best incision. An incision composed of multiple short stabs or slices is one that produces a considerable amount of damage and results in ragged and uneven edges that the body will have to try to repair during the healing process. The primary difference between these two incisional approaches is usually one of confidence of the surgeon and knowledge of the surgical procedure and the surgical anatomy involved.

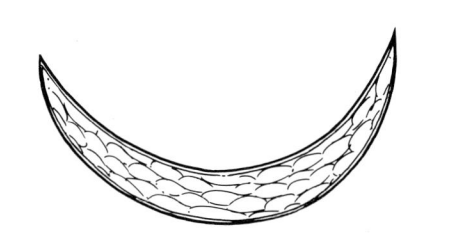

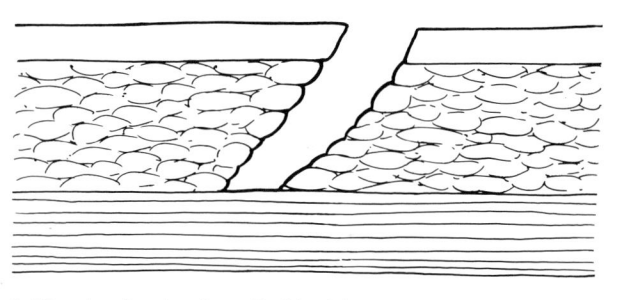

1.10 A scived or bevelled incision causes greater dermis injury and, when repaired, has an increased chance for necrosis and uneven scar formation.

1.11 Closure of a semicircular flap laceration (scived incision). Incorrect closure of a bevelled incision may result in a 'toilet seat' skin deformity. Correct preparation of the incision ensures a nicer scar.

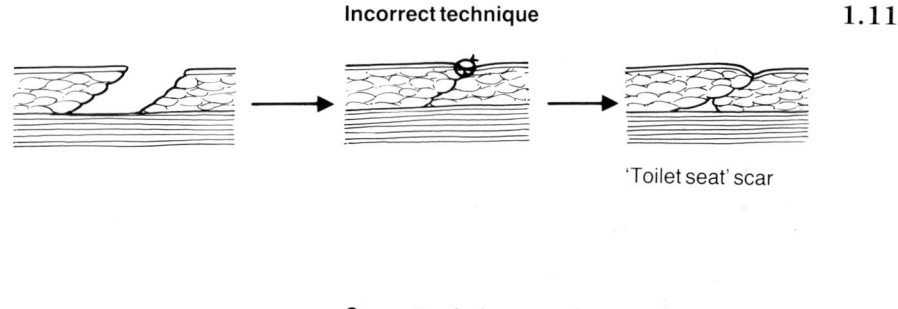

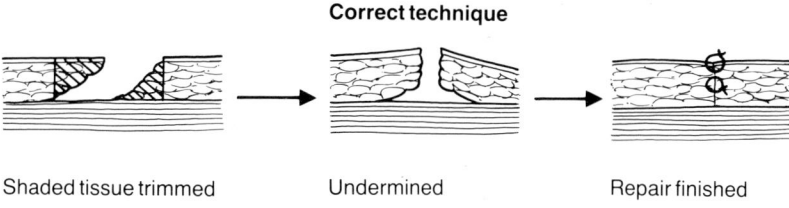

Incorrect technique

'Toilet seat' scar

Correct technique

Shaded tissue trimmed Undermined Repair finished

The deeper layer incision, through the subcutaneous tissue layer, will now expose the larger vascular structures, which should be identified and retracted, or isolated, clamped and either ligated or cauterized. Dissection through this region is best performed with blunt tissue scissors rather than with the surgical blade.

Once the subcutaneous layer has been opened, the skin can be safely undermined below this layer without much damage to the circulation of the overlying skin.

If the skin incision has been made on a bias or scived at an angle, it will be necessary to repair this prior to final closure (**1.11**). Trimming of the margins of the

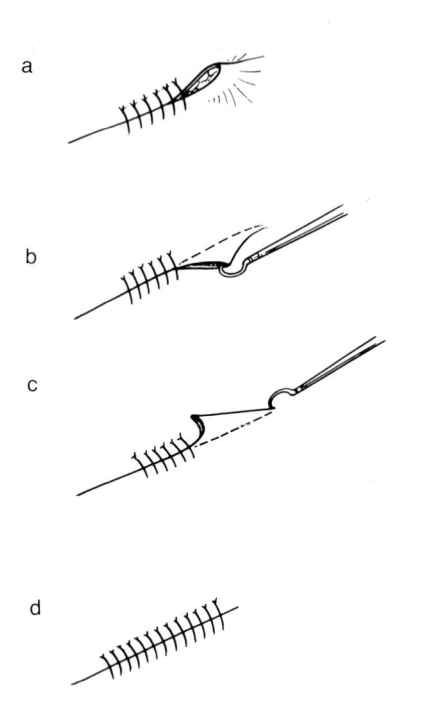

1.12 Correction of 'dog-ear' deformity in skin closure. (*a*) Excessive skin—dog-ear. (*b*) Skin hook to one side; incise, then undermine redundant skin. (*c*) Shift hook to end of new incision; excise overlapping skin. (*d*) Repair finished.

wound is followed by squaring the skin edges and, if necessary, undermining the skin before suturing the layers. This revisional treatment will prevent wound sloughing, excessive scarring, and the formation of the 'toilet seat' scar appearance.

When an incision is closed improperly or when there is excessive skin tissue on one side of the incision, the tissue may bunch-up and cause a 'dog ear' formation. This tissue may be overlapping or underlapping and may cause an unsightly scar to form. In general, it is advisable to remove medium-to-large dog-ear deformities at the time of original skin closure. One technique involves equalizing the arms of the incision by excising a wedge of tissue (**1.12**). When possible, the wedge should be placed in parallel with the relaxed skin tension line.

Special incisions

Z-plasty, V–Y-plasties, and S incisions

The Z-plasty procedure is frequently utilized in my practice and is one of the more useful techniques for tissue rearrangement. It consists mainly of the transposition of two corners of a Z incision, which creates a predictable lengthening effect. This makes the procedure particularly useful in treating linear contracture due to tight skin or scar tissue (**1.13**). The central or straight arm of the Z is placed in the line of contracture, along the previous scar, or in the direction in which increased length is needed. It is highly recommended that the Z-plasty be drawn out on the skin with a marking pencil prior to the incision being performed. The angle of the flaps should be 60°, which ensures sufficient vascular supply to the base of the flaps in most cases, and the arms of the Z should be equal in length (**1.14**). A pre-measured device is very helpful in confirming the proper angles (**1.15**). When the flap is planned properly, there will be an increase in length of 75% when the flap angles are cut at 60° (**1.16**). If the flap angles are smaller, i.e. 30°, then the increase is only 25%. In addition, the longer the length of the arms of the Z-plasty, the larger the overall increase in length.

Once the Z-plasty has been properly designed and the incision completed, the flaps should be adequately and deeply undermined, which enables them to easily transpose without tension (**1.17**, **1.18**). This incisional flap approach may be used over the lesser metatarsals to gain greater surgical exposure, prevent multiple incisions, and at the same time, decrease scar contracture (**1.19**, **1.20**).

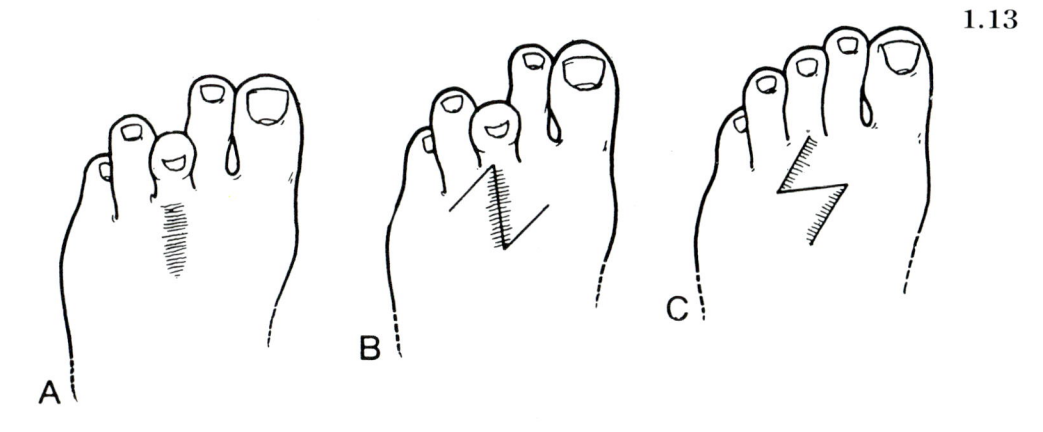

1.13 Use of Z-plasty to gain length and decrease scar contracture.

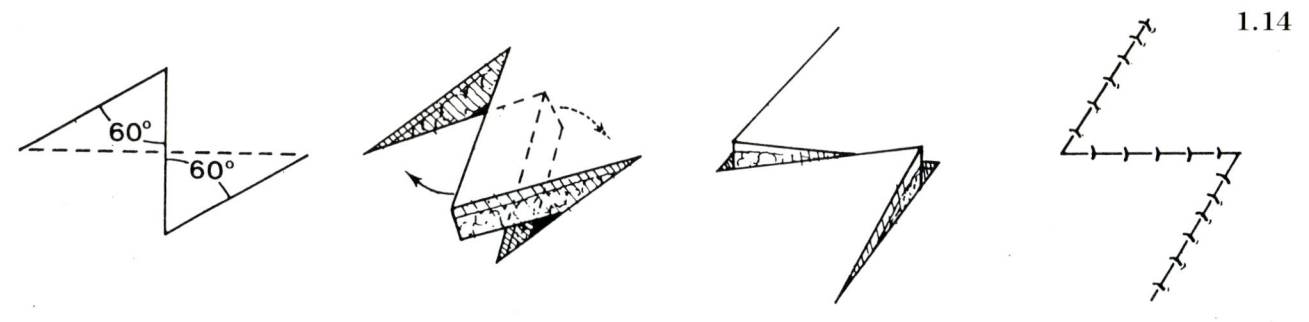

1.14 Creating the Z-plasty with equal-length arms allows proper transposition of the flaps.

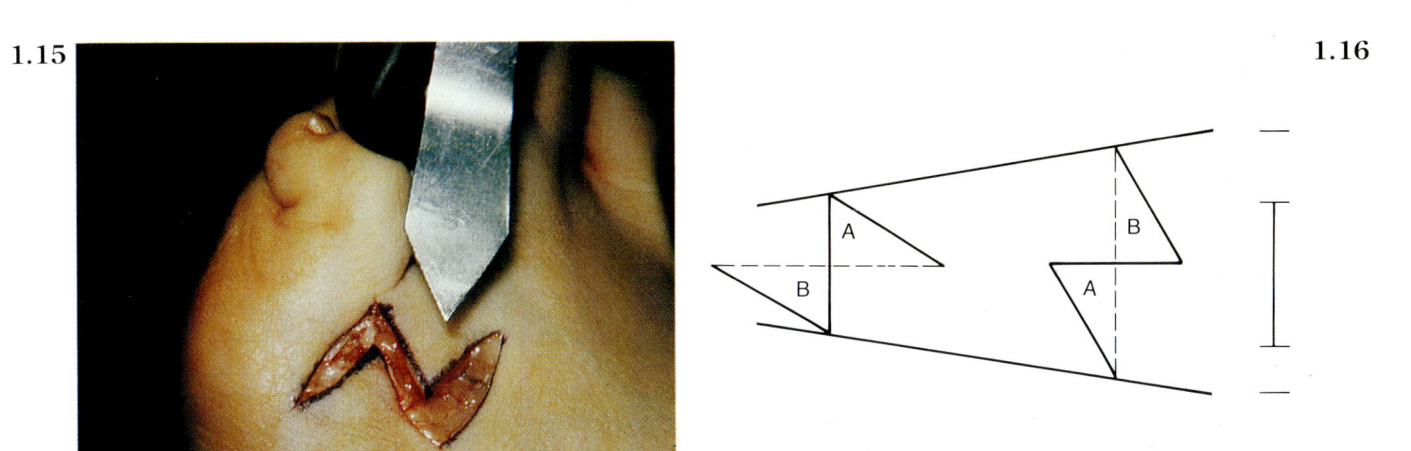

1.15 Using a pre-measured device, with the appropriate 60° angle, helps in making accurate Z-plasty corners.

1.16 An overall increase in length by 75% is achieved when two 60° flaps are transposed.

13

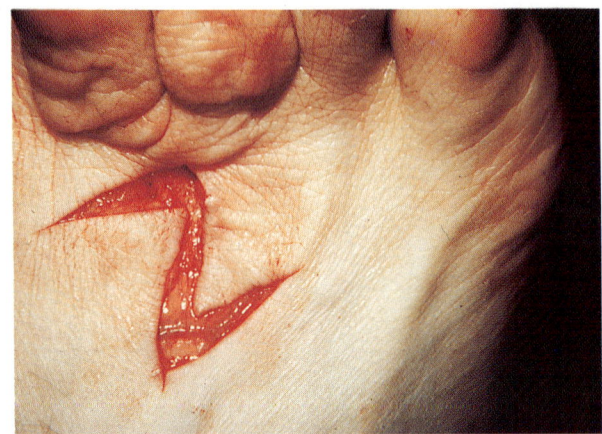

1.17 Correctly placed Z-plasty incision with adequate undermining.

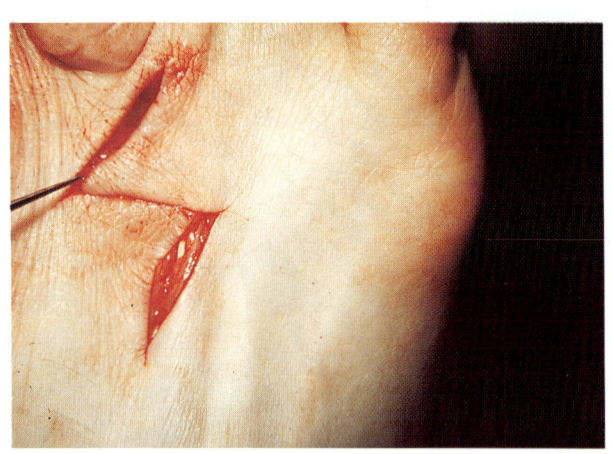

1.18 Transposition of the flaps is easily accomplished without adjacent tension on the skin edges or the flaps.

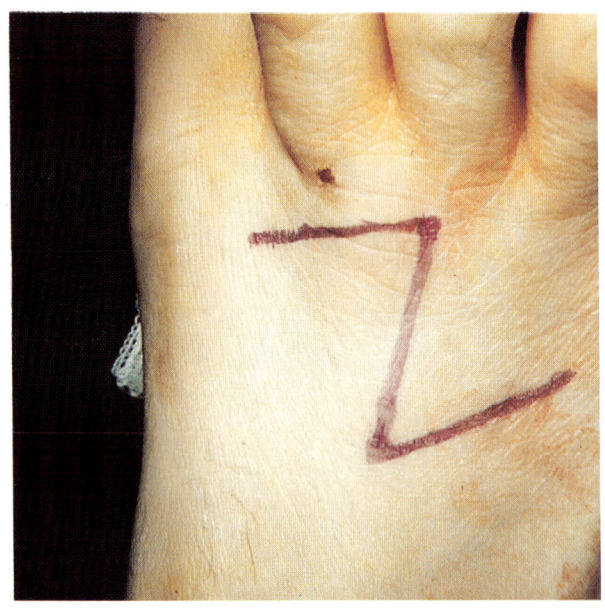

1.19 Large Z-plasty skin incision allows exposure to central metatarsals.

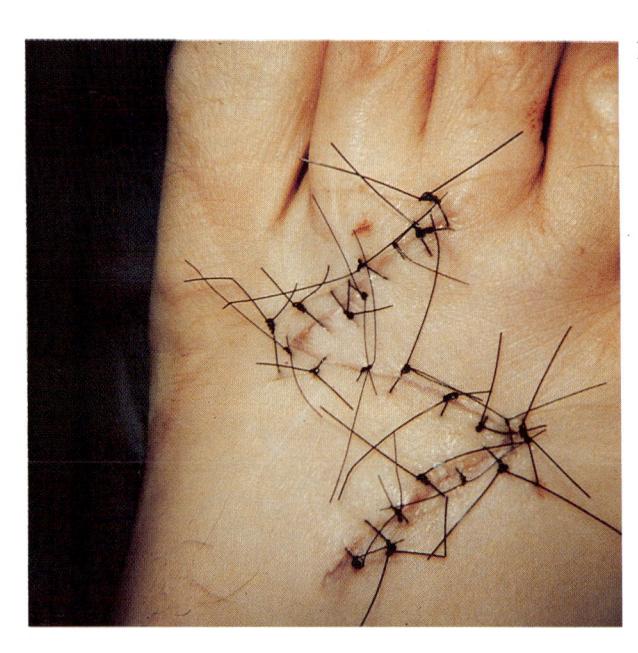

1.20 After final closure, there is decreased tautness of the dorsal foot skin and decreased potential for additional scar contracture.

To increase the survivability of this type of incision, avoid improper cutting of the edges, prevent scar tissue from forming across the base, keep the flaps thick and broad at the base, and decrease the tension on the flaps themselves. Another precaution is to handle the flap tips as little as possible and prevent pinching the skin with forceps or pickups during the procedure. Finally, use the correct suture technique during skin closure.

The V–Y-plasty procedure is very useful around the metatarsophalangeal joints of the foot (**1.21**). As with the Z-plasty technique, the incision should be full depth and the 'V' portion should be properly undermined so that it will move when placed on stretch. This will allow the formation of the 'Y' segment and create the new length pattern. The V–Y-plasty is one of the most commonly used lengthening techniques around the second and fifth digit areas (**1.22**, **1.23**).

1.21 V–Y skin plasty technique. V-incision is made (*a*), lengthens (*b*), and is converted to a Y-incision and sutured in place (*c*).

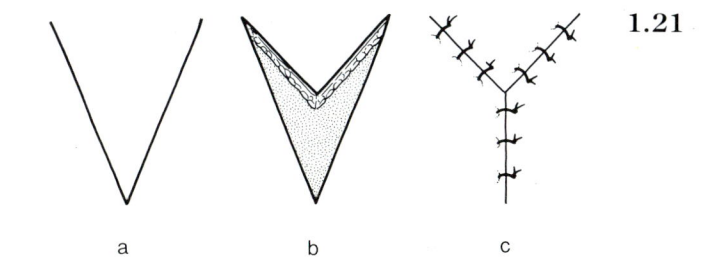

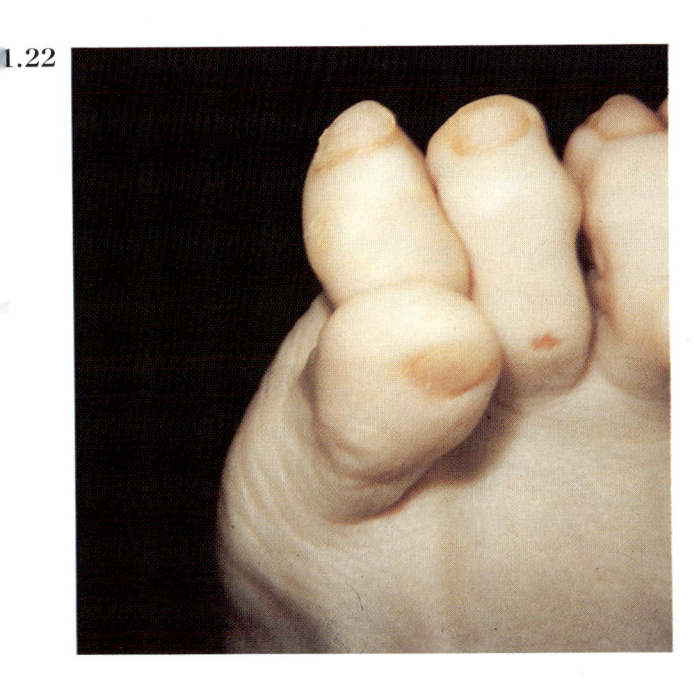

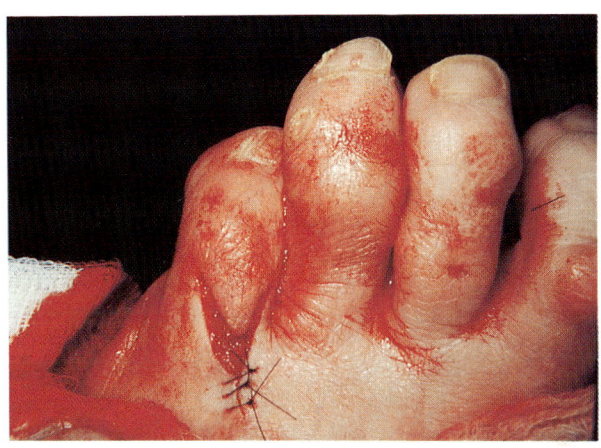

1.22 Clinical flexible contracture with elevated 5th digit.

1.23 V-incision converted to Y-incision, to decrease skin contracture. Additional procedures may include a dorsal tendon lengthening or tenotomy and joint capsulotomy.

The S incision is recommended whenever additional exposure is needed through the surgical site or in areas where linear incisions are known to form larger scars. In theory, the curved edges of the S incision tend not to draw back with contracture at the same rate as a linear incision, and linear scarring is therefore decreased. A local Seattle plastic surgeon, Virginia Scholl MD (personal communication), teaches that a correctly made S incision is *always* preferable to a straight linear incision.

As can be seen from the foregoing discussion, there should be no 'simple' incision, but rather a well-planned and executed 'uncomplicated' incision. We now turn our attention to the more complex issues of tissue coverage, skin grafts, skin flaps, and skin plasties.

Suture techniques

The type of suture and the techniques used to perform final closure of the incision or skin edges is almost as important to the overall results as the choice of incision.

As a general rule, it is best to use the least number of sutures as possible to adequately close each incision. Typically, the deepest layer (muscle, deep fascia, and capsule) is closed first, followed by the intermediate layer (deep subcutaneous and superficial fascia), and finally the skin layer. Failure to close the deep layers properly allows muscle or deep fascia retraction to occur, which encourages haematoma formation or separation of the layers; deep layer haematoma results in contraction, with resultant depression of the scar (**1.24**).

Personally, I do not like to place very many single absorbable sutures in the deep subcutaneous layer closure of wounds, preferring a running closure. This is because I have seen many deep-suture knot reactions when the deep layers were closed by simple interrupted knots. However, too many layers of running sutures may also cause tissue reaction and, eventually, scar formation or adhesions may occur. The exception to this is in the closure of joint capsules, which are best closed by the simple interrupted technique rather than the running style of closure: the joint capsule experiences a large amount of stress and motion, which necessitates a secure form of closure.

When the skin layer is closed by simple interrupted suture techniques, the sutures should be placed at equal distances from one another and the depth of the sutures should be into the subcutaneous layer. Evenly spaced and tied sutures prevent most problems of incision strangulation, uneven scarring, and inverted skin edges (**1.25**). Sutures placed too close to the skin incision edge cause uneven contact of the closed incision, bunching of the skin edge, and strangulation of the skin (**1.26**). Uneven suture technique does not lead to adequate healing, and the sutures may be very difficult to remove later.

The intradermal or subcuticular suture technique is employed frequently to close skin incisions on the foot and ankle (**1.27**). Intradermal sutures may be either absorbable or nonabsorbable, based upon surgeon preference. At the Waldo Podiatric Residency Training Program in Seattle, the nonabsorbable material is favoured for most linear and curvilinear incisions. This style of closure gives a very predictable fine scar in most patients and has the advantage of not needing to be removed. It is also easier to cover this type of closure with bandages for longer periods of time, such as under cast material, without the worry of suture-tract infections.

In many cases, skin incisions closed by the intradermal technique are supplemented by external steri-strip tape sutures. The sterile tape strips help to reduce tension across the incision area and therefore reduce the number of external sutures needed. Care must be taken to prevent increased skin pressure from applying the strips too tightly, and strips must not be used in patients with known tape allergies.

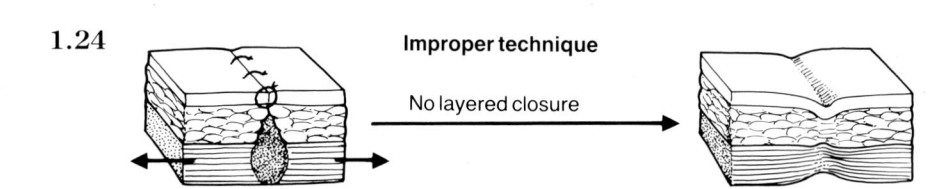

1.24

Improper technique
No layered closure

Muscle retraction allows haematoma formation and results in contraction with depressed scar

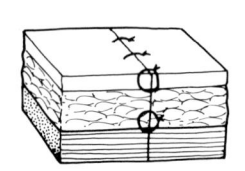

Correct technique
Layered closure
Skin, subcutaneous tissue and muscle properly apposed

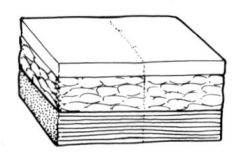

1.24 Layer closure prevents separation of deep layers and haematoma formation.

1.25 Incorrect suture placement and techniques. (*a*) Suture is too tight—the wound edges are blanched and pushed together. (*b*) Tissue is too heavy and there is too much of it. (*c*) Poor apposition—inverted skin results in a raised border.

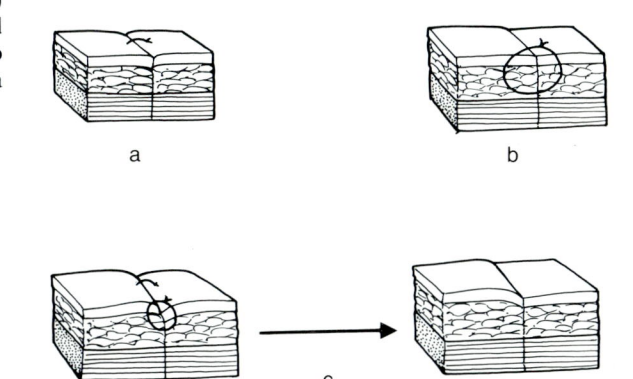

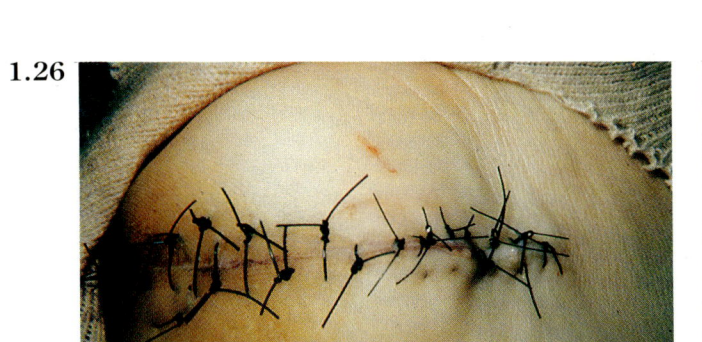

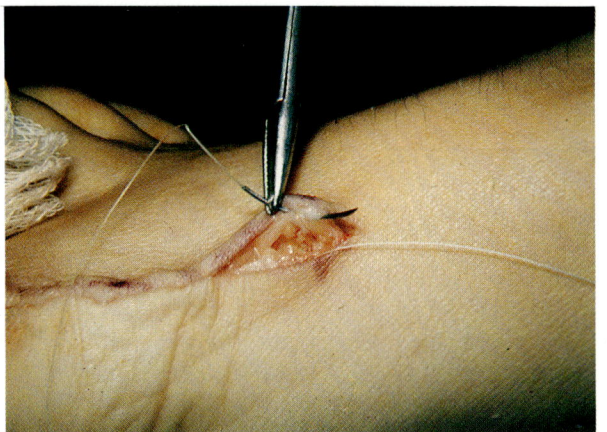

1.26 This incision was partially closed by the surgeon in an evenly spaced appropriate manner. The skin edges are equally apposed, with no tension. The remaining portion of the incision was closed by a trainee, who incorrectly placed the sutures. The incision is irregular, with strangulation of the tissue edges.

1.27 The subcuticular or intradermal suture technique decreases external suture scars and facilitates better looking incision scars in most cases.

For certain incisions, such as those with tension or movement across them, the external suture technique with nonabsorbable materials is preferred. Most flaps and grafts are sutured with nonabsorbable simple interrupted sutures. Two special suture techniques frequently utilized are the apical (or apex) stitch (**1.28**) and the side (or flap) stitch (**1.29**). The apical suture is commonly used for the corners of the V–Y-plasty and the Z-plasty flaps. The side stitch is used in rotation flaps and larger incisions to decrease the number of sutures in the actual skin edge of the flap.

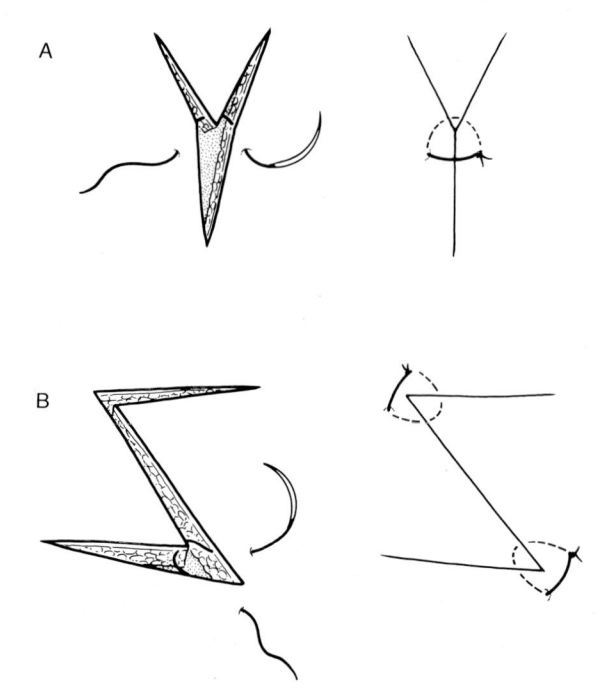

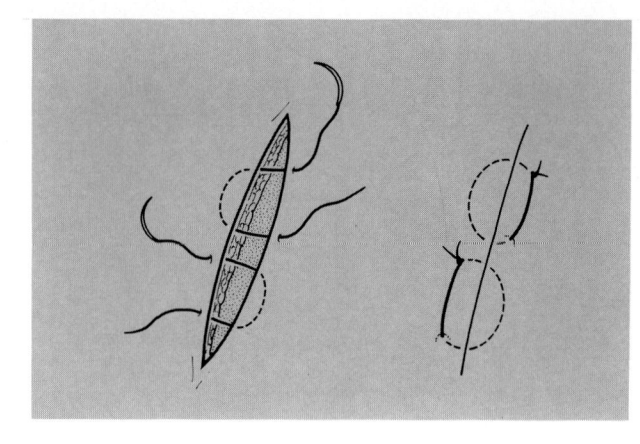

1.28 The apical or apex suture technique allows for closure of a flap tip without increasing the potential for strangulation of the tip. (A) V–Y apex stitch; (B) Z-plasty apex stitch.

1.29 The side or flap stitch is similar to the apical stitch and is used on flaps or longer incisions to decrease suture tension of the skin edges (see **1.6**).

Bandaging

Almost as important as the correct performance of the procedure and the prevention of fluid accumulation below the graft is the means of immobilizing the graft during the restoration process. Blood, serum, pus, and tissue fluids elevate the graft and interfere with the semipermeable membrane effect necessary for the diffusion of gases and nutrients to the living cell layer. During the restoration process motion also prevents the recipient area capillaries from penetrating the graft.

One method of stabilizing the graft that is commonly used, and frequently misused, is the stent dressing. In the stent fixation technique, the sutures that hold the graft in place are left long and tied over a sterile dressing fluff bolus. The purpose of using this dressing is to put pressure on the graft at the wound surface. In many cases, however, the surrounding skin is not sufficiently elastic or mobile (as around the foot and ankle region), and the pressure of the stent is greater at the edges of the graft than in the centre. The pressure effect is then dissipated within the hour, due to tissue creep, and this dressing is no better than any other standard dressing. For a correct stent dressing, the peripheral sutures actually draw the skin edges up and around the dressing, on top of the graft. The resilience of elasticity of the skin acts to continuously transfer mild pressure to the graft. In a correctly placed stent dressing, the level plane or slight convexity of the graft is converted to a slight concavity after the sutures are applied and secured.

Stent dressings are usually not recommended for free skin grafts on the lower legs or in areas where a free graft is used adjacent to a skin flap. Non-compressible conforming dressings are preferable in this situation. Flat 4 × 4 cotton sponges are moistened and flattened, and then cut to the size and shape of the free graft. Several layers are added until a non-compressible, firm dressing is created that rises above the level of adjacent skin of the flap. Regular dressings are then added, followed by sterile circular gauze and tape. It is possible to put too much pressure on free grafts and this occurs most readily over surfaces such as bone or tendons and prominent surfaces such as the anterior leg and the malleolar areas. Too much pressure can compress fragile proliferation capillaries and also decrease the fundamental process of tissue diffusion.

Skin grafts

Free skin grafts are of four main types: split-thickness (the most common), full-thickness, vascularized, and non-vascularized. The primary difference in these grafts is based upon the amount of dermis (thickness) taken for a graft and the vascular status of the graft.

Split-thickness skin grafts (STSGs) may be divided into three types, depending on the overall thickness of the skin: thin (0.20–0.31 mm), intermediate (0.33–0.38 mm), and thick (0.41–0.64 mm). The full-thickness skin graft (FTSG) includes the epidermis and the entire dermis but not the subcutaneous fat layer. Thin grafts, as a rule, take very easily, but contract quite a bit after healing and cause darker scarring to occur. Intermediate grafts are more durable but take longer to adhere and survive. Thick grafts, on the other hand, are even more durable, contract less, and are closer to normal skin in the final phase of healing. Unfortunately, they also have a higher failure rate, especially on the foot and ankle region, and for this reason, intermediate grafts are usually recommended.

STSGs usually leave the primary donor site with enough dermal elements to maintain its regenerative abilities. Re-epithelialization can then occur without contraction at the donor site, even though a slight increase in the pigmentation of the donor site may occur after final restoration is complete. In general, the thinner the graft, the greater the contraction of the graft itself once it has been transferred.

FTSGs are primarily used to cover areas where friction and pressure are greater, such as the malleoli, the heel, the metatarsal heads, and the plantar foot. Donor sites for the FTSG are from the inguinal region, the gluteal folds, and the dorsolateral aspect of the foot. Transfer of an FTSG leaves the subcutaneous fat layer exposed, and some provision must be made to close this defect or to cover the donor site. If the donor site area is in a relatively loose or redundant skin region, such as around the groin or gluteal fold area, the donor site may be closed primarily by direct suture. If the donor site skin is relatively tight or if the defect is larger than can be closed by direct suture of the skin edges, a graft from another site may be necessary.

After the FTSG has been harvested, it should be stripped of its fat layer and placed in the wound with the dermal side down. Only one or two pie-crust slits or drain holes are made in it and a mild compression dressing is applied. Because of the overall thickness of the FTSG, the ingrowth and revascularization to the graft takes longer than with an STSG, and fluid accumulation under the graft is more common. Consequently, survival of FTSGs is less predictable.[6,7]

Dressing grafts

In some cases of extensive soft tissue damage or traumatic wounds on the lower extremity, STSGs may be used as biological dressing grafts. Once these difficult wounds have been debrided of all devitalized tissue and foreign bodies, they may be covered with a thin STSG. A few well-placed sutures are needed to hold the graft in place, and a sterile topical dressing can then be applied. This technique allows the graft to 'take' over the adequately debrided wound surface. Contrary to popular belief, this dressing graft technique is no more occlusive than sterile gauze or petrolatum dressings. Even when the wound defect has not been properly debrided, take of the graft may produce a closed wound although degradation of deep necrotic tissue by scar replacement must still occur. This process may also prevent secondary wound infection from occurring, and in the presence of severe pre-existing infection, this wound covering graft does not normally increase complications. Overall, dressing grafts may greatly improve the healing of severe complicated wounds.

Pinch grafts

This special type of graft is essentially a relatively small FTSG that is harvested by lifting the donor site skin using standard atraumatic tissue forceps and cutting out one or several pieces using a surgical knife.[8] The free grafts are then placed upon the wound recipient bed in a random and spaced manner, and re-epithelialization occurs by secondary healing. Smaller pinch grafts may be obtained by inserting a needle into the dermal skin layer and, while using the syringe as a lever, lifting the needle to create a conical raised area.[9] This cone is then excised by a surgical knife, which results in a very small, 0.05–0.8 mm thick FTSG (**1.30**).

Free grafts are considered to be skin dressings or biological covers until they 'take' or survive by the re-establishment of circulation to the graft in its new location. Once the graft appears to adhere onto the new recipient surface, arterial connections begin to re-establish, and venous drainage begins. During this time, the graft becomes pink and blanches with intermittent pressure. Until these signs are evident, there is potential for failure: excessive movement of the graft area greatly increases the risk of devascularization and ultimate graft death. Underlying haematoma or serum collection, infection, or mechanical trauma may also interfere with this revascularization process, which is necessary for an adequate take of the graft.

Revascularization usually takes about four to five days before clinical evidence of successful function becomes evident. During this time, blood vessels in the recipient area develop afferent and efferent microconnections. Old vascular networks are also used by new sprouting capillaries and the old endothelial lining is replaced by new capillaries.[10]

As was stated earlier, the thickness of the free graft is important for ultimate survival. An extremely thin graft may not contain enough of the germinative epithelium, and the majority of the cells tranferred may be dead. Likewise, an FTSG has a thick layer of dermis that separates the germinal cells from the surface interface where revascularization occurs. Accumulations of serum, pus, or haematoma beneath an STSG may not result in loss of the graft; however, similar formation of fluids under an FTSG usually results in complete loss of the graft. In most cases, FTSGs are not usually recommended for resurfacing the foot and ankle region.

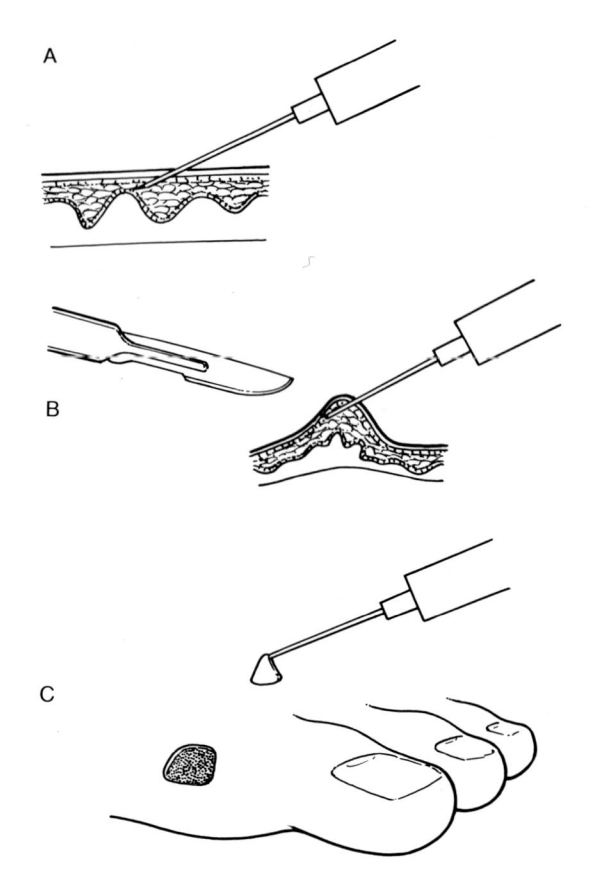

1.30 Technique for harvesting a pinch graft. The skin is lifted by using a 25-gauge needle which penetrates deep into the dermis (A); the cone is then lifted and cut using a scalpel (B), and transferred to the recipient site (C). (Redrawn from Saponara and Warren,[9] with permission.)

Instrumentation

Large hand-held manual dermatomes, such as the Humby and Blair knives, are available for harvesting large STSGs. The free-hand knife technique requires slightly more surgical skill and is used when smaller grafts are needed (**1.31**). Reese, Blair, Humby, Brown and many other mechanically powered dermatomes are now available. The removal of uniform STSGs from almost any site is much easier and more predictable with this technique. The mechanical, gas-powered dermatome produces STSGs of limited width, based on the width of the dermatome blade; however, in almost all cases on the lower extremity, the grafts are wide enough to completely cover the defect.

Commercial devices that mesh skin grafts to increase the surface size of the graft are not recommended unless a large area is to be covered (as in burns) or the graft simply is too small to cover the defect and additional donor grafts are not available. The resultant scars produced by meshing are cosmetically unacceptable and potential complications from multiple openings increase the risks. For the same reasons, we usually do not recommend multiple stab wounds or manual piecrust slits in skin grafts. A single or double small-slit incision in the central portion of the intact graft is all that is usually necessary to allow fluids to pass from below the graft to the over-dressings. We have seen much better cosmetic results in these intact forms of grafts than were seen when meshing was thought to be the only proper technique.

It is essential while using the mechanically powered dermatomes to keep the skin well lubricated with glycerine or heavy mineral oil and to provide an even, uniform pressure on the device. At the same time, it is important to keep equal tension on the adjacent skin as the graft is being harvested.

The location of the donor graft site must be considered. In most cases, the deformity created by taking skin from one area of the body should not create more of a physical or cosmetic problem than the original defect being covered. Grumbine found that females had a higher cosmetic- and overall patient-acceptance level of grafts from the arch of the foot as compared with grafts taken from the buttocks, the thigh, or the leg.[11]

Once the graft has been harvested, the donor site may be temporarily covered with gauze sponges moistened with epinephrine (adrenaline) solution to decrease free bleeding. This covering is then removed for final dressing coverings with either silk dressings or sterile petrolatum-based gauze dressings applied under dry, sterile gauze layers and evenly applied compression bandages.

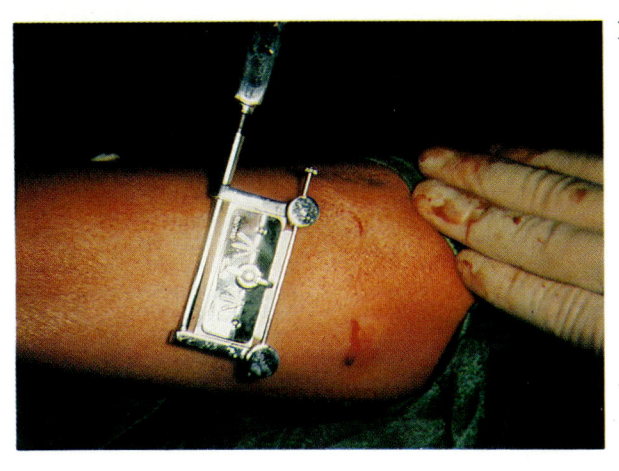

1.31 The hand-held dermatome gives a good STSG for smaller recipient sites, such as those needed for most foot surgery.

Skin flaps

Considerable forethought about the design of skin flaps and a sound understanding of the dynamics of their movement are necessary to obtain consistent success and to achieve cosmetically acceptable results. These principles, and skin flap design, are now discussed, and techniques are described for several different types of flaps.

In general, if a skin lesion can be completely excised within a fusiform (elliptical) segment of skin, whose long axis follows the RSTL, and the resultant skin defect can be closed by straight advancement of its skin borders following the lines of maximum extensibility (LME), then that is the procedure of choice (**1.32**).[12,13] However, this type of excision of a skin lesion from the leg, foot, or toe often produces a wound

1.32 Fusiform closure. The long axis of a fusiform (semi-elliptical) excision should follow the RSTL to close the defect without tension. Excising the lesion following the LME might jeopardize the skin closure and increase the thickness and size of the scar. (From: Dockery and Christensen,[6] with permission.)

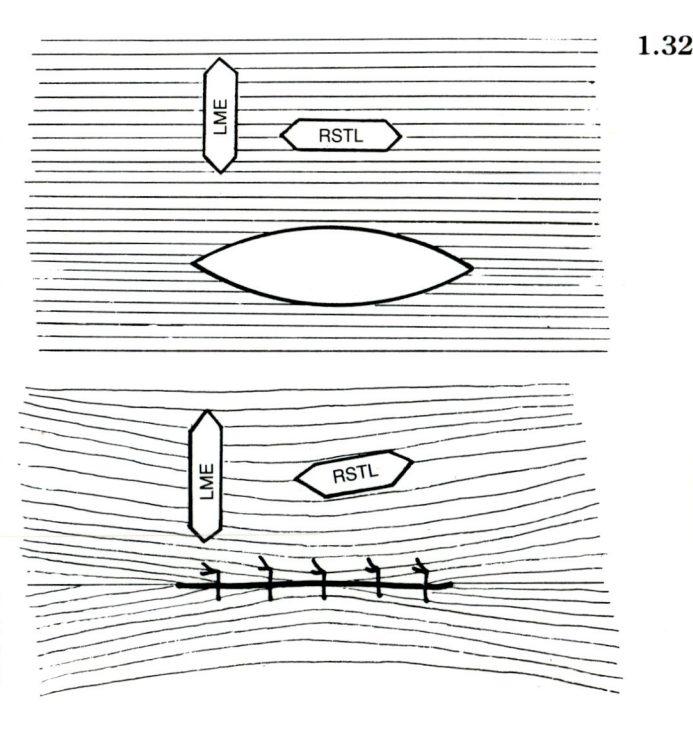

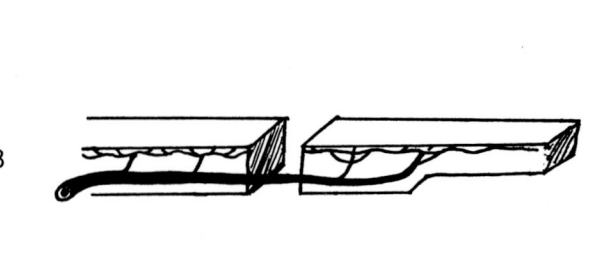

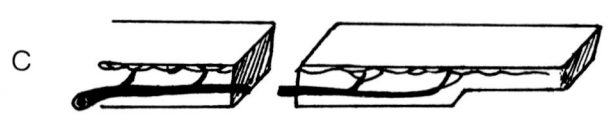

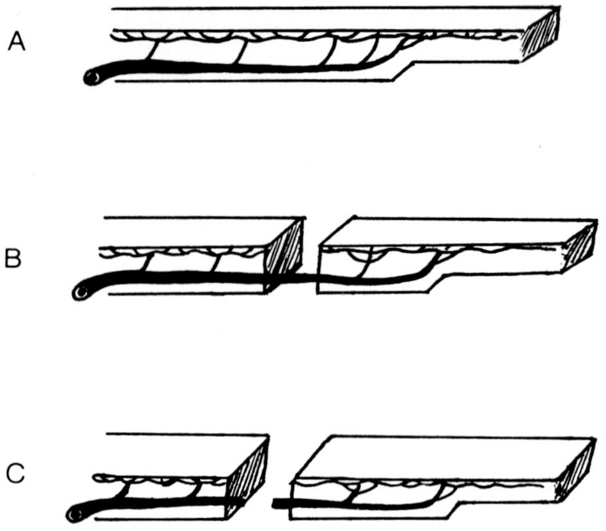

1.33 Random pattern flap. (From Dockery and Christensen,[6] with permission.)

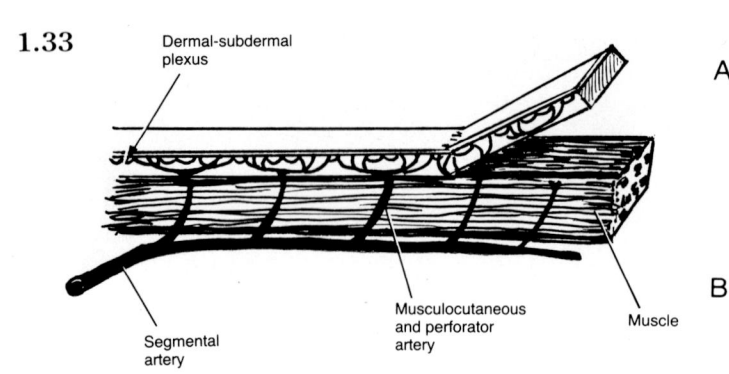

1.34 Axial pattern flaps. (A) Peninsular axial pattern. (B) Island axial pattern. (C) Free flap axial pattern. (From Dockery and Christensen,[6] with permission.)

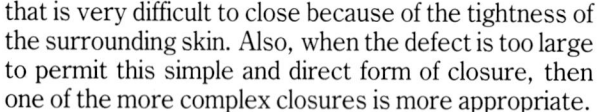

that is very difficult to close because of the tightness of the surrounding skin. Also, when the defect is too large to permit this simple and direct form of closure, then one of the more complex closures is more appropriate.

In the basic classification of skin flaps, there are two major categories:

- The type of blood supply to the flap.
- The shape and movement of the flap itself.

Classification according to blood supply is as important to the overall survivability of the flap as is the design and placement of the flap. McGregor and Morgan[14] first introduced the terms 'random pattern' and 'axial pattern' flaps in reference to the blood supply of flaps. The first type of blood supply is a random pattern (**1.33**), which refers to a non-specific blood supply such as a segmental artery and vein coursing deep to the muscle. This gives off perforator vessels that flow into the dermal–subdermal plexus of the skin. Musculocutaneous vessels, along with the perforators, have vast interconnections with the dermal layer to the skin flap. The second type of blood supply is the axial pattern (**1.34**), which has three subdivisions:

- The peninsular axial pattern, which has a direct cutaneous artery and vein that supply the dermal–subdermal plexus and run along the longitudinal axis of the skin flap.
- The island axial pattern, which is similar to the peninsular axial pattern; however, the flap is supported exclusively by the direct cutaneous vasculature supply because the flap has been dissected out.
- The free flap axial pattern, which is an island flap in which the blood supply has been divided from its base, prior to being moved to another site on the body.[15]

Additionally, consideration of the design, shape, and movement of particular flaps must also include the repair of the defect created in the donor site of the skin. Both repair of the original defect and the donor defect site must be planned to take place at the same surgical intervention. The movement of the flap itself onto a given defect should be thought of as *primary* and the movement of the skin around and adjacent to the flap and its pedicle as *secondary*.[16] The integration of primary and secondary movements and the ability to adjust them to attain maximum flexibility is most important for the success of flaps. Regardless of the combination of movements required in any given flap, one or possibly two carefully placed sutures will temporarily hold the freed portion of the flap in its new location. This placement of strategic securing sutures quickly tells the surgeon whether or not additional undermining or adjustments are necessary. At this point, the flap should be under very little tension and the outcome of the transfer should be visually apparent to the surgeon.

The following principles then are very important for the successful skin flap:[17]

- Complete understanding of the mechanism and the potential of movement of the flap.
- Proper selection and accurate design of the flap for the particular defect and its location.
- Consistent avoidance of tension on the suture lines.
- Adequate haemostasis and drainage in flaps for the first 48 h.

We now consider the design, shape, planning, and refining of advancement, rotation, simple transposition, and rhomboid flaps, as well as the double-Z rhomboid and reciprocal incisional approach for circular defects.

The advancement flap

The motion of this flap is directly forward, covering the defect without any lateral or rotational movement (**1.35**). The primary movement is so predominant that it may not be evident that the secondary movement may be equal to or at times greater than the primary movement. When the forward advancement flap produces 'dog ears' or puckers at the base of the flap, they may be excised. These corner excisions are termed Bürow's wedges (or triangles) (**1.36**) and they are cut out large enough to remove any excess tissue. They also aid directly in relieving some of the tension from the flap itself. In inelastic tissue, the wedge excisions may have to be large; however, in elastic tissue, they may be small or even unnecessary. Pantographic expansion (**1.37**), a modification of the advancement flap, aids in relieving tension on the graft without the need for Bürow's triangle excisions. When the defect appears too large to be covered with one flap, two adjoining advancement flaps may be utilized (**1.38**).

The major problem with this design is the potential for additional disruption of the blood supply to the flap. Since the majority of the advancement flaps are of the random pattern blood supply, failure to plan for secondary movement may result in more tension across the distal end of the flap, resulting in failure. It is rare that an advancement flap on the lower extremity has to be designed for primary movement only. The areas that require primary movement only are those in which the defects are on fixed structures that cannot be moved or distorted, such as over digits or the nail base. Areas that require mainly secondary movement are those in which the skin is inelastic but mobile (or mobilized by careful undermining), including the medial and lateral aspect of the heel, the posterior Achilles tendon area, and the medial and lateral malleolar region.

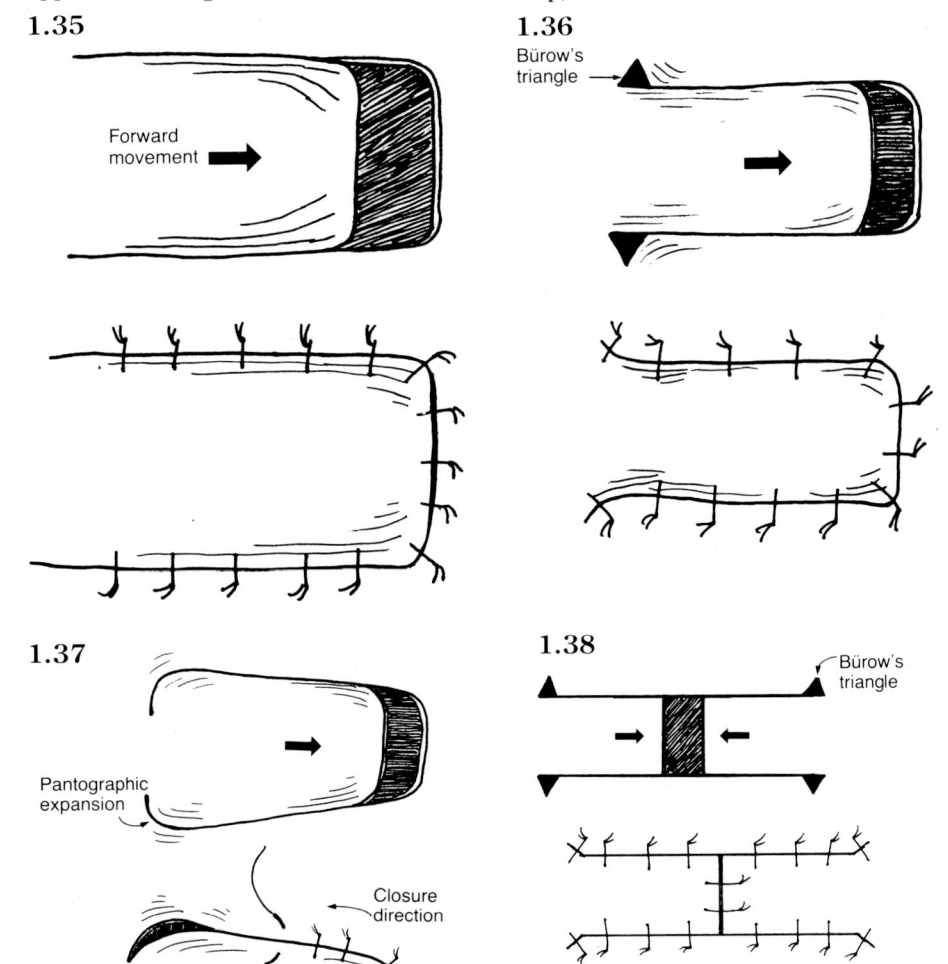

1.35 Basic advancement flap. (From Dockery and Christensen,[6] with permission.)

1.36 Bürow's triangles or wedges decrease tension on the ends of advancement flaps. (From Dockery and Christensen,[6] with permission.)

1.37 Pantographic expansion. (From Dockery and Christensen,[6] with permission.)

1.38 Adjoining advancement flaps. (Redrawn from Stegman;[16] from Dockery and Christensen,[6] with permission.)

Rotation flaps

The rotation flap used to close a circular defect (**1.39**) is usually a combination of both primary and secondary movements. The primary movement is the rotation and advancement of the flap itself over the defect: the secondary movement is the movement of the adjacent or surrounding skin in the opposite direction to the flap movement. The skin from the side of the defect opposite the flap moves over the defect more than the flap itself moves over the defect. This requires less rotation of the flap and creates less puckering at the flap pedicle. When puckers occur, they may be eliminated by cutting a Bürow's triangle in the usual manner.

The rotation flap used to close a triangular defect is usually a semicircular flap that rotates about a pivot point (**1.40**). The primary movement is of the flap itself and the line of the greatest tension extends from the pivot point towards the defect site. This distal tension point is the area of greatest vascular compromise.[18]

One type of local rotation flap that has great application for repair of plantar foot defects is the bilobed flap (**1.41**). As the name implies, this flap consists of two

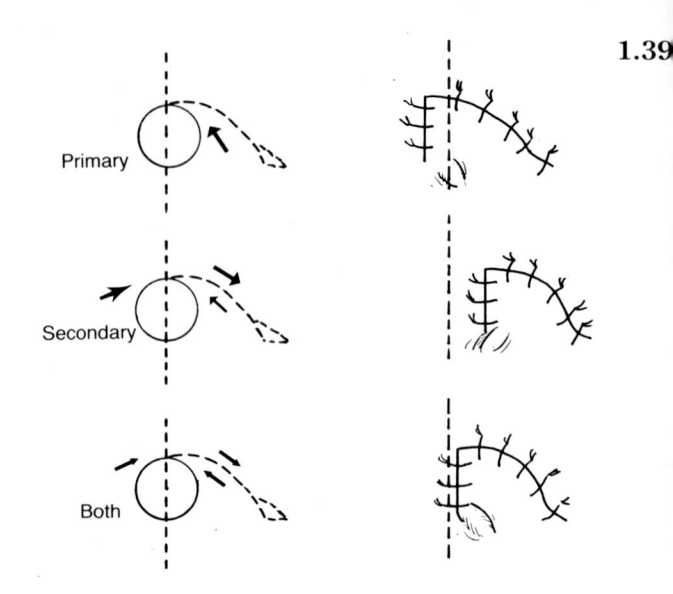

1.39 Rotation flap used to close a circular defect. All three movements are shown. (Redrawn from Stegman;[16] from Dockery and Christensen,[6] with permission.)

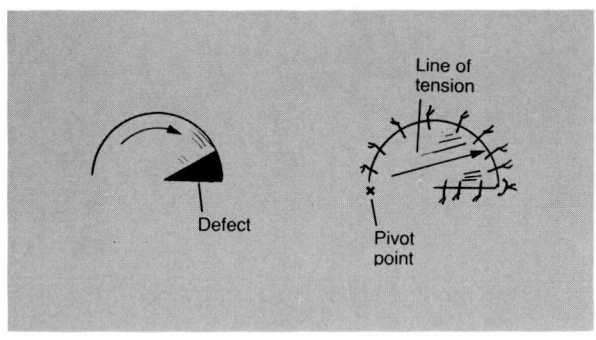

1.40 Rotation flap used to close a triangular defect. (From Dockery and Christensen,[6] with permission.)

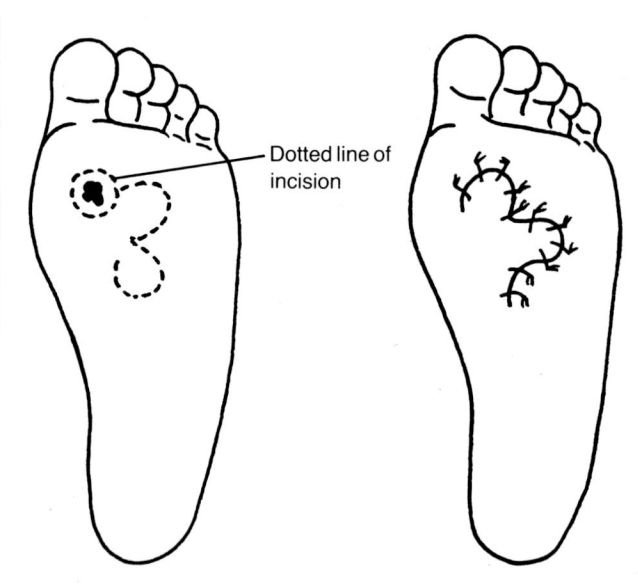

1.41 The local bilobed rotation flap and how it can be used to cover a plantar metatarsal defect. (From Dockery and Christensen,[6] with permission.)

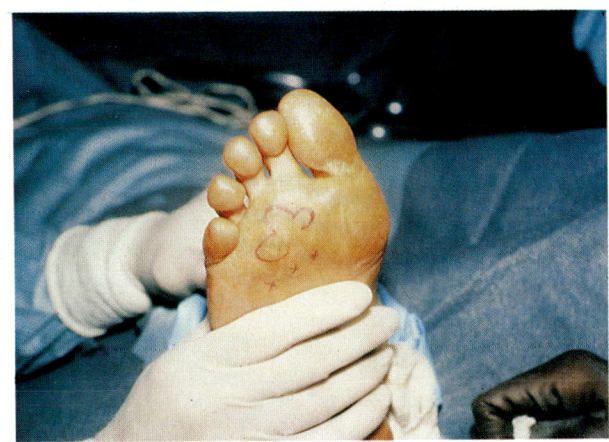

1.42–1.44 The bilobed flap used to remove a deep painful lesion and scar beneath the third metatarsal head. Bilobed flap is drawn out on the foot (**1.42**). Flap is transposed without tension (**1.43**). One-year post operative follow-up (**1.44**).

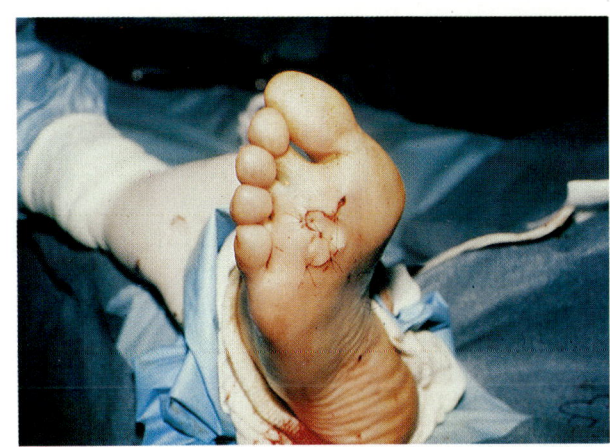

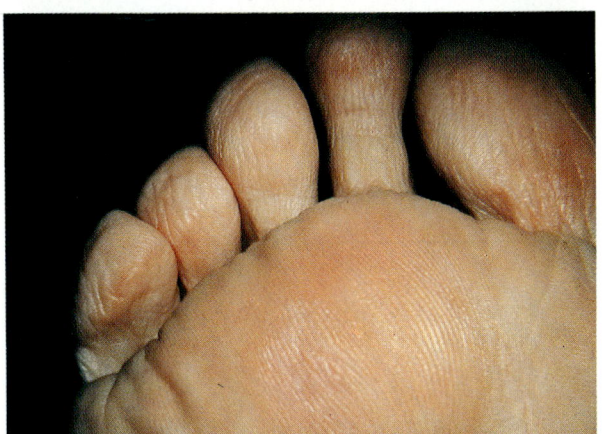

lobes separated by an angle and based upon a common pedicle.[19] The bilobed flap has been advocated for the repair of small circular defects over the plantar surface of the foot, in part because of the unique characteristics of the skin and subcutaneous tissue in that area of the body (**1.42–1.44**).[20] As with other local flaps on the plantar aspect of the foot, the donor site should not be taken from over an exposed prominence or weight-bearing surface that would make it more vulnerable to pressure and trauma.

A variation of the standard rotation flap designed by Schrudde[21,22] is a combination of a rotation flap and a transpositional flap, in which the flap employed to close the defect and the defect itself are cut to a round shape. Schrudde refers to this flap as a slide-swing plasty useful in closing circular defects and refers to three variants of the flap for general use (**1.45**). This approach possesses all of the advantages of local or rotational flaps and permits the use of unusually large flaps, because the principle guarantees sufficient vascularization and the normal relation between the length of the flap and its breadth of 1 : 1 can generally be exceeded (**1.46**). Additional advantages include:

- The similarity of the tissues employed. Subcutaneous tissue, and even muscle situated beneath it, can be used with the skin.
- Universal applicability, with reference to the size and location of the defect.
- Special resistance of the flap, resulting from the broad base which ensures a good blood supply.
- Avoidance of secondary defects or additional incisions.

This flap is also preferred for removing digital mucoid cysts (**1.47–1.51**) and small oval lesions (**1.52–1.55**). The resulting scars are cosmetically very pleasing and recurrence rates of the lesions are very low.

1.45

Type 1
Circular defect

Type 2
Oval defect

Type 3
Semicircular defect

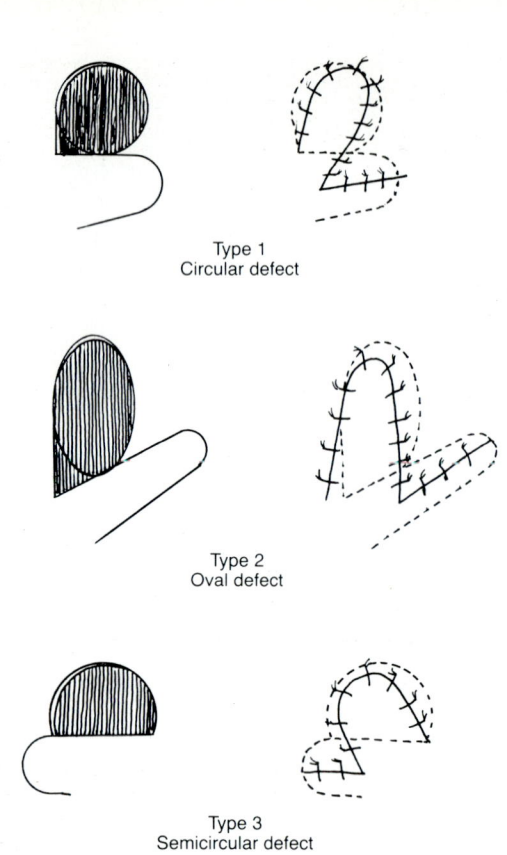

1.45 The Schrudde slide-swing plasty is a variation of a standard rotation flap which can be modified to close three differently shaped defects. (Redrawn from Schrudde and Petrovici,[22] with permission.)

1.46

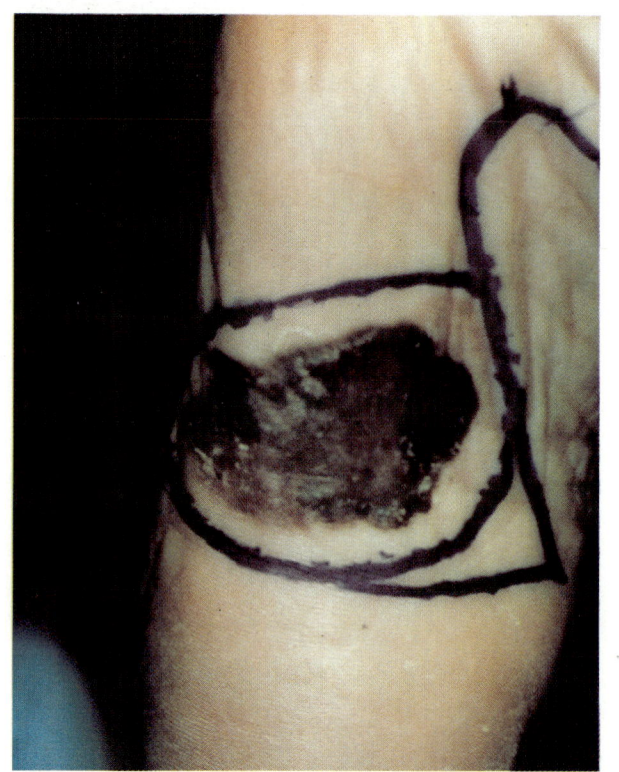

1.46 The use of a very large Schrudde slide-swing plasty to remove a lesion on the arch of the foot.

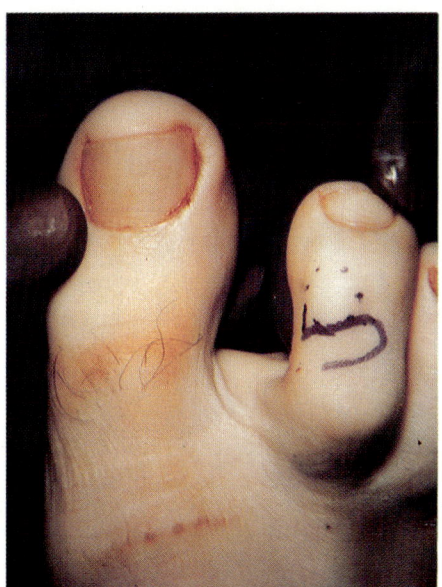

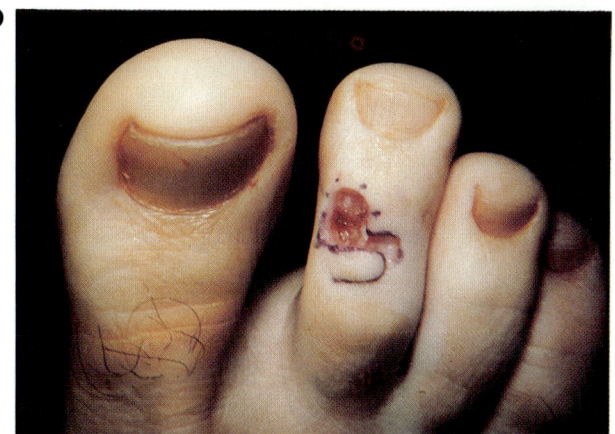

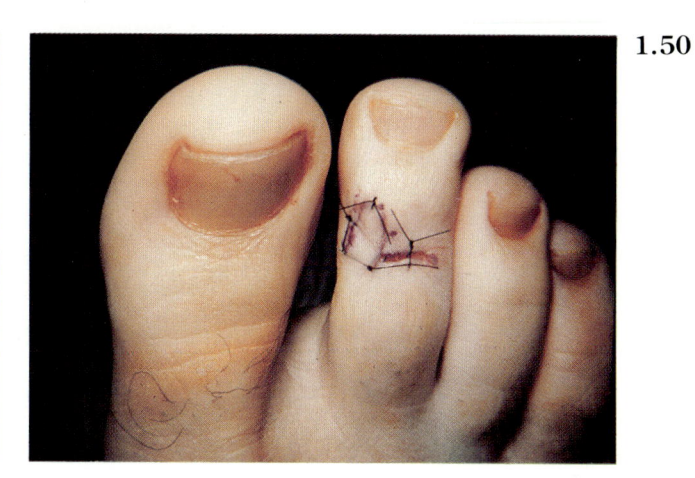

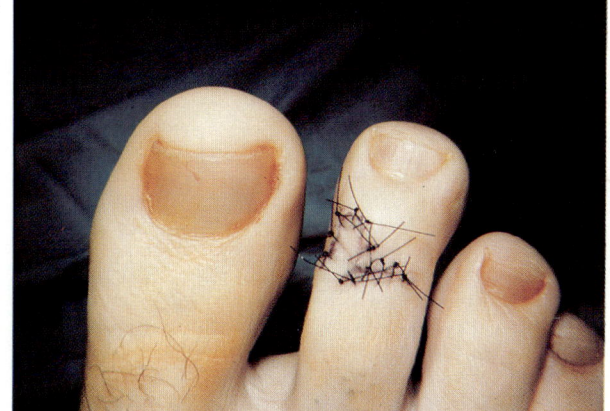

1.47–1.51 A type-1 Schrudde flap to remove a digital mucoid cyst. The cyst is marked (**1.47**). Schrudde flap drawn in (note placement to assure good blood supply) (**1.48**). Cyst excised and flap incised (**1.49**). Flap transposed without tension (**1.50**). Final closure (**1.51**).

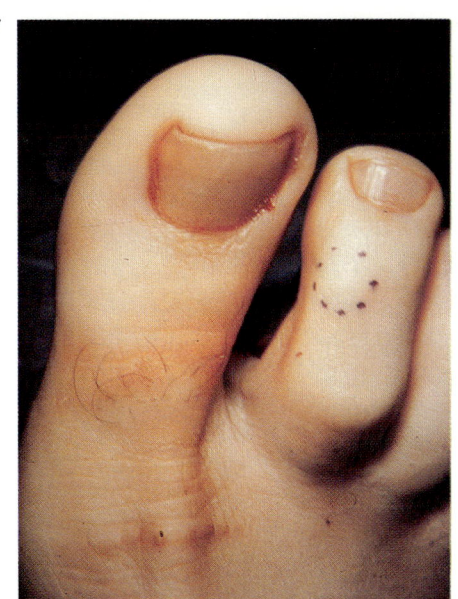

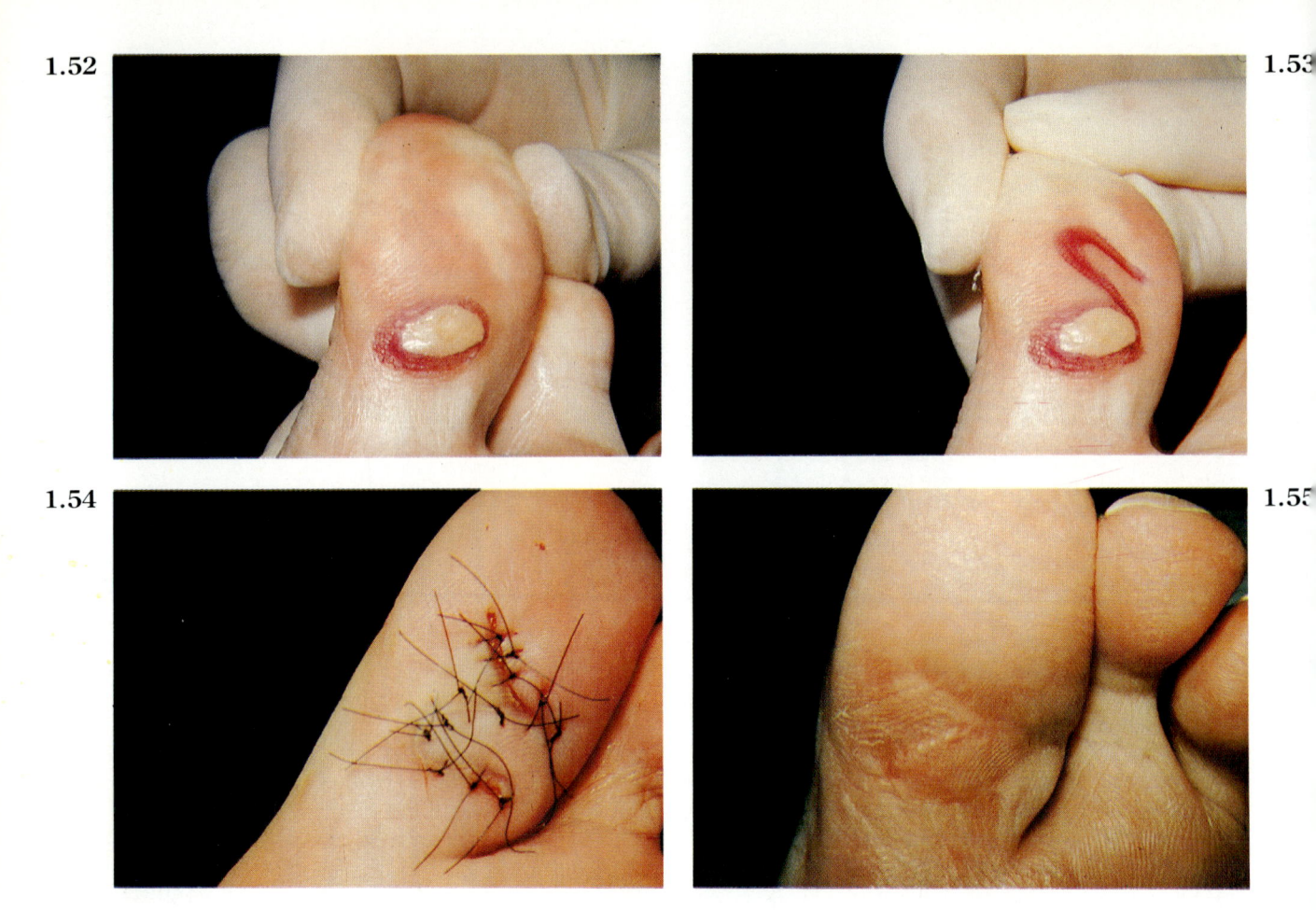

1.52–1.55 A type-2 Schrudde flap to remove an oval lesion on the plantar hallux.

Simple transposition flaps

The simple transposition flap (**1.56**) is usually thought of as a square or rectangular-shaped flap which, when closed, covers the original defect, leaving the secondary defect open. The primary motion allows the flap to be rotated about a pivot point into the immediate adjacent defect area. The resultant secondary defect is then covered with an STSG. One of the most important uses of this type of flap is in covering defects located over exposed joints or over bony prominences, such as the malleoli and posterior calcaneus. Many of the other flaps discussed in this chapter may be more suitable and eliminate the need for additional grafting.

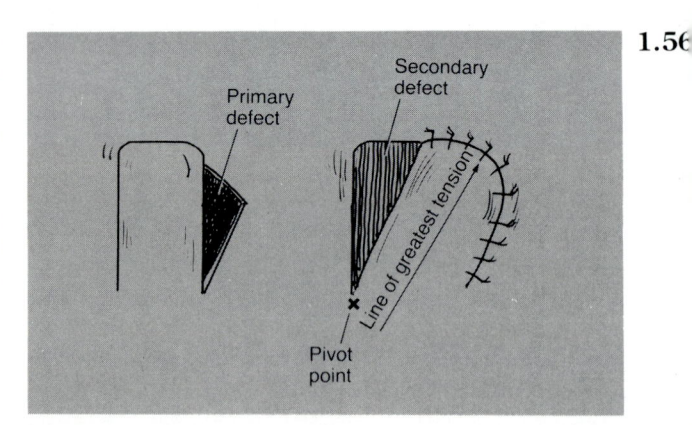

1.56 Simple transposition flap. Primary movement allows rotation at the pivot point to close the defect. (From Dockery and Christensen,[6] with permission.)

Rhomboidal or rhombic flaps

A rhombus is an oblique-angled equilateral parallelogram, which may be regarded as a fusiform shape with straight sides.[23] A rhomboid is an oblique-angled parallelogram with *unequal* adjacent sides;[13] therefore, a rhombic flap is one having the form of a rhombus. The rhomboid transposition flap, originally designed by Limberg[24,25] (**1.57**), has gained wide acceptance and popularity as an excellent-shaped flap for reconstruction of defects. This flap was designed for the closure of a 60° rhomboid defect, with angles of 60° and 120°. Its use of adjacent tissue in transfer and rotation to avoid tension make this rhomboid flap the preferred local pedicle flap in many cases on the lower extremity. This is also a very useful flap, because it can be rotated from any side over a defect and the broken-line scar that results is cosmetically favourable. With experience, a rhomboid flap can be designed and moved to cover circular, triangular, or other irregular defects.[12] Both primary and secondary motion should occur for maximum benefit with this flap. The primary motion is of the flap itself moving towards the defect site. The secondary motion is of the adjacent tissue to the defect moving towards the flap.

To minimize tension in the final closure, the original rhombic defect should be oriented so that its long diagonal is parallel with the LME and follows the natural skin creases, or RSTL. In so orientating the flap, tissue is taken from the LME, where it is plentiful, and transferred to the defect. Choosing the correct flap is done most easily if one simply visualizes the rhomboid shape around the lesion and orients it so that the distal point of the base of the flap is along the LME.

Difficulty in marking the Limberg rhomboid flap, due to the inability to visualize the relationship between the rhomboid about the lesion and the orientation of the adjacent flap with the proposed line of closure of the secondary defect, may be greatly reduced by a simplified technique described by Rossi and Jeffs.[26] They described the use of a 90° set square, made of metal, which could easily be sterilized and used in surgery. The 30° and 60° angles of the set square permit easy, rapid, and accurate marking.

The principles of design and placement of the rhomboid flap outlined by Monheit[27] include:

- A lesion should be excised in the shape of a rhombus (as an equilateral parallelogram with oblique sides).
- The flap should be designed along one of the four equilateral sides that is most convenient or feasible.
- Sufficient undermining of the recipient sites allows closure of defects with donor flaps that are slightly smaller than the defects themselves. (Undermining the base of the flap should not be done, and excising tissue from the flap itself is not recommended because this may severely compromise the blood supply to the flap.)
- The donor site should be closed first with anchoring sutures to take tension off the flap.
- The flap should not be stretched because that may compromise the blood supply. Dog-ears or pucker defects should be removed from the flap itself but away from its pedicle.
- As few sutures as possible should be used along the base of the flap to avoid constriction of blood supply.
- Excessive movement of the flap and pressure upon the graft should be avoided after surgery to prevent tissue death or haematoma formation.

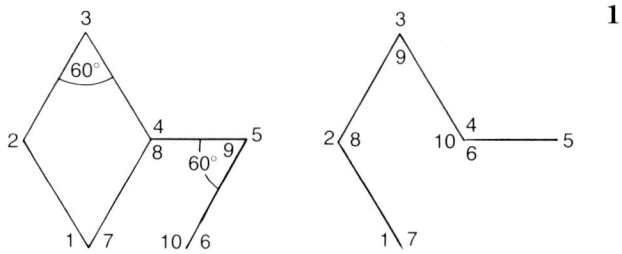

1.57 Limberg rhomboid transposition flap. (From Dockery and Christensen,[6] with permission.)

Because of the dynamics of the Limberg flap, there are certain limitations to its usage and additional problems may include excessive tension,[28] anatomical landmark displacement,[13] and trap-door deformity.[29] Excessive tension may be manifest along the line of closure of the flap donor site and at one or both of the tips of the advanced flap. Over one-half the total tension is located along the line of closure of the donor site, with the remainder being distributed at the tips of the advanced flap. Furthermore, since all of the tissue that is required to resurface the rhombic defect is borrowed from one area, and since the flap donor site is closed by advancement, the potential for anatomical landmark displacement exists. Tension at both tips of the advancement flap may result in blunting or rounding of the angles of the tips as they retract, which allows the leading edge and sides to assume a semicircular shape. The contracting forces of the semicircular scar may then produce the trap-door scar deformity.

In areas of tight skin where it is often difficult to rotate this flap into the rhomboid defect or to obtain a tension-free closure, Ashbell[30] recommends undermining the entire area, including the margins of the rhomboid defect and the base of the flap. This undermining, which must include the subcutaneous fat when the defect is deep, is continued until the flap can be transposed and the donor wound closed with only minimal tension.

Variations of the Limberg rhomboid flap

Dufourmentel [31] described a simple modification of the Limberg rhomboid flap (**1.58**). This flap was designed to close defects with any acute angle; however, the basic design of this flap is slightly more complicated than that of the Limberg flap. The short diagonal of the donor trapezium follows a direction closer to that of the short diagonal of the rhombic defect than it does in the Limberg flap. The Dufourmentel flap does not make use of the difference in tension between the LME and the RSTL to the extent that the Limberg flap does. The general direction of pull for the closure of the donor site is similar to that in straight-line closure of the original defect. We have already established earlier that a local skin flap is not used to cover a skin defect unless the feasibility of a straight-line closure (elliptical closure) has been ruled out. For this reason, if a local rhombic flap is to be used on the lower extremity to cover a skin defect, the flap designed by Limberg has greater usefulness than the flap design of Dufourmentel.

Webster et al.[32] further modified the Limberg rhomboid flap, which they termed the '30° transposition flap' (**1.59**). This technique created the use of a 30° flap instead of the traditional 60° flap. The inferior end of the rhomboid defect was then converted to an M-plasty, which effectively creates two 30° closures rather than one 60° closure. This preserves tissue and, because this flap is more narrow than the classic rhomboid flap, tension must be shared by the edges of the defect.

The Limberg, Dufourmentel, and Webster 30° transposition flaps were all reviewed by Bray,[33] who found that the Dufourmentel flap had no advantage over the Limberg flap for closure of the 60°/120°

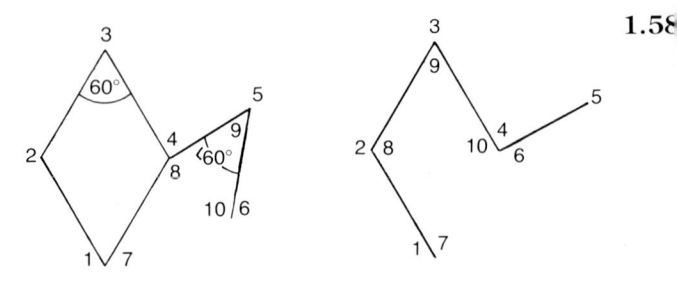

1.58 Dufourmentel rhomboid flap. (From Dockery and Christensen,[6] with permission.)

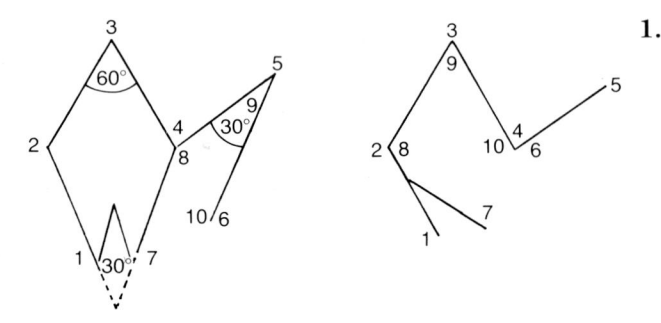

1.59 Webster 30° tranposition flap. (Redrawn from Webster et al.[32] with permission.)

rhombus defects. He also noted that the Limberg flap is much easier to create then the Webster flap, and it appears that there is less tension on the final transfer in the Limberg flap.

The double-Z rhomboid flap

In an attempt to overcome some of the difficulties of the Limberg flap, Cuono[34,35] developed a functionally and aesthetically satisfactory alternative procedure that he terms the 'double-Z rhomboid flap' (**1.60**). The design of the double-Z rhomboid flap incorporates two 60° Z-plasties generated on opposite sites of a standard 60°/120° equilateral parallelogram rhomboid defect. Closure of the original rhombic defect is effected by elevation and transposition of the four Z-plasty flaps. The amount of tissue required to close the defect is provided by borrowing equal amounts from each of the opposite sides of the defect. Once the defect has been excised, with adequate margins, to form a rhombic shape, there are two potential sets of double-Z

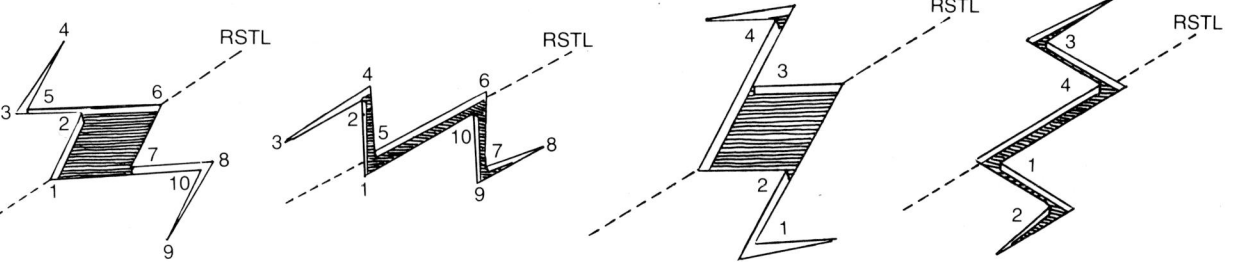

1.60 The double-Z rhomboid flap technique incorporates two 60° Z-plasties on opposite sides of an equilateral parallelogram rhomboid defect. (Redrawn from Cuono,[34] with permission.)

1.61 Once a rhombic defect has been created by excising the lesion, there are two potential methods of creating the double-Z rhomboid flap which will allow closure with minimum tension. The final line of closure must have three of the five segments of the double Z-plasty parallel with the RSTL. Compare with **1.60**. (From Dockery and Christensen,[6] with permission.)

rhomboid flaps that may be utilized (**1.61**).

Cuono[34] feels that the double-Z rhomboid technique is more reliable, more easily executed, and cosmetically superior to the Limberg flap. He also notes that the double-Z rhomboid flap is superior in situations in which the defect is in proximity to movable anatomical landmarks or on small joints, making this a procedure quite useful to foot surgeons.

Reciprocal incisions for circular defects

Alvarado[36] discussed the various methods that may be employed to repair circular defects, without first having to create rhomboid designs. He also suggests that the simplest and most practical approach is to make an elliptical incision along the minimal tension lines; however, this wastes sound skin that could be used to reduce tension at the suture line. Therefore, whenever the simplest closure cannot be performed on a circular defect, for whatever reason, an alternative closure technique may be used. He designed three different incisional approaches, which are well indicated in the closure of circular defects (**1.62**).

The first is the 'double-S incision', which may be used in areas where the defect is relatively small and the skin is fairly elastic. The second is the 'bow tie incision', which is used with intermediate-sized lesions in which the skin is quite elastic. The third incision is the 'combined-V incision', which is valuable for large defects in which the skin is fairly elastic. Also, no additional adjacent tissue is wasted with this procedure because only the defect tissue is excised.

Alvarado's combined-V incision also borrows tissue from opposite sides of the defect, as does the rhomboid flap. However, the length of each limb of each V in this incision is only equal to the radius of the circular defect,

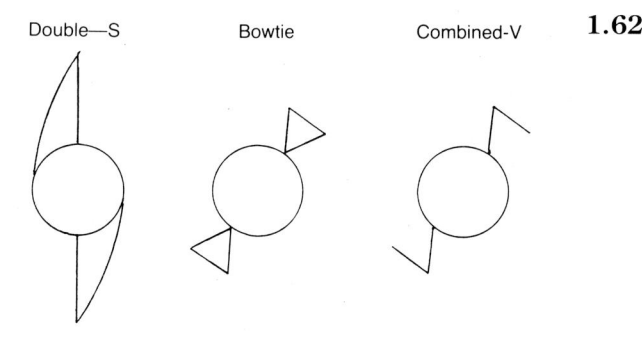

1.62 The three reciprocal incisions of Alvarado for closure of circular defects: the double-S incision, the bow tie incision, and the combined-V incision. (Redrawn from Alvarado,[36] with permission.)

which means that the combined area of the flaps is small in relation to the total area of the circular defect. Therefore, a significant amount of direct advancement must be accomplished in order to close a wound. For practical purposes, since the main problem is that the resultant circular defect may prove to be very difficult to close, the use of reciprocal incisions for closing circular defects on the lower extremities is limited.

Post-operative care

The immediate post-operative period is critical for proper wound healing, and several factors may influence the overall appearance of the incision and survivability of the flap or skin graft. Initially, I recommend using a mild compression dressing on all incisions. During the first five to seven days, the bandage is not removed or adjusted unless there are problems. If there is swelling, staining, stench (or smell), or the surgeon is at all suspicious, then the bandage may be inspected or replaced. The patient is instructed to refrain from allowing motion to occur at the incision site in most cases. Additionally, it is very important to keep the bandages dry and clean.

At the first post-operative visit, some or all of the retention skin sutures may be removed and a new compression sterile dressing applied. At this visit, the first time the patient sees the incision area, the physician can explain the procedure again and emphasize the importance of the post-operative instructions. The next visit is usually scheduled one week later and, at that time, alternating simple interrupted sutures may be removed. On the third visit (14–21 days post-operative), the final remaining sutures may be removed. This programme is guided by the incision's appearance: if there is slight wound dehiscence early on, the sutures are left in slightly longer. At any visit, steri-strip tape sutures may be used to reduce tension across incisions. Most external skin sutures should be removed by three weeks, to prevent suture track scars from forming.

For skin flaps and grafts, I like to keep a mild elastic compression bandage in place most of the time for 8–12 weeks after surgery. This tends to make the flaps flatter and softer, with less discoloration. At four weeks post-operative, I also recommend massage of the area with lotion or cream.

Summary

Making well thought-out skin incisions, utilizing the correct suture materials and techniques of wound closure, and applying the proper principles of skin grafts and tissue flaps are very important surgical concepts for foot surgeons. Successful and appropriate use of these principles in the lower extremities can be rewarding and can provide the surgeon with powerful tools to use in reconstructive lower extremity procedures.

Equally important is the distinction that must be made between tissue movability and tissue elasticity when considering tissue movement with the hope of predicting good results. Tissue movability is either inherent, as on the back of the thigh, or is created by undermining, back-cutting, or cutting out Bürow's triangles. The elasticity of skin is inherent everywhere and is difficult to accurately predict. Elastic tissue will gape when cut, whereas inelastic tissue will not. Finally, elastic tissue will rotate with little puckering, but inelastic tissue will form large dog ears when rotated.

For these reasons, as soon as the decision has been made to use a flap, it is important to 'pre-think' the dynamics of flap movement and decide which type of flap to use and what is to be accomplished. If consideration is given to which flap will best allow proper transfer of tissue and at the same time give the best cosmetic result, the task is usually simpler. By further considering the secondary movement of surrounding tissues (as well as the primary movement) the number of potential techniques and designs is greatly increased.

References

[1] Converse, J.M., McCarthy, J.G., Brauer, R.D., et al. Transplantation of skin: Grafts and flaps. In Converse, J.M. (ed.), *Reconstructive Plastic Surgery,* 2nd edn. Philadelphia, W.B. Saunders, 1977, pp.152–239.

[2] Miller, S.J. The art of making incisions. *Clin. Podiatric Med. Surg.,* **3**: 223–233, 1986.

[3] Borges, A.F. Relaxed skin tension lines (RSTL) versus other skin lines. *Plast. Reconstr. Surg.,* **73**: 114–150, 1984.

[4] Cibella, V.G., Smith, L., Haas, M., Green, A. and Stewart, J. Skin blade versus deep blade: a vehicle of contamination in podiatric surgery? *J. Foot Surg.,* **29**: 44–45, 1990.

[5] Fairclough, J.A., Mackie, I.G., Mintowt–Czyz, W. and Phillips, G.E. The contaminated skin knife: a surgical myth. *J.B.J.S.,* **65**B: 210, 1983.

[6] Dockery, G.L. and Christensen, J.C. Principles and descriptions of design of skin flaps for use on the lower extremity. *Clin. Podiatric Med. Surg.,* **3**: 563–577, 1986.

[7] Marcinko, D.E. Plastic surgery in podiatry (simplified illustrated techniques). *J. Am. Podiatric Med. Assoc.,* **27**: 103–110, 1988.

[8] Baerg, R., Beal, W. and Cohen, M. The use of large pinch graft technique in a traumatic foot wound. *J. Am. Podiatric Med. Assoc.,* **77**: 92, 1987.

[9] Saponara, G.C. and Warren, A.M. Pinch grafts—Applications in podiatric wound closure. *J. Foot Surg.,* **27**: 111–115, 1988.

[10] Dockery, G.L. Skin grafting techniques. In Jay, R.M. (ed.), *Current Therapy in Podiatric Surgery.* Toronto, B.C. Decker, 1989, pp.1–17.

[11] Grumbine, N.A. Free split thickness skin grafts. *Clin. Podiatric Med. Surg.,* **3**: 269–275, 1986.

[12] Borges, A.F. Choosing the correct flap. *Plast. Reconstr. Surg.,* **62**: 542, 1978.

[13] Borges, A.F. The rhombic flap. *Plast. Reconstr. Surg.,* **67**: 458–466, 1981.

[14] McGregor, J.A. and Morgan, R.G. Axial and random pattern flaps. *Br. J. Plast. Surg.,* **26**: 202, 1973.

[15] Christensen, J.C. and Dockery, G.L. Flap classification and survival factors: current concepts. *Clin. Podiatric Med. Surg.,* **3**: 579–588, 1986.

[16] Stegman, S.J. Principles of design and the dynamics of movement of flaps. *J. Dermatol. Surg. Oncol.,* **6**: 182–186, 1980.

[17] Abdel-Fattah, A.M.A. Local skin flaps in reconstruction following excision of basal cell carcinomas of the cheek and temple. *J. Surg. Oncol.,* **21**: 223–229, 1982.

[18] Grabb, W.C. and Smith, J.W. (eds). *Plastic Surgery.* Boston, Little, Brown, and Co., 1979, pp.36–70.

[19] Miller, S.J. The bilobed skin flap rotation. *Clin. Podiatric Med. Surg.,* **3**: 253–258, 1986.

[20] Zimany, A. The bi-lobed flap. *Plast. Reconstr. Surg.,* **11**: 424–434, 1953.

[21] Schrudde, J. Primary soft tissue plastic operations following removal of malignant tumors. Proceedings of the First Annual Meeting of the Swiss Society of Plastic and Reconstructive Surgeons, Locarno, April 1965. *Excerpta Medica, Int. Congress Ser. Nr.,* **98**: 40, 1965.

[22] Schrudde, J. and Petrovici, C. The use of slide-swing plasty in closing skin defects: A clinical study based on 1308 cases. *Plast. Reconstr. Surg.,* **67**: 467–481, 1981.

[23] Lister, G.D. and Gibson, T. Closure of rhomboid skin defects: The flaps of Limberg and Dufourmentel. *Br. J. Plast. Surg.,* **25**: 300, 1972.

[24] Limberg, A.A. *Mathematical Principles of Local Plastic Procedures on the Surface of the Human Body.* Leningrad, Medgriz, 1946.

[25] Limberg, A.A. Design of local flaps. In Gibson, T., (ed.), *Modern Trends in Plastic Surgery,* 2nd edn. London, Butterworths. 1966, pp.38–61.

[26] Rossi, A. and Jeffs, J.V. The rhomboid flap of Limberg—a simple aid to planning. *Ann. Plast. Surg.,* **5**: 494–496, 1980.

[27] Monheit, G.D. The rhomboid transposition flap re-evaluated. *J. Dermatol. Surg. Oncol.,* **6**: 464–470, 1980.

[28] Larrabee, W.F., Trachy, R., Sutton, D. and Cox, K. Rhomboid flap dynamics. *Arch. Otolaryngol.,* **107**: 755, 1981.

[29] Austin, A. The 'trap-door' scar deformity. *Clin. Plast. Surg.,* **4**: 255, 1977.

[30] Ashbell, T.S. The rhomboid excision and Limberg flap reconstruction in difficult tense-skin areas. *Plast. Reconstr. Surg.,* **4**: 724, 1982.

[31] Dufourmentel, C. Le fermeture des pertes de substance limitées le lambeau de rotation en losange. *Ann. Chir. Plast.,* **7**: 61–66, 1962.

[32] Webster, R.C., Davidson, T.M. and Smith, R.C. The thirty degree transposition flap. *Laryngoscope,* **88**: 85–94, 1978.

[33] Bray, D.A. Clinical applications of the rhomboid flap. *Arch. Otolaryngol.,* **109**: 37–42, 1983.

[34] Cuono, C.B. Double Z-plasty repair of large and small rhombic defects: The double-Z-rhomboid. *Plast. Reconstr. Surg.,* **71**: 658–666, 1983.

[35] Cuono, C.B. Double Z-rhombic repair of both large and small defects of the upper extremity. *J. Hand Surg.,* **9A**: 197–201, 1984.

[36] Alvarado, A. Reciprocal incisions for closure of circular skin defects. *Plast. Reconstr. Surg.,* **67**: 482–491, 1981.

Further reading

Banks, A.S. and McGlamry, E.D. 'Z' incision and surgical access to the plantar aspect of the foot. *J. Foot Surg.*, **27**: 134–138, 1988.
Becker, F.F. Rhomboid flap in facial reconstruction. *Arch. Otolaryngol.*, **105**: 569–573, 1979.
Cantanzariti, A.R. and Wehman, D. Rotational skin flap for treatment of hypertrophic plantar scars. *J. Foot Surg.*, **27**: 124–126, 1988.
Dintcho, A.S. Plastic surgery techniques of the foot. *Arch. Podiatric Med. Foot Surg.*, **4**: 1, 1977.
Dobbs, B.M. Arthroplasty of the fifth digit. *Clin. Podiatrics Med. Surg.*, **3**: 29–39, 1986.
Fenton, C.F. Wound healing in podiatric surgery. *J. Foot Surg.*, **27**: 99–102, 1988.
Grumbine, N.A. Split thickness skin grafts from the junctional skin of the arch. *Clin. Podiatric Med. Surg.*, **3**: 259–267, 1986.
Monaco, A. and Grumbine, N.A. Lines of minimal movement. *Clin. Podiatric Med. Surg.*, **3**: 235–239, 1986.
Sullivan, J.D. Approaches to the ankle region. *Clin. Podiatric Med. Surg.*, **3**: 289–302, 1986.
Webster, R.C. M-plasty techniques. *J. Dermatol. Surg.*, **2**: 393–396, 1976.

2 Local anaesthetics

ROGER BUTTERWORTH

Introduction

Any agent that, when applied to nerve tissue, is capable of preventing conduction in the neurone, can be called a local anaesthetic. This definition encompasses a wide range of active substances. Clinically useful local anaesthetic agents must induce a reversible block to conduction.

Discovered in the late nineteenth century, cocaine was the first local anaesthetic isolated. It was used in the then new field of ophthalmic surgery, for which an anaesthetic was essential. The topical anaesthetic potency of cocaine is equalled by very few agents. However, its toxicity, action on the central nervous system and the addiction of many of the early researchers led others to split the molecule in their search for a true local anaesthetic. Tropocaine and eucraine resulted (**2.1**).

Subsequent research showed that less complex molecules could induce very effective anaesthesia when infiltrated in the region of the nerve. Procaine and the ester group of local anaesthetics resulted directly from these studies. Lignocaine (Lidocaine), now the most widely used agent, was discovered in 1943 in research into the cause of haemorrhage in young cattle fed on spoilt hay.

2.1 Isolation of local anaesthetic activity of cocaine.

Pharmacology

Chemically, local anaesthetics possess an aromatic, lipophilic group and a hydrophilic group linked through a chain. This classical shape is found extensively in pharmacologically active substances and is associated with an amphoteric character and surface activity. Most of the clinically active compounds are linked with either an ester (COO–) or amide (NH.CO–) group (**Table 2.1**). These links give rise to the major families of local anaesthetics, the esters and amides, for which procaine and lignocaine, respectively, are the parent compounds (**2.2**).

The electrical impulse is transmitted along the neurone by the depolarizing effect of the sudden influx of sodium ions into the axon. This changes the potential

Table 2.1 Clinical information on some commonly used local anaesthetics

Anaesthetic	Group	Max. safe dose for 70 kg* adult	Max. safe dose per kg body weight	Latency	Duration of anaesthesia
Bupivacaine (Marcaine, Marcain)	Amide	150 mg or 30 ml of a 0.5% solution	2 mg/kg	30 min	8 h
Lignocaine (Duncaine, Lidocaine, Xylocaine)	Amide	200 mg or 20 ml of a 1% solution	3 mg/kg	5–10 min	1.5–2 h
Mepivacaine (Carbocaine, Meverin)	Amide	400 mg or 55 ml of a 0.5% solution	5 mg/kg	Rapid	Slightly longer than lignocaine
Prilocaine (Citanest Distanest, Propitocaine, Xylonest)	Amide	400 mg or 55 ml of a 0.5% solution	10–16 mg/kg	Varies with site	Similar to lignocaine
Procaine (Ethocaine, Neocaine, Novocain, Planocaine)	Ester	1000 mg or 100 ml of a 1% solution	–	Rapid	0.5 h

* The values quoted are for local anaesthetic solutions injected *without* a vasoconstrictor agent. When vasoconstrictors are used the maximum safe dose can be increased as the agents remain more localized. It is good practice in all drug therapy to use the *lowest* effective dose.

from the resting level, -70 mV to $+40$ mV at the maximum action potential. Local anaesthetics have been shown to act at a receptor in the sodium channel. The impulse is gradually blocked and conduction lost in the nerves according to their size. Large, myelinated nerves are the most difficult to block as the local anaesthetic can only gain access to the plasma membrane of the axon at the nodes of Ranvier. Full conduction block is only achieved in these neurones when two or more consecutive nodes are affected. Conduction proximal and distal to the point of application remains normal in all conductive tissues.

Pain is carried on small non-myelinated neurones, which are easily blocked by the local anaesthetic. The sensations of pain and temperature are very rapidly lost when an anaesthetic is applied. Thus, selective sensory loss can be achieved by careful adjustment of the concentration and site of infiltration of the local anaesthetic. Motor function is usually retained but the autonomic nerves are often affected, resulting in vasodilation. The traditional term 'local anaesthetic' has been replaced by 'local analgesic' in some recent texts as the latter is a more accurate reflection of the clinical use of the drugs; anaesthesia implies loss of motor and sensory impulses, whereas analgesia is the suppression of pain.

Conduction on the neruone returns in reverse order; motor function is only affected for very short periods of time. The last sensation to reappear is pain. Patients can experience prolonged analgesia in the post-operative period, which is psychologically beneficial.

Procaine (ester-linked)

Lignocaine (amide-linked)

2.2 Chemical structures of procaine and lignocaine.

Local anaesthetics have pK_a values between 7 and 9 (**Table 2.2**). Therefore, they are weak bases, present as both ionized and un-ionized drugs at physiological pH values. The ionized form is active at the sodium channel but the agents diffuse through lipid layers as the free, un-ionized bases. An amphoteric character and a pK_a close to physiological pH are essential to the potency and pharmacology of these agents.

Local anaesthetic free bases are relatively insoluble in water; therefore, they are formulated as solutions of a water-soluble salt that dissociates on contact with physiological buffers. Traditionally, the hydrochloride is used, but recently trials have been carried out using carbonated agents. The carbonate dissociates more rapidly than the hydrochloride, depositing the local anaesthetic quickly at the nerve. The latent period is therefore shorter and the block more intense. However, the products are more expensive and not marketed worldwide at present.

There is no evidence to suggest that local anaesthetics interfere with wound healing, whether administered with or without vasoconstrictor agents.

Table 2.2 Pharmacological information

Anaesthetic	pK_a	Primary metabolic pathway and route of elimination
Bupivacaine	8.2	Metabolized in the liver, some unchanged drug and N-dealkylated metabolite found in urine
Lignocaine	7.86	Metabolized by oxidases and amidases in liver, excreted in urine, some unchanged; excretion enhanced in acid urine
Mepivacaine	7.8	Some metabolized in liver and excreted in urine; excretion enhanced in acidic conditions; not metabolized in neonates
Prilocaine	7.9	Metabolized in liver, kidney, and lungs, partly by amidases, more rapidly than lignocaine; may account for the increased incidence of methaemoglobinaemia seen; very little excreted unchanged in urine
Procaine	8.9	Metabolized throughout tissues and plasma by various esterases; metabolites found only in urine

Clinical considerations

The ideal characteristics of local anaesthetic agents have been summarized as follows:[1] complete reversibility; low systemic toxicity; action confined principally to nerve tissue; short onset time and a duration sufficient to facilitate the required procedure without unnecessarily prolonging the recovery period; solubility in saline and water; sterilizability and storability without deterioration; compatibility with vasoconstrictor drugs and non-irritability to the tissues.

It is also necessary to remember that local anaesthetics function best in a substrate that is neutral or has a slightly alkaline pH. An acidic substrate, such as inflamed tissue with its accompanying acidosis, will prejudice their efficacy.

Adrenaline and other vasoconstricting agents

The use of vasoconstrictors in local anaesthetic solutions is advocated for three reasons: they produce a bloodless field in local infiltration; the constriction of the blood vessels slows the absorption of the drug and minimizes the risk of a toxic reaction; and they prolong the time of analgesia by ensuring that the solution is not washed away or metabolized.

Over the years, however, a convention has developed which dictates that vasoconstrictors should not be used in conjunction with local anaesthetic solutions in the vicinity of the digits, because the consequent (profound?) vasoconstriction will result in development of gangrene. Many authorities now challenge this view, and are able to produce evidence to support their arguments. It is also true that almost all the papers on this subject relate to injections into the fingers rather than the toes, and that in many cases the conclusion is based on incomplete evidence. Additionally, these papers relate almost exclusively to epinephrine (adrenaline).

According to Bradfield,[2] 'Forty-one cases of this complication (gangrene of the finger) have been reported in the literature. Three have been added to this number as a result of personal communications. In studying these cases it has been difficult to come to very definite conclusions because much of the information is missing concerning the factors which may have been responsible for the development of gangrene. Unfortunately the facts available in the articles reporting the occurrence of gangrene are too scanty to be much help in all but the . . . use of adrenaline and the presence of a tourniquet.' Bradfield summarises these findings in **Table 2.3**. He concludes that 'It is accepted as axiomatic today that adrenaline must not be present in the anaesthetic solution for digital blocks. It is not certain, however, whether it is safe to use a tourniquet . . . there are 2 cases of gangrene which occurred in the absence of both adrenaline and a tourniquet.'[2] Bradfield also raises the possibility of factors other than adrenaline and a tourniquet being responsible for adverse reactions and lists volume of anaesthetic solution injected, time taken for the procedure, and the presence of peripheral vascular disease (Raynaud's phenomenon) as being possible causes of an ischaemic reaction.

Professor Mercado,[3] commenting specifically on the foot is less compromising: 'There seems to be a well-ingrained belief that the use of (adrenaline) epinephrine in local anaesthetics used for digital blocks will cause permanent damage to the blood vessels and hence cause gangrene. Where this began, it is hard to tell, but it is certainly lacking in clinical research. Kaplan and Steinberg, reporting their individual findings of thousands of well-documented cases, emphatically disagree with this antiquated truism. The use of epinephrine (adrenaline) in healthy patients with patent circulation is recommended whenever its action is desirable.'

Dagnall[4] offers further insight into the origins of this dispute by pointing out that in the not too distant past local anaesthetic solutions were mixed with adrenaline immediately before injection, with very little control over the accuracy of the dosage, and with consequent massive adrenaline overdose, leading to profound vasoconstriction and gangrene.

Table 2.3 Gangrene of the finger following digital block anaesthesia (from Bradfield[2])

	Tourniquet+	Tourniquet−	Tourniquet?
Adrenaline+	3	6	11
Adrenaline−	1	2	3
Adrenaline?	7	9	2

One must conclude that the use of a 1:200,000 concentration of epinephrine (adrenaline) in conjunction with local anaesthetic solutions is only contraindicated by pathologies such as vascular disease, that vasoconstriction in digital (especially nail) surgery is better achieved by tourniquet, and that where vasoconstrictors are used they should still be used with discretion.

Felypressin (Octapressin) and other recently developed vasoconstrictors would appear to offer a much safer alternative, producing fewer undesirable reactions, especially if vascular disease is present. Their main advantage is that '. . . they act directly on the smooth musculature without causing sympathetic stimulation.'[5] 'Although Felypressin (Octapressin) is a perfectly adequate vasoconstrictor for enhancing local anaesthetic potency and duration, it appears to provide poor control of haemorrhage during surgery because it does not constrict arterioles effectively. In describing a vasoconstrictor similar to Felypressin, however, Lindorf[6] suggests that this observed deficiency may be merely the result of time lag in the vasoconstrictor response.'[7]

Monoamine oxidase inhibitors (MAOIs) increase the susceptibility to adrenaline. Local anaesthetic solutions containing adrenaline are therefore contraindicated in patients taking MAOIs.

Complications and contraindications

The remote nature of the foot and the relatively small doses of local anaesthetic needed to achieve analgesia serve to minimize the possibility of complications as well as making contraindicators less significant, but this does not mean that the potential dangers of these drugs can be ignored: deaths do occur from the direct and indirect effects of local anaesthetics. Complications arising from the use of local anaesthetics are local, general, or psychogenic.

Local complications develop in the proximity of the injection and fall under five headings.

- Infections, which by definition are the result of a breakdown in procedure, particularly inadequate skin preparation.
- Tissue reaction, due to the deposition of metallic ions and other contaminants.
- Needle injuries causing haematoma, thrombosis, or nerve damage (with a resultant paraesthesia), which are unavoidable, and loss of a needle in the tissues. The effects of traumatic paraesthesia may last several weeks, and both the surgeon and the patient should be aware of the fact.

- Chemical vasoconstrictors producing profound reaction, and the consequent onset of gangrene. Vasoconstriction may also occur spontaneously as an idiosyncratic reaction to an anaesthetic (and some are recognized as having the potential to cause vasoconstriction as a side-effect). In this latter case, however, the effect is not so profound and may be mitigated by blocking the nerve trunk serving the area with another anaesthetic, so inducing a sympathetically moderated vasodilation in the area.
- Toxic solutions inadvertently injected into the area in mistake for the anaesthetic!

General complications, with the exception of allergic reactions, should not be seen when correct doses are properly administered for foot surgery. These reactions are most likely to occur where doses at or above the advised maxima are used intravenously, or following spinal and epidural anaesthetics. Systemic reactions fall into three major categories:

- Central nervous system reactions: these are preceded by restlessness, yawning, nausea, and vomiting, and followed by convulsions and respiratory failure.
- Cardiovascular reactions—these can result in a fall in blood pressure (mimicking syncope) and myocardial depression, leading to arrhythmias and cardiac arrest.
- Allergic reactions—these can combine features of both the above but may be of more rapid onset. They include bronchospasm, urticaria, and oedema. Contact dermatitis and all allergic reactions are more likely to occur with the ester-linked drugs; hence the preference for amide-linked agents to which allergy is rare.

Any systemic reaction to a local anaesthetic must be regarded as extremely serious. The initial response is to cease the administration of the drug. If an overdose is suspected, a tourniquet should be applied to the limb to prevent further absorption of the local anaesthetic into the general circulation. Place the patient horizontal, elevating the legs, and assist respiration with oxygen. If the patient suffers respiratory failure or cardiac arrest, external massage must be commenced. Then send for an ambulance.

Psychogenic reactions and syncope will both arise from stress brought on by the anticipation of surgery, and it is wisest not to commence procedures using local anaesthesia if the patient appears unduly agitated. If the patient has a history of anxiety, this may be moderated by a pre-operative sedative. Syncope is treated by placing patients horizontal and elevating their legs. Although not strictly necessary, the post-syncope symptoms in patients are most readily alleviated by giving the patient oxygen.

All local anaesthetics are contraindicated in cases of epilepsy, myasthenia gravis, impaired cardiac conduction, and liver damage. Ester-linked local anaesthetics antagonize the sulphonamide antibacterial agents and may increase the risk of infection in some applications. Amide agents do not pose this problem. Similarly, the ester-linked agents are contraindicated in patients known to have low plasma esterase levels as they may experience prolonged anaesthesia and toxicity due to reduced metabolism. These contraindications, together with the higher incidence of allergic reactions, have made the amide-linked agents the more widely used local anaesthetics.

Patient preparation and positioning

Experience suggests that it is most convenient to complete all local anaesthetic procedures prior to commencing the preparation of the patient for surgery. Not only does this avoid complicating, and possibly prejudicing, the pre-operative routine, but it also allows the patient to be prepared for surgery while the practitioner is awaiting the onset of the anaesthetic. The skin may also be sterilized with an alcohol swab, independently of the surgery. When commencing the anaesthesia it is advisable to place any posterior ankle blocks first, with the patient lying prone, and then to turn the patient to a supine position if anterior ankle blocks or dorsal infiltrations are necessary. Carrying out the procedures in this way minimizes moving the patient and allows one to settle the patient before the pre-operative routine. The provision of a personal stereo for the patient during procedures, especially those in an operating theatre, not only helps to divert the patient's attention from the surgery but also allows the surgeon to speak more freely to his colleagues without fear of causing the patient additional anxiety.

Administration of local anaesthetics

Although the percutaneous administration of local anaesthetics is a rapidly developing area, the use of such substances is confined to specific, relatively superficial, procedures. Local anaesthetic solutions remain the conventional approach to most procedures and are administered by a hypodermic syringe, through a carefully prepared skin.

The choice of applicator and needle must be a personal decision. In principle, the finer the gauge of the needle, the less discomfort it will cause the patient, and it is the compatibility of the finer gauge 25 or 27 needle that may ultimately determine the choice of applicator. All modern needles have a bevelled tip (**2.3**) and good practice requires that the bevel is situated uppermost as the needle is inserted into the slightly stretched skin with a quick jab. Some practitioners advocate the raising of a small wheal at the site of the injection as a basis from which to make further injections. It is also important to use a needle of sufficient length and never insert it to its 'hub'.

One of the less appreciated complications of any injection is that of a needle breaking at the point where it joins the hub. If this should occur while the needle is fully inserted into the patient it will be lost, and can then only be recovered by surgery, which is often surprisingly difficult.

It is hardly necessary to add that syringes must always be sterile and that the sterility of the needle must be maintained throughout the injection. To this end, needles should be changed after the filling of the syringe (where cartridges are not being used), and before re-using a half-filled syringe. This last point is especially important, since the process of attempting to restore a needle to its sheath to maintain its sterility is the one that most commonly results in the surgeon sticking the needle into his own finger (needlestick injury). Care must also be taken to eliminate all air from the syringe before injecting the patient. In practice, it is often easiest to use 2, 3, or 5 ml disposable applicators that can be thrown away after using once.

Before injecting the solution, practitioners should always aspirate the syringe to ensure that they are not injecting into a blood vessel or cavity. Perhaps the only exception to this requirement is when the point of the needle is moving constantly through the tissue in infiltration techniques. Should the effect of aspiration be to fill the syringe with blood (**2.4**), then it is advisable to remove the needle and re-inject with an uncontaminated solution.

For most patients, the worst part of the anaesthetizing process is not the 'jab' as the needle penetrates the skin but the infiltration of the solution into the tissues, which frequently produces an intense stinging sensation, either from the use of a solution below body temperature[8] or from the fluid forcing the tissues apart. This is almost entirely avoided by using solutions at room or body temperature and by either minimizing the pressure applied to the plunger in the applicator and, therefore, the pressure at which the solution enters the tissues or by using a smaller applicator. In most cases a 2 ml applicator is quite sufficient and reduces interstitial pressure, which is especially important in younger patients in whom the tissue tone is good. The tissues of older patients accept the solutions much more easily. The anaesthetic process therefore requires time, and this means that the practitioner should rest comfortably and is not stressed by bending over or standing at a difficult angle.

If, during the injection process, a sudden resistance develops, the needle should be withdrawn slightly and

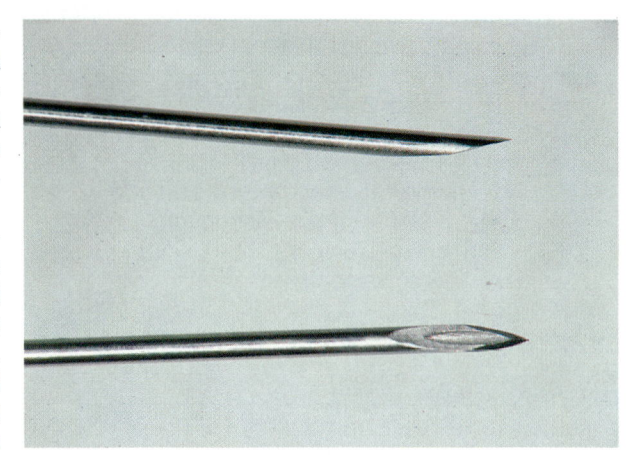

2.3 Bevelled needle tip.

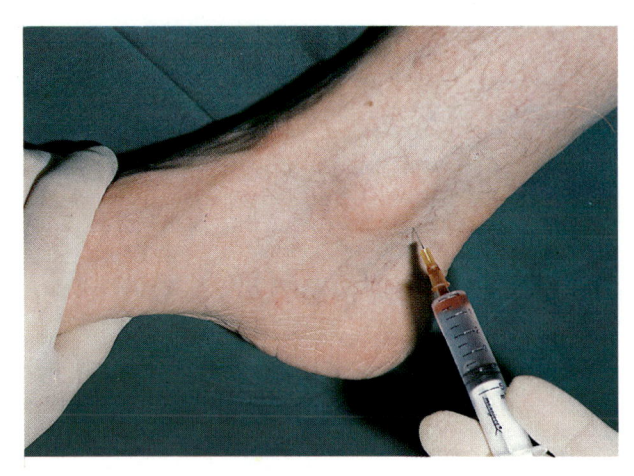

2.4 Aspiration, demonstrating the withdrawal of blood.

re-inserted at a different angle. There is evidence to suggest that pockets formed by 'fascio-septal compartments'[9] will act to inhibit the infiltration of the solution, especially in the toes, and the practitioner will have to move the tip of the needle out of these 'pockets'. Conversely, if the resistance to the solution rapidly decreases, the process should also be suspended and the point of the needle moved to another location, since such a decrease in pressure usually indicates that the needle has penetrated a body cavity, or more seriously, a blood vessel.

Local anaesthetics must be administered with care: not only because of the systemic potential but also because of the damage that can be caused to soft tissue, especially nerve trunks and occasionally blood vessels, by the carelessly executed injection. The use of these anaesthetics in conjunction with adrenaline or other vasoconstrictor drugs has already been discussed, but it should never be forgotten that vasoconstrictors may further modify the pharmacology of the solutions.

There will always be a delay between the injection of an anaesthetic and the onset of its effects: this period of latency varies with patient and with anaesthetic. The same principle also applies to the potency and duration of different anaesthetics (**Table 2.1**). Clinically, these features can also be combined to provide post-operative analgesia for the patient in procedures which experience shows to be accompanied by an unreasonable amount of post-operative pain. The most common example is the combination of Lidocaine and Bupivacaine.

Two less welcome effects of the unpredictability of both the anaesthetic and the way in which the patient reacts to it are that occasionally one may come across a patient who appears to be unaffected by the drug, or conversely, a patient exhibits an expected but exaggerated response. In the first case, the practitioner will have little choice but to switch to an alternative drug; in the second, the response to watch out for is from those anaesthetics that are known to have a mild vasoconstrictor effect and which, for idiosyncratic reasons, produce an exaggerated or prolonged response in the patient.

Before commencing surgery the effect of the anaesthetic can be tested with a disposable needle by lightly stabbing the operative area with either end, and asking the patient to identify the sensation as being 'sharp or blunt' (or absent). However, do not place too much importance on such tests; they do not take the problem of trespass into consideration and are, at best, rather subjective.

As with the administration of most drugs, common sense dictates that only the lowest effective dosage at the lowest effective concentration should be used, and that the maximum safe dosage should never be exceeded. Since dosages tend to be given by weight, whereas solutions are measured by volume, a small calculation is needed to ensure that the dose relates accurately to the patient, who is defined by 'adult body weight' (**Table 2.4**).

Although local anaesthetics will act in a slightly acidic environment, the latency will be significantly prolonged and the potency severely diminished. The drugs diffuse to the plasma membrane as free bases which are not present in acidic conditions. Local anaesthetics are not administered to inflamed areas as the buffer capacity of such tissues is significantly impaired. Injection into infected tissue is irresponsible, as it can only spread the infection and prejudice healing.

'Given suitable patients and lots of practice, total anaesthesia of the foot can be obtained with as little as 2 ml of anaesthetic solution. This is possible because all the nerves to be blocked can be visualized or palpated as they cross the ankle, thereby making it possible to deposit the anaesthetic solution in close proximity to each individual nerve fibre'[10].

Table 2.4 Calculating the 'maximum safe dosage' for local anaesthetic solutions

The maximum safe doses for local anaesthetics are given in the literature in mg for a 70 kg individual. A calculation must be made to convert this information to the volume of solution of given concentration.

The maximum safe dose D (ml) of a solution of concentration $Z\%$ (w/v) is

$$D = \frac{X \times 100}{Z}$$

Where X is the maximum safe dose.

Consider a 2% solution of lignocaine: the maximum safe dose is 200 mg (0.2 g) for a 70 kg individual, so the maximum advised adult dose is

$$D = \frac{0.2 \times 100}{2} = 10 \text{ ml}$$

The maximum safe dose (D) for a *young child* or *small adult* is calculated as

$$D = \frac{X \times Y \times 100}{70 \times Z}$$

Where Y is the weight of the child in kg.

The calculation is simplified by using the maximum safe dose per kg body weight. (V g/kg). The equation then becomes

$$D = \frac{V \times Y \times 100}{Z}$$

Example: The maximum safe dose of a 2% lignocaine solution for a child weighing 35 kg is

$$\frac{0.003 \times 35 \times 100}{2} = 5.25 \text{ ml}$$

When calculating by this method the result is slightly higher than if the adult doses were divided. This is because the dose per kg body weight is quoted to the nearest whole number.

Recording the volume of anaesthetic solution administered

It is inevitable that in the filling of syringes, the elimination of air bubbles and the administration of the anaesthetic solution, some of the solution will be wasted. It is therefore impossible to say with absolute accuracy how much solution is injected into the patient. When recording the volume of solution administered, it is recommended that the maximum possible dosage be described, so as to avoid any ambiguity; that is, if two 5 ml vials of solution are opened during the administration of a local anaesthetic, the dose recorded should be 10 ml.

Administration of local anaesthetics

Prepare emergency resuscitation equipment. Prepare skin with antiseptic of choice, clean with 70% alcohol, and dry.

Select a syringe compatible with the volume of solution to be injected. The larger the syringe, the greater the hydrostatic pressure and, consequently, the greater the potential for pain.

Personally identify the anaesthetic agent and its concentration. Use at room/body temperature. Cold solutions cause pain.

Calculate the maximum safe dosage, having regard for the physique and age of the patient. Special considerations apply with children, the aged, and the ill.

Use the minimal volume of solution at the minimal effective concentration.

Select a needle of smallest practical gauge and length.

Inject slowly and aspirate frequently.

Carefully observe the reactions of the patient during and after the injection; be prepared for adverse reactions.

Innervation of the foot and ankle

Apart from the saphenous nerve (**2.5, 2.6**), a terminal cutaneous branch of the femoral nerve which supplies the medial side of the leg and ankle, the innervation of the foot and ankle derives from the sciatic nerve (**2.7**) through its two major branches: the larger tibial nerve (**2.7**) and the smaller common peroneal nerve (**2.7**).

The tibial nerve (**2.8**) and its derivatives, the sural nerve (**2.6, 2.7**), medial and lateral plantar nerves, and plantar digital nerves (**2.9**), innervate the muscles of the back of the leg and the sole of the foot and are cutaneous to the back of the leg and the plantar surface of the foot.

The common peroneal nerve (**2.7**) divides above the popliteal fossa to give a communicating branch to the sural nerve, and then passes along the medial border of biceps femoris, lateral to the gastrocnemius. The nerve lies above the tendon of biceps femoris as it inserts into the head of the fibula. Before winding around the neck of the fibula, the common peroneal nerve divides to give a sensory branch to the skin and the lateral cutaneous sural nerve. Distal to the head of the fibula, it divides into its two terminal branches, the superficial (**2.6**) and deep peroneal nerves.

The superficial peroneal nerve (**2.10**) supplies the peronei and is cutaneous to the lower part of the front of the leg before dividing to form the medial and intermediate dorsal cutaneous nerves and the dorsal digital nerves, which innervate the skin of the dorsum of the foot and toes (**2.11**).

The deep peroneal nerve supplies all the muscles in the anterior compartment of the leg together with extensor digitorum brevis muscle. Most important, it is cutaneous to the contiguous sides of the first interdigital space (**2.12**).

The innervation of the digits derives as a fairly complex hierachy from the tibial and common peroneal nerves (**2.11**), the only exception being the medial border of the foot to the first metatarsal phalangeal joint, which is innervated by the saphenous nerve.

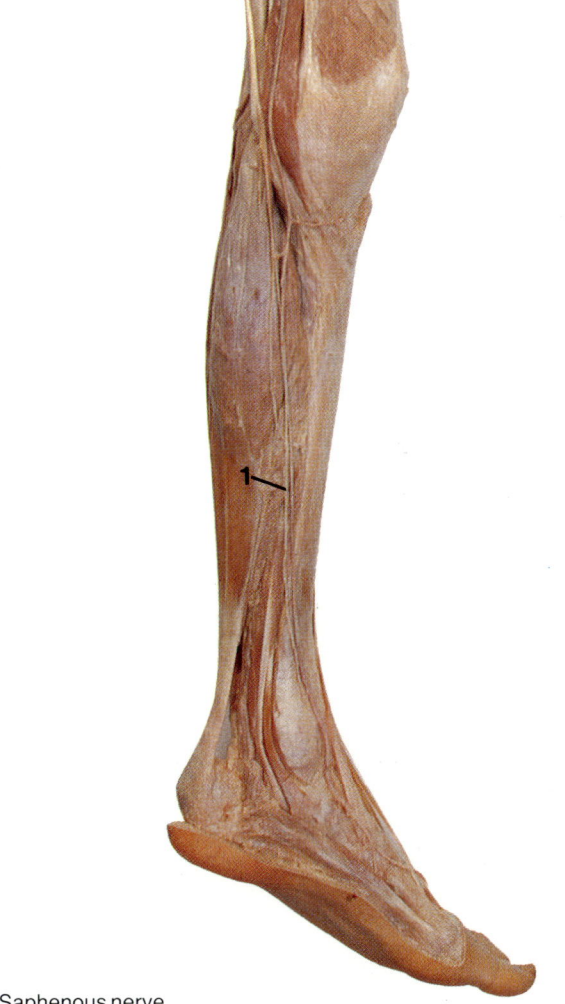

2.5

1 Saphenous nerve

2.5 Dissection of the lower limb, demonstrating the saphenous nerve. (From McMinn et al.,[11] with permission.)

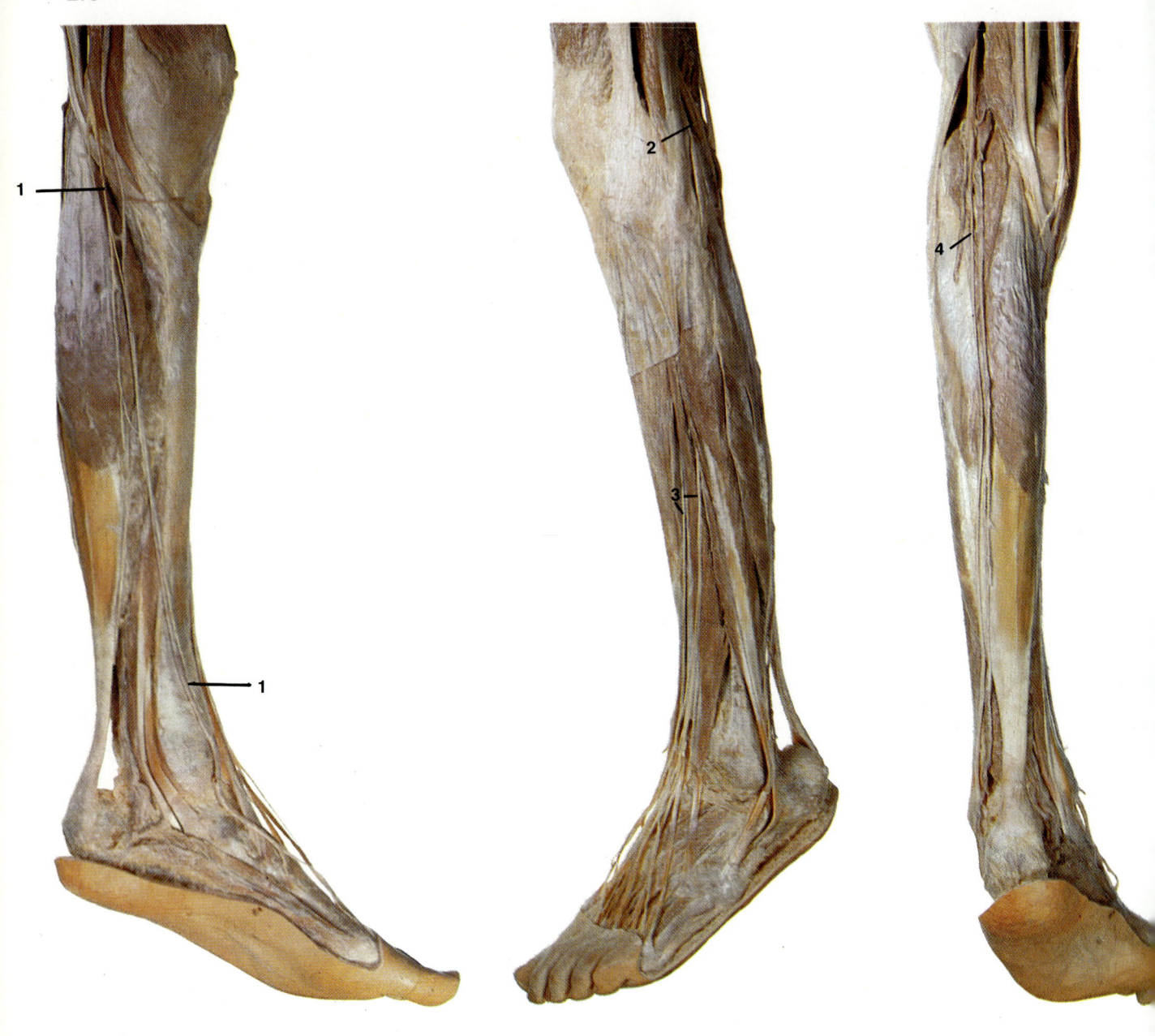

1 Saphenous nerve
2 Common peroneal nerve
3 Superficial peroneal nerve
4 Sural nerve

2.6 Dissection of the leg and foot, demonstrating the saphenous, common peroneal, superficial peroneal, and sural nerves. (From McMinn et al.,[11] with permission.)

The basic organization of the digital innervation is that each toe derives two dorsal and two plantar digital proper nerves (medial and lateral) from the common dorsal and plantar digital nerves, respectively, each of the proper nerve branches supplying contiguous sides of the digits. The one exception to this formula is the first digital interspace, the contiguous sides of which are supplied by the deep peroneal nerve.

The distribution of the nerves in the lower extremity may be variable, in the position, the bifurcation, and the areas of the foot the nerves supply. The problem of trespass is an ever-present difficulty for those attempting to anaesthetize the foot, and especially the toes. In foetal nail development, the primary nail field develops on the apex of the toe before migrating dorsally to the adult position. In doing so, it would appear to take its innervation with it and, in consequence, the nail bed itself frequently derives its nerve supply from the plantar digital proper nerves.

Another consequence of these variations is that the bifurcation of the nerve may occur proximal to its expected position, which results in a correctly positioned nerve block with incomplete anaesthesia. This is a problem most frequently encountered in the superficial peroneal nerve.

1 Sciatic nerve
2 Tibial nerve
3 Common peroneal nerve
4 Sural nerve

2.7 Dissection of the lower limb, demonstrating the sciatic, tibial, common peroneal, and sural nerves. (From McMinn *et al.*,[11] with permission.)

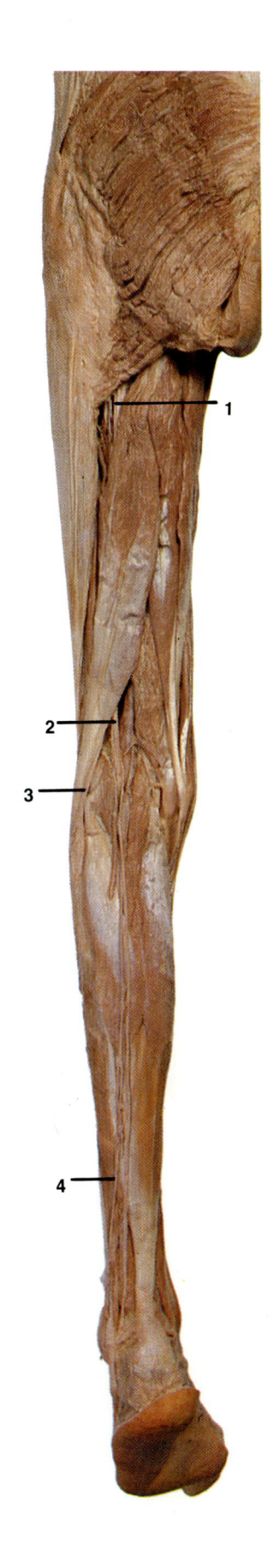

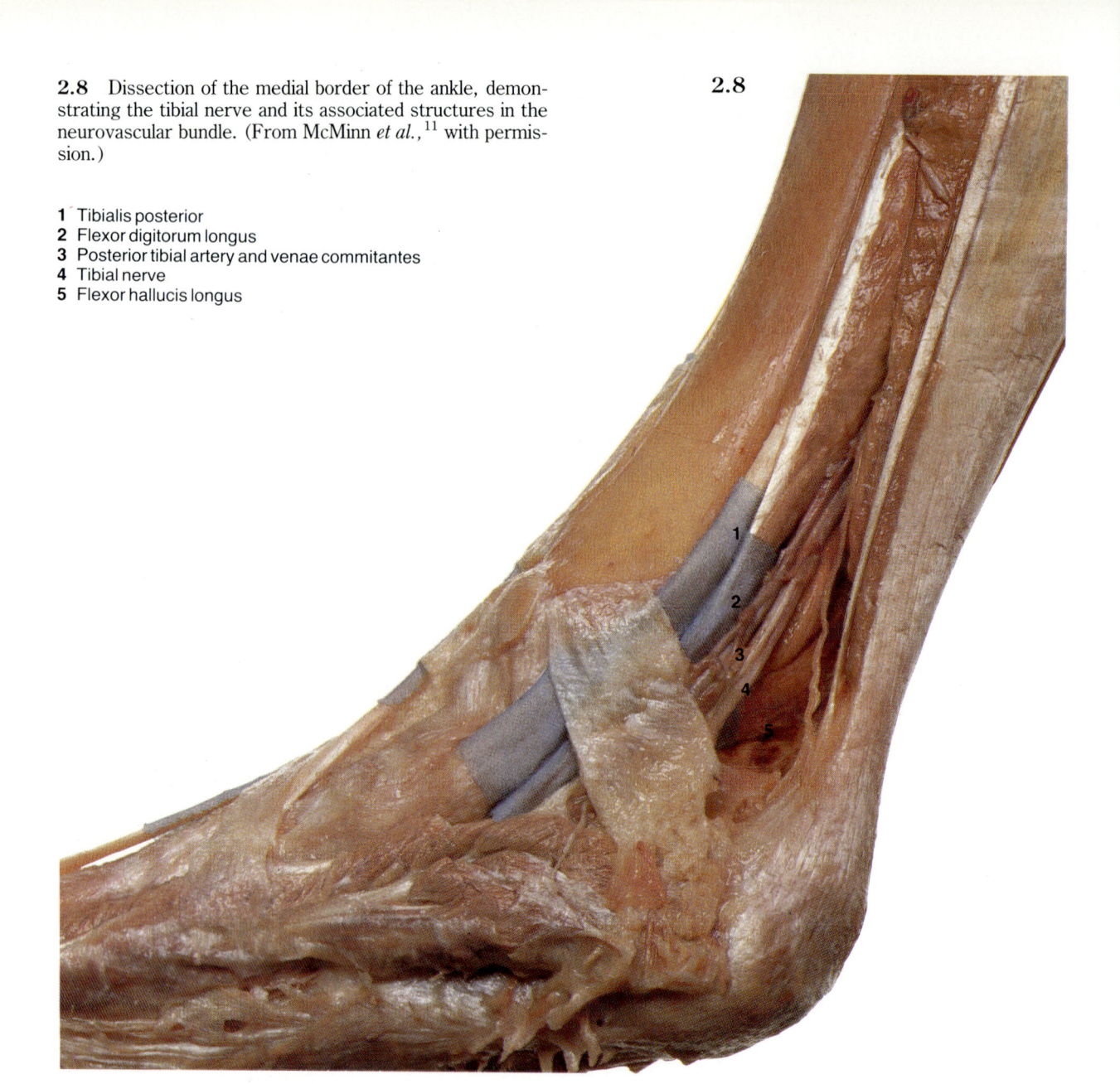

2.8 Dissection of the medial border of the ankle, demonstrating the tibial nerve and its associated structures in the neurovascular bundle. (From McMinn et al.,[11] with permission.)

1 Tibialis posterior
2 Flexor digitorum longus
3 Posterior tibial artery and venae commitantes
4 Tibial nerve
5 Flexor hallucis longus

2.9

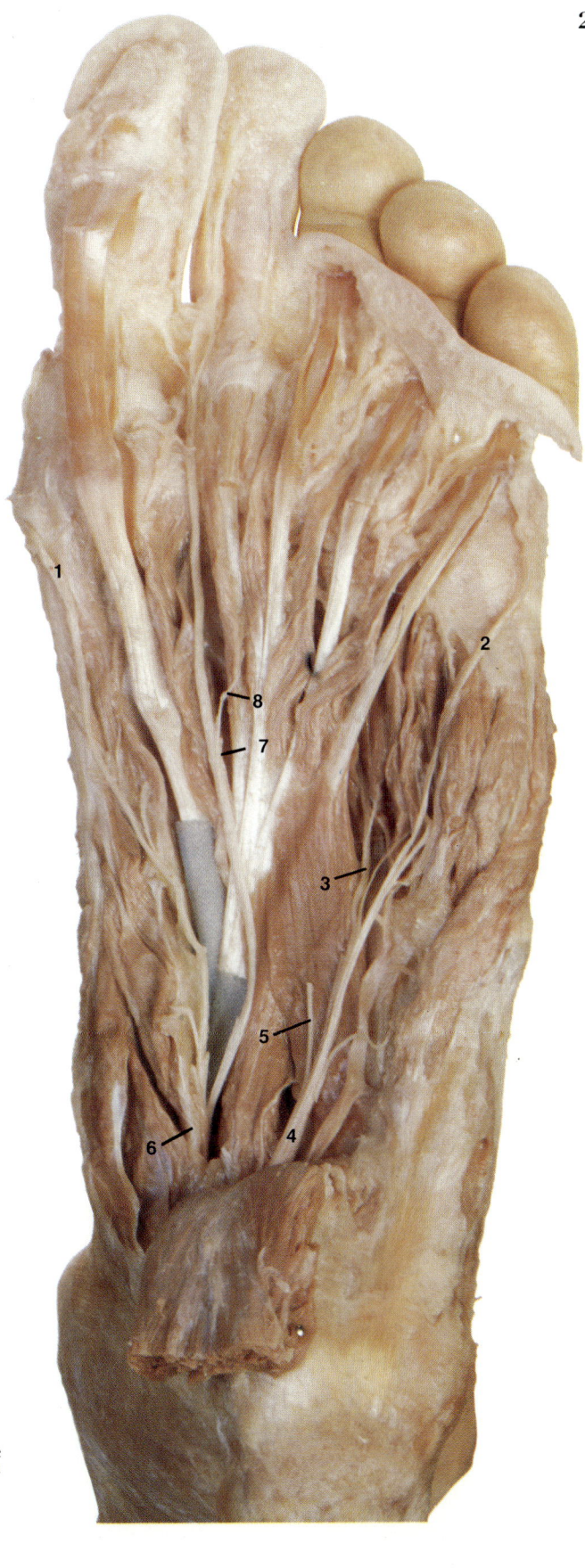

1 Proper plantar digital nerve of great toe
2 Proper plantar digital nerve of fifth toe
3 Deep branch of lateral plantar nerve
4 Lateral plantar nerve
5 Fourth common plantar digital nerve
6 Medial plantar artery overlying nerve
7 First common plantar digital nerve
8 Nerve to first lumbrical

2.9 Dissection of the sole of the foot, demonstrating the distribution of the plantar nerves. (From McMinn *et al.*,[11] with permission.)

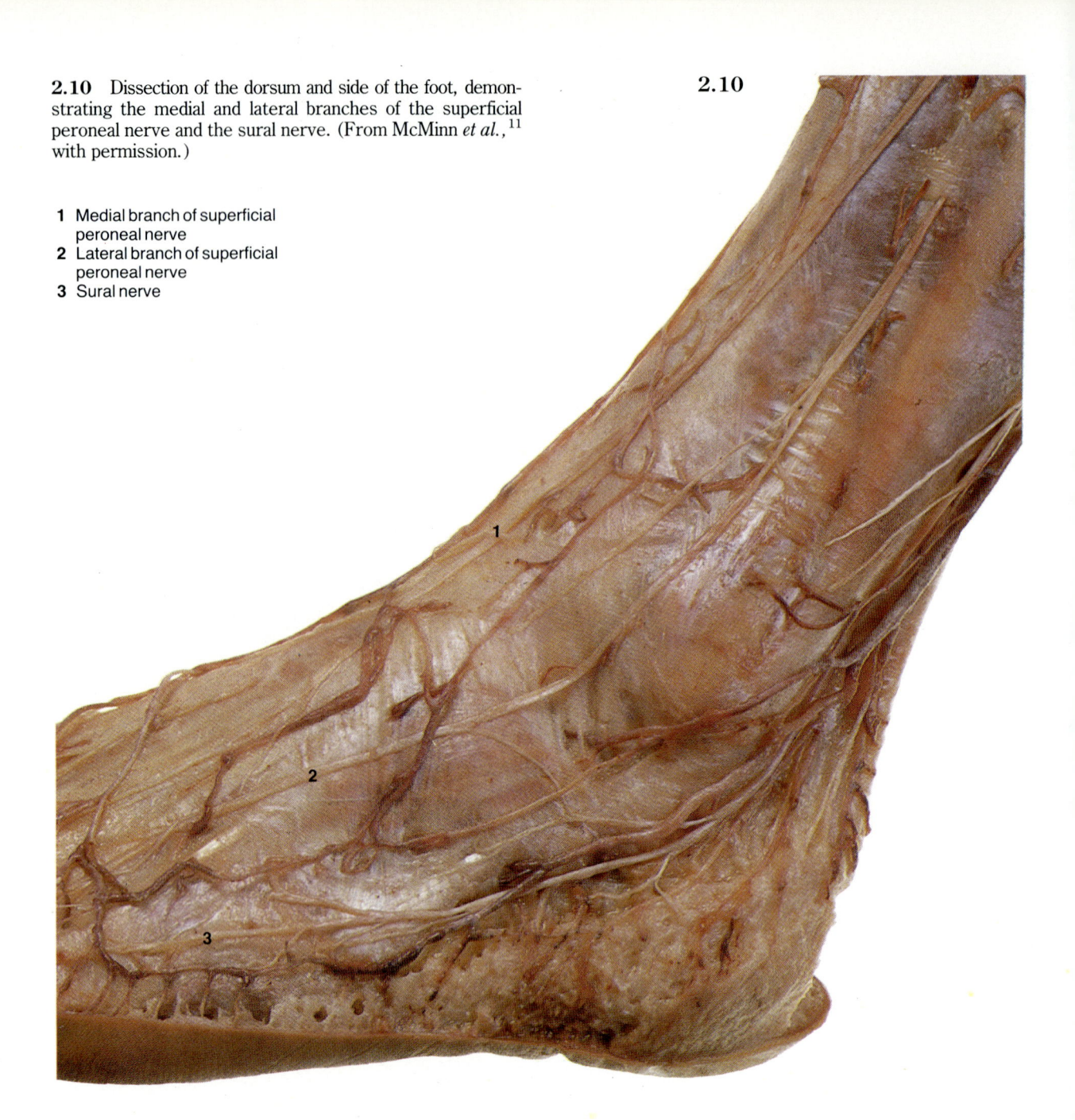

2.10 Dissection of the dorsum and side of the foot, demonstrating the medial and lateral branches of the superficial peroneal nerve and the sural nerve. (From McMinn et al.,[11] with permission.)

1 Medial branch of superficial peroneal nerve
2 Lateral branch of superficial peroneal nerve
3 Sural nerve

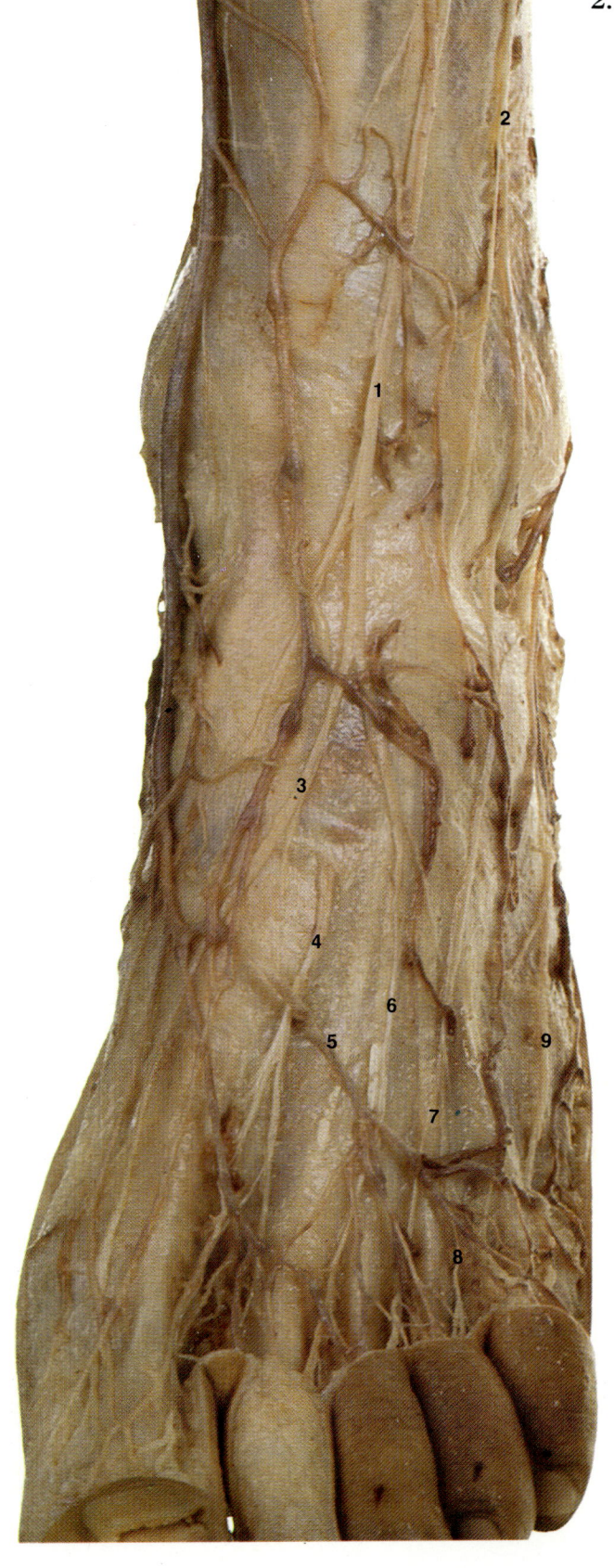

1 Medial branch of superficial peroneal nerve
2 Lateral branch of superficial peroneal nerve
3 Proper dorsal digital nerve of great toe
4 Medial terminal branch of deep peroneal nerve
5 Dorsal venous arch
6 Dorsal digital nerve to second cleft
7 Dorsal digital nerve to third cleft
8 Dorsal digital nerve to fourth cleft
9 Sural nerve

2.11 Dissection of the dorsum and sides of the foot demonstrating the distribution of the dorsal digital nerves. (From McMinn et al.,[11] with permission.)

2.12 Dissection of the dorsum and sides of the foot demonstrating the deep peroneal nerve and its medial terminal branch. Note its distribution to the contiguous sides of the first digital interspace. (From McMinn *et al.*,[11] with permission.)

1 Deep peroneal nerve
2 Medial terminal branch of deep peroneal nerve

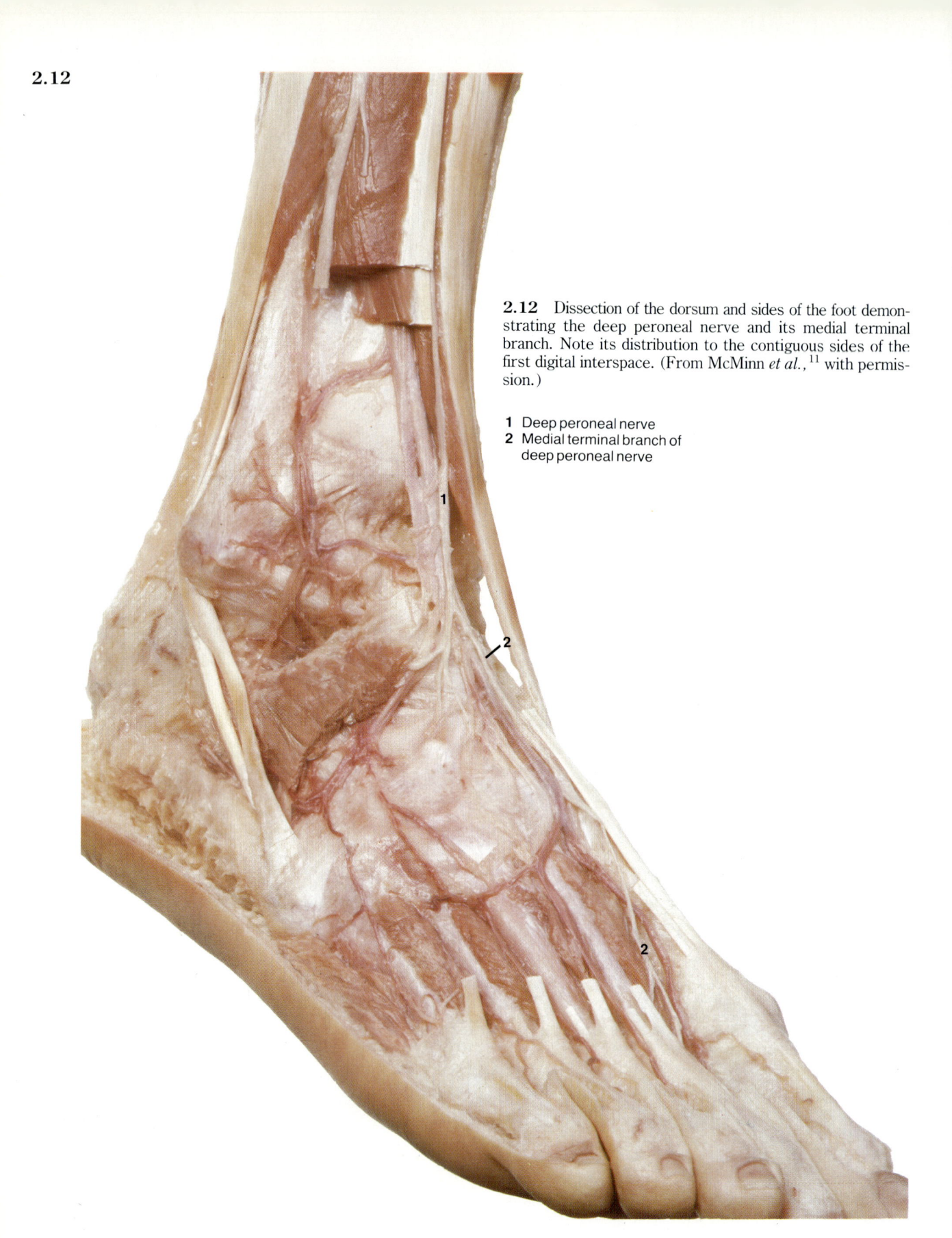

Specific procedures

Procedures for anaesthetizing the lower limb can be divided into three groups: percutaneous anaesthesia, used for desensitizing the skin and superficial tissues; nerve blocks, which block sensory (and motor) impulses through a nerve trunk; and infiltration techniques, including digital and Mayo blocks.

Percutaneous anaesthesia

Topical formulations of local anaesthetics were developed alongside the parenteral applications. The first use of cocaine was as a topical anaesthetic, but none of the more recently synthesized agents have been as effective when applied to membranes. Many are well absorbed when applied to mucous membranes and are used in a wide range of topical formulations, including cough lozenges, haemorrhoid creams, and anaesthetic sprays. Absorption of the local anaesthetic from such products can vary considerably, and accidents have occurred when individuals have absorbed doses equivalent to intravenous injections after applications of sprays to mucous membranes. None of the products used on mucous membranes are effective when applied to intact skin.

Many minor surgical procedures, particularly in the fields of dermatology, plastic surgery, and chiropody/podiatry, involve only the superficial layers of the skin. Often the most painful part of such an operation is the infiltration anaesthetic injection(s), particularly in plastic surgery where large areas of skin may be involved, (e.g. in skin grafting). Adults can be counselled on the necessity of the injection and, when informed of the stinging, will cooperate. Children and young infants pose a very different problem. Studies have shown children fear needles most of all the invasive procedures performed in or out of hospital. Young children are often given a general anaesthetic, which is considerably more dangerous, to avoid the unpleasantness of the needles.

Although much research has been carried out in the field of percutaneous anaesthesia over the past 30 years, few products have reached the market and most of these have either contained unacceptably high concentrations of drug or penetration-enhancing agents that are detrimental to the skin.

EMLA, a product based on lignocaine and prilocaine, is being marketed in Europe to reduce pain of venepuncture. After an application time of 60 min. under occlusion, reliable analgesia is reported to have been achieved in around 80% of patients. The most recent research uses sedated infants in the pre-operative period, the analgesic being used to reduce the stress of the intravenous anaesthetic. This test removes the subjectivity of analgesic testing, as the children do not wake on insertion of the needle.

EMLA and similar products have been tested as analgesics for taking split-skin grafts, superficial biopsy, and dermabrasion, with some reported success. Most reports note a reduction in the pain, and any infiltration analgesic can be administered with reduced discomfort. EMLA is currently under testing for a range of chiropody/podiatry applications, but the results are unpublished.

Nerve blocks

The efficacy of a local anaesthetic solution is not entirely pharmacological; it also depends on the proximity of the solution to the nerve. Around the knee and ankle, the superficiality of the nerve trunks facilitates the process of analgesia and several of the nerves can be palpated or visualized and even a paraesthesia elicited by pressure. Where palpation is not possible, the position of the nerve trunk may be sufficiently consistent for paraesthesia to be elicited by moving the needle from side to side after insertion, and before injection. Where more than one block is being used, particularly if the whole foot is to be anaesthetized, the blocks should be placed at different levels to reduce the risk of circulatory complications. For example, the saphenous nerve may be blocked at the level of the knee, rather than the ankle, and the superficial peroneal nerve can be blocked by anaesthetizing its derivatives, the medial and intermediate dorsal cutaneous nerves.

The efficacy of nerve blocks can be established by lightly pricking the skin of the area the nerve supplies, and (sometimes) by observing the reactive hyperaemia produced by the effect of the drug on the sympathetic fibres.

The common peroneal nerve

The common peroneal nerve can be palpated as it passes behind the lateral condyle of the femur or the head of the fibula and on the posteriolateral side of the neck and the fibula (**2.6**). It is at this latter point that the anaesthetic solution can be introduced. The needle is inserted vertically above the posterior edge of the fibula head and advanced about 1 cm. At this point, it should be possible to elicit paraesthesia, and after aspiration, 1–3 ml of solution can be injected into the area (**2.13, 2.14**).

This nerve block will desensitize the lateral border of the leg and the dorsum of the foot, and is particularly suited to superficial procedures in this area and to lateral ankle surgery.

Injury to the common peroneal nerve as it passes around the head of the fibula is not uncommon, and the impaired function of the lateral and anterior muscle compartments of the leg, together with the desensitization of the overlying skin, enables the clinician to visualize the effects of anaesthetizing this nerve.

2.13

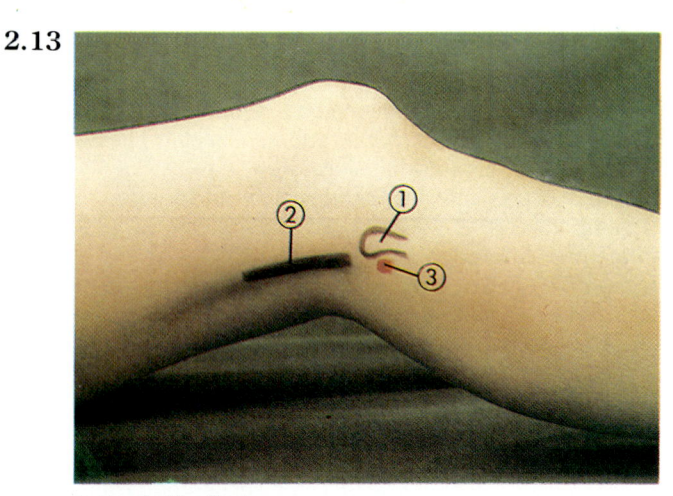

1 Head of the fibula
2 Tendon of the biceps femoris muscle
3 Point of entry (peroneal block)

2.15

2.14

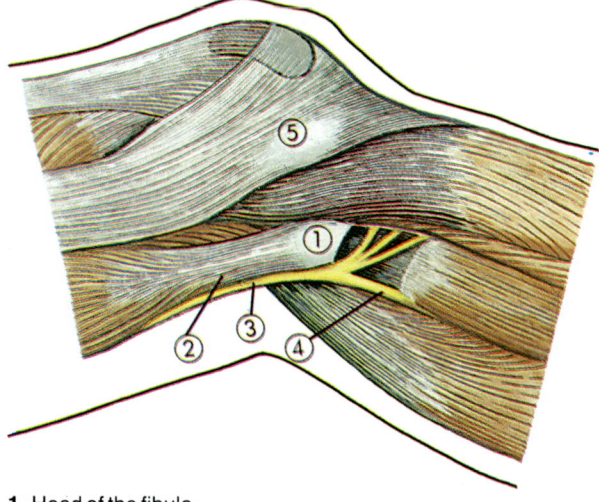

1 Head of the fibula
2 Tendon of the biceps femoris muscle
3 Common peroneal nerve
4 Lateral sural cutaneous nerve
5 Tibial tubercle

2.13, 2.14 Plotting the site of injection for a block on the common peroneal nerve. (From Hoerster et al.,[12] with permission.)

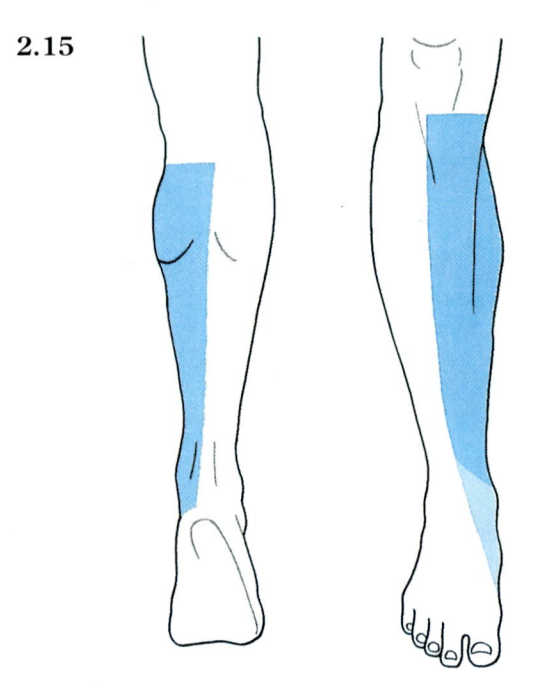

2.15 Dermatomes of the saphenous nerve. (From Hoerster et al.,[12] with permission.)

The saphenous nerve

The saphenous nerve (**2.6**) is a terminal sensory branch of the femoral nerve and descends through the sub-sartorial canal before passing deep to become subcutaneous below the insertion of sartorius. Here it joins the great saphenous vein subcutaneously, and together they travel down the medial border of the leg, to which the nerve provides a cutaneous supply (**2.15**). The nerve, which is not readily palpable, is blocked by subcutaneous infiltration around the great saphenous vein.

The block can be placed just below the knee, on the anterio-medial aspect of the leg, by subcutaneous infiltration of the area from the medial aspect of the tibial tuberosity over the medial condyle of the tibia (**2.16, 2.17**).

More accurately, a block can be placed above the medial malleolus (**2.18**) where the subcutaneous tissues overlying the tibia are thin. The exact location of the saphenous nerve at this point can be found by identifying the great saphenous vein. The foot is dorsiflexed to create a sulcus between anterior tibial tendon and the medial malleolus, and through the

2.16

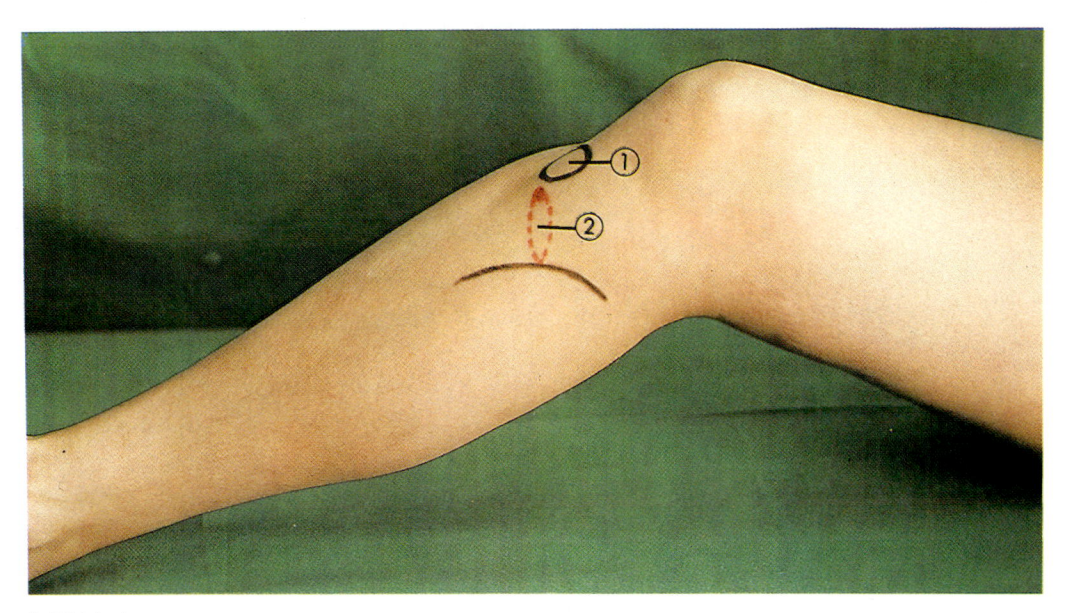

1 Tibial tuberosity
2 Subcutaneous infiltration

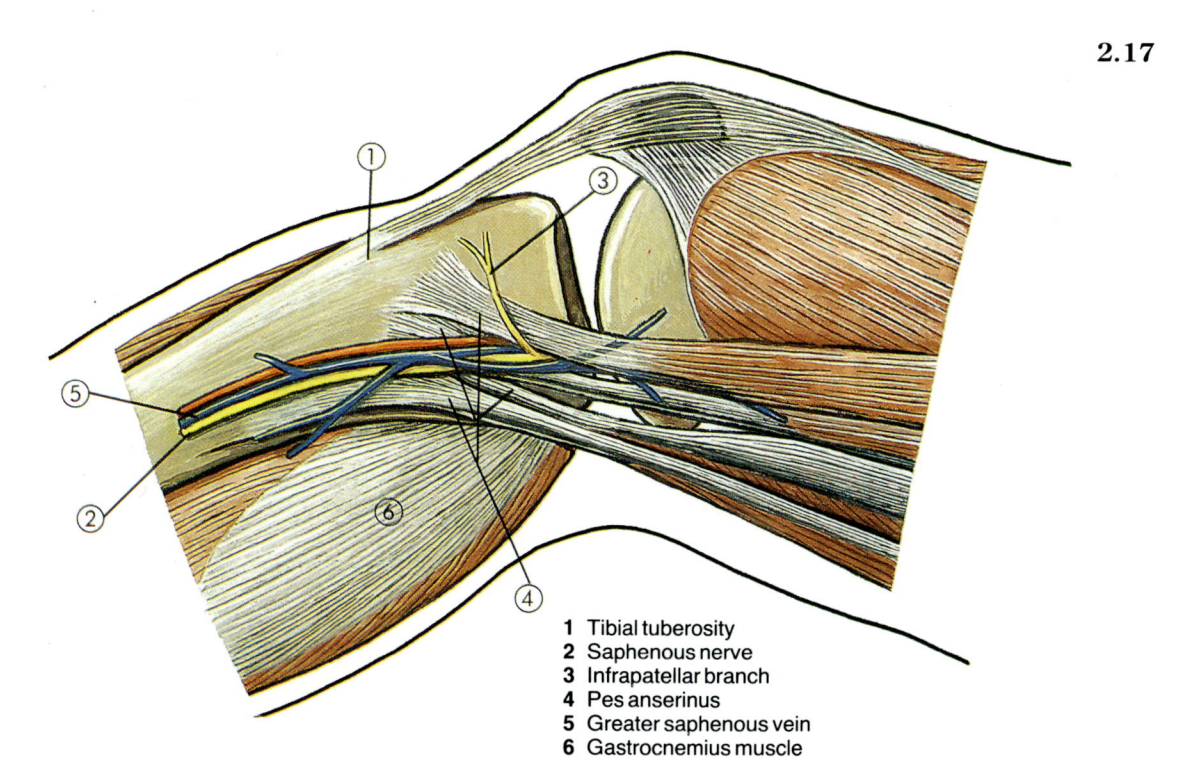

2.17

1 Tibial tuberosity
2 Saphenous nerve
3 Infrapatellar branch
4 Pes anserinus
5 Greater saphenous vein
6 Gastrocnemius muscle

2.16, 2.17 Plotting the site of injection for a (proximal) block on the saphenous nerve. (From Hoerster *et al.*,[12] with permission.)

53

2.18

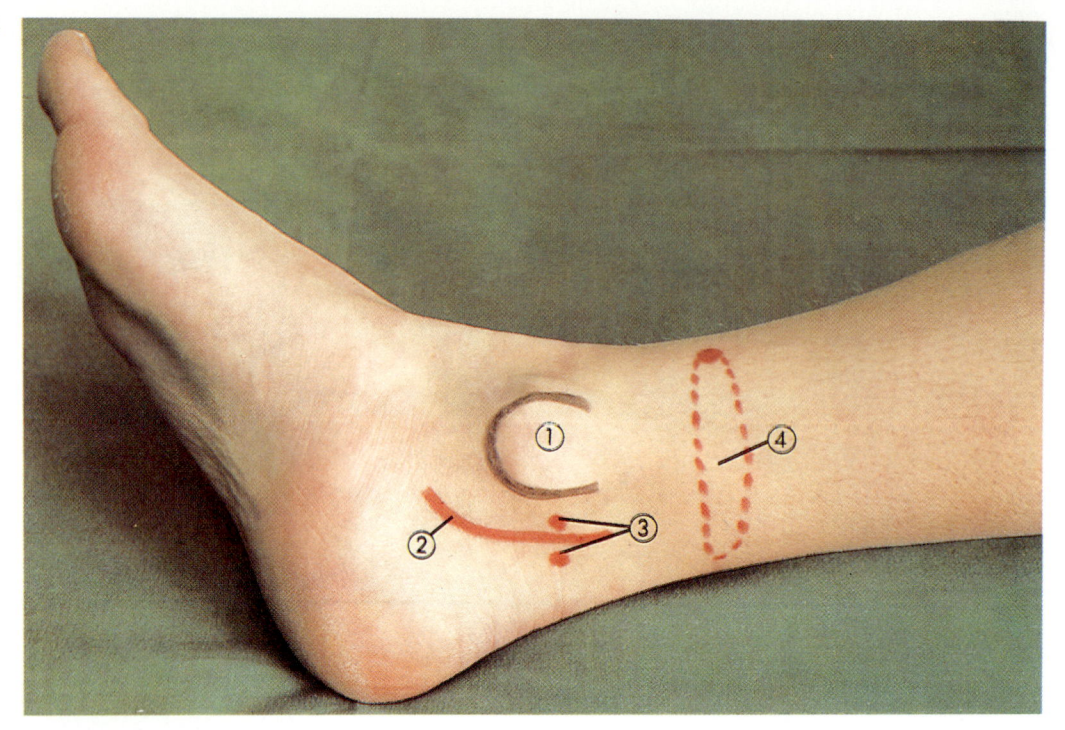

1 Internal malleolus
2 Tibial artery
3 Point of entry (tibial block)
4 Subcutaneous infiltration (saphenous block)

2.18 Plotting the site of injection for a (distal) block on the saphenous and tibial nerves. (From Hoerster et al.,[12] with permission.)

centre of this sulcus the great saphenous vein is readily visualized. It is at this point that the solution is infiltrated (**2.18**). This latter is probably the block of choice, but is contraindicated if used in conjunction with a tibial block, or if varicosity is present. Indeed, the risk of intravenous injection in varicosity is sufficient to preclude the administration of this block altogether.

At either level the block is effected by infiltrating the area around the great saphenous vein with up to 3 ml of 0.5% or 1% solution, taking care to aspirate before injecting.

The tibial nerve

The tibial nerve longitudinally bisects the popliteal fossa (**2.19, 2.20**) and should be blocked at the proximal corner of the fossa, as it emerges between the hamstrings, above the division of the sural nerve.

Because the nerve accompanies the popliteal artery and vein, and is surrounded by fat and connective tissue, the placing of the injection must be plotted very carefully (**2.19**). The patient is placed prone, the medial and lateral epicondyles of the femur are palpated and a line drawn between them. The needle is introduced vertically at the mid-point of this line, and progressed downwards for some 2–3 cm until paraesthesia can be elicited. The syringe is then aspirated, and up to 5 ml of solution is injected into the area. The depth of this nerve, and the difficulty in placing the injection with absolute accuracy, usually requires that the solution is fanned out slightly, aspirating prior to each injection.

This is one of the least pleasant injections for the patient, and it is advisable to have an assistant hold the ankle to stop the patient flexing the knee during the operation. However, one injection at this level can obviate multiple additional injections distally.

From the popliteal fossa the tibial nerve descends between the deep and superficial posterior muscle compartment of the leg, becoming superficial on the

2.19

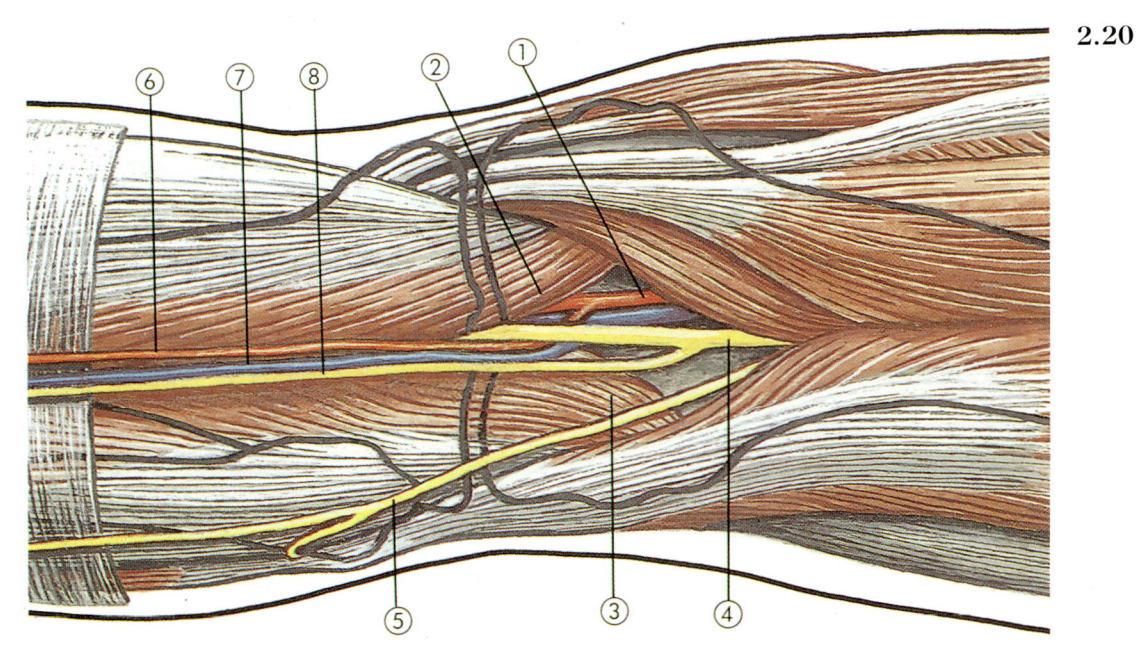

1 Popliteal artery

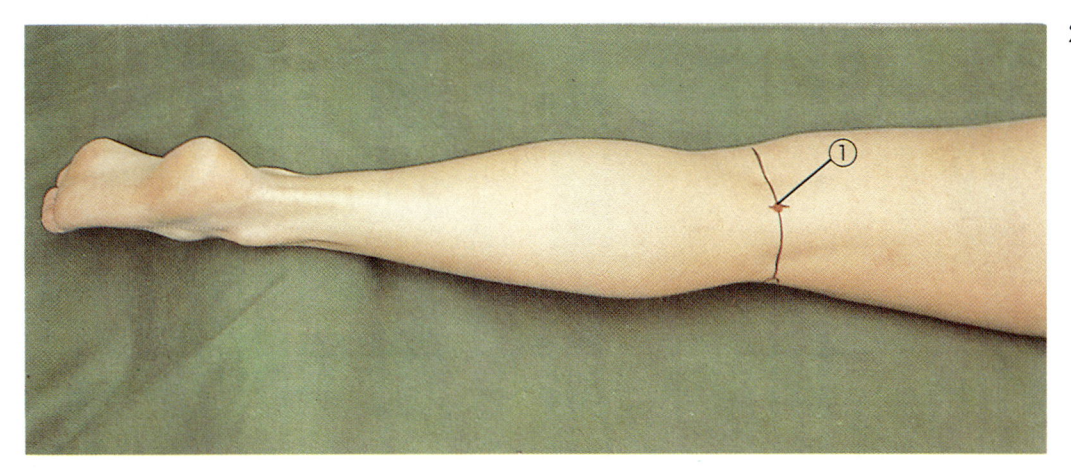

2.20

1 Popliteal artery	5 Common peroneal nerve
2 Medial head of the gastrocnemius muscle	6 Sural artery
3 Lateral head of the gastrocnemius muscle	7 Lesser saphenous vein
4 Tibial nerve	8 Sural nerve

2.19, 2.20 Plotting the site of injection for a (proximal) block on the tibial nerve. (From Hoerster *et al.*,[12] with permission.)

medial side of the ankle midway between the tibial malleolus and the tendo calcaneus. It lies immediately behind, and parallel to, the posterior tibial artery, the pulse of which gives a good indication of the position of the nerve. At this point the tibial nerve can also be blocked (**2.18**).

This lower block can be effected with the patient either prone or supine. In the first case, the patient is prone, with the ankle either supported by a pillow or the foot hanging over the edge of the table, so avoiding dorsiflexion of the foot and increased tension in the structures surrounding the ankle. The needle is then introduced to the medial side of the tendo calcaneus, immediately above the malleolus (**2.21**), and progressed downwards. The needle is taken as far as the posterior border of the tibia, and then withdrawn about

2.21

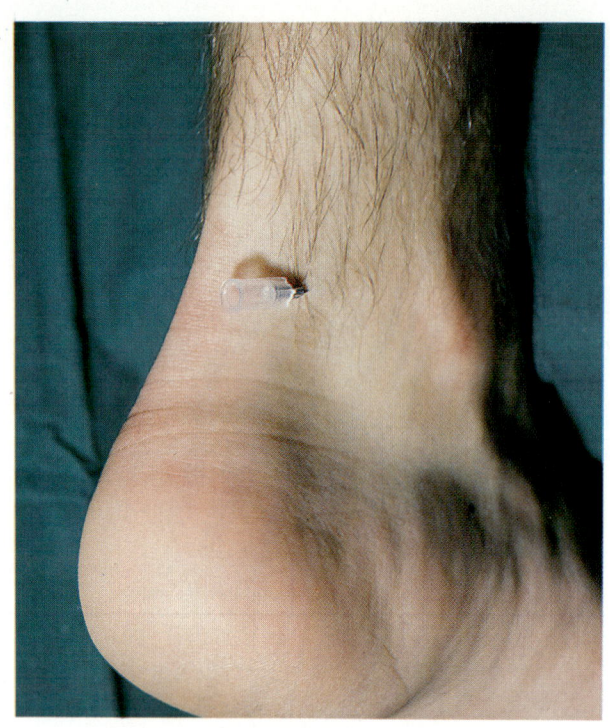

2.21 Distal tibial block, posterior approach.

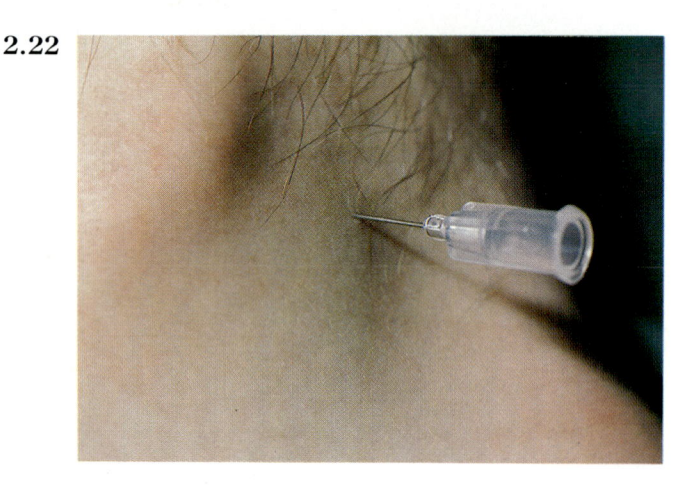

2.22

2.22 Distal tibial block, medial approach. Note neurovascular bundle.

an inch before aspiration and infiltration of the solution. Paraesthesia can frequently be elicited during the insertion of the needle, especially if the needle is moved from side to side, in which case it is not necessary to insert the needle further before injecting the anaesthetic. The advantage of placing the patient prone while introducing this block is that it facilitates the placing of a sural nerve block either in conjunction with, or as a supplement to, the tibial block. It is, of course, necessary to use a needle of sufficient length in this technique, and wise to have an assistant hold the leg to prevent flexion.

An alternative, and usually preferred method of obtaining this lower tibial block is to either place the patient prone, as described above, or in a sitting or supine position, with the leg laterally rotated and the foot slightly inverted from a neutral position. This inversion of the foot will make the neurovascular bundle behind and below the malleolus more prominent, and the nerve can then be palpated by placing the fingers just below the posterior tibial pulse and compressing the structures until the nerve is felt like a thin cord, which can be rolled between the fingers and the underlying bone. The needle is then inserted at right angles above the nerve (**2.22**), and it should be possible to elicit paraesthesia of the forefoot by gently moving the needle from side to side before aspiration and injection. The nerve can be blocked with 1 ml of 1% anaesthetic solution.

Sarrafian et al.[13] describe yet another technique, which is to be recommended where more extensive surgery is being carried out. With the patient supine, 'The foot is extended to 90° relative to the leg and is externally rotated with its lateral border resting on sheets which firmly support and elevate the foot. This provides easy access for the injection. Flexing and supporting the knee facilitates the positioning of the foot. At two finger breadths proximal from the tip of the medial malleolus, a line is drawn perpendicular to the tibial long axis (**2.23**). This indicates the level of penetration of the needle (25 gauge, 3.8 cm (1.5 inches) in length). The needle is inserted tangential to the medial border of the Achilles tendon, perpendicular to the tibia, at the level of the traced line (**2.24**). The needle is advanced until touching the tibia, withdrawn about 2 mm, and 7–10 ml of bupivacaine 0.5% are injected after an initial aspiration to assure that the needle tip is not within a vessel. No attempt is made at producing paraesthesia within the territory of the posterior tibial nerve. The injection aims at filling the neurovascular tunnel with anaesthetic agent . . . The regional block provided excellent analgesia in 94% and good in 6%. The method also has the advantage of avoiding the use of (systemic, post-operative) analgesics for a period of 10 to 25 hours post-operatively.'[13]

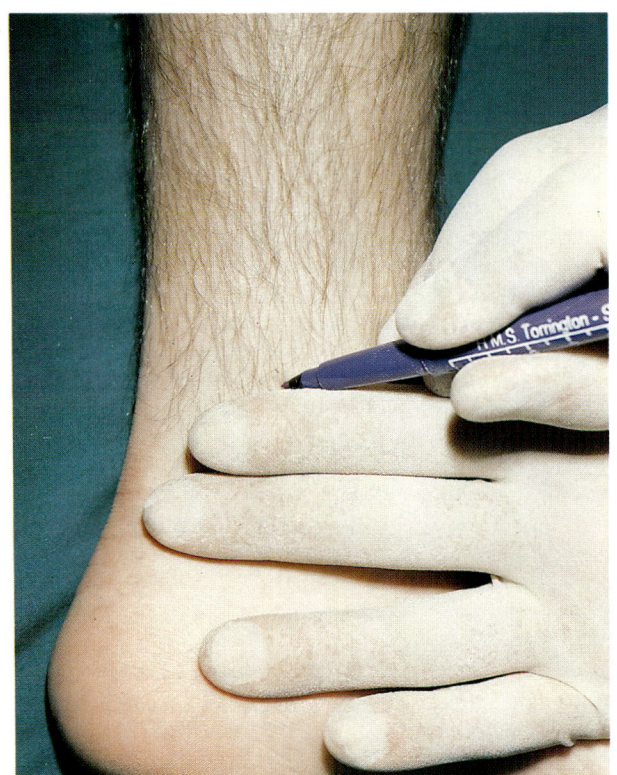

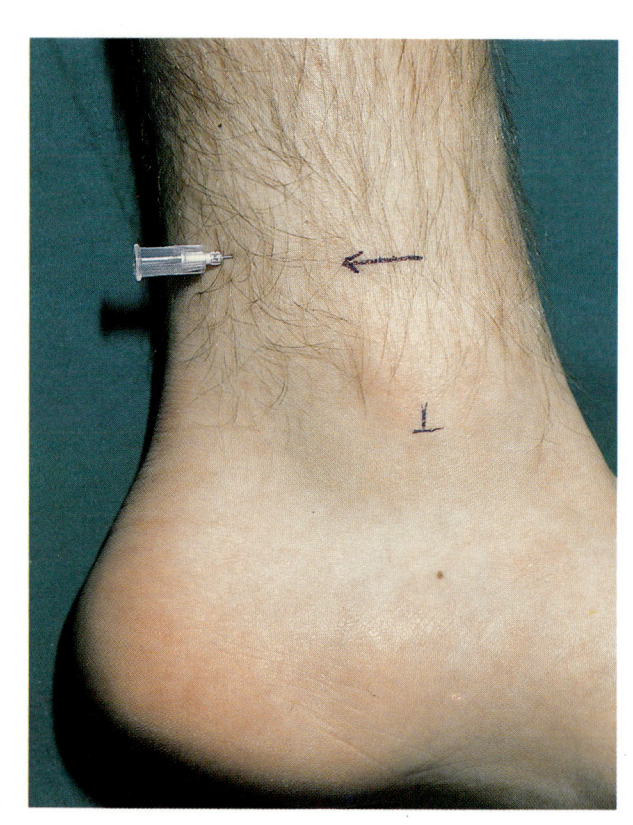

2.23, 2.24 Tibial block through an infiltration of the neurovascular tunnel, as described by Sarrafian *et al.*[13]

The sural or lateral dorsal nerve

The sural nerve arises from the tibial nerve in the popliteal fossa, and descends down the back of the leg becoming superficial half-way down and just above the point at which it is joined by the communicating branch of the common peroneal nerve. From this point it accompanies the small saphenous vein to the lateral border of the foot, passing behind the lateral malleolus, where it can be anaesthetized.

The foot should be slightly adducted and dorsiflexed, so identifying the small saphenous vein which is intimately applied to the sural nerve at this level. Finger pressure to the vein at this point readily elicits the cord-like structure of the nerve, around which the solution can be infiltrated (**2.25**): 1 ml of 0.5% or 1% solution are sufficient for the purpose of blocking the sural nerve at this point. Take care to differentiate the vein and peroneal tendon sheath from the nerve before aspirating and injecting.

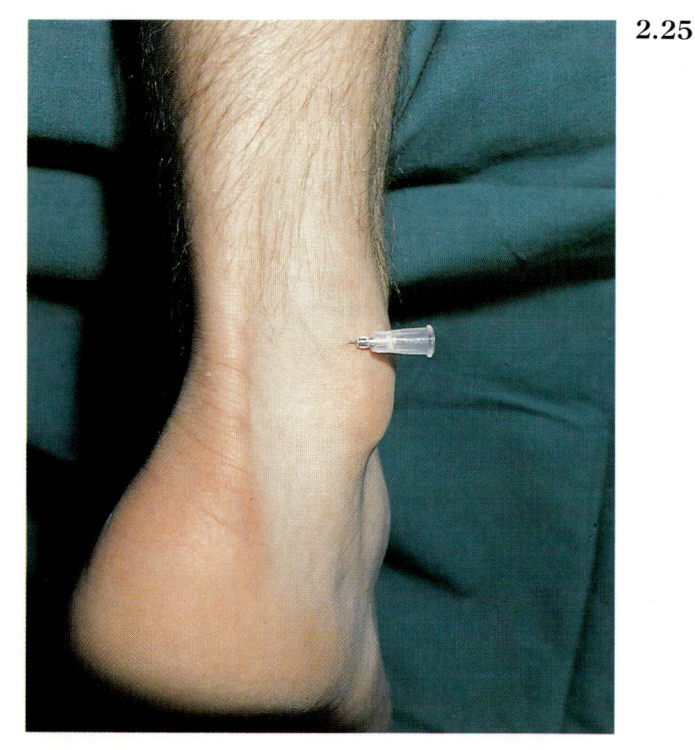

2.25 Sural nerve block.

2.26

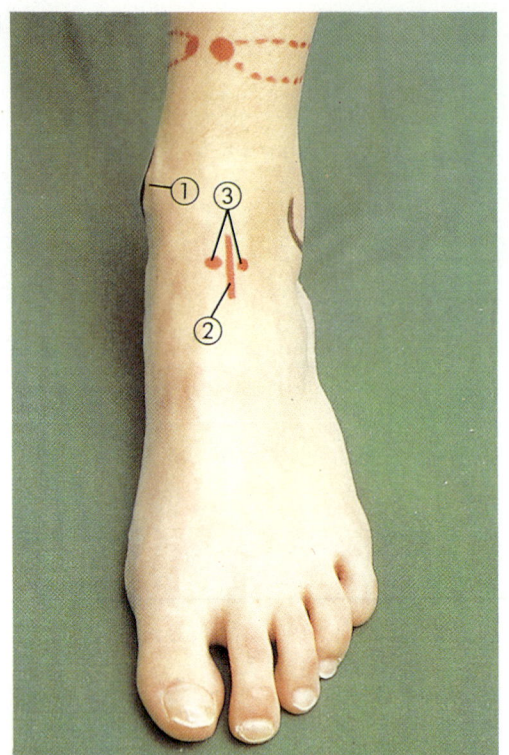

1 Internal malleolus
2 Dorsalis pedis artery
3 Point of entry (deep peroneal block)

2.27

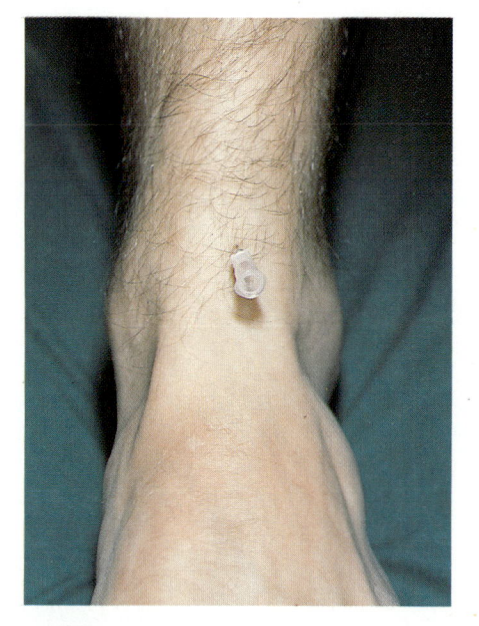

2.26, 2.27 Deep peroneal nerve block. (**2.26** from Hoerster et al.,[12] with permission.)

The deep peroneal nerve

The deep peroneal nerve descends through the anterior muscle compartment of the leg on the interosseous membrane, becoming superficial with the anterior tibial/dorsalis pedis artery at the front of the ankle. Its position at this point is easy to locate, lying directly between the extensor hallucis longus and the extensor digitorum longus tendons, above the extensor flexure lines of the ankle and with the anterior tibial artery placed laterally. Anaesthesia is elicited by placing the injection directly between the two extensor tendons, angling the needle slightly towards the medial border. The needle is inserted as far as the tibia and then withdrawn slightly before aspiration and injection (**2.26, 2.27**). Of all the nerve blocks around the ankle, this is the most accurate, and paraesthesia is so readily elicited that the solution can be deposited with great accuracy. Rarely is it necessary to use more than 2 ml of 1% solution to achieve anaesthesia.

Alternatively, the nerve can be blocked at the level of the dorsalis pedis pulse, with which it is intimately associated (**2.28**). Again, finger pressure to the pulse will enable the cord-like nerve to be palpated before aspiration and injection. The problem with this second method, however, is that it may be difficult to palpate the nerve in those 18% of patients who do not present with a dorsalis pedis pulse.

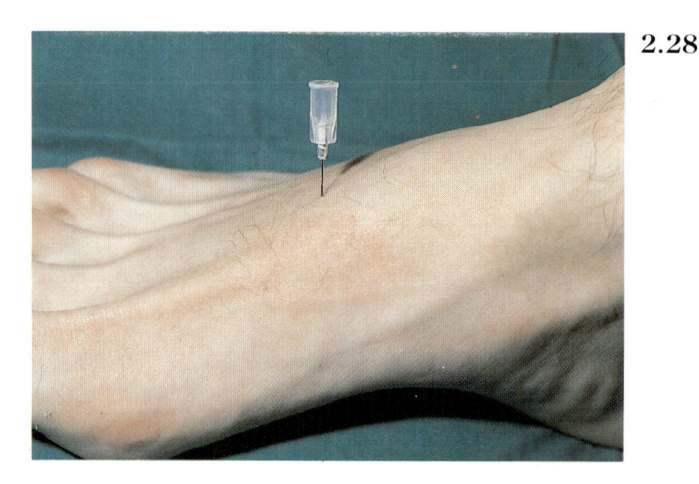

2.28 Deep peroneal nerve block at the level of the dorsalis pedis pulse.

58

The superficial peroneal, medial and intermediate dorsal cutaneous nerve

The superficial peroneal nerve descends through the peroneal or lateral muscle compartment of the leg, becoming superficial at the front of the leg between peroneus brevis and extensor digitorum longus. It is at this point that the block may be effected by a subcutaneous infiltration from the anterio-lateral border of the tibia to the lateral malleolus (**2.29**). Even if paraesthesia is elicited in this process, the infiltration should be completed because of the variable level of branching in this nerve. Lemont[14] describes a more precise variation of this procedure, which can be used in those patients in which the superficial peroneal nerve is readily palpated. 'Visually identify the intermediate dorsal cutaneous branch of the superficial peroneal by plantarflexing the foot. Trace the nerve proximally over the sinus tarsi to a point where the nerve loses its prominence . . . Inject 2 × 1 ml xylocaine peroneally.'

Greater accuracy can be attempted by blocking both the derivative nerves of the superficial peroneal nerve if they can be palpated. These are the medial and intermediate dorsal cutaneous nerves. The foot should be plantarflexed and slightly adducted, and the intermediate branch should be blocked first. It can be palpated just medial to the fibular malleolus. The medial branch lies 1 to 2 cm medial to the intermediate branch, but cannot be satisfactorily palpated by rolling beneath the fingers. It is identified by rolling between the index finger and thumb.

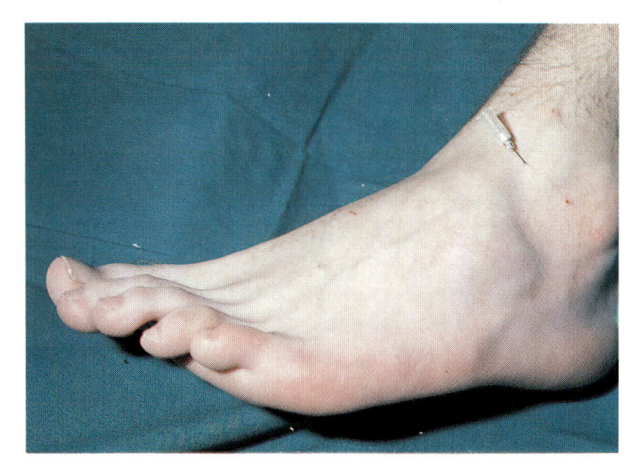

2.29 Plotting the infiltration to block the superficial peroneal nerve.

In practice, the superficial peroneal nerve and its derivatives are the most difficult nerves to palpate because they are also the most anatomically variable. For this reason they are all better treated as subcutaneous infiltrations, and anaesthetized with not more than 2 ml of 0.5% or 1% solution (**Table 2.5**).

Local infiltration

Local-infiltration techniques diffuse anaesthetic solutions throughout an area of tissue; the innervation pattern of the lower limb necessitates that this area be proximal to the area to be anaesthetized, although it usually includes the target area itself. These techniques can be used most effectively to anaesthetize small areas of relatively superficial tissue, especially when percutaneous anaesthesia is not suitable.

V-blocks

The initial injection is made just proximal to the target area and the solution is then 'fanned' out through the subcutaneous tissues, constantly moving the needle backwards and forwards. In practice, one is unlikely to penetrate blood vessels and body cavities in this situation, but it is necessary to ensure that the anaesthetic is spread evenly throughout the tissues. These blocks are sometimes called V-blocks, and can be built into a hierarchy by moving the initial injection proximally, and then placing further V-blocks at the lateral borders of the anaesthetized field. In this way, quite a large area of tissue can be anaesthetized without the necessity of a nerve block.

Probably the most common mistake in infiltration is that too high a concentration of solution is used in too great a volume simply because time is not afforded for the drug to achieve its effect.

Table 2.5 Minimal dose regional ankle block (From Carter.[10])

Nerve	Anatomical position	Sensory innervation	Identification of nerve	Methodology
Intermediate dorsal cutaneous	Lies medial to the fibular malleolus, crossing the ankle close to the midline	Central portion of the foot, lateral dorsum of the third toe, dorsum of the fourth toe, and medial dorsum of the fifth toe	Visualized by plantar flexion of the foot, with slight adduction	Inject lateral to the nerve, advance needle to the nerve, and slowly deposit 0.3 ml of solution
Medial dorsal cutaneous	Lies 1 to 2 cm medial to the intermediate dorsal cutaneous nerve as it crosses the dorsum of the foot	Medial dorsum of foot, medial side of the first MPJ and hallux plus adjacent sides of second and third toes. Does not innervate the first interspace	The proper manipulation of the nerve requires it to be rolled by the finger tips, as when rolling a pencil while keeping one's fingers on the pencil	Inject lateral to the nerve, advance needle to the nerve, and slowly deposit 0.3 ml of solution
Lateral dorsal cutaneous or sural	Passes from the lateral leg to the lateral foot, crossing the ankle with the small saphenous vein behind the fibular malleolus	Lateral aspect of the foot and the fifth toe, sometimes communicates with intermediate dorsal cutaneous nerve	Best visualized with slight adduction and dorsiflexion of the foot, Identification is the small saphenous vein, which is intimately applied to the nerve	Deeper than other dorsal cutaneous nerves, but with exacting technique the needle can be placed accurately; 0.2 ml of solution
Saphenous	Crosses the ankle between the medial malleolus and the anterior tibial tendon	Medial aspect of the foot	Identification of the nerve depends on the saphenous vein. Dorsiflex foot to form sulcus between anterior tibial tendon and medial maleolus where the vein can be easily palpated	Inject the region of the long saphenous vein; take care to aspirate before injecting 0.2 ml of solution
Tibial	Travels in the neurovascular bundles, with the posterior tibial artery and veins, lying deep to the vascular components	Divides into the medial and lateral branches, giving innervation to the entire plantar surface of of the foot	Can be palpated between the medial malleolus and the Achilles tendon. First palpate tibial pulse, and then inject behind it, after aspiration. Adduction of the foot will make the neurovascular bundle more prominent	Initial penetration over the nerve through flexor retinaculum. Aspirate and deposit 0.25 ml of solution either side of the nerve
Deep peroneal	Crosses the ankle in the neurovascular bundle on the dorsum of foot with the dorsalis pedis artery	Dorsal aspect of the first digital interspace, adjacent sides of the hallux and the second toe. Also, short extensors of the toes	Easily palpated with the dorsalis pedis pulse. Can be rolled beneath finger tips, producing paraesthesia to the first interspace	Palpate the dorsalis pedis artery, insert the needle to either side of the nerve and advance to the periosteum. Aspirate and deposit 0.2 ml of solution

Field blocks

Where a more extensive, usually deeper, field of anaesthesia is required than can be achieved by infiltration, the technique can be extended to form a field block. These blocks are of two types. In the first, the initial injection is made close to the centre of the field to be desensitized, and the solution is then fanned out through 360°. In the second, a V-block is placed distally as well as proximally to the target area.

Digital blocks

Digital blocks provide an exception to the general rule of 'lowest possible volume at the lowest possible concentration'. The restricted volume available within the diameter of the digit, and the amount of solution necessary to be effective, requires that the volume of anaesthetic be kept to a minimum at the expense of increasing the concentration of the solution. It is therefore vitally important that the dosage of the drug be monitored, especially if more than one toe is to be anaesthetized. Although the use of 'half blocks' for either side of the toe is sometimes recommended, in practice the peculiarities of digital innervation usually necessitate a total block, and even if the use of a 'half block' is proposed, its possible extension to a full block should always be anticipated.

Digital blocks are administered with the surgeon sitting with the back to the patient and leaning over the patient's extended leg, so as to inhibit any sudden movement of flexion in response to the insertion of the needle. The foot is held firmly in one hand, the digit to be anaesthetized being held between the forefinger, resting under the toe, and the thumb. The initial injection is made at the base of the toe, parallel to the interdigital webbing (**2.30**). The anaesthetic is slowly injected into the tissues in such a way as to ensure that the solution is projected ahead of the constantly moving needle. This enables the surgeon to feel the distension of the tissues as the needle approaches the ventral surface of the toe. Not only will this reduce the patient's discomfort, but too rapid a penetration of the tissues may result in the needle passing right through the toe and into the surgeon's finger. If the insertion of the needle into the dorsal skin of the toe is painful its passage out through the ventral skin is excruciatingly so, and presents serious dangers of cross-infection to both parties if the needle should also penetrate the finger of the surgeon. (The author once worked with a colleague who contracted syphilis in just this way. Today it might be hepatitis or AIDS.)

Once the ventral surface of the toe is reached, the needle should be withdrawn slightly and the solution fanned out a little to ensure an effective block of the plantar digital nerve. The needle may then be withdrawn, and in a large or 'fleshy' toe, partially repeated. Once the solution has been dispersed into one side of the toe, the needle should be withdrawn to a point at which the tip rests just below the skin. It is then turned sideways and more solution introduced across the dorsal surface of the digit (**2.31**), (the needle passing under the relaxed? extensor tendon). Care should be taken to deposit a small amount of the solution just beneath the skin at the extremity of the injection to

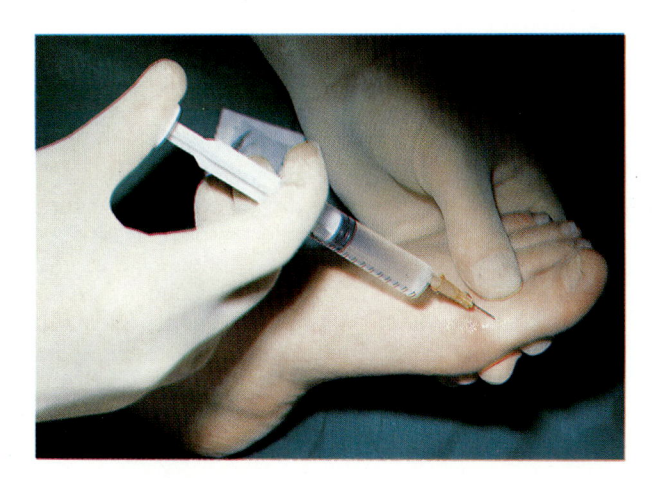

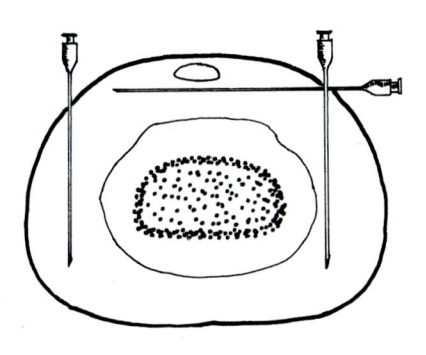

2.30 Effecting a digital (total ring block) on the hallux: medial digital infiltration.

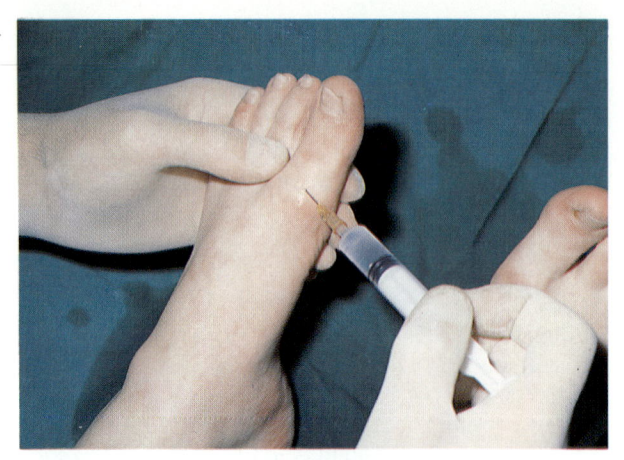

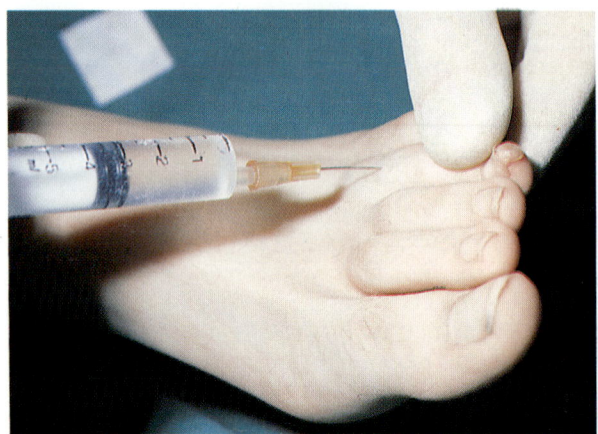

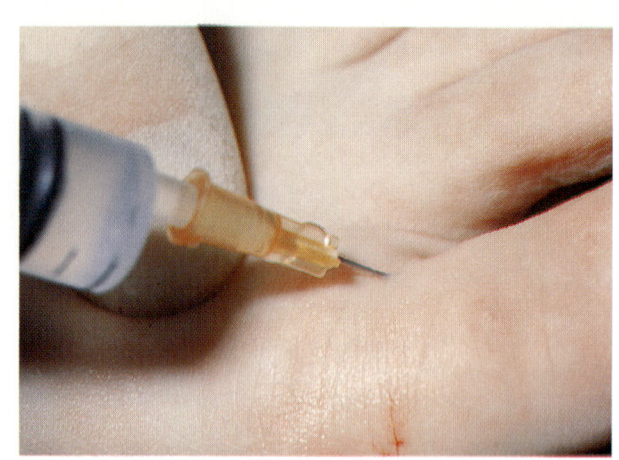

2.31 Effecting a digital (total ring block) on the hallux: dorsal infiltration.

2.32 Effecting a digital (total ring block) on the hallux: lateral infiltration.

2.33 Effecting a digital block on a lesser toe.

facilitate a second injection blocking the other side of the toe. The process is then repeated on the other side of the toe (**2.32**).

A variation of this technique can be use on the lesser toes whose relative narrowness and tissue elasticity allows one to place the injection in a centralized position on the dorsal surface. The solution can then be infiltrated around the side of the extensor tendon and down each side of the toe without the necessity to withdraw the needle (**2.33**).

Mayo block

The Mayo block is a technique in which the anaesthetic solution is infiltrated around the proximal metatarsal shaft, so as to densensitize the metatarsal head area and its corresponding digit. In practice its use is confined to first or fifth metatarsal ray surgery, where the innervation derives from the medial border only, and the problem of trespass is less likely to arise, or is more easily coped with.

The surgeon positions himself as if effecting a digital block. The forefoot is held in one hand, with the thumb dorsally. The fingers are spread over the plantar surface of the foot in the area of the injection, so as to feel any swelling of the tissue as the solution is expressed from the needle. In this way the surgeon can be sure that the needle will not penetrate the plantar skin. As with other infiltration techniques, the point of the needle should be moved constantly throughout the injection, since aspiration is not feasible, and the solution fanned throughout the intermetatarsal space. The Mayo block is ideal for small procedures, such as 'lumpectomies', in the region of the first and fifth metatarsal heads.

References

[1] Robbins, G.M. (ed.). *Clinical Handbook of Podiatric Medicine,* 2nd edn. Ohio College of Podiatric Medicine, 1983, pp. 1–5.
[2] Bradfield, W.J.D. Digital block anaesthesia and its complications. *Br. J. Surg.*
[3] Mercado, O.A. *An Atlas of Foot Surgery, Vol. 1. Forefoot Surgery.* Illinois College of Podiatric Medicine, 1980, p.3.
[4] Dagnall, J.C. Personal communication.
[5] Tarkkanen, L. and Shrala, U. Effect of adrenalin, noradrenalin and Octapressin on bleeding and circulation in ear operations. *Acta Oto-Laryng. Stockholm,* **59**: 1–19, 1965.
[6] Lindorf, H.H. Investigation of the vascular effects of newer local anaesthetics and vasoconstrictors. *Oral Surg.,* **48**: 292–297, 1979.
[7] Jastak, J.T. and Yagiela, J.A. Vasoconstrictors and local anaesthesia. *J.A.D.A.,* **107**: 623–630, 1983.
[8] Arndt, K.A., Burton, C. and Noe, J.M. Minimizing the pain in local anesthesia. *Plast. Reconstr. Surg.,* **72**: 676–679, 1983.
[9] Smidt, L.A. The deposition of local analgesics in the foot. *Chiropodist,* **30**: 177, 1975.
[10] Carter, C.A.H. Minimal dose regional ankle block. *Podiatry Assoc. J.,* **2**: 8, 1985.
[11] McMinn, R.M.H., Hutchings, R.T. and Logan, B.M. *Foot and Ankle Anatomy.* London, Wolfe Medical Publications, 1982.
[12] Hoerster, W., Kreuscher, H., Niesel, H. Chr. and Zenz, M. *Regional Anesthesia,* 2nd edn. St. Louis, Mosby–Year Book, 1990.
[13] Sarrafian, S.K., Ibrahim, I.N. and Breihan, J.H. Ankle–foot peripheral nerve block for mid- and forefoot surgery. *Foot and Ankle,* **4**: 86–90, 1983.
[14] Lemont, H. A simplified nerve block to control postoperative foot pain. *J. Am. Podiatry Assoc.,* **68**(3): 193, 1978.

Further reading

Technical data on local analgesics

Atkinson, R.S. *et al. Anaesthesia,* 9th edn. John Wright & Sons.
British National Formulary, **12**: 124, 1986.
Eriksson, E. *Illustrated Handbook of Local Anaesthesia.* 2nd edn. Copenhagen, Sorensen, 1980, p.13.
Laurence, D.R. and Bennett, P.N. *Clinical Pharmacology,* 6th edn. London, Churchill Livingstone, 1987.
Martindale: The Extra Pharmacopoeia, 27th edn. London, The Pharmaceutical Press, 1977, p.861.

Percutaneous anaesthesia

Cooper, X., *et al.* EMLA cream reduces the pain in venepuncture in children. *Eur. J. Anaesthesia.* **4**: 441–448, 1987.
Juhlin, L. *et al.* Lidocaine–prilocaine cream for superficial skin surgery and painful lesions. *Acta Derm. (Stockholm),* **60**: 546–554, 1980.
McClelland, K.H. Studies on percutaneous local anaesthesia. PhD thesis, Queens University Department of Pharmacy, Belfast, 1986.

3 Nail surgery

ROGER BUTTERWORTH

Structure and growth of the human nail

The very catholic nature of that epidermal appendage known as the nail serves to disguise its clinical significance and it is only when the nail becomes troublesome or deformed that its possessor becomes concerned with its economy. Nails are an early acquirement of the digitate vertebrate.[1] The primary nail fold appears early in foetal life:[2] this area of nail formation is situated nearer the tip of the foetal toe than is the nail of an adult, and moves relatively further back along the dorsal surface of the toe to assume the position of the adult nail. The migration may be associated with the dorsal distribution of ventral nerve twigs.[1] Once this 'adult' position is assumed, the nail undergoes rapid development, and by the eighth month cuts through the overlying eponychium, which shrinks back to form the cuticle and hyponychium of the mature nail. The forward growth of the cornified nail plate continues throughout foetal life, and by full term the tips of the nails have grown to reach the end of the digit.

The normal anatomy of the nail unit[3] is shown in (3.1) and (3.2), and comprises the proximal nail fold, the matrix, the nail bed, and the hyponychium. Together these structures form the nail plate, comprising close-packed, adherent, interdigitating cells that lack nuclei or organelles.[3] The edges of the nail plate are protected by lateral nail grooves. The growth and morphology of the nail plate has not been fully defined, but it is accepted that it is formed exclusively by the matrix under normal conditions,[3] and that the existence of a ventral nail plate is probably indicative of pathological changes.[4] Important characteristics of nail unit structure are the smooth dorsal surface and the irregular ventral surface of the plate, where the longitudinal striae of the plate interface with the nail bed, and which indicate the axis of growth of the nail plate. This interface is further characterized by the formation of parakeratotic material. The ventral surface of the

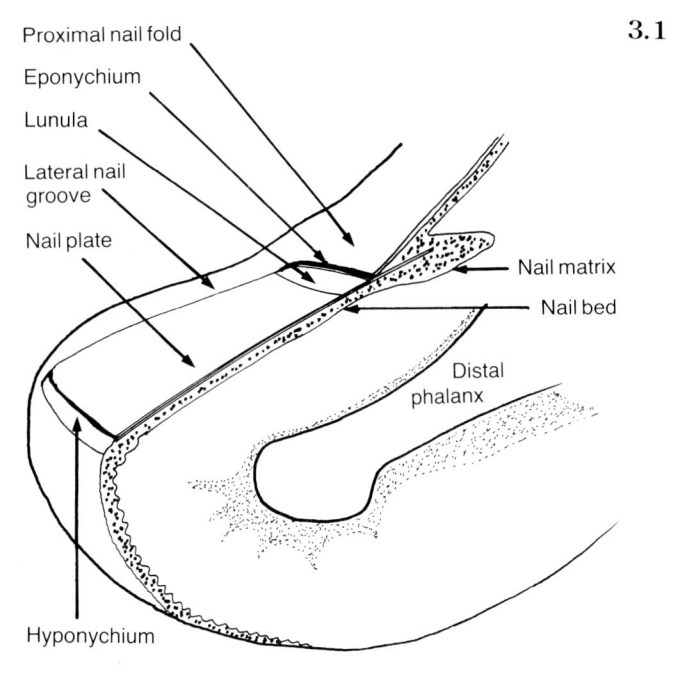

3.1 The nail unit.

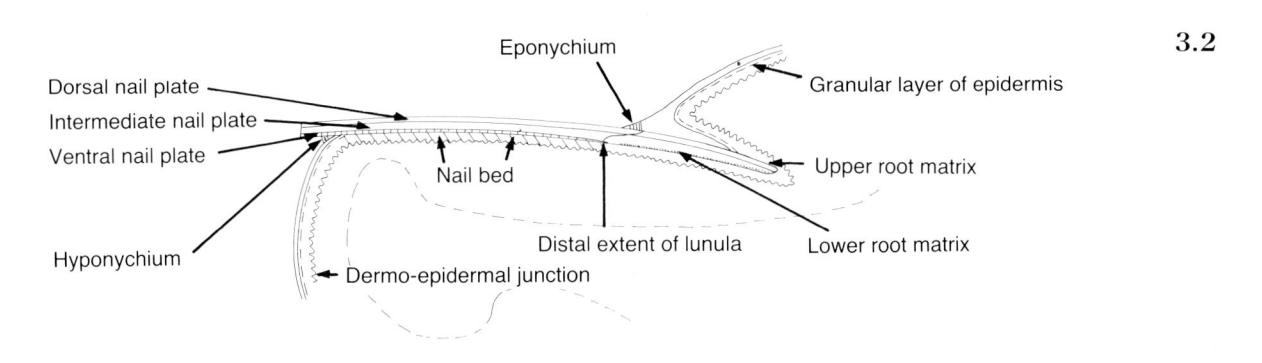

3.2 Longitudinal section of the nail unit. (After Rayner[5].)

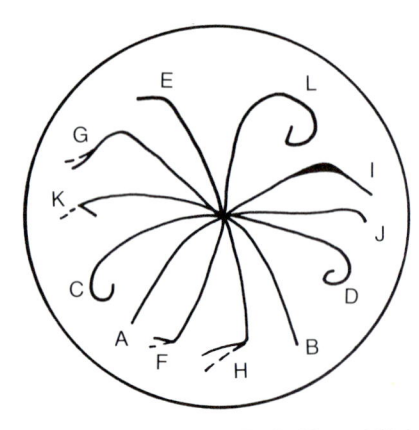

3.3 Nail shapes: borders E, F, G, H, and K demonstrate involution, where the edge of the nail plate is presented to the sulcus; borders C, D, and L demonstrate convolution, where the nail plate doubles back on itself. (After Krausz.[6])

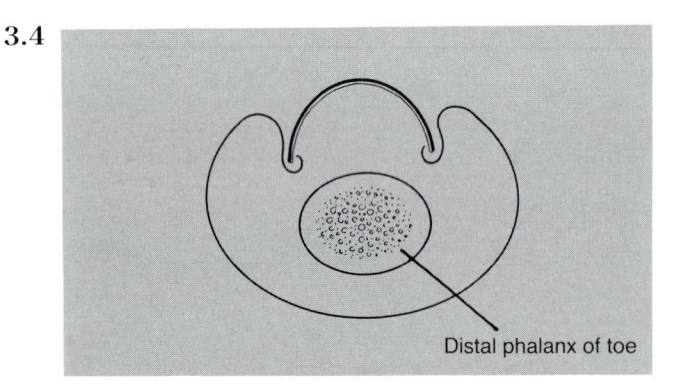

3.4 Involuted nail plate.

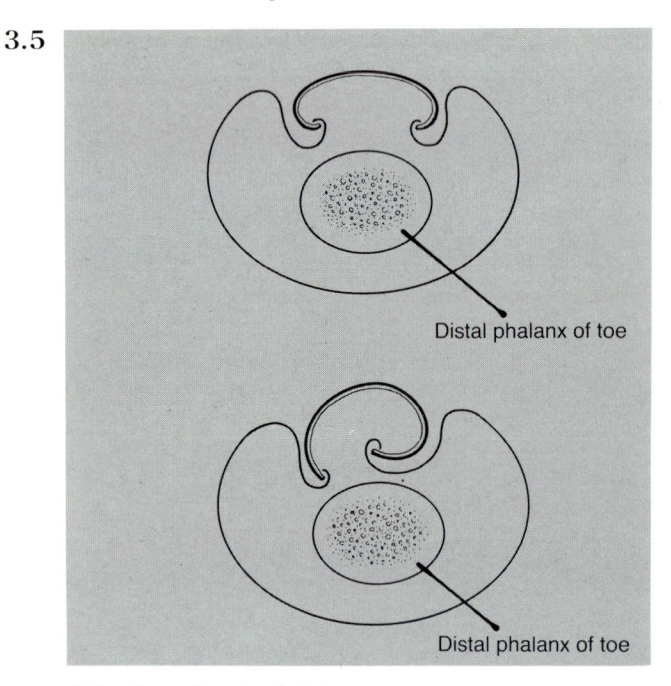

3.5 Convoluted nail plate.

proximal nail fold is adhered to the nail plate at the cuticle or eponychium, via the perionyx[1] or nail vest[5] situated at its distal margin.

The lateral curvature of the nail plate is very variable and has been described by Krausz[6] (**3.3**). It is also important to differentiate between the anatomical curvature of the nail plate, determined by the curvature of the nail matrix, and an acquired curvature of the distal portion of the nail plate that gives rise to the involuted (**3.4**) and convoluted nail (**3.5**). Natural curvature is symptom-free,[7] whereas acquired curvature is invariably painful and will not readily respond to palliation or correction, ultimately requiring surgery. Various hypotheses have been promoted to explain this increasing curvature,[8–11] to which must be added the possibility of the diseased nail, with its ventral nail plate behaving like a laminate. The continued development of this acquired curvature after surgery must be considered as one of the more intransigent of complications.

There is one final feature that should be mentioned. Whenever the author has surgically resected the lateral border of a nail it has been possible, indeed desirable, to remove an epithelial lining which invests both the lateral nail folds of the nail unit as well as the nail matrix. Only McGlamry[12] references this structure in the literature and any consideration of its anatomical function must be somewhat speculative. Microscopic examination would suggest that this 'lining' may be a vestige of the embryonic eponychium, as are the cuticle and hyponychium with which it is continuous, and that it serves a protective function. Microscopic examination further reveals that chronic nail groove pain is characterized by hyperplasic changes and sensory innervation of this epithelial 'lining', which correlates with the work of Fitzgerald *et al.*[13]

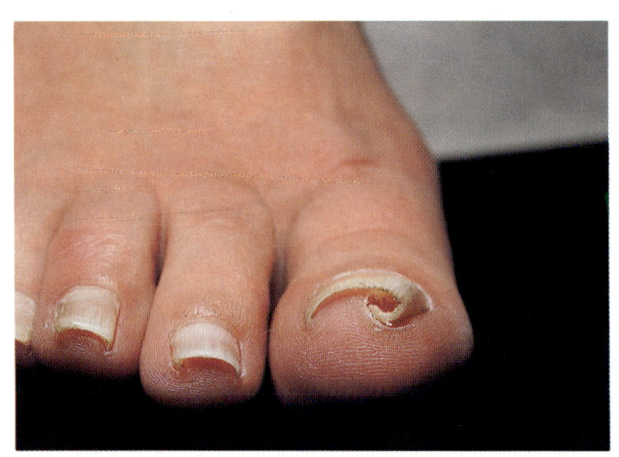

Nail pathology

Nail pathology may occur for a great variety of reasons. Pardo-Castello and Pardo[14] list some 50 separate conditions, and in a survey of patients attending their dermatology clinic identified 41% as having one or more abnormalities of the nails. Frost[15] references 46 factors as giving rise to nail conditions requiring surgery, and in a survey of 12,000 chiropody/podiatry patients, Krausz[6] identifies 61% as suffering from disorders of the nails; it is probably not coincidental that 45% sought treatment for conditions that are readily identified as being symptomatic. It is this latter group of nail conditions that are most amenable to surgery. While more conservative treatments will alleviate the symptoms, they rarely afford permanent relief.

There are two groups of surgical procedures to be recommended for the alleviation of painful nails: non-incisional techniques such as partial and total matrix sterilization; and incisional techniques, which are reserved for conditions involving the periungual tissues or where the condition is complicated by a subungual exostosis.

Non-incisional techniques

The decision as to which non-incisional technique to adopt as being most appropriate remains a matter of debate, and there are no absolute guidelines. Dagnall,[16] in his definitive analysis of nail matrix phenolization, commented that in Britain there is a tendency to perform more partials (often with minimal nail removed) than totals, whereas about 80% of his cases were totals. He stated that a partial should only be decided on when it is considered that the residual plate will never cause problems, even under unfavourable conditions, and that any separation of the plate from the bed of the nail that remains is a contraindication to a partial.

McGlamry,[12] summarizing his own position, stated that onychogryphosis was a typical nail condition in which it was desirable to destroy the entire nail. However, whenever a reasonable nail could be preserved, it was more desirable to remove and sterilize the lateral sections than to remove the entire nail, as lateral margin (sterilizations) produce considerably less tissue shock and heal more quickly. In addition to onychogryphosis, and the other more obvious candidates for total matrix sterilization such as onychauxis and some cases of onychomycosis, McGlamry also lists two less obvious conditions. The first is the 'tent' nail (**3.6**), in which the nail is incurvated from the very centre of the nail plate. No matter how much the nail may be narrowed on the lateral margins it still tends to ingrow or create pressure at its new lateral margins. The second condition is the nail that is shaped something like the bowl of an inverted spoon (**3.7**), and in which the distal tip of the nail ingrows distally;[12] in this second condition, McGlamry also offers the alternative solution of resection of the distal digital structures into which the nail is growing.

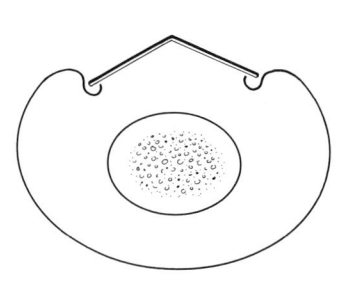

3.6 McGlamry's 'tent nail'.

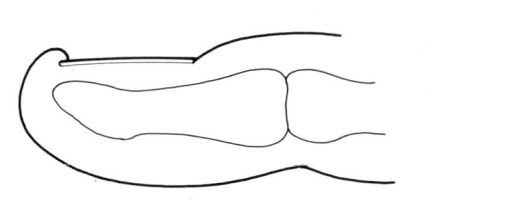

3.7 Inverted spoon or embedded nail.

Pre-operative assessment and preparation

Little pre-operative preparation is necessary, or indeed possible, for some nail conditions, especially where the object of the exercise is the relief of an acute nail condition. It is always advisable to bring infection and severe inflammation under control by the use of saline footbaths, antiseptic dressings and antibiotic therapy before operating, since puncture of the periosteum underlying the nail matrix area is a frequent occurrence and too extensive an inflammatory reaction can prejudice analgesia.

With chronic and non-inflammatory nail conditions, a more careful evaluation should be undertaken as a basis from which to anticipate post-operative results. An examination of the nail on weight-bearing and walking should be made, as well as a consideration of biomechanical influences, deformities such as hallux valgus, and footwear. The toe should also be X-rayed if enlargement or deformity of the underlying phalanx (such as an exostosis) is suspected.[12] Thinning of the nail plate and salicylic acid nail packs have been advocated as means of facilitating the removal of hyperkeratotic periungual tissues and the fibrous lining of the nail sulcus.

Historically, toe nail surgery has been characterized as being difficult and generally unsuccessful, frequently leaving the toe shortened, disfigured, and with a painful keratotic plaque where the nail has been removed. In addition, nail spicules and scarring have complicated post-operative recovery. This was certainly the outcome of the most popular procedures, such as that described by Zadik.[17] In 1945, Boll[18] described a technique for the partial ablation of the nail plate that has become a standard procedure, not only because of its technical superiority but also because it is cosmetically acceptable to the patient. Furthermore, it is a technique that can be extended to the ablation of the whole nail plate.

Partial nail matrix removal

Boll's technique must owe its popularity to its simplicity. It is carried out on an exsanguinated toe, using local analgesia and within an antiseptic field. It is suitable to both acute and chronic nail pathologies, and there are few systemic contraindications to its use.

The instruments needed for nail procedures are relatively few, and most practitioners keep comprehensive nail surgery packs, suitable for all types of nail work, independent of other surgical packs.

Technique

First, the nail plate is trimmed back closely to the hyponychium to simplify the splitting of the nail plate. Exsanguination of the toe is then effected by use of a narrow Esmarch bandage, secured proximally with large mosquito forceps. The nail is then exposed by unwinding the more distal part of the bandage to a level below the interphalangeal joint (**3.8–3.11**).

Separation of the dorsal nail fold from the (lateral) portion of the nail plate to be removed is effected with a spatula, or a similar flat, blunt instrument. Some force may be needed, since the attachment can be quite strong. The toe is held between the thumb and index finger of one hand and the end of the spatula handle is placed in the palm of the other hand. The spatula is then placed flat against the nail, parallel to the long axis of the toe, and pressure applied in a proximal direction until the separation is achieved. The direction of the pressure can be guided by the index finger of the hand holding the spatula. Care should be taken to ensure that the separation of the nail fold from the plate is carried to the lateral edge of the nail plate. Should the analgesic block be incomplete it will become evident at this point and the procedure should not continue until the situation is remedied.

The lateral portion of the nail can then be separated from the main nail plate with a chisel or sterile No. 62 Beaver blade. Holding both the toe and the chisel in the same way as when using the spatula, and again 'guiding' the chisel with the index finger, the nail plate is split longitudinally. This is done by starting at the free distal border and working proximally and by gently increasing the force applied through the chisel (**3.12, 3.13**). It is most important that this should be a 'controlled' movement and that the chisel should not be allowed to slip and pierce either the dorsal nail fold or the operator's hand! The edge of the chisel should pass under the cuticle and be progressed proximally until the matrix is divided (**3.14**). This final division cannot, of course, be seen by the operator, but is felt as a reduction in the resistance to the chisel (as it penetrates the softer matrix area), followed by a sudden final resistance as the chisel embeds itself in the dorsal proximal condyle of the underlying phalanx. The chisel can then be removed.

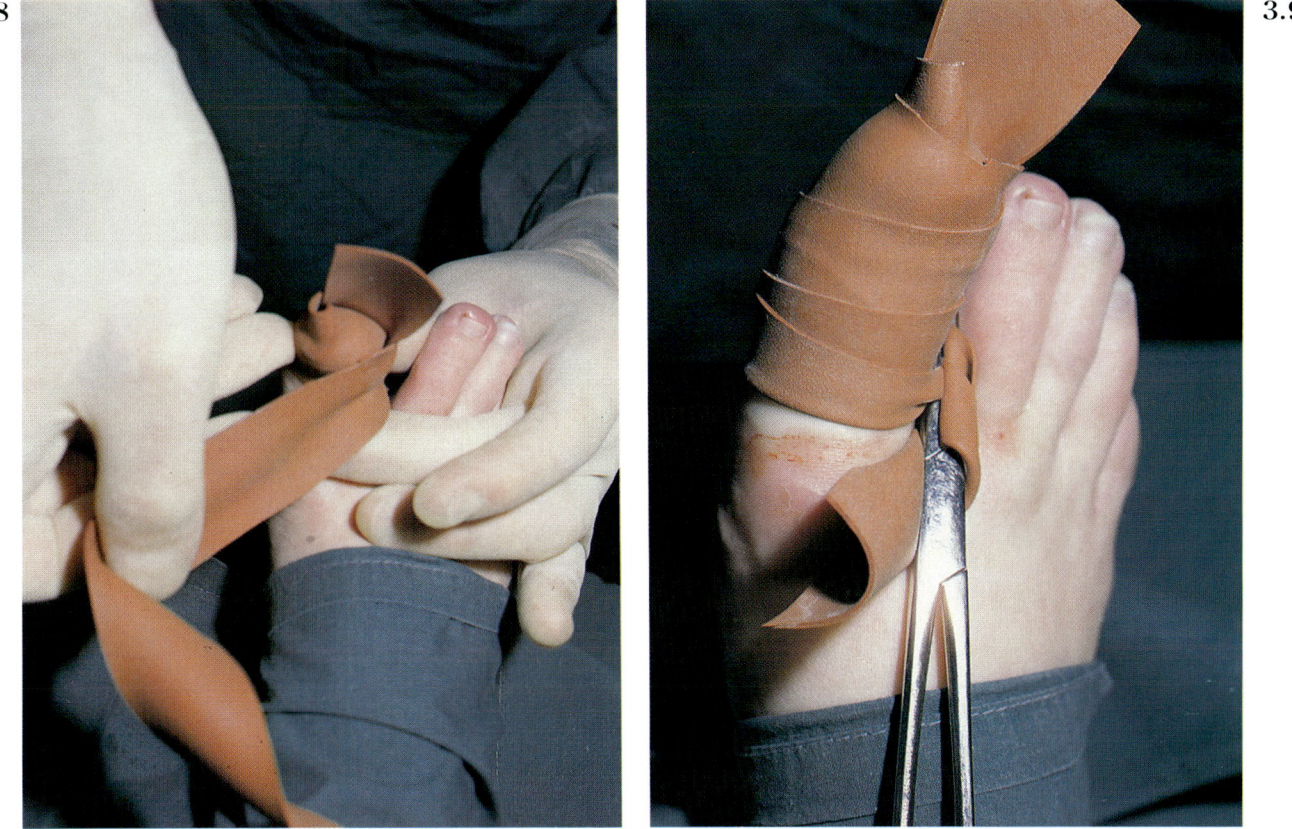

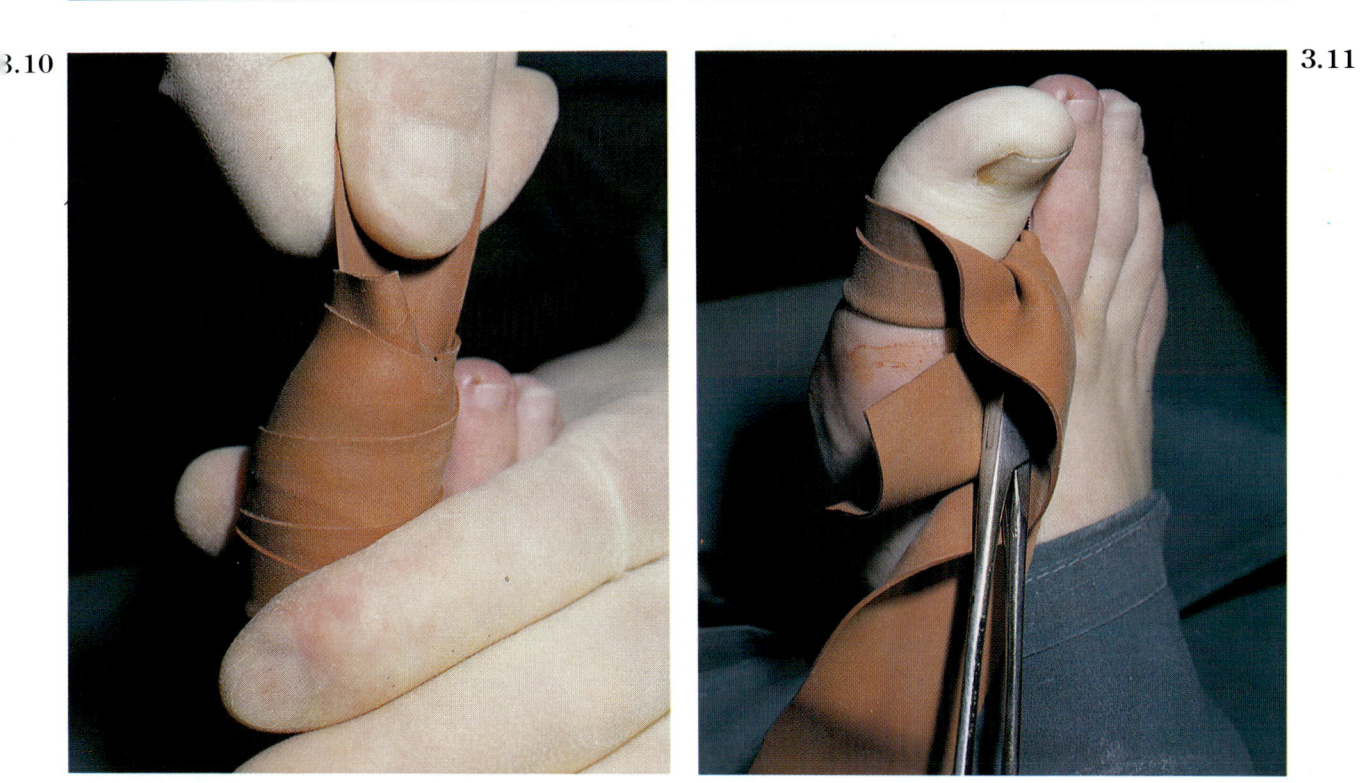

3.8–3.11 Exsanguination of the toe.

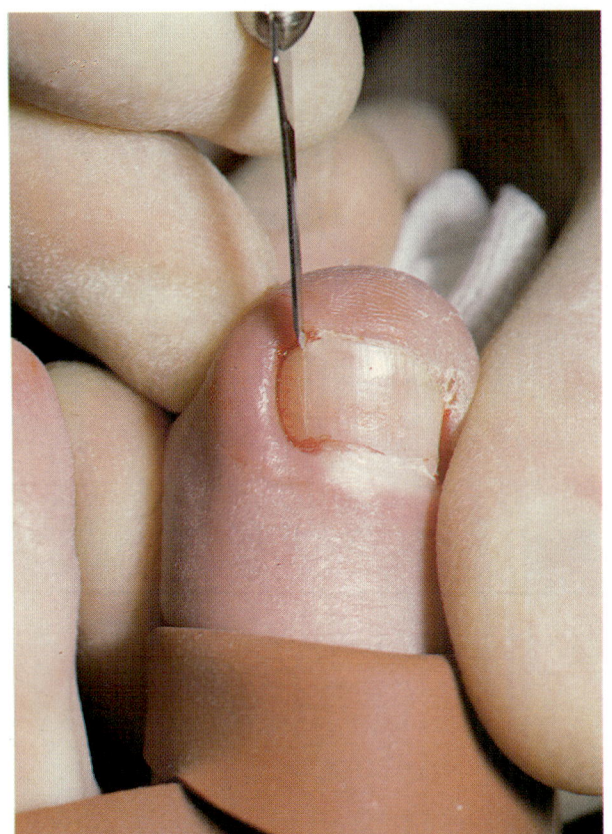

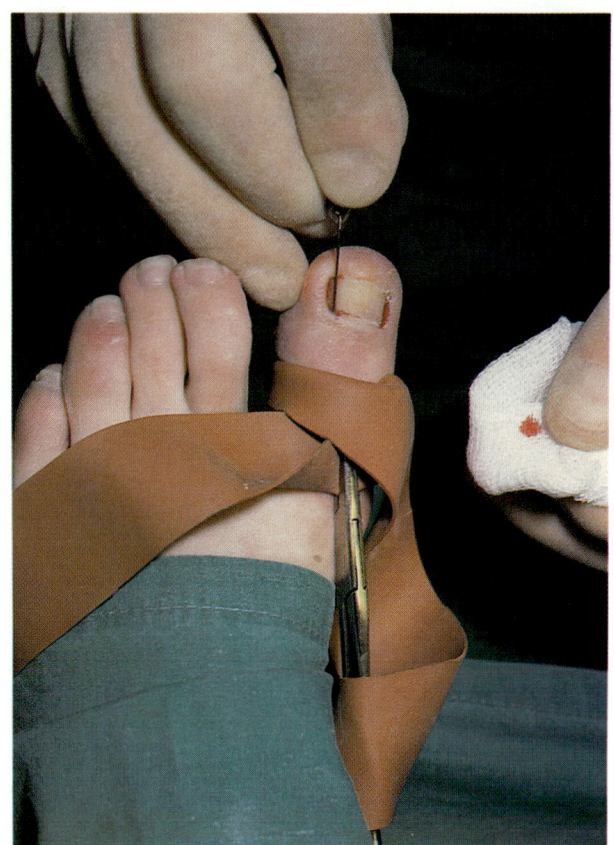

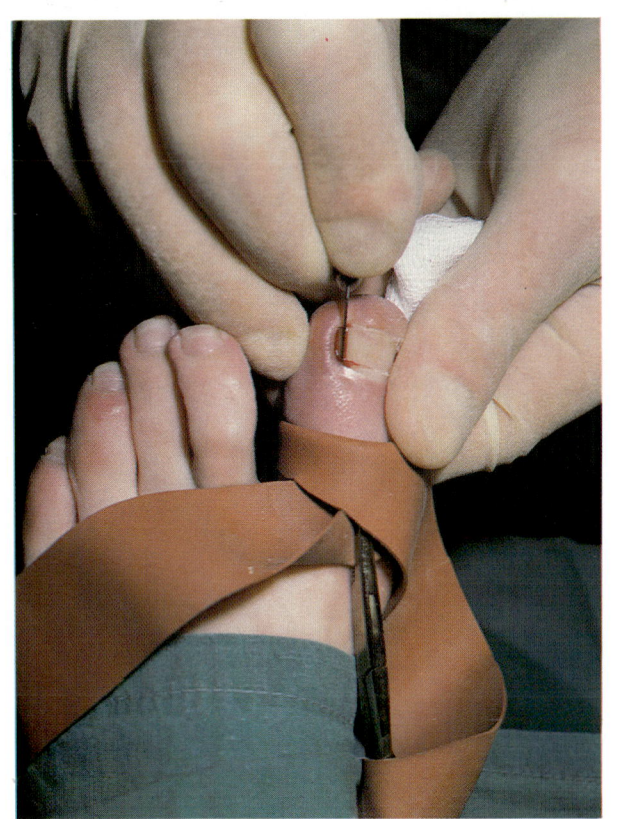

3.12, 3.13 Longitudinal division of the nail plate border.

3.14 Division of the nail matrix, taking care not to damage the eponychium.

70

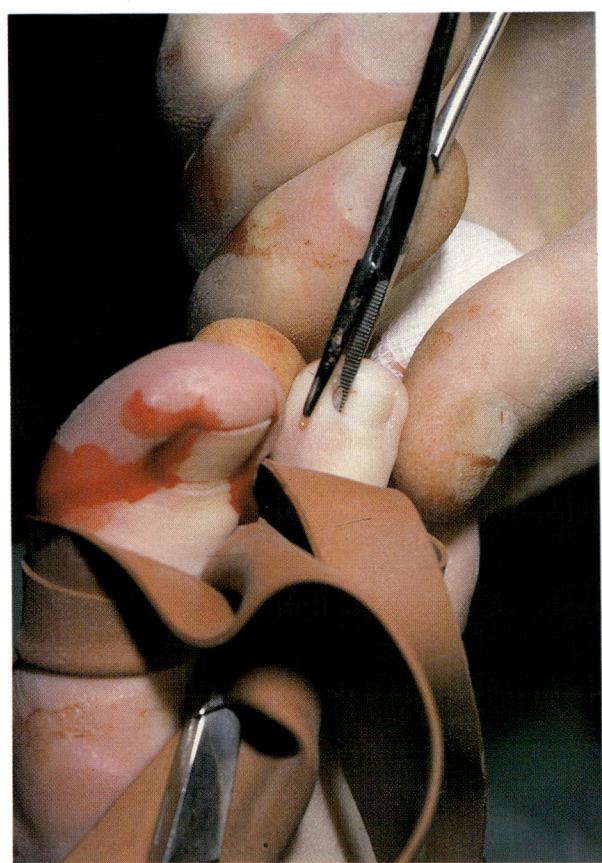

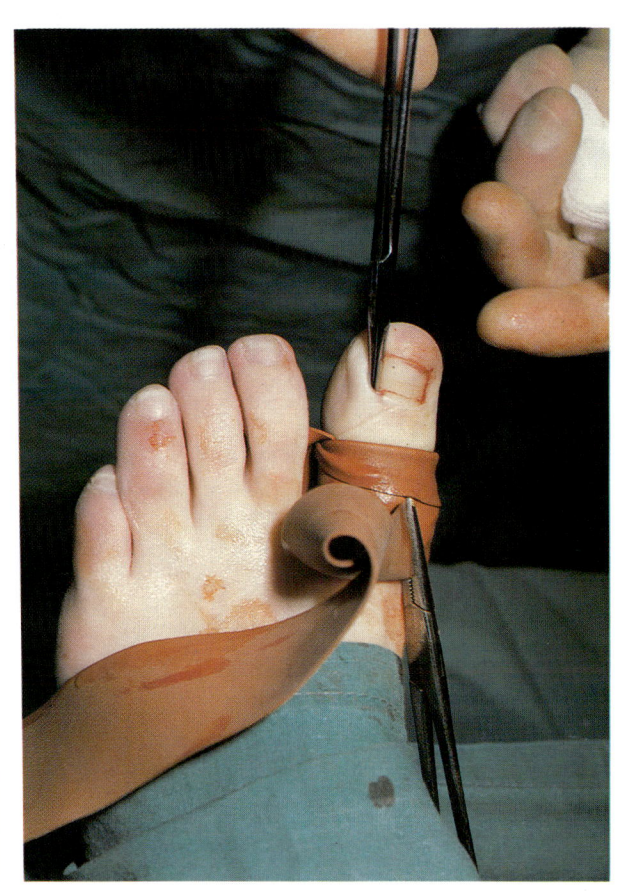

3.15, 3.16 Use of the haemostat to clamp the resected border of the nail.

With thicker nail plates it may be necessary to start this process with straight-edged nail nippers; usually, however a chisel will suffice. Avoid using unnecessary force, and take great care to ensure that the split closely follows the longitudinal striations of the nail plate so the nail width will not widen or narrow during post-operative growth. If such accuracy is impossible, the section should deviate as little as possible towards the mid-line of the toe so that the width of the nail will decrease slightly during subsequent growth. A section of nail at least 1/16th of an inch wider than is considered necessary should be removed. The section of the nail is then clamped with appropriately sized haemostats, the lower jaw of which is used to separate the nail section from its underlying nail bed. The upper jaw is eased under the dorsal nail fold as the haemostat is slipped forward to achieve maximum grip as it clamps the nail section (**3.15, 3.16**).

Keeping the long axis of the haemostat parallel with that of the toe, the instrument can be gently rotated, laterally and medially, to loosen the section from the toe (**3.17, 3.18**). Once sufficient freedom is achieved, the section is rotated medially until it separates from the nail unit (**3.19, 3.20**). It is vitally important that this process be carried out gently and with care, because as the section comes away it should retain its attachment to the fibrous sheath, which not only invests the sulcus, but also the matrix area. So long as this sheath retains its investment of the matrix area the surgeon can be confident that all the nail matrix cells have been removed with the section, which makes cauterization much easier (**3.21, 3.22**).

Before cauterization, the sulcus should be examined carefully for any remaining debris, especially for remnants of the fibrous sheath, all of which must be stripped away by curettage if necessary.

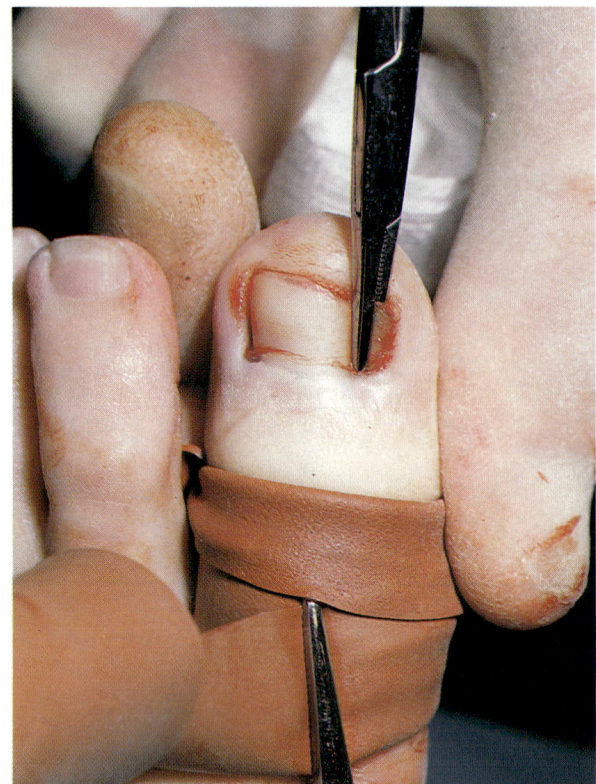

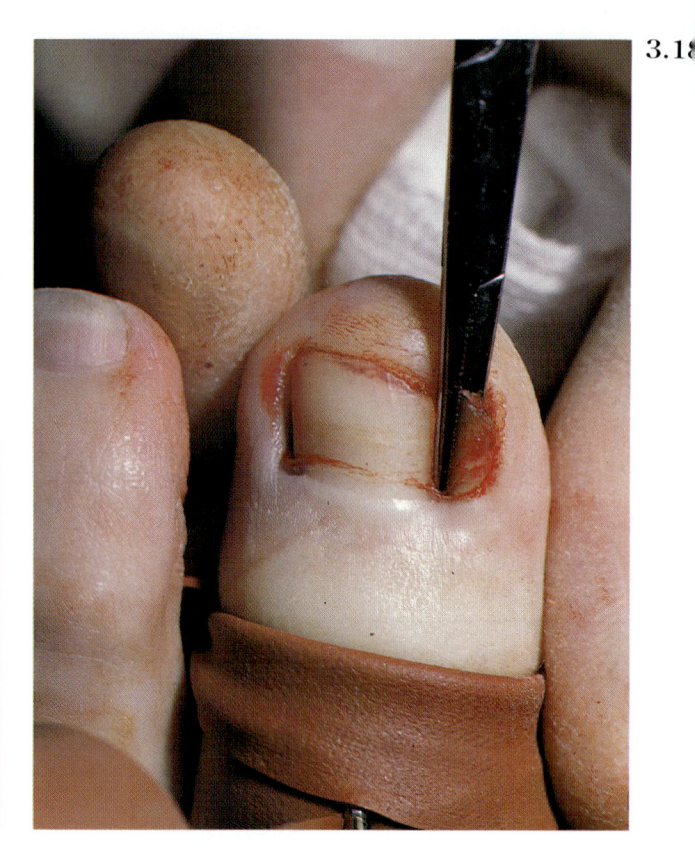

3.17, 3.18 Loosening the resected nail border by rotating the haemostat.

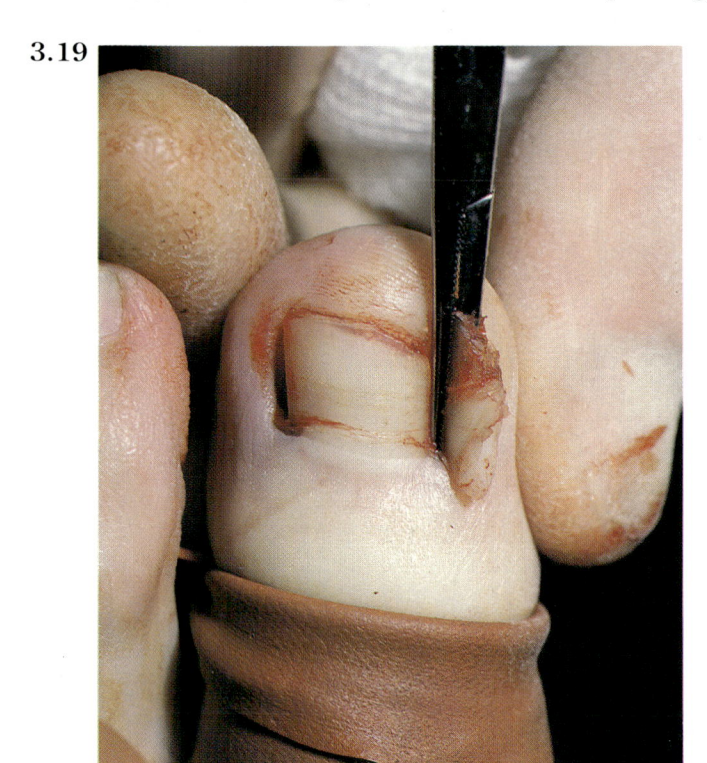

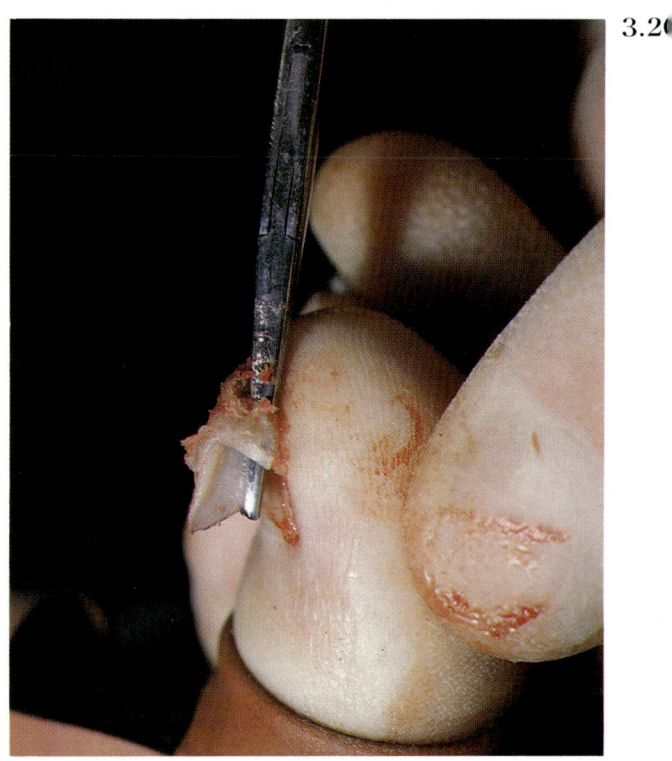

3.19, 3.20 Removal of the resected nail.

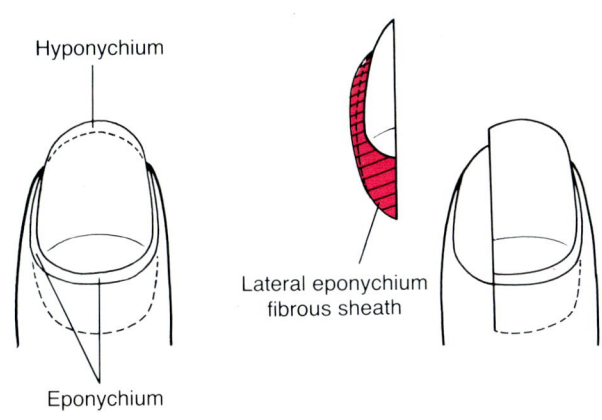

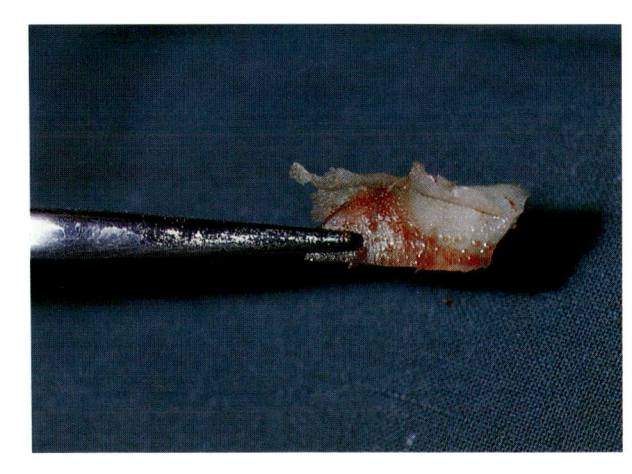

3.21 Diagrammatic representation of nail section and fibrous sheath.

3.22 Resected nail section and fibrous sheath.

Cauterization of the generative nail tissue

Cauterization of the nail matrix and nail bed are as important to the success of the procedure as the surgery itself. Failure to adequately destroy the former risks post-operative spicule formation, while failure to cauterize the latter will effect an unsightly parakeratotic plaque which will snag hose and can be intrinsically irritating.

The two most common forms of cauterization are by phenolization and negative galvanism, although Travers and Ammon[19] also advocate the direct application of 10% sodium hydroxide as a variant of the negative galvanic technique. Phenolization has the advantage of simplicity, but by definition results in a chemical burn which may be contraindicated in some patients. Negative galvanism is a more complex procedure, and more difficult to use, but minimizes tissue damage. The author's preference is for phenolization because of its ease of use and because experience suggests that the greater inflammatory reaction produced is accompanied by a more extensive fibrosis, which in turn gives a firmer post-operative structure to the periungual tissues. The process of cicatrization also appears to play its part in improving the post-operative appearance of the toe. Robertson and Crawford[20] disagree, stating that the long-term cosmetic results were slightly better on patients treated with negative galvanism, compared with phenol, as there appeared to be less fibrosis in the sulcus.

Phenolization

Phenolization should be commenced only when the area to be cauterized is dry and, in particular, free of blood. If the toe has not been exsanguinated, bleeding points (**3.23**) can be stopped with ferric chloride solution.

Although some maintain that phenol which has changed colour is none the less effective, it is probably wise to use a relatively fresh and colourless solution. The alternative is to make up small quantities from crystals. In the United Kingdom, liquefied phenol (*B.P.*), 80% (w/w) in water, is used. In the United States, liquefied phenol (*U.S.P.*), contains not less than 89% (w/w) in water. The higher strength used in the United States is unlikely to produce any significant difference in the outcome of the procedure, but a comparative study would be worthwhile. Phenol should be stored in a brown glass bottle, ideally with a glass stopper (plastic caps and washers are affected by phenol and can contaminate the solution), kept in a cool dark cupboard, and shaken before use. A small amount should be poured into something like a watch glass for use, and any left over discarded.[16]

The application of the phenol may be effected by a variety of methods, including a 'cotton wool bud', Black's file, glass rod, or pipette; but whatever method is chosen, the phenol must not be spilt on the adjacent tissues. It therefore makes sense to keep the source of the phenol distal to the foot and to introduce the liquid into the sulcus from over the end of the toe (**3.24**).

The length and manner of application of the phenol are the aspects of the technique that give rise to argument and most often raise doubts in the mind of the operator. The duration of applying the phenol should not be according to an arbitrary period of time but dep-

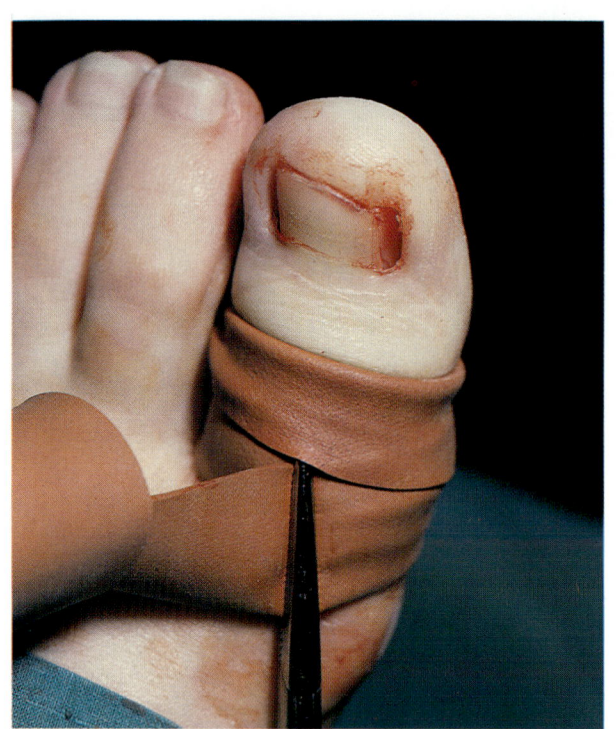

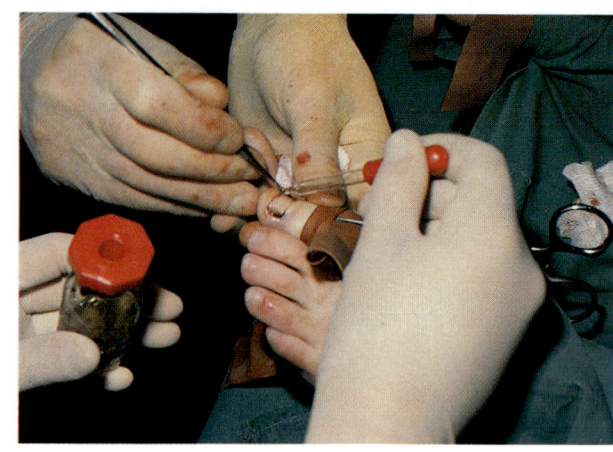

3.23 Toe nail after the nail section has been removed.

3.24 Application of phenol prior to cauterization.

endent upon the changes in the matrix tissue, since the thickness and area of the matrix vary considerably.[18]

This required 'change in the matrix tissue' is felt rather than seen; although the effect of the phenol is to turn the tissues white, the operator is really concerned in feeling for the change in which the periungual tissues of the matrix and nail bed alter from a tough fibrous texture to a softer, almost mushy texture. This process is facilitated by scarifying the tissue with a Black's file. Although not necessary in theory, the author also prefers to dry the sulcus halfway through the cauterizing process, and apply fresh phenol, before finally drying off the surplus phenol once the described change in the germinative areas of the nail is achieved. Nyman[21] observes that phenol precipitates proteins because of a change in solvents and not because of a definite chemical combination with the protoplasmic constituents of the tissues, and therefore its action is self-limiting. In practice, the application of phenol will take at least a minute, and usually significantly longer, depending on the thickness and the area of the matrix. Special care should be taken to scarify the proximal and lateral borders of the groove, since experience demonstrates that it is from these areas that spicules will most commonly form post-operatively.

Opinions vary as to whether it is sufficient to dry the phenol in the nail groove before dressing or whether it should be diluted with alcohol or glycerin. Greenwald and Robbins,[22] in an informed commentary, point out that a key step in the performance of the chemical matricectomy is the removal of the caustic agent at the end of the procedure, the so-called neutralization step. Since no chemical reaction occurs between phenol and alcohol, neutralization really refers to a dilution, and secondary spreading of the phenol will most assuredly be involved. This will increase the area of tissue necrosis and the resulting inflammatory response, prolonged drainage being the ultimate expression.[22]

The hygroscopic effect of the glycerin will also precipitate post-operative maceration and delay healing. The author's preference is to dry the sulcus well and leave it at that.

Surplus phenol should be carefully discarded, and all containers thoroughly rinsed immediately after use. Phenol burns can be treated with Ichthammol in glycerin (*B.P.C.*).

Negative galvanism

From the viewpoint of electrotherapy, the human body may be viewed as a bag of skin holding a solution of NaCl in dissociation, the sodium being positively charged (Na^+) and the chloride carrying a negative charge (Cl^-). Galvanic current is a direct current, the flow of which through a solution containing the above-described ions causes Na^+ to migrate towards the cathode and Cl^- towards the anode. This process is known as iontophoresis. Another process proceeds at the same time: the anode frees available oxygen at its site, whereas the cathode liberates available hydrogen. Our concern is with the cathode: in the presence of a negative galvanic charge we might expect hydrogen to be liberated from the cellular material with which this charge comes into contact. This combines with sodium to form sodium hydroxide.[23] Alkali burns produce a crust that is soft, moist, penetrating, and white. Its action is to liquefy protein substances. Liquefaction necrosis results from the action of powerful enzymes, which literally digest the cell and transform it into a proteinaceous fluid.[19]

Negative galvanic current producing cauterization of the germinative tissue of the nail by liquefaction necrosis is both a simple and safe procedure if carried out correctly, and is dependent upon the establishment of a galvanic current between a positive, dispersive or indifferent electrode and a negative or active electrode used in the cauterization process. It was first described in the literature by Polokoff,[24] who used it in conjunction with the reduction of hypertrophied nail lip, because this condition is usually concomitant with the chronic ingrown toe nail. Abbott and Geho[25] in a recent, comprehensive review of the procedure characterize it as having two advantages; little or no post-surgical pain and a very low infection rate. They describe the procedure as follows: addressing the exposed nail groove and bed, it is generally found that there is a hyperkeratotic formation in the groove. This must be removed, since it can cause post-operative discomfort: it is removed by curettage. The bed is also curetted. Before the foot is prepped and draped, a flat, square dispersive electrode is secured to the posterior aspect of the leg with a rubber strap. It has been soaked in saline solution and a wet sponge is placed between the leg and the electrode. The negative electrode (2.5×24 mm^2) is applied to the cavity created by the nail evulsion. After the electrodes are in contact with the tissue, the current from the galvanic unit is turned on. If the current is turned on before the electrode is applied, the patient will feel an uncomfortable shock. A current of 8 mA is applied for 3 min. Sometimes the patient will experience a burning feeling where the positive electrode is placed. When this happens, the amperage should be decreased and the time of application extended. This change is determined by how much discomfort the patient experiences. The greater the discomfort, the greater the change. The negative electrode is pressed against the matrix and the phalanx. It is not pressed against the top part of the cavity. If this is done, blistering can occur. The electrode is moved from medial to lateral in a side-to-side motion, with particular attention being directed towards the corner. When the 3 min are up, the current is turned off and the electrode is removed. The effect of the current on the tissues is reflected in the release of hydrogen bubbles from the negative electrode, producing a fine white foam that can be flushed away with an antiseptic solution.

Abbott and Geho[25] reiterate much of Polokoff's[24] original description, stating that the operation is an ambulatory, routine office procedure with minimal postoperative difficulty. They differ, however, in advocating the application of the positive electrode to the leg; Polokoff proposed its application to the foot. In this respect, all recent authors are unanimous in advocating the application of the positive electrode to the calf of (either) leg, and the application of the electrode to the foot may have been the basis of Polokoff's warning of 'sensitivity under the wet electrode' when applied to the plantar surface of the foot. All authors agree that wherever the positive electrode is applied it should be securely bound to the limb and should not overlie abrasions or other lesions which might be irritated.

Whether or not the positive electrode should be soaked in warm water or saline solution before application appears to be a matter of personal choice, with no advantage apparent either way. Gardner[23] advises that the patient should be warned about the sensation he describes as '... formication, the feeling of slight tickling or the sensation of crawling ants', when the current is switched on.

The major discussion with this technique really revolves around the questions of the strength of the current and length of application. Polokoff[24] advocates 8 or 10 mA for approximately 10 min for one nail side and warns of the danger of undertreatment. Gardner[23] found that 5 mA applied for 10 min is the usual current application required to destroy the nail cellular tissue of the great toes; less time is required for the lesser toes. He also emphasizes the influence of the tissues on both the speed of the cauterization process and the resistance to the current, and their interrelationship. Robertson and Crawford[20] are even more precise, stating that a negative galvanic current of 6 mA was used via either a 3 mm or 5 mm wide electrode for 6 min. Abbott and Geho[25] found a positive correlation between the length of application and the rate of success in cauterizing nail matrix tissue at a standard current strength.

In practice, there can be no absolute criteria for determining when cauterization of the germinative nail tissue has taken place; experience suggests that the operator will have to judge when the necessary changes have taken place from the feel of the tissues.

Electrodesiccation

Although phenolization and negative galvanism are probably the two most commonly accepted methods of cauterizing germinative nail tissue, a variety of other procedures have been described. In 1982, Kerman and Kalmus[26] described a method of partial matricectomy by electrodesiccation, which, although not widely adopted, is a technique used by those practitioners having access to equipment capable of discharging a monopolar high-frequency, high-voltage current.

A high-frequency, high-voltage current discharging from one outlet or terminal to the patient is variously described as monoterminal, monopolar, or as an Oudin current. A monoterminal technique in which the electrode is held in surface contact or inserted into the tissues, is described as desiccation.

The technique of electrodesiccation, which utilizes a high-voltage, low-amperage current, causes dehydration and superficial destruction of tissues. The tissue destruction consists of coagulation necrosis and carbonization of cells. The coagulum will further degenerate to a state of liquefaction necrosis and be removed via a combination of enzymatic degradation and phagocytosis.

The eletrocautery unit is set at a minimal voltage, and beginning at the proximal end of the exposed nail bed, the whole of the germinative area of the nail is scarified by the needle, taking particular care to cauterize the proximal corners of the nail fold. Too high a voltage will allow the current to penetrate deep to the periosteum of the underlying phalanx. In practice, the penetration of the tissues by the tip of the needle and the physical debridement of the tissue with the needle are an integral part of the procedure. Kerman and Kalmus[26] reported the results (**Table 3.1**) of a survey of 100 patients.

Table 3.1 Survey of electrodesiccation (Kerman and Kalmus[26])

	Minimum (days)	Average (days)	Maximum (days)
Healing	6	16	37
Drainage	1	4	24

Regrowth, partial	4 days
Regrowth, complete	0 days
Infections	8 days
Granulomas	2 days

The two most important factors contributing to satisfactory correction with minimal complications are a thorough knowledge of the anatomy by the physician and the willingness of the patient to cooperate. These two factors combined, result in a procedure that is safe, fast healing, and extremely effective.

Total nail matrix removal

Where a partial nail matrix removal is considered to be unsatisfactory, the technique can be extended to removal of the complete nail plate by dividing the nail down its centre and removing the two halves separately. Some authorities advocate the removal of the complete nail plate, but such arguments tend to ignore the delicacy required for a successful outcome to the procedure.

Rather more preparation is required for this procedure than is necessary for the partial removal of the nail plate. If the nail is thickened, it must be reduced prior to surgery. This can be effected with a burr and drill, or manually with a scalpel. In this latter procedure, the nail plate should be softened with 5% potassium hydroxide solution (though some clinicians prefer to use 20% salicylic acid nail packs), and the nail plate material carefully pared away with a scalpel, taking care not to drag on the nail.

Of the two procedures the latter is the more difficult, but probably the preferred technique since it is important not to thin the nail plate too much. Additionally, the keratolytic action of potassium hydroxide facilitates removal of the periungual debris prior to surgery. Indeed, all that is really necessary is to remove the harder dorsal surface of the nail plate so as to facilitate the splitting of the nail prior to removal. If the plate is thinned too much it will disintegrate during removal, and this is particularly the case with onychmycotic nails. Preparing the nail for total removal is better completed before the appointment for surgery.

Once the toe has been anaesthetized and the patient prepared for surgery, the whole of the cuticle should be detached from the nail plate with a spatula or similar flat, blunt instrument. The spatula is most easily inserted under the eponychium at its lateral border, where it separates from the nail plate to form the sulcus. From this position it can then be moved across, under the eponychium.

It is also necessary to separate the nail plate from the nail bed before commencing removal, and this can be effected with either the same spatula used to detach the cuticle from the plate, or a more substantial instrument, such as a small periostial elevator.

The nail plate is now split down its centre, preferably with straight-edged nail nippers, and the two halves clamped with large haemostats and carefully removed by the twisting action described in the partial nail matrix removal section. Again, great care should be taken to retain the investment of the nail matrix tissue by the fibrous lining. In reality, this is much more difficult if the nail is thickened, and the operator may have to carefully curette away the remnants of the nail before cauterizing the whole of the germinative area of the nail.

By definition, the process of cauterization after total nail removal will be far more extensive than after partial removal, and although phenolization might appear to be the preferred method, negative galvanism will produce less tissue shock and must therefore be the method of choice where healing might be prejudiced. Whichever method is chosen, particular care must be taken to destroy the whole of the nail bed. Frequently, clinicians take care to destroy the matrix area, forgetting that the exposed nail bed will form a heavy parakeratotic crust that is both unsightly and irritant if it is not also destroyed.

Post-operative management of non-incisional nail procedures

The post-operative care of non-incisional nail surgery can be regarded as standard for all techniques and comprises the following steps:

- Ensure that adequate circulation has returned to the toe; this is readily assessed by watching the return of colour to the toe once the tourniquet is removed, and by evidence of bleeding from the wound.
- Control post-operative bleeding by the discrete use of haemostatic and non-adhesive dressings and light pressure from tubular bandages. The patient should be advised that a certain amount of bleeding will be apparent through the dressing, and indeed is an indication that the dressing is not occlusive. It should be noted, however, that post-operative bleeding after negative galvanic cauterization is minimal, since some coagulation of the capillaries takes place.
- Elevation of the affected limb(s) for some 30 min after completion of the procedure to ensure that post-operative bleeding is not excessive and that the patient has fully recovered from the procedure.

The patient may then be sent home with instructions to keep the limb(s) elevated as much as possible for the rest of the day. The immediate initiation of soaking, 2–3 h post-surgery, and wound hygiene are very important factors in the reduction of the inflammatory response and post-operative drainage.[22] Footbaths are most easily effected with warm saline solution; some authorities advocated magnesium sulphate, but this produces too vigorous an action if used immediately after surgery. Post-operative pain, which is usually minimal, can be controlled by paracetamol or similar analgesics. Patients should be provided with a contact telephone number in case of emergencies, and re-appointed within 24 h for a post-operative review. At the 24-h post-operative review, the wound is thoroughly cleaned to ensure that it is draining properly, and the patient is advised to continue the use of saline footbaths and to dress the wound with povidone iodine[27] or antiseptic creams until the wound has healed. Ointments and pastes are contraindicated because they tend to interfere with drainage. In the absence of complications, post-operative reviews should be conducted after 7, 28, and 56 days, at which time the patient can usually be discharged.

Post-operative healing times

It is important to tell patients that the toe will often look as if it is getting worse and that they should not regard the long period of drainage as a disadvantage but as an essential part of the treatment.[23] Healing times following partial nail avulsion would appear to be greatly influenced by the level of post-operative activity of the patient and should possibly be given greater consideration in the pre-operative evaluation.[28]

Healing rates will also vary with the procedure adopted for the cauterization of the germinative nail tissue, with the patient's age, and possibly with the choice of post-operative dressing. On average, drainage of the site may continue for up to 28 days, and it may be 56 days before any resultant eschar sloughs away. Post-operative improvement in the appearance of the toe will continue for up to 6 months, during which time any post-operative sensitivity will decrease. Indeed, post-operative assessment of the procedures should not be routinely attempted until a 6-month period has passed.

Post-operative complications

Post-operative complications fall into four categories: infection, restricted drainage, swelling, and regrowth. By definition, the process of cauterization results in an almost infection-free post-operative wound; any infection that occurs can only be as a result of a breakdown in post-operative procedures—usually the failure of the patient to follow instruction as to footbaths and dressings. Such eventualities can be resolved by the restoration of the correct post-operative regime. Rarely is the infection so serious as to require antibiotic therapy. Abbott and Geho[25] give an incidence of post-operative infection averaging 9% over a five-year survey of patients receiving cauterization by negative galvanism, while Robertson and Crawford,[20] in a retrospective analysis of both phenol and negative galvanic cauterizations, report that no patient was found to have a definite infection post-operatively. Gardner[23] gives an incidence of 0.57%.

Failure to establish and maintain drainage of the wound is potentially the most serious complication of non-incisional surgery and will rapidly lead to abcess formation. Generally, it arises from the application of an occlusive dressing immediately after surgery, though it may also result from the patient's failure to maintain drainage through regular footbaths.

Post-operative swelling of the toe is the most frequent, and most painful complication and, in the absence of compromised drainage of the wound, invariably arises from the failure of the patient to adequately elevate the foot after surgery. The restrictive nature of the toe's circumference means that even a limited amount of swelling will produce a rapid increase in the interstitial pressure of the tissues and, consequently, pain. Relief can only be obtained by elevation of the foot and analgesics, and it behoves all practitioners to advise their patients accordingly.

The incidence of regrowth is very low, and usually correlates with the care and experience of the surgeon. Abbott and Geho[25] record an incidence of 5.6% and Gardner[23] an incidence of 5.7% in patients treated by negative galvanism. Morkane *et al.*[29] demonstrated a regrowth of 7.4%, Robertson and Crawford[20] no recurrence and Shapiro[30] an incidence of less than 4% in patients treated by phenolization.

Nor should it be assumed that all regrowths will be symptomatic; this is frequently not the case. Indeed, the necessity to repeat the procedure usually relates more to the need to remove post-operative spicules than to the recurrence of pain. However, patients should be warned of this eventuality, prior to surgery.

Incisional techniques

Removal of nail plate material by non-incisional techniques, while popular and straightforward, has its limitations. Chief of these is the resolution of those conditions involving the periungual tissues, either through excessive curvature of the lateral margins of the nail and consequent involvement of the soft tissues of the nail groove, through hypertrophied ungualabia, or both. In these cases, incisional techniques are to be preferred; indeed, some authorities indicate a general preference for such procedures. While there is nothing wrong with these non-incisional techniques, they do not give the consistently good results that can be obtained with a well-executed Winograd procedure (see the following section).[31]

Incisional techniques invariably involve wound closure and should therefore be carried out within a sterile field, and in the absence of infection. If, in an emergency, these conditions are not available, antibiotic cover must be provided.

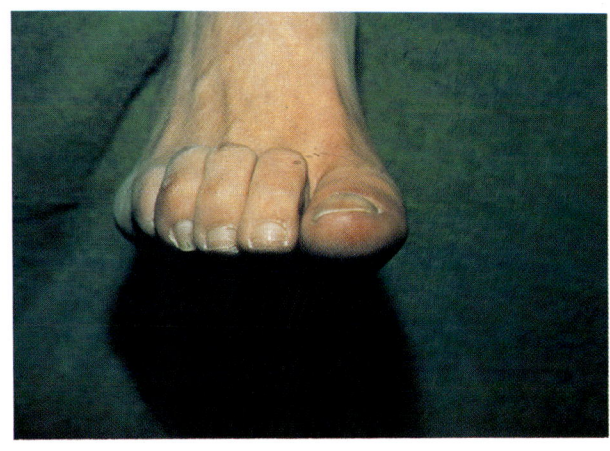

3.25 Pre-operative illustration showing periungual involvement.

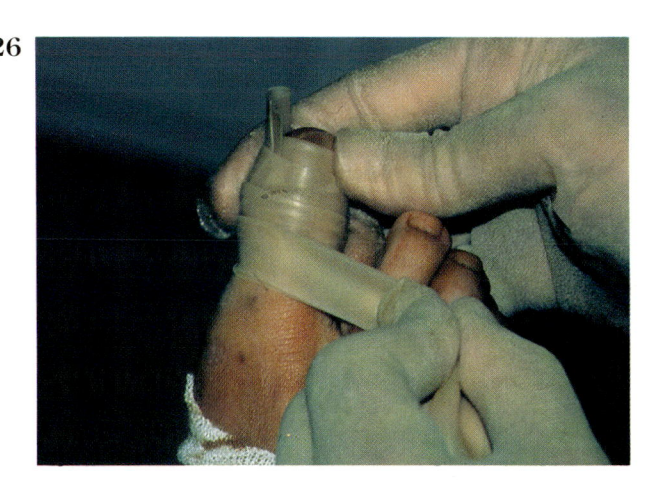

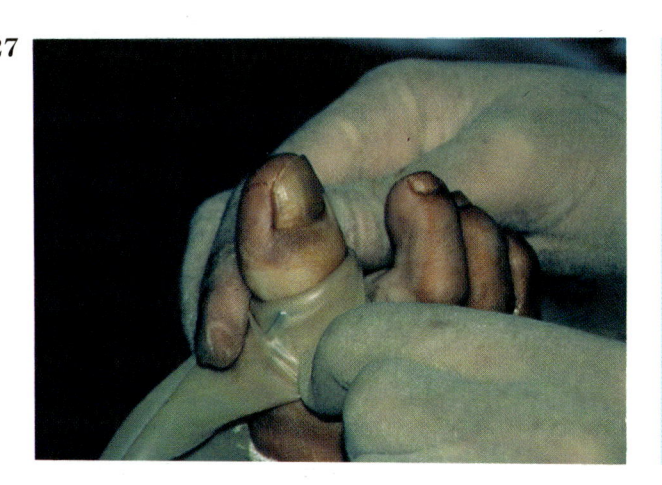

3.26, 3.27 Exsanguination of the anaesthetized toe.

The Winograd procedure

This procedure was first described by Winograd[32] in 1929 as an alternative to existing procedures, which he described as being unnecessarily elaborate and contraindicated in the 'usually inflamed and frequently infected condition of the flesh'.

Today, the technique is used for the removal of the involuted lateral nail plate with soft tissue hypertrophy, either in the form of hypergranulation tissue (proud flesh) or enlarged ungualabia, and has been slightly modified from Winograd's original description (**3.25**).

The toe is anaesthetized, sterilized, and exsanguinated (**3.26, 3.27**). The nail plate is then split (with a chisel) through to its matrix, and the division extended with a scalpel incision into the eponychium and nail fold to about 1 cm. It is then taken deep to the underlying phalanx, and extended forward to split the hyponychium (**3.28**).

A second, semi-elliptical incision is then made lateral to the first incision and also taken down to the phalanx, in such a way as to create a 'pie wedge' section that will allow resection of the offending nail plate, nail bed, nail matrix, and hypertrophied soft tissue. It is important to place this second incision very carefully, so as to ensure that the whole of the nail matrix area is included in the section. Greater control can be exerted by using a sawing motion of the (D15) blade, which will insure an even cut and prevent accidental slipping and cutting of good tissue. Any remaining nail matrix tissue should be curetted away from the phalanx. Mercado even advocates the 'rasping' of the surface of the phalanx to ensure complete removal of the matrix.[30]

The remaining ungualabia is then remodelled against the remaining edge of the nail, and the wound closed with sutures and steri-strips (**3.29–3.21**).

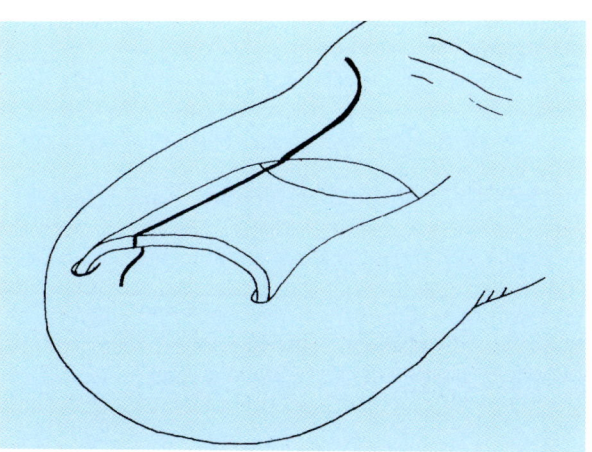

3.28 Diagrammatic representation of the Winograd procedure.

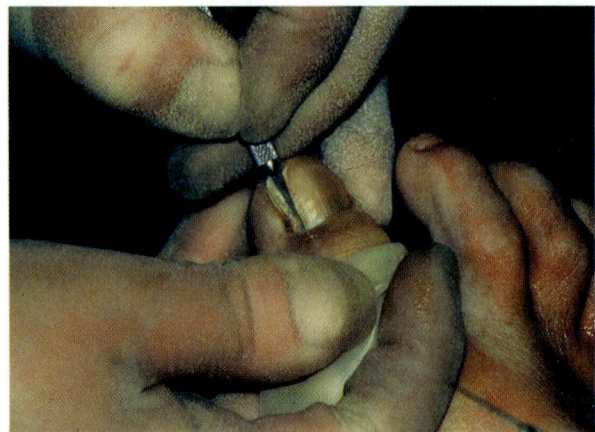

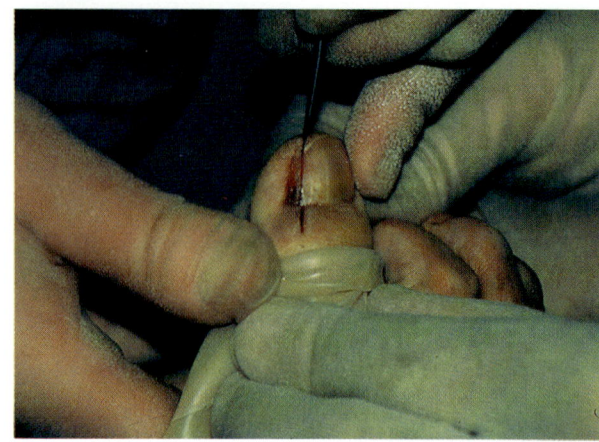

3.29–3.31 Sequence showing Winograd procedure.

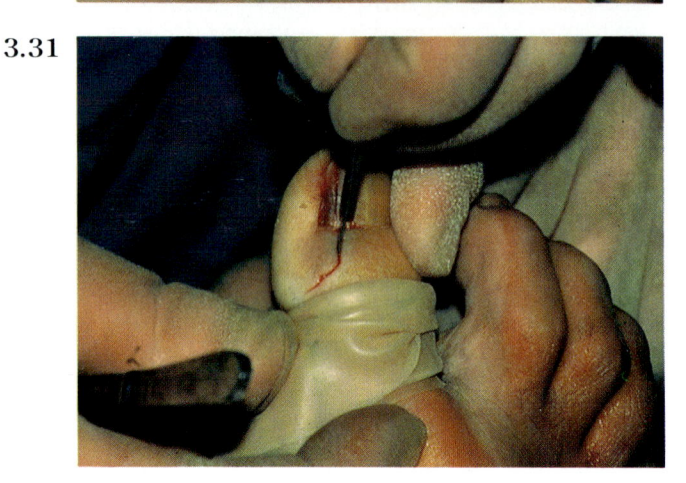

The Frost procedure

It is interesting that both Frost and Zadik should have published papers on the surgical treatment of ingrowing toe nails in the same year (1950) and that both should have been motivated by the unsatisfactory prognosis of existing procedures. Zadik's[17] solution, total avulsion of the nail unit, though the more radical, has failed to stand the test of time, and it is Frost's more conservative approach[15] that is now used for the partial avulsion of the convoluted nail border when there is little involvement of the ungualabia (**3.32**).

The toe is anaesthetized, sterilized and exsanguinated. The incision, an inverted 'L' (**3.33**) through the long axis of the nail, is carried out 1/16th inch beyond the distal end of the nail (and about 1 cm proximal of the eponychium). It is vertical, and is carried down to, but not into, the phalanx. This incision is medial to the imbedded portion of the nail and is gauged to remove the offending curvature of the nail, leaving the free edge almost horizontal.[15]

The base of the 'L' is an incision just through the dermis, down to, but not into, the nail root. Sharp dissection of the skin off the nail root provides a flap for later replacement. The nail root is recognized by its white, glistening, fibrous appearance (**3.34–3.36**). Be certain that none is left attached to the flap, for this could be a source of recurrence. If the flap is of insufficient thickness, sloughing will occur.[15] The skin flap is then retracted and a second incision made lateral to the first.

The nature of this second incision is a matter of some debate. In his original description, Frost described the second incision as being parallel to the first but deeper, so as to ensure that it extended below the level of the sulcus. He described it as beginning beneath the retracted flap of skin and only becoming semi-elliptical at its distal end, so as to join the first incision. More recently, it has been suggested that both ends of the second incision should be semi-elliptical and that the resultant segment can be removed as a 'pie wedge'. In practice, this latter procedure tends to defeat the purpose of the exercise in that it fails to isolate the whole of the offending sulcus before excision.

The distal portion of the segment that is to be removed is then grasped with mouse-toothed forceps to facilitate its removal. Using curved Mayo scissors, dissection is carried close to the phalanx. The dissection is

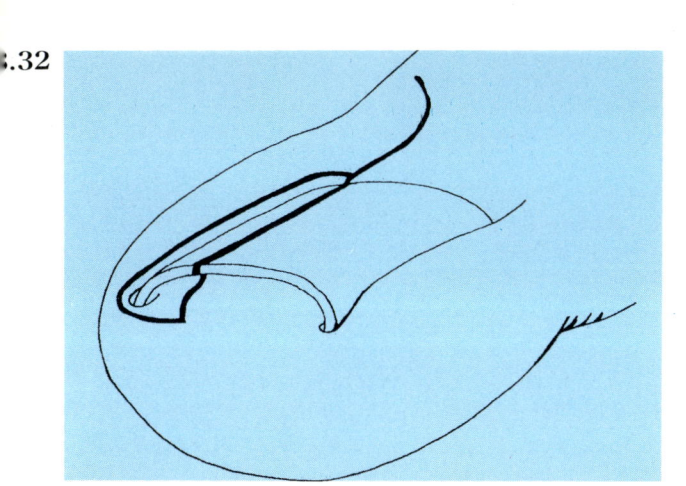

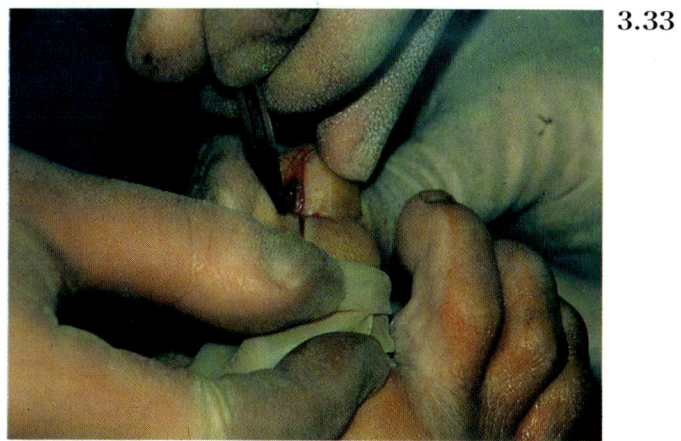

3.32, 3.33 The Frost procedure, initial incision.

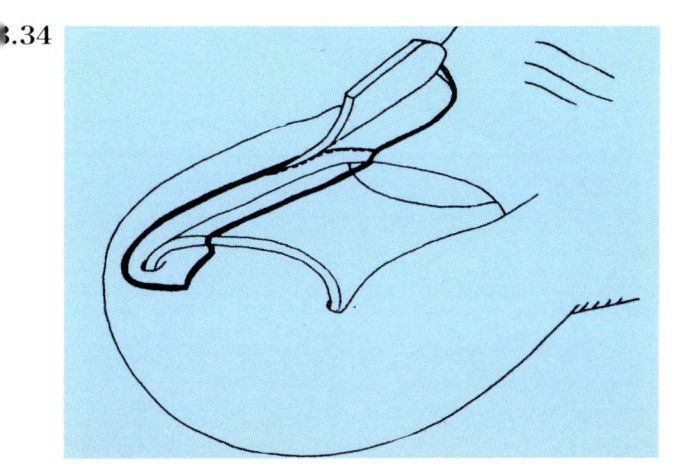

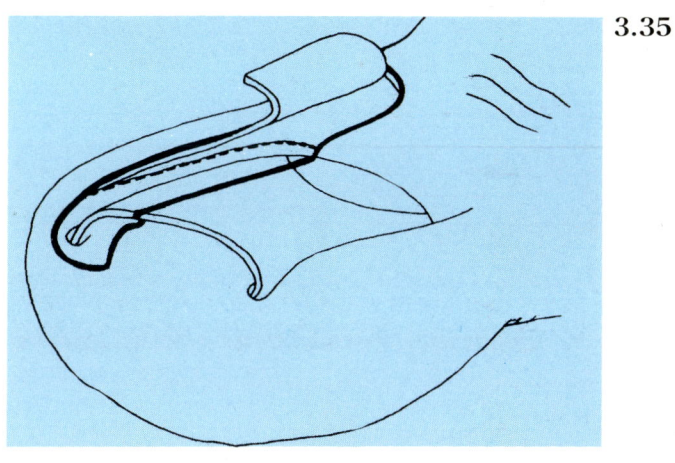

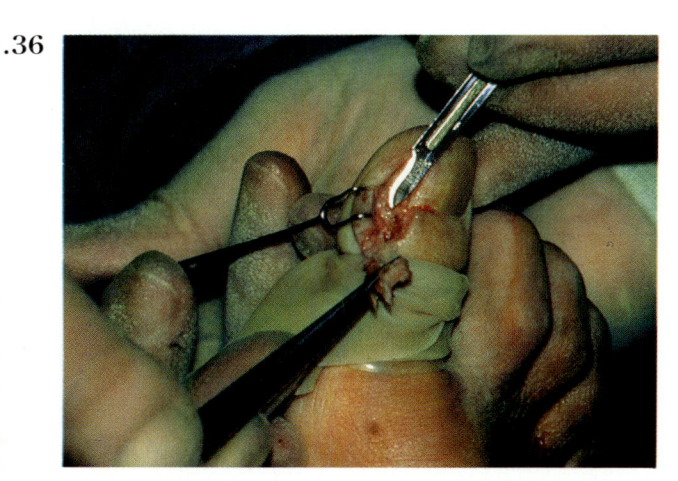

3.34–3.36 The Frost procedure, dissection of the skin off the nail root providing a flap for later replacement.

3.37–3.39 The Frost procedure, dissection of the nail border.

3.40 The Frost procedure, showing resected tissue.

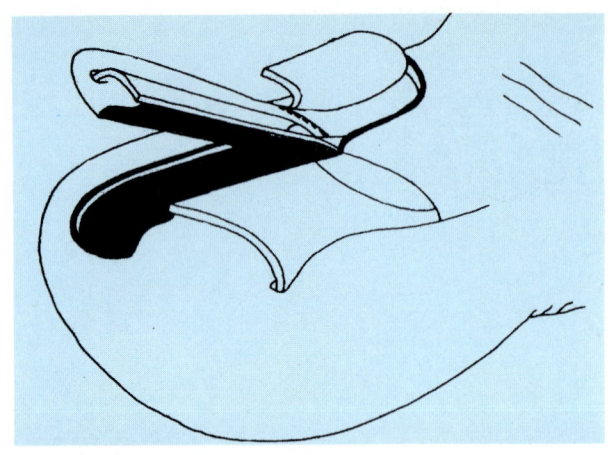

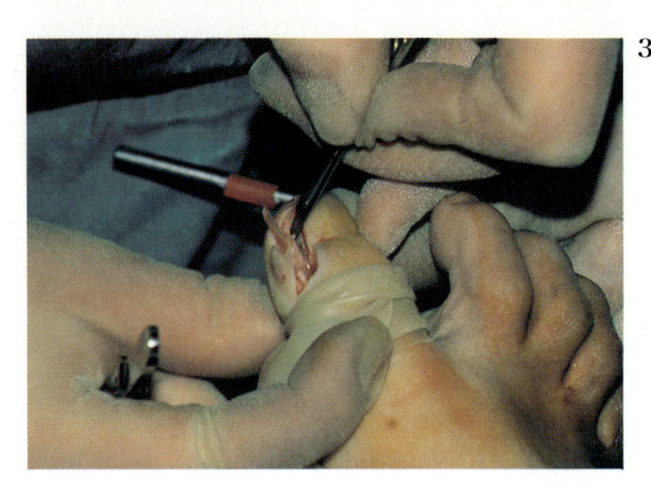

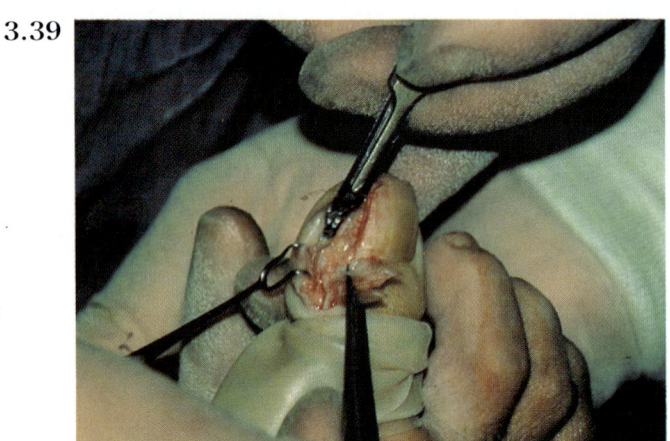

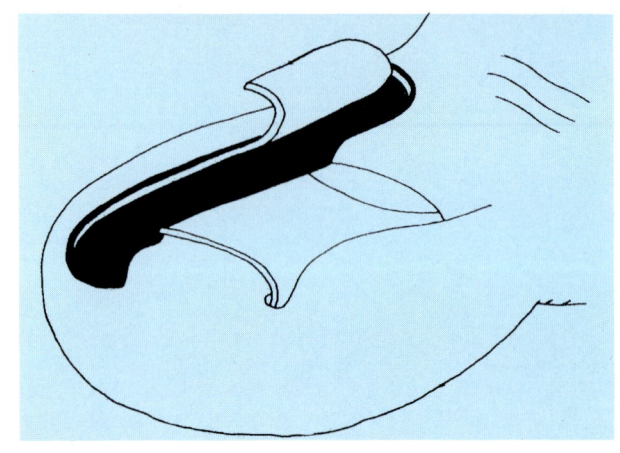

carried back onto the base of the phalange until this portion of the nail root is free. Careful inspection is then necessary to determine if any root particles remain (**3.37–3.39**).[15]

Frost[15] further advocates care, so as not to injure the periosteum, while Mercado[31] contradicts this opinion, stating that the periosteum of the phalanx is rasped to expose the bone. Mercado also advises that care be exercised, so as not to carry the flap incision too far plantarly as this could cause localized ischaemia (**3.40**). The flap is then replaced over the wound and secured.

Frost[15] also deprecates the use of sutures, stating that they tend to interfere with the blood supply in the flap, thereby causing sloughing. He advocates the use of a firm bandage, which he says controls haemorrhage and holds the flap *in situ*. Again Mercado disagrees, stating that the 'L' shaped flap is then repositioned to its original site and sutured. Current practice holds that the wound should be closed with fine sutures and/or steri-strips.

Post-operative management of incisional techniques

The sterile nature of the incisional nail procedures minimizes the risk of post-operative infection, although there always remains a possiblity that contamination may occur from the nail sulcus. It is, therefore, rarely necessary to apply more that a non-adhesive post-operative dressing, lightly secured by a conforming bandage, over the wound. In some cases the wound might be dressed with an antiseptic cream. As with non-incisional techniques, post-operative elevation of the foot is a necessity, and a period of 24–48 h is recommended. The dresssing should be replaced after that time, and healing will be complete in a couple of weeks (**3.41–3.46**).

If the nature of the nail and its sulcus are such as to lead the surgeon to expect wound contamination and some post-operative infection, antibiotic cover should be provided, and a fine Penrose drain inserted into the distal edge of the wound to facilitate drainage. This drain can be removed at the first post-operative redressing, if no obvious infection has occurred.

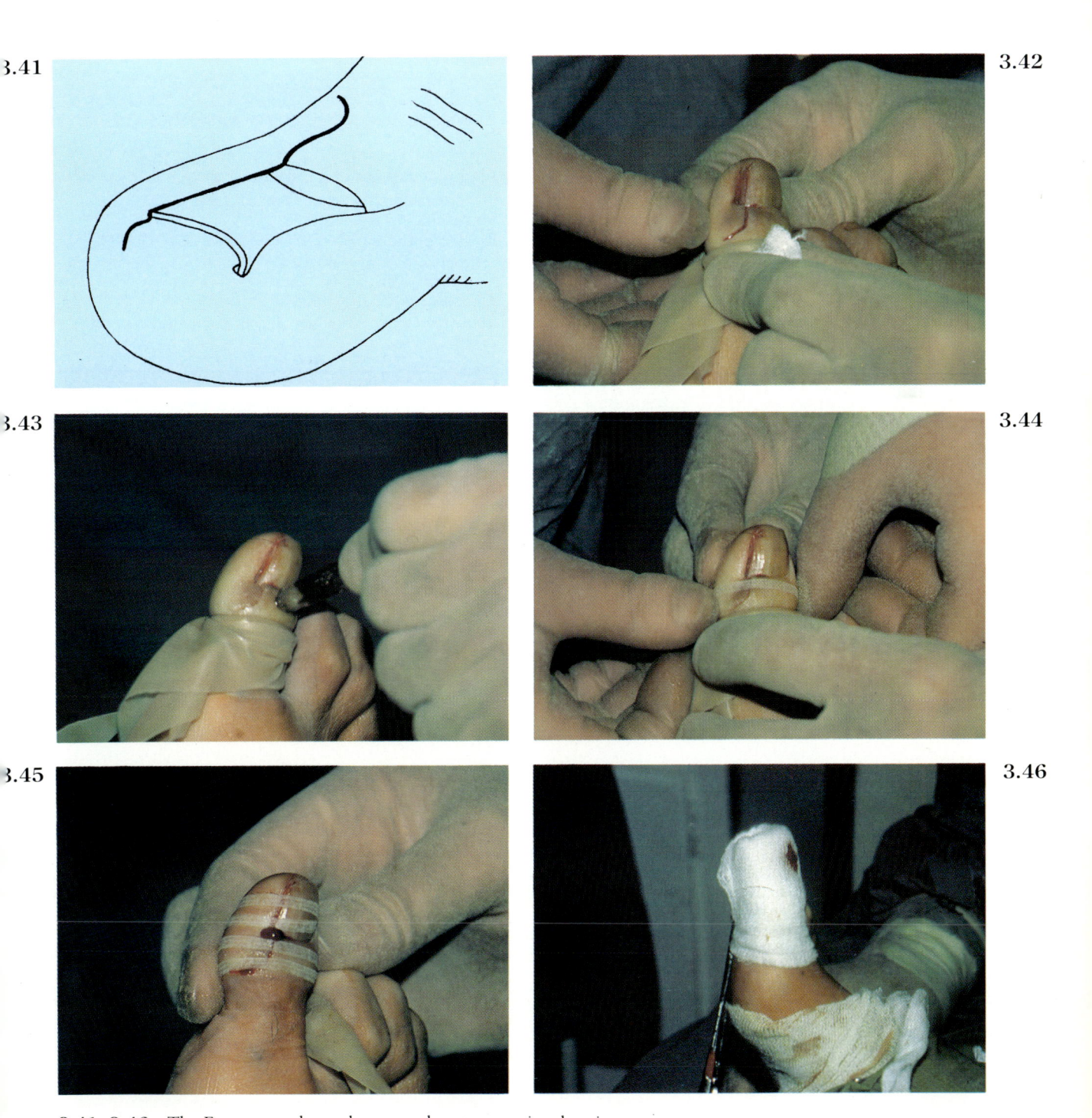

3.41–3.46 The Frost procedure, closure and post-operative dressings.

83

References

[1] Jones, F.W. *Principles of Anatomy as Seen in the Hand*. J & A. Churchill, 1920, p. 93.
[2] Zaias, N. Embryology of the human nail. *Arch. Dermatol.*, **87**: 37–53, 1963.
[3] Fleckman, P. Anatomy and physiology of the nail. *In* Daniel, C.R. (ed.), *Dermatologic Clinics*. Philadelphia, W.B. Saunders, 1985, pp. 373–381.
[4] Samman, P.D. The ventral nail. *Arch. Dermatol.*, **84**: 192–195, 1961.
[5] Rayner, V.R. An investigation into nail hypertrophy. *Chiropodist.*, **28**: 294–302, 1973.
[6] Krausz, C.E. Nail survey, 1942–1979. *Br. J. Chiropody*, **44**: 208, 1979.
[7] McKay, J.S. The Ross–Fraser nail brace. *Chiropodist*, **18**: 324–338, 1963.
[8] Lake, N.C. *The Foot*. Bailliere, Tindall & Cox, 1935.
[9] Ross-Fraser, A.R. Personal communication, 1979.
[10] Orr, C.M.S. and Photious, X. *Hospital Update*, **3**: 465, 1977.
[11] Bird, S. Correspondence. *Br. Med. J.*, 4th November 1978, p. 1297.
[12] McGlamry, E.D. Nail matrix phenolisation. *Br. J. Chiropody*, **43**: 221, 245, 1978; ibid. **44**: 55, 57, 81, 105, 1979.
[13] Fitzgerald, M.J.T. *et al.* Innervation of hyperplastic epidermis. *J. Investig. Dermatol.*, **64**: 169–174, 1975.
[14] Pardo-Castello, V. and Pardo, O.A. *Diseases of the Nails*, 3rd edn. Springfield, Charles C. Thomas, 1960, p. 23.
[15] Frost, L.A. Root resection for incurvated nail. *J. Natl. Assoc. Chiropodists*, **40**: 19–28, 1950.
[16] Dagnall, J.C. The history, development and current status of nail matrix phenolisation. *The Chiropodist*, **35**: 315–323, 1981.
[17] Zadik, F.R. Obliteration of the nail bed of the great toe. *J. Bone Joint Surg.*, **32B**: 66–67, 1950.
[18] Boll, O.F. Surgical correction of ingrowing nails. *J. Natl. Assoc. Chiropodists*, **35**: 8–9, 1945.
[19] Travers, G.R. and Ammon, R.G. The sodium hydroxide chemical matricectomy procedure. *J. Am. Podiatry Assoc.*, **70**: 476–478, 1980.
[20] Robertson, K. and Crawford, S. Nail wedge resections, a retrospective analysis. *The Chiropodist*, **30**: 225–228, 1976.
[21] Nyman, S.P. The phenol alcohol technique for toenail excision. *J. New Jersey Chiropodists Soc.*, **5**: 4, 1956.
[22] Greenwald, L. and Robbins, H.M. The chemical matricectomy. *J. Am. Podiatry Assoc.*, **71**: 388–389, 1981.
[23] Gardner, P. Negative galvanic current in the surgical correction of onychocryptotic nails. *J. Am. Podiatry Assoc.*, **48**: 555–560, 1958.
[24] Polokoff, M. Negative galvanic current used to destroy nail matrix. *J. New Jersey Chiropodists Soc.*, 1935.
[25] Abbott, W.W. and Geho, H. Partial matricectomy via negative galvanic current. *J. Am. Podiatry Assoc.*, **70**: 239–243, 1980.
[26] Kerman, B.L. and Kalmus, A. Partial matricectomy with electrodesiccation for permanent repair of ingrown nail borders. *J. Foot Surg.*, **21**(1): 1982.
[27] Dagnall, J.C. Povidone iodine and nail matrix phenolisation. *Br. J. Chiropody*, **50**: 213–216, 1985.
[28] Lavis, G.J. An investigation of wound healing and tissue zinc levels in patients undergoing partial nail avulsions. BSc thesis, Polytechnic of Central London, Project Report No. 86/2, 1986.
[29] Morkane, A.J., Robertson, R.W. and Inglis, G.W. Segmental phenolization of ingrowing toenails: a randomized controlled study. *Br. J. Surg.*, **71**: 526–527, 1984.
[30] Shapiro, S.L. Observations on the phenol technique of nail matrix eradication. *Curr. Podiatry*, 18–21, 1969.
[31] Mercado, O.A. *An Atlas of Foot Surgery, Vol 1: Forefoot Surgery*. Illinois College of Podiatric Medicine, 1979, pp. 19–22.
[32] Winograd, A.M.A. Modification in the technique of operation for ingrown toe-nail. *J. Am. Med. Assoc.*, **92**: 229–230, 1929.

Further reading

Bouché, R.T. Matricectomy utilizing negative galvanic current. *Clin. Podiatric Med. Surg.*, **3**: 449–456, 1986.
Dockery, G.L. Common toenail conditions. *Todays Jogger*, **2**: 57–59, 1978.
Dockery, G.L. Nails: fundamental conditions and procedures. *In* McGlamry, E.D. (ed.), *Comprehensive Textbook of Foot Surgery*. Baltimore, Williams & Wilkins, 1987, pp. 1–37.
Scher, R.K. and Daniel, C.R. *Nails: Therapy, Diagnosis, Surgery*. Philadelphia, W.B. Saunders, 1990.

4 Subungual (periungual) exostectomy

ROGER BUTTERWORTH

Introduction

Exostoses may occur in any bone that is preformed in cartilage; in rare cases, they may occur as an inherited condition, with systemic consequences.[1] They usually form in the foot as a result of localized acute or chronic insult—the most common sites being the posteriodorsal surface of the calcaneum,[2] the anterior plantar margin of the calcaneum (calcaneal spur),[3] the dorsal tarsal surface,[4] the medial surface of the first metatarsophalangeal joint in conjunction with hallux valgus,[5,6] and the phalanges.[7] Digital exostoses are usually regarded as subungual lesions, but this is not necessarily the case. Exostoses of the phalanges have a different pathology to other exostoses and, interestingly, can also be found on the digits of the hands. The term subungual exostosis may be misleading as to the nature of the lesion. In some instances, the tumours are not subungual; that is, they are not below the nail. The lesions can be present on the periungual area, with no disturbance to the nail itself.[8] They are not related to conventional exostoses (osteochondromas) seen in other parts of the skeleton, nor are they found in patients with multiple hereditary exostoses. Subungual exostoses do not arise adjacent to the epiphyseal growth plate, which is basal in the distal phalanx.[7]

Morphology and situation

Although periungual exostoses occur most commonly as subungual lesions, whose position and shape can vary considerably, they have occurred symptomatically as spurs on both the plantar[9] and lateral[10,11] borders of the hallux. The varying morphology and situation of these lesions is illustrated in **4.1, 4.2**.

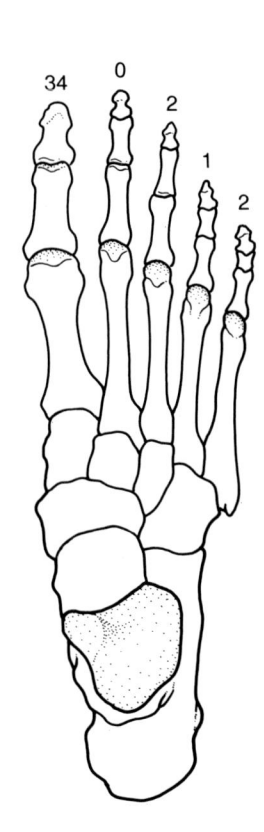

4.1 The varying morphology and situation of periungual exostoses. Distribution of periungual exostoses in 39 patients (after Landon et al.[7]).

4.2

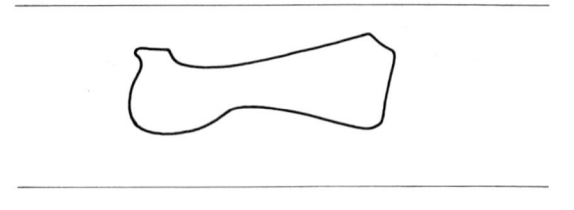

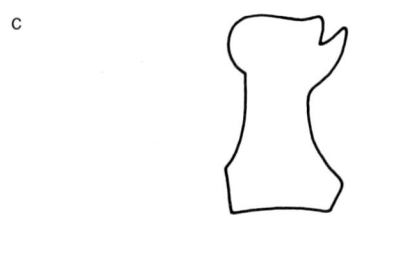

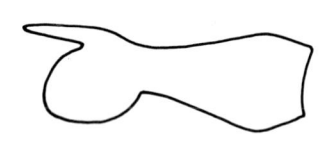

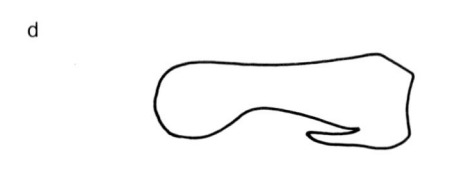

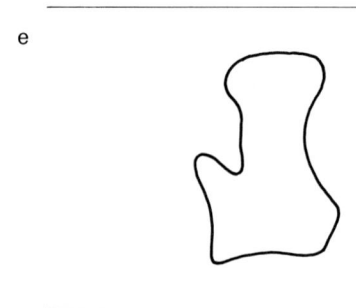

a

b

c

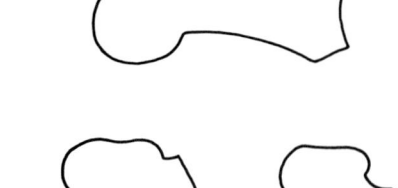

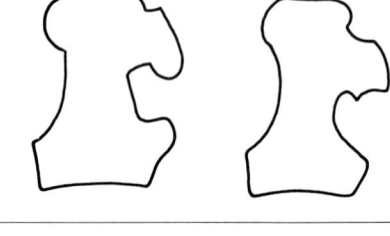

d

e

4.2 Morphology of periungual exostoses. After Cohen *et al.*[12] (*a*); after Evison and Price[11] (*b*); after Shaffer[8] (*c*); after Houle[9] (*d*); after Chinn and Jenkin[10] (*e*).

Clinical features

The clinical features (**4.3**) of the subungual exostosis were first recognized by Dupuytren in 1817 and published by him in 1839. He wrote, 'It occasionally happens that the upper surface of the ungual phalanx of the great toe presents a swelling, which has been commonly mistaken for a disease of the nail . . . . I discovered that such was not the case, and that the disease was an exostosis in the situation above indicated.'[13]

Although discussed at regular intervals in the literature since Dupuytren's first description, the clinical features remain ambiguous, probably because of their variable presentation. Indeed, authors are more united in their agreement over the need to differentiate a subungual exostosis from other lesions than in the clinical features of the lesion itself. The differential diagnosis may include subungual verruca, granuloma pyogenicum, glomus tumour, carcinoma of the nail bed, melanotic whitlow, kerato-acanthoma, subungual epidermoid inclusions, and endochondroma, according to Cohen;[12] subungual coagulum, according to Bodine;[14] subungual exostoses can and have been mistaken pathologically for malignant tumours, according to Landon *et al.*[7]

The characteristics of the condition (as described by various authors) are summarized in Table **4.1**. Although the extrapolation of information in this manner is not very satisfactory, it does afford an objective basis from which to derive a diagnosis. Typically, subungual exostosis presents as a solitary, unilateral lesion (99%) on the medial (tibial) border of the hallux (88%). It affects women more than men, in a ratio of 3:2 (3:1, if Landon *et al.*'s[7] figures are excluded), and arises most frequently (but not exclusively) during the second or third decade of life (72%). In a significant minority of patients the nail is elevated (25%), painful (30%), and demonstrates secondary clinical characteristics such as inflammation, infection, or ulceration (31%). Clinically, the information evidences to a pink or red coloration of the lesion under the nail, together with 'cornification or fibrosis'. Not all authors agree with this description, however;

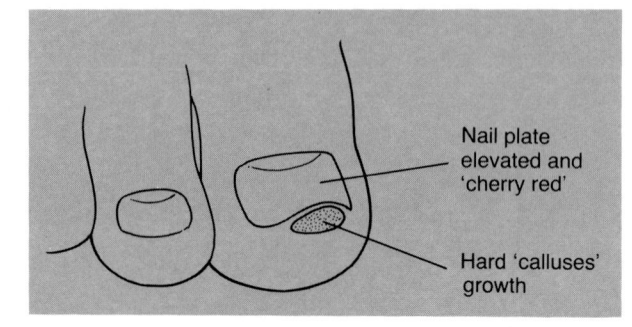

4.3 Clinical features of subungual exostosis.

Nail plate elevated and 'cherry red'

Hard 'calluses' growth

Johnston[16] describes 'The pearly mass growing through the nail.' Perhaps the best guide to the initial diagnosis is to always bear the possibility of an exostosis in mind.

Table 4.1 Characterization of the clinical features of subungual exostoses as described by various workers

	Dupuytren[13]	Cohen et al.[12]	Evison and Price[11]	Landon et al.[7]	Kurtz[15]	Shaffer[8]	Totals
Date of publication	1847	1973	1966	1979	1926	1933	
No. of patients in sample	5	7	20	44	42	4	122 (=100%)
Hallux	3	3	15	34	1	–	107 (=87%)
medial border of apex	2	2	8	–	39	4	
Lesser toes	–	2	3	5	2	–	13 (=11%)
Fingers	–	–	2	5	–	–	11%
Unilateral/solitary lesion + bilateral lesion	5	+	20	44	+	4	121 (=99%)
Number of males:females	0:5	2:5	6:14	30:14	–	1:3	
Ratio:patients				1:3	1:3	2:3	
Nail							
elevated	1	3	–	+	+	1	25%
brittle or broken	–	–	–	–	–	–	
painful	2	3	–	15	+	1	30%
colour, pink or red	–	1	–	–	+	3	–
cornification/fibrosis	–	1	–	–	–	2	–
inflamed, infected superating bleeding, or ulcerated	3	+	4	15	12	2	31%
Antecedent trauma	1	2	2	9	28	–	35%
Matricectomy/crytosis	–	–	–	–	12	–	29%
Pigmentation	–	1	–	+	–	–	–
Occurring during the second or third decade of life	5	4	13	+	+	4	72%

Notes: + Indicates that this worker recognizes this feature as a clinical characteristic
– Indicates an absence of affirmative information in the text
( ) Indicates an estimate or implicit recognition of the characteristic.

Radiological features

Most authors reference the use of X-rays to confirm the diagnosis of exostosis, and it is therefore suprising that Evison and Price[11] appear to be the only radiologists to have published a paper on the subject. Not suprisingly, their paper defines most clearly the almost classical radiographic features of the lesion. They describe the lesion as an outgrowth of trabeculated bone from the dorsal or dorso-medial surface of the terminal phalanx, beneath the nail. It may be broadly based, tapering a little before finally expanding at the summit, or the base may be fairly narrow, with the width increasing gradually. The summit of the growth is usually flattened or cupped, occasionally domed. The margin of the summit may be clearly demarcated or it may appear as an ill-defined edge that merges with the adjacent soft tissue shadow. The growth is capped with fibrous tissue or fibrocartilage, which is radiolucent.

The clarity of definition of the summit may depend to some extent on the radiographic projection, appearing clear cut when the incident ray is tangential. Lack of definition of the upper margin of the growth may also be present when soft tissue infection has occurred, but none of the cases in the present series, which showed poorly defined upper margins radiologically, had any histological evidence of chronic inflammation. The trabecular pattern of cancellous bone can be distinguished throughout: however, there is no defined cortex, though the margins of the growth are clear cut. All the lesions appear benign radiologically. No evidence of soft tissue calcification can be detected.[11] In an interesting case history, Rubin[17] evidences to the narrowness of the base of the exostosis by reporting the case of a patient whose exostosis fractured.

Aetiology and pathology

The relatively low incidence of antecedent trauma reported by most authors (**Table 4.1**) should not disguise the fact that irritation of the periosteum is the most probable cause of subungual exostosis. The histology suggests a response to chronic irritation, according to Campbell,[18] while Katz[19] considers the periosteum to be a sleeve of soft tissue surrounding the bone, which if irritated by any stimuli, will lay down bone matrix that will eventually be mineralized. Evison and Price[11] say that it seems likely that the majority of subungual exostoses represent an ossifying form of fibrocartilagenous metaplasia, arising in response to chronic stimulation, the exact nature and cause of which remain obscure. Landon et al.[7] state that these lesions are uniformly benign, and cautions against diagnosing them as sarcoma: the rapidly proliferating cartilagenous cap may mimic sarcoma in much the same way as does a fatigue fracture or hypertropic bone formation; however, one should note the lack of true anaplasia and the overall orderly maturation to trabecular bone.

The variable and remote nature of the periosteal irritation frequently obscures the nature of the cause. Nail surgery[10], onychocryptosis,[15,21] having the toe trodden upon during dancing or in crowded places or having weighty objects fall on the toe,[8,12,13,15] local injury,[12] 'a great deal of walking ... but there was no definite injury,'[8] and cauterization of a wart[13] are all listed as causes of the lesion by different researchers. Evison and Price[11] produce circumstantial evidence to suggest that footwear, particularly in women, is another probably cause. All the women in their study presented a similar radiological and histological picture, and the lesions all occurred on the dorsal or dorso-medial surfaces of the toes—12 of the 14 lesions studied were on the hallux. The development of an exostosis as a secondary factor to instability of the long arch of the foot is one pathology that is not considered, but given the tendency for some patients to activate the 'windlass effect'[20] in an effort to stabilize the foot, and in so doing to dorsiflex their hallux against the toe box of the shoe, such an eventuality should be considered, and treated before surgery is commenced.

Treatment

Although paring of the nail, palliation, and shoe modifications can all be used to relieve the initial discomfort of the condition, the only satisfactory treatment for symptomatic periungual exostosis is surgical removal. In those rare cases where the condition is further complicated by a pathology such as osteomyelitis, surgery may necessitate a terminal or partial Symes procedure, but in the great majority of cases removal of the exostosis itself is sufficient, and the only question that arises is which procedure to adopt. If the literature is ambiguous about the clincial features of the exostosis, it is almost universally dismissive of the details of treatment: excision;[13] excision or curettage;[16] removal of sufficient nail to allow the protuberance to be completely nibbled away;[5] avulsion of the toe-nail, longitudinal incision through the nail bed, isolation of a structure, and its removal with an osteotome;[21] radiation, cauterization, or even amputation of the great toe of a patient whose tumour was considered to be a sarcoma;[7] the nail is cut away, the growth peeled from its bed, the cavity is painted with pure phenol followed by alcohol.[15] Only Landon et al.[7] and Campbell[18] emphasize the need to protect the nail unit. Lapidus[22] recommended complete removal of the nail and amputation of the distal half of the phalanx.

Analysis of these various proposals would indicate that traditionally the surgical procedures adopted have involved the partial or complete avulsion of the nail plate and an approach to the lesion through the nail bed with consequent post-operative nail deformity. Mercado's[23] solution to this problem is to approach the exostosis through an apical 'fish mouth' incision in the apex of the toe, White[24] advocates osteotripsy through a similar, though smaller incision, while the author's own preference is through a modification of a Winograd or Frost procedure of the nail, followed by a careful undermining of the nail bed so as to elevate the whole of the distal nail unit to expose the exostosis. Mercado's 'fish mouth' incision and the modified nail procedure are the procedures considerd in this text. The main criteria in the procedure, other than the removal of the exostosis itself, should be to preserve the integrity of the nail unit and to remove the exostosis in such a way as to leave a concavity in the underlying phalanx, the effect of which is to obviate a recurrence of the lesion. According to Shaffer,[8] there is uniform acceptance of total excision as the best method of treatment; if the tumour is simply removed to the normal level of the bone, it usually recurs, whereas if it is peeled out of the bone leaving a cavity with some surrounding condensation of bone, it never recurs.

Mercado's 'fish mouth' incisional approach (4.4)

This approach is used when the nail plate is normal, except for the underlying exostosis. The incision is placed within a papillary ridge on the distal (anterior) surface of the toe, below the level of the sulci, and extending beyond the sulci, so as to allow the elevation of the complete nail unit. The incision is deepened to the bone, and the dorsal surface of the bone and its exostosis are exposed. The nail unit is very carefully elevated to provide exposure of the exostosis, which is then resected using small rongeur bone forceps. It is important that this resection is carried out in such a way as to leave a concave surface at the site of the exostosis and so minimize the risk of the exostosis reforming as the bone heals. The wound can then be closed with 5-0 nylon sutures and dressed. In describing this procedure Mercado emphasizes the placing of the fish-mouthed incision inside a papillary ridge to ensure almost scar-free healing. Care should be taken when retracting the dorsal portion of the wound, and Mercado advocates the use of skin hooks, as these will not damage the fragile nail plate.

4.4

— Incision

Incision widened and deepened to expose phalanx and exostosis

— Incision closed

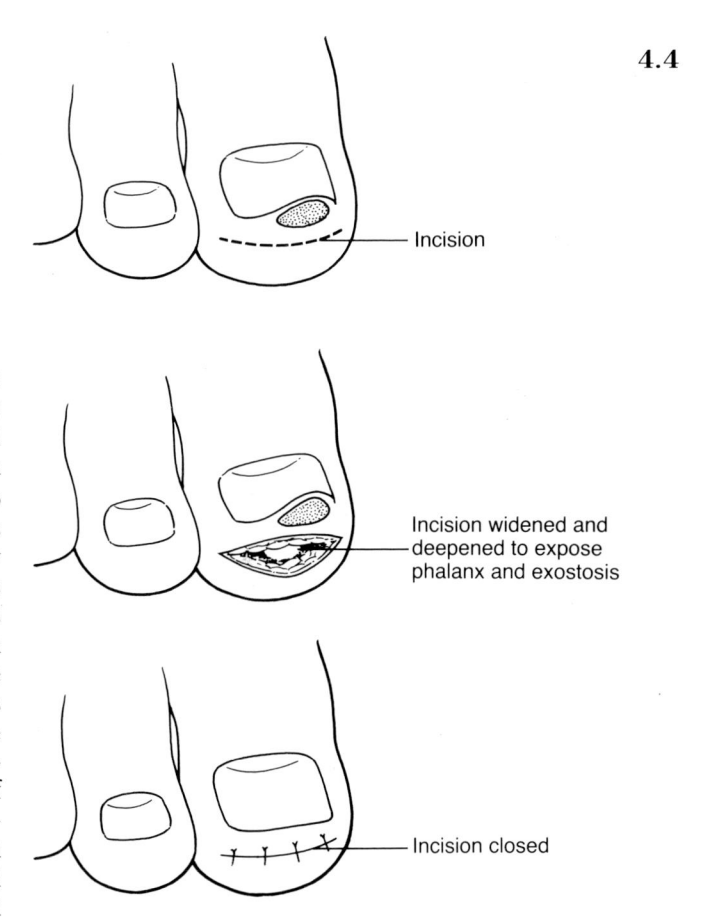

4.4 Mercado's 'fish mouth' incisional approach.

4.5

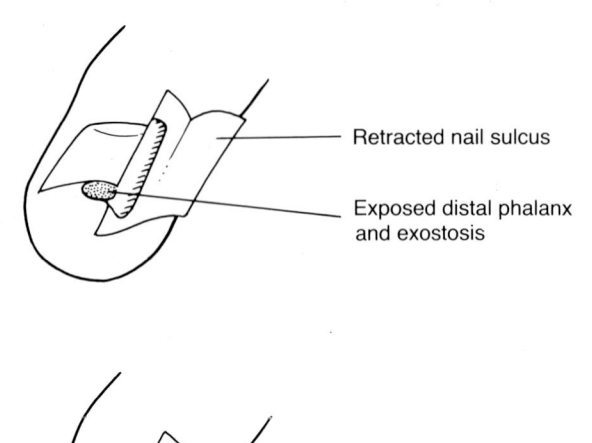

- Retracted nail sulcus
- Exposed distal phalanx and exostosis

- Nail plate/bed and exostosis is surgically undermined and the exostosis removed

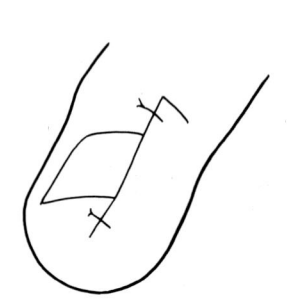

4.5 Modified Frost approach.

Modified incisional nail approach (4.5)

This approach involves either a Frost or Winograd procedure to remove the lateral border of the affected nail unit on the side closest to the exostosis, which can then be exposed by gently undermining and elevating the nail unit. The exostosis is removed with small rongeur bone forceps, and in such a way as to leave the concavity described in the Mercado technique. The wound can then be closed using 5-0 nylon and dressed. The advantages of this technique are that it minimizes postoperative scarring, providing an aesthetically acceptable result, and most important, it facilitates the resolution of associated nail groove pathology.

Complications

The only common complication of an exostectomy is that of regrowth. Again, little is made of this possibility in the literature, although Landon et al.[7] reported that after initial treatment of the tumour, 11% of patients had local recurrence. The five patients underwent subsequent local excision, with no additional recurrence.

Nor is the possibility of malignant changes developing in an exostosis, or as a result of an exostectomy, really considered. Landon et al.[7] report that 'None of the 44 tumours underwent malignant change', and one must assume that where neoplastic changes are found, there has been an initial mistake in the diagnosis of exostosis.

References

[1] Solomon, L. Hereditary multiple exostoses. *J. Bone Joint Surg.*, **45**: 292, 1963.
[2] Bateman, J.E. The adult heel. *In* Jahss, M.H. (ed.). *Disorders of the Foot, Vol. 1*. Philadelphia, W. B. Saunders, 1982, pp. 764–775.
[3] Costello, M. and Gibbs, R.C. *The Palms and Soles in Medicine.* Springfield, Charles C. Thomas, 1967, p. 510.
[4] Jahss, M.H. Disorders of the anterior tarsus and Lisfanc's joint. *In* Jahss, M.H. (ed.), *Disorders of the Foot, Vol 1*. Philadelphia, W. B. Saunders, 1982, pp. 711–726.
[5] Edgar, M.A. Hallux valgus and associated conditions. *In* Klennerman, L. (ed.), *The Foot and Its Disorders,* 1st edn. Oxford, Blackwell, pp. 83–130.
[6] Kelikian, H. *Hallux Valgus, Allied Deformities of the Fore-foot and Metatarsalgia.* Philadelphia, W.B. Saunders, 1965.
[7] Landon, G.C., Johnson, K.A. and Dahlin, D.C. Subungual exostoses. *J. Bone Joint Surg.*, **61A**: 256–259, 1979.
[8] Shaffer, L.W. Subungual exostoses. *Arch. Dermatol. Syphilol.*, **24**: 371–379, 1933.
[9] Houle, R.J. Spur-shaped phalangeal exostosis. *J. Am. Podiatry Assoc.*, **57**: 21, 1967.
[10] Chinn, S. and Jenkin, W. Proximal nail groove pain associated with an exostosis. *J. Am. Podiatric Med. Assoc.*, **76**: 506–508, 1986.
[11] Evison, G. and Price, C.H.G. Subungual exostosis. *Br. J. Radiol.*, **39**: 451–455, 1966.
[12] Cohen, H.J., Frank, S.B. and Minkin, W. Subungual exostosis. *Arch. Dermatol.*, **107**: 431–432, 1973.
[13] Baron Dupuytren, *On the Injuries and Diseases of Bones* (translated and edited by F. Le Gros Clark). Sydenham Society, 1847, London, p. 408.
[14] Bodine, K.G. Subungual coagulum. *J. Am. Podiatry Association.*, **57**: 377–378, 1967.
[15] Kurtz, A.D. Subungual exostosis surgery. *Gynecol. Obstetr.*, **43**: 488–490, 1926.
[16] Johnston, J.O. *In* Mann, R. (ed.), *DuVries's Surgery of the Foot*, 4th edn. St Louis, C.V. Mosby, 1978, p. 436.
[17] Rubin, L.M. Fracture of a subungual osteoma. *J. Am. Podiatry Assoc.*, **57**: 334–335, 1967.
[18] Campbell, C.J. Tumors of the foot. *In* Jahss, M.H. (ed.), *Disorders of the Foot, Vol. 1*. Philadelphia, W.B. Saunders, 1982, pp. 979–1013.
[19] Katz, F.N. Bone tumor diagnosis. *In* McGlamry, E.D. (ed.), *Reconstructive Surgery of the Foot and Leg.* Intercontinental Medical Book Co., 1974, pp. 83–96.
[20] Hicks, J.H. The mechanics of the foot II: The plantar aponeurosis and the arch. *J. Anatomy,* **88**: 25–32, 1954.
[21] Stern, J. Removal of subungual exostosis and subsequent removal of needle. *J. Am. Podiatry Assoc.*, **60**: 406–407, 1970.
[22] Lapidus, P.W. Complete and permanent removal of the toe nail in onychogryphosis and subungual osteoma. *Am. J. Surg.*, **19**: 92–94, 1933.
[23] Mercado, O.A. *An Atlas of Foot Surgery, Vol. 1: Forefoot Surgery.* Carolando Press, 1980, pp. 33–34.
[24] White, D.L. Minimal incision techniques for digital deformities. *Clin. Podiatric Med. Surg.*, **3**: 105–106, 1986.

Further reading

Brenner, M.A., Montgomery, R.M. and Kalish, S.R. Subungual exostosis. *Cutis,* **25**: 518, 1980.
Chesler, S.M. and Basler, R.S.W. Subungual exostosis. *J. Am. Podiatry Assoc.*, **68**: 732–734, 1978.
Dockery, G.L. Nails: fundamental conditions and procedures. *In* McGlamry, E.D. (ed.), *Comprehensive Textbook of Foot Surgery.* Baltimore, Williams & Wilkins, 1987, pp. 1–37.
Fuselier, C.O., Binning, T., Kushner, D., *et al.* Solitary esteochondroma of the foot: an in-depth study with case reports. *J. Foot Surg.*, **23**: 3–24, 1984.
Kehr, L.E. Onychocryptosis due to subungual exostosis. *J. Foot Roentgenol.*, **3**: 7, 1965.

5 Sesamoidectomy

ROGER BUTTERWORTH

Introduction

The interest shown in the sesamoid bones of the first metatarsal head by ancient physicians and mystics[1] is not reflected in modern medical literature, and those few articles which have been published only serve to emphasize this neglect. Helal writes,[2] 'Although largely ignored by orthopaedists the sesamoid bones of the great toe received considerable attention in ancient times.'

This recent neglect is probably due to a failure to recognize that discrete pathologies can affect the sesamoids in isolation of other affections and must be treated as such. They may be treated conservatively, but frequently require surgery. According to Kaiman,[3] 'When one considers the vast array of afflictions to which the human body is subjected in the course of a lifetime, it is not unusual that sesamoid pathology is discussed infrequently. The ills to which the diminutive structure plays host are many and they may lend themselves to conservative therapy. Should the patient not respond and the condition prove debilitating, surgical intervention then becomes the treatment of choice.'

Distribution and morphology of sesamoids in the forefoot

The distribution of sesamoid bones in the forefoot is potentially quite extensive and is illustrated in **Table 5.1**, although those underlying the first metatarsal head are the only ones that could be considered a constant feature.[4] Jahss[5] considered the medial and lateral sesamoids (of the first metatarsal) to be constant bones, in that very rarely were either one congenitally absent. In such cases, there is usually no deformity, the conjoined tendon being functionally normal. DuVries,[6] however, does report a congenital absence of the tibial sesamoid associated with secondary clawing.

The consistency with which the sesamoids of the first metatarsal are found in the foot contrast with their integrity. The reported incidence of bipartite and multipartite sesamoids in the literature varies considerably (**Table 5.2**) as does their configuration (**5.1**). Gallocher[12] refined these figures to show that the incidence of multipartite bones is highest in the 10–12 years of age group, and after that there is a very marked fall in the incidence of multipartite bones in people over 30 years of age. The greatest fall in incidence is in the over-40 age group. The fall in incidence of multipartite sesamoids is greater in men than in women. As seen in **Table 5.3**, multipartite bones tend to unite with increasing age. As ossification comes about by calcification and then ossification of existing cartilage, this may be the reason for the belief that sesamoids that have been fractured heal without callous formation. The few cases of callous formation recorded in the literature then become of greater significance and are a truer indication of the rarity of fracture as a cause of pain in the region.[12]

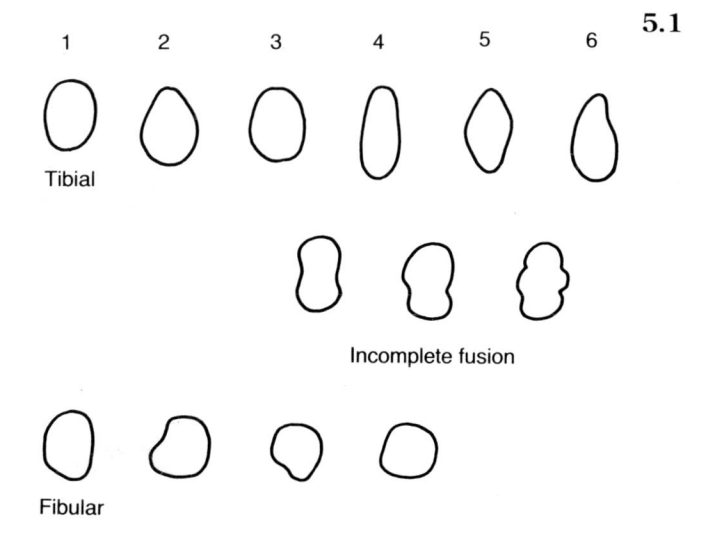

5.1 Normal sesamoids of the great toe in descending order of frequency. (After Kewenter.[7])

Table 5.1 Percentage distribution of sesamoid bones in the (adult) foot

	Hallux Tibial	Hallux Fibular	Hallux Interphalangeal	Second toe Tibial	Second toe Fibular	Third toe Tibial	Third toe Fibular	Fourth toe Tibial	Fourth toe Fibular	Fifth toe Tibial	Fifth toe Fibular
Burman & Lapidus[51]	100	100	13.1	3.4	0.0	0.4	0.0	0.7	0.0	16.3	2.9
Pfitzner	100	100	50.6	1.6	0.0	0.0	0.0	0.0	0.0	6.2	5.5
Bizzaro[4]	100	100	5.0	1.0	0.0	0.0	0.0	2.0	0.0	10.0	0.0
Kassatkin	100	100	m—53.3 f—57.8	4.2	0.2	0.7	0.0	1.4	0.6	12.2	10.1

Table 5.2 The incidence of bipartite sesamoids of the first metatarsal reported in the literature

	Number of feet surveyed	Incidence of bipartitism (%)
Kewenter[7]	1588	33.5
Inge and Ferguson[8]	1025	10.7
Freiberg[9]	1000	1.0
Francis[10] Male:	100	33.0
Female:	90	28.0
Scranton and Rutkowski[11]	45	11.1

Table 5.3 Incidence of appearance of sesamoids and incidence of division[13]

	Males Medial Per cent of appearance	Males Medial Per cent of divided	Males Lateral Per cent of appearance	Males Lateral Per cent of divided	Females Medial Per cent of appearance	Females Medial Per cent of divided	Females Lateral Per cent of appearance	Females Lateral Per cent of divided
Age								
7	0.1	—	—	—	1.8	33.3	3.5	—
8	—	—	—	—	13.3	19.0	12.0	—
9	2.1	—	2.1	—	33.1	28.2	26.3	—
10	15.2	36.7	16.2	6.25	71.9	25.8	67.4	9.2
11	46.0	45.0	43.1	16.0	88.6	41.5	91.0	1.3
12	69.5	36.7	68.0	2.9	97.9	41.9	99.1	3.9
13	83.8	31.0	82.0	7.7	99.6	33.0	100.0	0.9
14–15	97.5	27.0	96.5	5.0	100	39.0	100	0.6
16–19	100	22.1	100	3.9	100	36.2	100	0.5
20–29	100	11.8	100	1.3	100	32.1	100	0.2
30–39	100	11.7	100	—	100	11.1	100	—
40 plus	100	5.6	100	0.6	100	11.0	100	0.7

Structure and function of the first metatarsal sesamoids

Embryologically, the first metatarsal sesamoids begin to differentiate about the eighth week of foetal life,[8] but will not ossify until the eighth to tenth year of life.[10] The process of ossification occurs from multiple centres, which may or may not fuse, and it is this failure to unite that is believed to give rise to partite sesamoids[14] (**5.2**). The sesamoids often develop from multiple centres of ossification, failure of fusion resulting in partite sesamoids.[5] Failure of fusion occurs in the medial sesamoid of the great toe much more frequently than in the lateral sesamoid.[8] Gallocher points out that bipartite sesamoids tend to unite later in life.[12] The functional consequences of partite sesamoids appear limited, however, unless there is an associated pathology. There is usually a firm fibrocartilagenous union between the two bones, which appear as one bone to the naked eye.[15] Very rarely, a sesamoid may fail to ossify.[16]

Sesamoid bones, so called because they are shaped like sesame seeds, develop within tendons. One surface of the bone is covered with hyaline cartilage and is in apposition to the articular cartilage of the bone with which it articulates. All other aspects of the sesamoid are firmly attached to the tendon of which it is part.[15]

The normal contour of (first metatarsal) sesamoids is a convex transverse surface superiorly and an even convexity of the main part of the bone. The main convexity longitudinally is even, and slightly longer than the transverse, and the superior surface is slightly concave. Alterations in outline are significant when they affect the even convexity of the inferior surface, and are usually seen as an increase in the depth of the bone, giving a more acute convexity to the outline. In a few cases this is seen on radiographs as an almost triangular, or pyramidal, outline on axial views, with the apex directed towards the plantar tissues.[12]

The structure of the first metatarsophalangeal joint and its sesamoids have been described by Haines and McDougall[17] (**5.3, 5.4**); Sarrafian and Topouzian[18] elaborated on that original description. The two sesamoids underlying the first metatarsal head articulate with the two corresponding plantar grooves of the metatarsal and are an integral part of the structure of the first metatarsophalangeal joint (**5.5, 5.6**).[19] There are grooves in the metatarsal head for the sesamoids rather than facets, because the metatarsal head rotates over the fixed sesamoids in the propulsive phase of gait. There is a joint-like relationship between the sesamoids and the head of the metatarsal, and synovium and synovial fluid are present at their articulation.[20] Conventionally they are accepted as lying within the bifurcated head of the flexor hallucis brevis muscle, but this picture is a little simplistic. Many of the fibres of the muscle insert through the sesamoids, but so do some of the muscular fibres of the adductor and abduc-

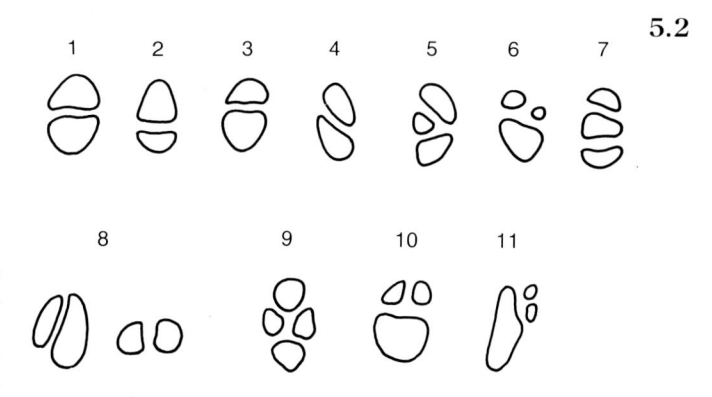

5.2 Developmental variations of the partite sesamoids of the great toe in descending order of frequency. (After Kewenter.[7])

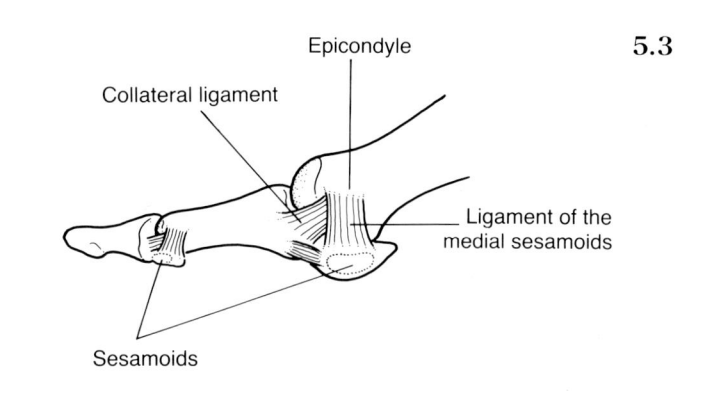

5.3 Medial view of the first metatarsophalangeal joint and hallux, demonstrating the sesamoids. (After Haines and McDougall.[17])

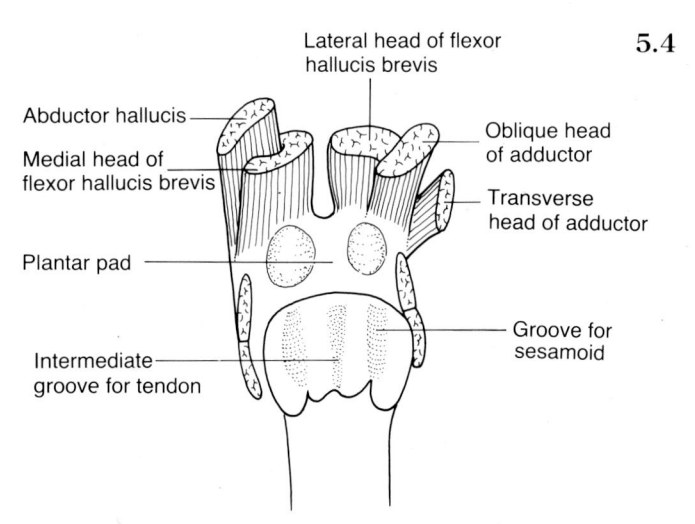

5.4 Dissection of the first metatarsophalangeal joint to demonstrate sesamoids and related structures. (After Haines and McDougall.[17])

5.5

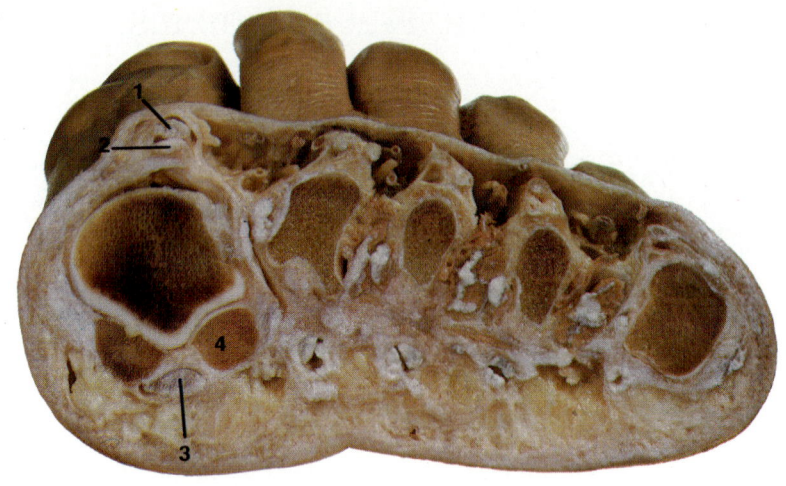

1 Extensor hallucis longus
2 Extensor hallucis brevis
3 Flexor hallucis longus
4 Sesamoid bone

5.5 Section through the heads of the metatarsal, demonstrating the relationship of the sesamoids to their surrounding structures. Note the position of the flexor hallucis tendon. (From McMinn *et al.*,[19] with permission.)

5.6 The hallucal sesamoids and related structures. Sagittal section of the right foot through the medial part of the talus, sustentaculum tali and the great toe, from the lateral side. (From McMinn *et al.*,[19] with permission.)

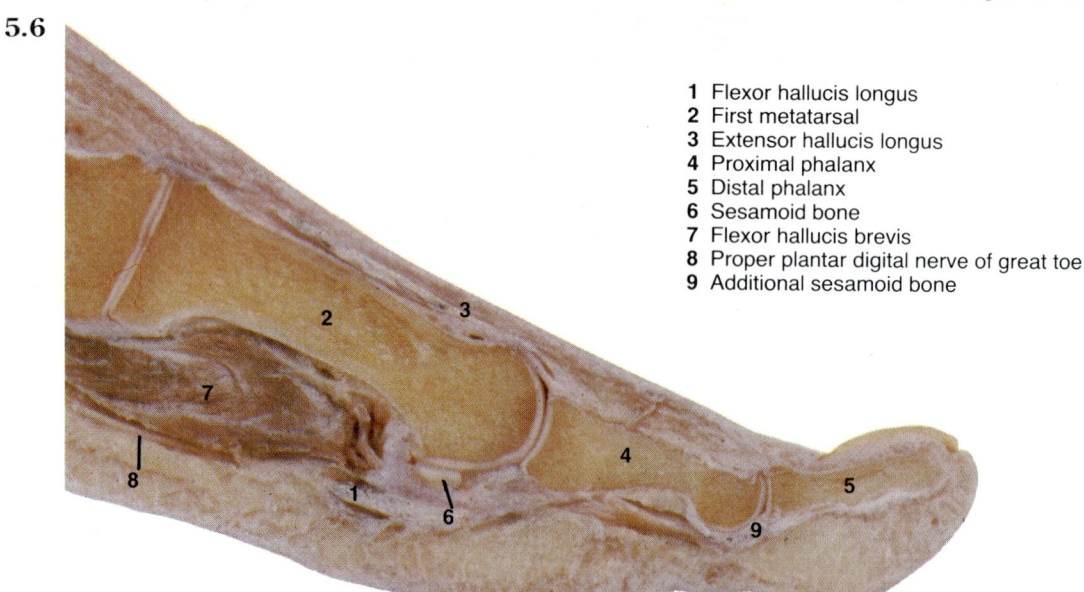

1 Flexor hallucis longus
2 First metatarsal
3 Extensor hallucis longus
4 Proximal phalanx
5 Distal phalanx
6 Sesamoid bone
7 Flexor hallucis brevis
8 Proper plantar digital nerve of great toe
9 Additional sesamoid bone

tor of the great toe, and so also a very strong band of plantar aponeurosis.[17]

According to Inge and Ferguson[8]: 'In the human adult there are constantly present two osseous sesamoid bones at the metatarsophalangeal joint of the great toe; each is enclosed around the margin of its superior facet by the capsule of the joint and invested throughout the remainder of its surface by the corresponding tendon of the flexor brevis hallucis. These tendons are inserted into the proximal end of the first phalanx of the great toe, and are the only effective plantar flexors of the metatarsophalangeal joint; their fibres bite into the roughened non-articular surface of the sesamoids, there being no smooth periosteum; hence the difficulty in shelling these bones out of their tendons. The sesamoids articulate with, and rest under, the first metatarsal head, the cartilage of the latter being prolonged proximally for this purpose. From above and in profile they have a characteristic smooth shape. Though joined together by the strong bands of the joint capsule, (a stout, thick intermetatarsal ligament[21]), they are separated from each other by the tendon of the flexor longus hallucis on its way to insertion into the distal phalanx of the toe, and their corresponding articular facets on the metatarsal head are separated by a bony ridge; this ridge is not high enough to prevent dislocation of the medial sesamoid laterally in severe hallux valgus. Between the sesamoids and the skin there is normally only the thick fibrous pad of the 'ball' of the foot, through which the two small bones can sometimes be palpated. Not infrequently a bursa is interposed between the sesamoids and the skin surface.'[8] There is a constant bursa on the plantar aspect of the sesamoid on the tibial side.[2]

Notwithstanding the accepted view of the sesamoids as being invested by the bifurcated heads of the flexor hallucis brevis, Acton, reviewing the surgical anatomy of the foot, argues that the sesamoids should be considered as lying within the plantar pad of the first metatarsal for purposes of surgery. The deep transverse metatarsal ligament of the metatarsophalangeal joint of the great toe differs from that of the corresponding joint in the thumb. In the great toe this ligament contains two sesamoid bones, whereas in the thumb the sesamoids are within the substance of the conjoined tendons related to the respective sides of the joint. Thus, in the foot, the flexibility and mobility of the thumb give way to stability and weight bearing, both of which are furthered by the sesamoids being within the fibrocartilagenous plate.[22]

Gallocher found in all specimens that a pronounced thickening of the joint capsule formed a fan-shaped ligament, which arose in an oblique line from the plantar surface of the neck of the metatarsal and the plantar tubercles and ran in an anterio-lateral direction and plantarward to the posterior and lateral edges of the sesamoids.[12]

On either side of the metatarsal head, as it tapers proximally, is an epicondyle that serves as the origin for the medial and lateral collateral and sesamoid ligaments.[23] The latter two ligaments and the anterior medial and lateral sesamoidal ligaments bind the sesamoids to the metatarsal head and plantar aspect of the base of the proximal phalanx, respectively. Proximally, they are attached by the plantar portion of the metatarsophalangeal joint capsule to the neck of the first metatarsal.[5,24] Three of the four intrinsic muscles that insert into the base of the hallux are involved with the sesamoids by way of the conjoined tendon mechanism. The extensor hallucis brevis, flexor hallucis brevis, adductor, and abductor hallucis muscles in the normal foot produce no more than 15° of lateral deviation of the digit.[20] Hawkins points out that the four intrinsic muscles, particularly the adductor and abductor hallucis, stabilize the hallux and influence rotation and transverse plane deviation when they are not in balance.[26] Even in the normal foot, the long flexor and two extensors are somewhat obliquely placed, so as to abduct the hallux towards the second toe, in addition to their main actions. Particularly when the toe is already abducted, the ligaments are stretched; this bowspring effect is significant.[3,24] This tendency is further enhanced because the extensor wing is thicker on the fibular aspect than on the tibial aspect of the hallux.[22]

The destabilizing effect of this bowstringing is further enhanced by the intrinsic instability of the first metatarsal head itself. No muscle inserts into the head of the metatarsal, leaving it dependent for its stability on those extrinsic muscles (tibialis anterior and peroneus longus) having their insertion in the base of the metatarsal, and the indirect influence of those muscles inserting directly or indirectly into the proximal phalanx of the hallux. In effect, the metatarsal is supported in a hammock, and according to Kelikian,[27] the base of the proximal phalanx may be likened to the controlling post of a hammock. The joint capsule, the collateral ligaments and the sesamoid pad form a shallow hammock that is reinforced laterally by the adductor obliquus (oblique head of the adductor hallucis) and medially by the abductor hallucis. When the proximal phalanx deviates towards the outer border of the foot, subluxates, and everts, the hammock moves from under the metatarsal head.[27] The sesamoids move with the hammock.

Helal[2] and Gallocher[12] emphasize the close relationship between sesamoids and the corresponding metatarsal with which they articulate, and Scranton and Rutkowski[11] describe the range of motion of the sesamoids. The average angular excursion of the sesamoids ($71.9 \pm 11°$) is quite large. It is less than that of the great toe (91°), but this is probably a result of some degree of elasticity in the tendon of the flexor hallucis brevis. With extension of the hallux, sesamoids are drawn distally, approximately 1 cm to the distal end of the metatarsal head, and tilt dorsally.[5] Gallocher[12] draws attention to the limitations in the range of motion of the first metatarsophalangeal joint due to soft tissue pathology of the perisesamoidal structures. Hass[28] further emphasizes the significance of this range of motion for foot pathology. The position of the hallucal (first metatarsal) sesamoids, as seen on an anterioposterior X-ray, may indicate the position of the first metatarsal in the sagittal plane. If the sesamoids appear at the first metatarsophalangeal joint level, the first metatarsal may be plantarflexed: if the sesamoids appear more proximal at the metatarsal neck level, the first metatarsal may be dorsiflexed. The seamoids lie at a constant distance from both the second metatarsal[12] and the proximal phalanx of the hallux, the latter distance being determined by the length of the head of the flexor hallucis brevis and designed to ensure that the sesamoids always lie beneath the metatarsal head when the hallux is plantigrade. The two ossicles move as one, the sesamoids moving with the hallux.[27] In all specimens, the plantar pad and sesamoids have a very strong series of attachments on the lateral aspect, which has the effect of ensuring a fairly constant relationship of the sesamoids and the second metatarsal.[12] This characteristic is an important consideration when taking X-rays of the sesamoids.

The presence of these bones as 'true sesamoids' (as opposed to accessory bones) is now accepted,[4,29] and their functional and pathological analogy to the patella[11,30] evidences to their importance in the function of the foot and in its pathology. According to Helal,[30] 'These little bones lie like small kneecaps on the metatarsal heads and suffer much the same diseases as the patella.' Sesamoids appear where changes in the direction of pull of a tendon occur. They provide protection for the tendon, as well as giving a mechanical advantage. The great toe sesamoids also protect the long flexor tendon and give lift to the metatarsal head, an important feature in the biomechanics of the forefoot[2] (**5.7**). The relatively acute angle found between the long axis of the first metatarsal and the ground means that even a slight elevation of the metatarsal head will extend the line described by the long axis of the first metatarsal considerably. Providing this elevation of the metatarsal is stabilized by adequate support, it must follow that the 'functional length' of the metatarsal is also increased. Gallocher[12] also showed that, because the relationship between the hallux and the sesamoids is stable, the 'functional length' of the metatarsal is preserved at all times.

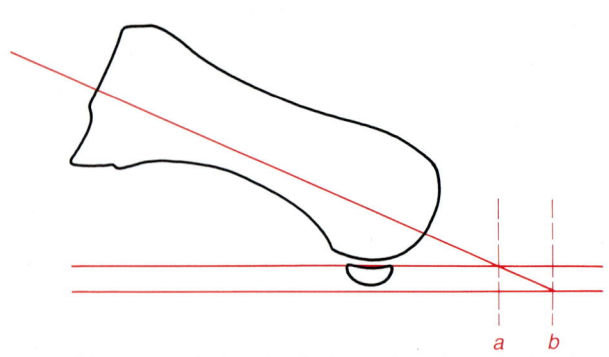

5.7 Diagrammatic longitudinal section through the first metatarsal to demonstrate the influence of the sesamoids in increasing the functional length of the metatarsals from *a* to *b*.

Radiographic projections

The diminutive size of the sesamoids, together with the masking effect of the first metatarsal head, requires that radiography of the sesamoids be carried out with care and precision. Although medial/lateral and oblique projections are sometimes useful, and anterior/posterior (dorsal/plantar) views are frequently and effectively used, they both suffer from the problems of masking by other tissues. The visualization of the plantar aspect of the sesamoid metatarsophalangeal area on a radiograph was difficult, with no consistent means of preventing the superimposition of the digits and the soft tissue over the metatarsal heads.[31] This problem was solved by Gamble and Yale,[32] who first elaborated the 'plantar axial/sesamoid view' in 1966. Downey and Dorothy refined the technique by developing a positioning device to elevate the rearfoot and the digits, thus preventing soft tissue and osseous interference in the visualization of the plantar aspect of the forefoot.[31] Fuson *et al.*[33] improved the technique further by developing a radio-opaque sponge axial orthoposer. Whereas the standard axial orthoposer allows visualization of anatomical shapes of the metatarsal heads and evaluation of the cristae (intersesamoidal ridge) and the sesamoids, it has rarely satisfactorily allowed evaluation of the relationships of the metatarsals to the transverse plane.[33] This is most important when evaluating plantar-declinated metatarsals. Because visualization of the sesamoids roentgenologically is so difficult, it is advisable to take multiple views, including routine anterior-posterior, lateral and sesamoid views along with a slight medial oblique for the lateral sesamoid and a slight lateral oblique for the medial sesamoid.[5] The tibial sesamoid position as seen on an anterior-posterior radiograph is determined by relative position to a line bisecting the dorsal longitudinal axis of the first metatarsal (**5.8**). This is measured on a scale from 1 to 7, from medial to lateral planes. The normal tibial sesamoid position is 1 and 2. As the hallux drifts laterally, the sesamoid apparatus moves from a medial to lateral position under the first metatarsal head. When the tibial sesamoid is in a position of 3 or greater, it is being jammed against the middle crista (intersesamoidal ridge) on the plantar aspect of the first metatarsal head. The position of the tibial sesamoid is used as an indicator for determining whether or not to remove the fibular sesamoid. Generally, the fibular sesamoid should be removed when the tibial sesamoid is in a position of 4 or more. In this position, the sesamoid is resting on or over the crista of the first metatarsal and causing degenerative joint disease and articular destruction of the dorsal surface of the tibial sesamoid. The fibular sesamoidectomy procedure in bunion surgery is no longer in vogue and sesamoid relocation procedures are generally recommended in most cases (see Chapter 10). It should be noted, however, that a frontal plane rotation of the metatarsal will invalidate this indicator; therefore, this sesamoid position must be correlated with a plantar axial radiographic view.[28]

In radiographic evaluation of the sesamoids, it is also important to evaluate the metatarsus adductus angle,[32,34] the metatarsus primus adductus angle[32,34] and the hallux abductus angle[32,34] to ensure that a full hallux abducto valgus procedure is not indicated. The angle of declination[32] of the first metatarsal should also be assessed to ensure that the first ray is not flexed, contraindicating sesamoid surgery.[35]

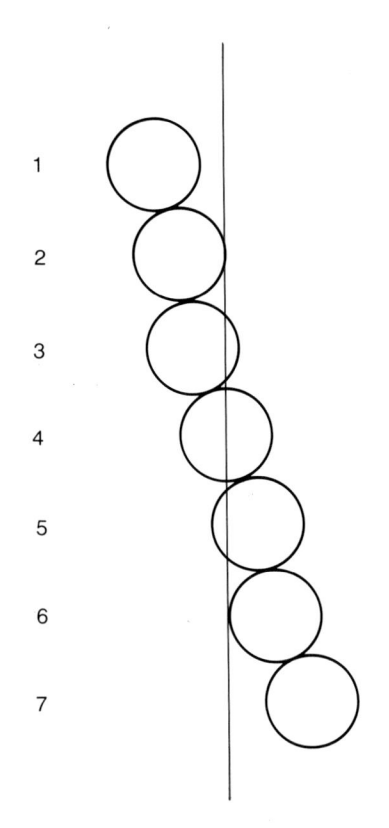

5.8 The right tibial sesamoid position as seen on an anterior-posterior radiograph. The normal tibial sesamoid position is 1. When the fibial sesamoid is in position 3 or greater, it is being jammed against the intersesamoidal ridge.

Causal relations

The aetiological significance of different forms of stress in the development of sesamoid pathology evidences to the interrelationship between the sesamoids and the structural integrity of the foot, and makes an examination of those relationships a necessary precursor to the consideration of surgery.

Evidence has already been drawn to the angle of declination of the first metatarsal and its significance for the position and range of motion of the sesamoids and also to the importance of the sesamoids for the functional length of the first metatarsal. Less readily appreciated is the inherent instability of the first ray, dependent as it is on the indirect influence of those muscles inserted into the base of the proximal phalanx. In all intrinsic foot pathologies that give rise to pronation the forces on the first metatarsal head area during propulsion will be increased by a factor of up to three.[36] This amount of stress, when imposed on a regular basis, will lead to a stretching and eventual rupture of the medial collateral ligament of the first metatarsal joint,[27] allowing the metatarsal head to move medially and periarticular structures to be displaced laterally. The resultant muscular corruption is recognized as a major influence in the development of hallux abducto valgus. Implicit in this process is the lateral displacement of the sesamoid pad relative to the metatarsal,[12] which may undergo axial rotation,[6,15,27] placing the tibial sesamoid beneath the intersesamoidal ridge of the first metatarsal and allowing the fibular sesamoid to move into the intermetatarsal space. This process may be regarded as pathognomic of incipient hallux abducto valgus. According to Fielding,[37] 'If the fibular sesamoid lies in the first metatarsal interspace, one can promise the patient that the hallux abductus deformity, which may be only in its early stages, will continue to increase.' Nor is the emphasis on hallux abducto valgus an unneccessary affectation since it defines the deformity as occurring in the frontal and transverse body planes, as well as in the sagittal plane, a process characterized by rotation of both the hallux (medially) and metatarsal, though there appears to be some debate as to whether the axial rotation of the metatarsal is in a medial[27] or lateral[15] direction. Lipsman and Frankel[20] relate the rotation of the metatarsal to its range of motion and mobility. Stability of the first metatarsal is necessary in the propulsive phase of gait. The first ray plantarflexes and rotates over the sesamoids. The extensors create a rigid beam so that the hallux may be stabilized against the ground by the flexors. The short flexors, through their sesamoid fulcrum, stabilize the base of the proximal phalanx to the ground. The abductor hallucis and the adductor hallucis provide medial and lateral stability of the first metatarsophalangeal joint. The motion of the first ray normally occurs as dorsiflexion, inversion and adduction above the transverse plane and plantarflexion, eversion and abduction below the transverse plane. In the propulsive phase of gait, the first metatarsal plantarflexes as it rotates over the sesamoids. The position of the sesamoids is important for stabilization of the hallux. When there is hypermobility of the first ray, the metatarsal is dorsiflexed, inverted, and adducted and displaced from the sesamoids. The sesamoids appear to have moved laterally, but it is the metatarsal head that has moved.[20] This rotation of the metatarsal will itself disturb its relationship with sesamoids and related structures, producing degenerative changes.[28]

It should not be imagined, however, that the sesamoids play a purely passive role—the relationship is really a cyclical one. The heads of flexor hallucis brevis, acting through their corresponding sesamoids, possess strong rotational influences on the hallux[26] as well as contributing to its frontal plane displacement, which should be recognized since they may influence the prognosis. The additional leverage afforded the flexor hallucis brevis by the sesamoids has already been evidenced, and it must follow that if the sesamoids are displaced then the balance of power between the two heads of the hallucis brevis muscle will be upset. The power of the muscle will then be greater on one side of the hallux than on the other and, given the oblique insertion of the muscle, the influence will be to rotate the hallux in the direction of the greater force.[15] The second effect of the imbalance in the force applied through one or other of the heads of the flexor hallucis brevis is to modify the 'functional length' of the respective heads, so their linear influences are also varied, and will in turn influence the alignment of the hallux on the metatarsal, irrespective of their rotational influences.[15] Hawkins[26] endorses this argument, and develops it by considering the influences of the extensor hallucis brevis, adductor hallucis, and abductor hallucis, which he rightly considers to be equally significant for the stability of the first metatarsal segment.

Pes cavus, forefoot valgus, plantarflexed first ray, and similar conditions can predispose to sesamoid pathology. If one then superimposes activities such as athletics[20] or ballet,[5] unsuitable footwear, or systemic disease on such a situation, it is hardly surprising that the patient develops problems. Nor can one overlook the consequence of more direct trauma such as direct impact or dislocation of the hallux.

The tibial sesamoid apparently bears more weight than the fibular sesamoid, since it is more frequently fractured by direct force[38] as well as by the repeated stress that occurs in activities such as ballet and long-distance running. In metatarsus primus varus, the tibial sesamoid bears excessive weight, effaces the sesamoid ridge and develops osteoarthritic spurring, while the fibular sesamoid lies lateral to the metatarsal head in the first interspace. Interruption of the lateral conjoined tendon may lead to hallux varus, while interruption of the medial tendon results in hallux valgus. The latter complication is not as common since the abductor hallucis often partially or totally inserts into the plantar medial base of the proximal phalanx, independent of the medial sesamoid. Interruption of the conjoined tendons is most often iatrogenic, secondary to bunion surgery or sesamoid excision, but may also be caused by trauma, collagen disease, or psoriasis. Interruption of one of the conjoined tendons, but more often both, results in a 'cocked up' hallux[8] through loss of the powerful action of the flexor brevis.[5]

Less commonly, there may be a luxation of the tibial sesamoid to the tibial side of the first metatarsal head. This is usually only seen after an overcorrection of a hallux abducto valgus problem. Such a luxation would convert the flexor hallucis brevis into a very powerful adductory component, adding to the hallux overcorrection. Fractures of the hallucal sesamoids frequently occur and failure to heal usually produces considerable pain, requiring surgical excision of the sesamoid.[37]

Pathology

The various pathologies indicative of surgical intervention are detailed in **Table 5.4**, and although statistical evidence is lacking it would appear that chondromalacia, degenerative changes and hypertrophy, bursitis and, most of all, fractures, are the most common pathologies giving rise to surgery in the absence of hallux valgus and other deformities. The sesamoids of the great toe are involved in a number of disease processes, including subluxations, dislocations, various forms of fracture, chondromalacia, involvement in de-

Table 5.4 Classification of sesamoid pathology (excluding hallux valgus), indicating surgical intervention and sesamoidectomy

	Apley[19]	Bizzaro[38]	Gordon[40]	Helfet[11]	Helal[2]	Hubay[14]	Ilfeld[42]	Inge[8]	Jahss[5]	Kaiman[3]	McGlamry[15]	Rowe[43]	Smith[44]	Speed[45]
Chondromalacia/'sesamoiditis'	+			+				+						+
Congenital variations								+	+					
Degenerative changes/osteoarthritis			+				+		+	+				
Fractures		+		+	+			+		+				
Luxation/displacement/prolapse					+			+	+		+			
Osteochondritis				+		+		+	+					
Osteomyelitis		+		+				+	+				+	+
Parasesmoidal bursitis				+			+	+	+					
Conjoined tendon									+					
Neurological			+					+	+					
Systemic disorders								+	+					
Tumours/cysts, etc.				+				+	+					

Table 5.5 Comparison of the distribution of partite[8,51] and fractured[38] sesamoids

	Number of patients	Sesamoids		
		Tibial	Fibular	Both
Partite sesamoids				
Inge and Ferguson[8]	110 (100%)	101 (92%)	3 (2.7%)	3 (5.3%0
Burman and Lapidus[51]	78 (100%)	72 (92.3%)	6 (7.7%)	—
Fractured sesamoids				
Bizzaro[38]	60 (100%)	52 (86.6%)	7 (11.7%)	1 (1.7%)

generative as well as other forms of arthritis, and there may be inflammation of the presesamoid bursa.[2] It is perhaps significant that, with the exception of Inge and Ferguson,[8] only Helal,[2] Jahss,[5] Haines and McDougall,[17] and Seder[46] attach significance to the luxation and chronic injury of the tibial sesamoids. Gallocher[12] had difficulty in identifying specific diseases of the sesamoid bones: they are so intimately connected with the surrounding tissues that it is impossible to consider them as isolated structures.

The variety of conditions to which the periarticular structures of the first metatarsal phalangeal joint are susceptible make differential diagnosis important. They include gout,[2] rheumatoid arthritis,[2] Reiter's disease,[47,48] giant xanthomatous tumours,[49] loose bodies,[50] psoriasis, Charcot's joint, sub-sesamoidal bursitis, and inclusion cysts.[5] Of greatest significance must be the differentiation between partite and fractured sesamoids.

Table 5.5 extrapolates and compares the (rather ambiguous) findings of Inge and Ferguson,[8] and those of Burman and Lapidus,[51] with those of Bizzaro,[38] and supports the argument of Inge and Ferguson that unilaterality cannot be trusted as a criterion of fracture.[8] Burman and Lapidus[51] point out that callus will unite the fragments of a fractured sesamoid, as in all fractures, which is a definite criterion in the differential diagnosis from developmental division. Conversely, Inge and Ferguson suggest that in the case of congenitally divided bones, the articular cartilage is seen to dip down between the two segments, an appearance not at all suggestive of a fracture. The periosteum is indistinguishable from the investing tendinous fibres, which insert deeply into the rough plantar surface.[8] Para[52] finds that a pathognomic symptom in fractures of the sesamoids of the foot is that no matter what type of conservative treatment is tried, the pain from the fracture will persist.

Gallocher[12] discusses the pathology underlying hypertrophy of the tibial sesamoid, while Mercado[35] emphasizes the need to further evaluate such patients. According to Mercado, the procedure for resection of the medial sesamoid is indicated whenever there is an intractable plantar keratosis on the first metatarsophalangeal joint with an associated hypertrophic medial sesamoid. Initially it is important to ascertain that the first metatarsal ray is not plantiflexed. If the ray is plantiflexed, the medial sesamoidectomy procedure will not work—the technique of choice would then be a dorsiflectory wedge.

The non-invasive treatment of sesamoid pain

Non-invasive treatment of sesamoid pain involves three processes: the adoption by the patient of low-heeled shoes for all routine activities; palliation of the plantar sesamoid area of the foot; and intralesional injection.

Most cases of painful sesamoids are relieved by such conservative measures as a metatarsal pad or bar, massage, and anti-arthritic treatment, with only 40% of the cases requiring operation.[8]

Para describes a case: 'Treatment first was instituted by taping and bandaging the foot and a series of diathermy treatments. One week later because of persistent pain, infiltrations of procaine were tried. These were followed by intraarticular Hydrocortisone injections . . . . The treatment of choice in the fracture of the sesamoids of the foot is excision.'[52]

Surgery

Sesamoiditis, while usually indicative of sesamoid pathology, may also be symptomatic of a plantarflexed first metatarsal ray. If this is the case, a wedge osteotomy of the first metatarsal may be the procedure of choice. If a plantarflexed first metatarsal is accompanied by sesamoid pathology, removal of the sesamoid with or without the osteotomy may be indicated. The criteria for surgery fall under four main headings:

- Excision of the sesamoids in cases of specific systemic pathology.[2,3,5,8,17]
- Excision of the sesamoids in the event of continuing symptoms that remain unrelieved by palliation.[3,6,8]
- Excision of fractured sesamoids.[8,52]
- Excision of the (fibular) sesamoids as a prophylactic measure in incipient hallux abducto valgus.[15,20]

It is also necessary to decide whether or not to remove one or both sesamoids. In those cases in which the pathology affects both sesamoids,[3,5,31] the question does not arise—but what if only one sesamoid is affected? Speed[45] was of the opinion that both should be removed, for if one was left without its companion support it would soon become the source of irritation on account of its localized pressure. Para[52] also appears to remove both sesamoids: to avoid foot imbalance at the anterio-medial point of support of the foot and to obviate the possibility of another fracture. Most recent authors[2,5,15,53] disagree. Speed[45] claimed that if excision was to be performed, then both bones should be removed, but this is wrong . . . . In the best and most complete survey of the subject, Inge and Ferguson[8] concluded that both sesamoids should not be removed if at all possible. McGlamry[15] and Mann and DuVries[53] have elaborated this argument in their discussions of both the biomechanical and post-operative consequences of the indiscriminate removal of both sesamoids. Only one sesamoid should ever be excised at a time,[53] and indeed in some cases of incipient hallux abducto valgus a successful prognosis may in part depend upon the remedial effects of the retained tibial sesamoid.[15]

Finally, one has to decide on where to place the incision. Helal[2] advocates the most direct approach, writing that personal experience has shown that by far the best approach is through a longitudinal incision on the sole directly over the bone to be excised; rarely, if both need removal, is the approach through the midline between the two sesamoids. It is now common knowledge that incisions on the sole of the foot are remarkably trouble-free.[2] The lateral sesamoid is most readily removed through a vertical plantar incision, lateral to the metatarsal head. It is virtually impossible to excise the lateral sesamoid through a vertical dorsal incision when it lies normally under the head of the first metatarsal, according to Jahss.[54]

Not all authors would agree, Viladot[55] states categorically that a direct plantar incision must never be made. Viladot,[55] Mann,[53] Inge and Ferguson,[8] and McGlamry[15] all use a medio-dorsal or medio-inferior longitudinal incision over the first metatarsophalangeal joint, avoiding surfaces that will bear weight or be rubbed by the shoe,[8] for access to the tibial sesamoid.

Only Inge and Ferguson[8] specifically advocate the

use of the medial incision for the removal of the fibular sesamoid. They used the same operative technique in all cases: exposure through a medial longitudinal incision. In 25 feet, both sesamoids were removed; in 15 feet, only the medial; and in 1 foot, only the lateral.[8] It may well be that other workers also use the medial approach to remove the lateral sesamoid, but this is not clear in the perfunctory accounts they offer of their procedures. Some workers appear to regard the fibular sesamoid as being of no consequence.

The only detailed account of a fibular sesamoidectomy using a dorsolateral approach to the joint capsule is offered by Lipsman and Frankel,[20] although McGlamry reviews the implications of this procedure for the prognosis of hallux abducto valgus, writing that sesamoidectomy of the fibular sesamoid, while more common than removal of the opposite member, is rarely performed as an isolated procedure. Fibular sesamoidectomy is accomplished by careful, sharp anatomical dissection along the (dorso-) lateral aspect of the first metatarsophalangeal joint, through the subcutaneous tissues and into the interspace.[20]

The question of haemostasis during surgery on the sesamoids is not addressed by most authors, although haemostasis is implicit in many of their comments. Only Inge and Ferguson[8] and Mann and DeVries[53] specifically advocate the use of haemostasis. Inge and Ferguson write that the use of a tourniquet is essential, and that the bursa underlying the sesamoids is usually not removed.

The reader will appreciate the close parallels that exist between the incisional approaches to the sesamoids and those used to gain access to an intermetatarsal neuroma, and is referred to Chapter 8 on this latter procedure for elaboration of the argument.

Plantar incisional approach

As with any plantar incision the main concern must be the formation of post-operative scarring, and while this may usually be obviated by taking care to place the incision between the papillary ridges, the extensive whorl formed by these ridges under the first metatarsalphalangeal joint must make this technically impossible. Nevertheless, careful attention to this principle will reduce post-operative scarring considerably.

The initial longitudinal incision is placed immediately over the sesamoid to be removed or, if both are to be removed, equidistant between them,[2] and deepened by blunt and sharp dissection. The fibro-fatty plantar pad makes this approach more difficult than may be anticipated, and great care must be taken not to damage structures adjacent to the sesamoid bone. Once the plantar pad has been dissected and the flexor hallucis brevis muscle exposed, the exact position of the sesamoid can be located by placing a finger in the wound and flexing and extending the hallux. This allows the surgeon to palpate the precise position of the sesamoid. The sesamoid is then dissected away from the flexor hallucis brevis tendon which invests it, through a small longitudinal incision. It is imperative to hug bone and avoid disrupting its conjoined tendon. The defect in the tendon is closed with an absorbable suture.[54] Full weight-bearing should not be resumed for at least three weeks to minimize scarring, which can be further minimized by intralesional injections of steroids.

Medial approach

The medial approach to sesamoidectomy is the one advocated by most authors,[45] although the majority are only concerned with removal of the medial sesamoid or are carrying out the sesamoidectomy in conjunction with hallux abducto valgus surgery.[2,5,15,27] A major advantage of this approach is that it facilitates an accompanying inverted-V capsulotomy, which is sometimes indicated in incipient hallux abducto valgus or dorsiflexion of the hallux,[15] and flattening of the plantar surface of the metatarsal head if both sesamoids are to be removed. This last procedure reduces, but does not eliminate, pressure on, and consequential degeneration of the flexor hallucis longus tendon.

The procedure described is the one advocated by Mann and DuVries.[53] A semi-elliptical incision is made along the medioplantar border of the metatarsophalangeal joint of the hallux, placed immediately dorsal to the level of the medial sesamoid in its anatomical position, and above the level of the abductor hallucis, which will have usually been displaced in a plantarward direction, especially if the hallux is abducted. In this position the incision should lie between and parallel to the neurovascular bundles supplying the medial side of the toe. The incision itself should extend from the middle third of the metatarsal to the middle of the proximal phalanx. The incision is carried directly down to the joint, and the skin flaps, together with their immediately inferior structures, are retracted. The surgeon can then insert his index finger beneath the joint and palpate the medial sesamoid while flexing and extending the toe. Having accurately assessed the position of the medial sesamoid, a 1 cm incision is made into the joint capsule along the dorso-medial aspect of the sesamoid. In this way the surgeon will avoid compromising the abductor hallucis by avoiding the problem of unnecessarily weakening its insertion into the hallux, which the abductor hallucis should help to stabilize.[3] The abductor hallucis is essentially not only an abductor of the big toe but also a flexor of the metatarsophalangeal joint and an extensor of the interphalangeal joint (through its insertion into the extensor hood ligament).[18] Once the capsule is opened, the medial sesamoid is readily identified and can be removed by sharp dissection, using its own outline as a guide.[53] In practice, once the edges of the sesamoid have been separated from the tendon it can be grasped with Allis' forceps; this facilitates the process. The roughened plantar surface of the sesamoid provides for a very firm attachment between the tendon and the bone and the actual separation of the sesamoid can be quite difficult. If the process of removal damages the tendon significantly it should be reinforced with absorbable sutures before closure. Should it be necessary to remove the fibular sesamoid either in association with the tibial sesamoid, or by itself, the same procedure can be used except that access to the sesamoid may be facilitated by plantarflexing the hallux, thus reducing tension on the joint capsule to a minimum. In practice, fibular sesamoidectomy through a medial incision is very difficult (the author has never attempted it himself), especially if it is bipartite. Displacement of the fibular sesamoid to the intermetatarsal space must render this approach impractical. The capsule may be closed with interrupted catgut sutures, particularly reinforcing the medial colateral ligament, and the skin closed in layers.

In practice, the closure of the capsule can have important implications for the prognosis. If the hallux demonstrates a tendency to hyperextend, and inverted-V capsulotomy may be incorporated into the procedure[15] (**5.9**), and if it presents as an incipient hallux abducto valgus a 'Washington monument' capsulotomy[37] (**5.10**) may be used to great effect. Tenoplasty of the extensor hallucis longus and tendonectomy of the extensor hallucis brevis are further associated procedures that can be used to compensate for the weakening effect of (medial) sesamoidectomy on the flexor hallucis brevis.[15]

5.9 McGlamry's inverted-V capsulotomy for hyperextension of the hallux.

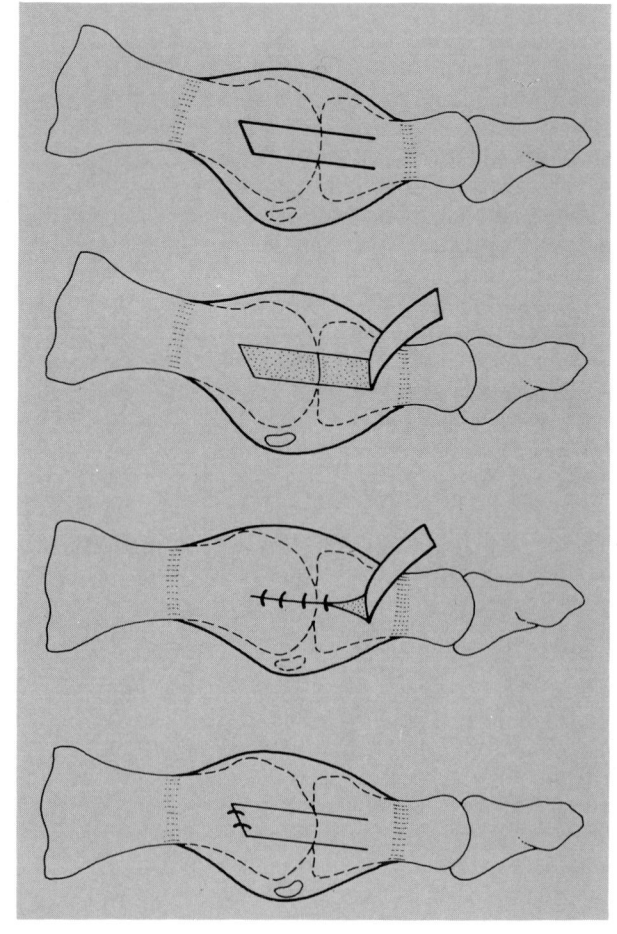

5.10 The 'Washington monument' capsulotomy procedure for correcting an abduction of the hallux.

Apart from scarring, the main complications associated with this procedure arise from damage to associated structures. In the absence of calcification there should be no damage to the flexor hallucis longus tendon, and if the flexor hallucis brevis is inadvertently divided it should be repaired efficiently, otherwise a 'trigger' deformity of the hallux will result.[2,6,54]

Dorso-lateral approach

The procedure described is that advocated by Lipsman and Frankel.[20] The initial dorsal incision is made on the dorso-lateral surface of the first metatarsophalangeal joint, midway between it and the second metatarsophalangeal joint, and deepened through the subcutaneous tissue into the interspace. Blunt dissection is used to deepen the wound until the joint capsule, adductor hallucis muscle, and the other transverse structures that insert through the metatarsophalangeal joint complex, are exposed. A self-retaining retractor is then placed between the first and second metatarsal heads. The displacement of the sesamoid into the interspace is accompanied by a corresponding degree of distortion of the joint capsule, which, while tending to obscure the sesamoid itself, facilitates the incision into the capsule, which is opened by a sharp dissection just dorsal to its attachment to the adductor hallucis. This frees the lateral collateral and the lateral sesamoidal ligaments, and the lateral aspect of the joint capsule and the sesamoid is exposed in the interspace by the pull of the adductor muscle. The sesamoid is undermined by a sharp dissection from a lateral inferior direction and released posteriorly from the flexor hallucis brevis. The anterior lateral sesamoid ligament is then cut, leaving the sesamoid attached only by the intersesamoidal ligament. The final cut takes place as follows: if you are right-handed, working on the left foot, push the sesamoid laterally and inferiorly and cut proximal to distal. The sesamoid is now free.[20] This process may be assisted by Allis' forceps, and, as is the case with the medial sesamoid, the difficulty in dissecting out the sesamoid should not be underestimated.

Ferris *et al.*[56] have described a technique to facilitate the extirpation of the fibular sesamoid, which Cavolo[57] found extremely helpful in mobilizing the sesamoid apparatus into the interspace for excision. Removal of the fibular sesamoid bone can be difficult even in experienced hands, chiefly because of an inability to securely grasp the sesamoid or soft tissue attachments while dissecting the bone free. A threaded 0.062-inch Kirschner wire has been used to maintain a secure grasp of the bone while it has been dissected free, either by an isolated procedure or in conjunction with bunionectomy. The wire is driven into the sesamoid with a wire driver after dorsal exposure via the first intermetatarsal space, care being taken not to penetrate the plantar cortex too deeply if a cartilage knife is used in the dissection. Manipulation in all planes is possible during the dissection. This method permits the surgeon to grasp the fibular sesamoid firmly during its dissection, minimizing surgical trauma to surrounding tissues and reducing the risk of cutting the flexor hallucis longus tendon. The technique has been useful in 30 sesamoidectomies. It is less effective where a severely osteoporotic sesamoid or a partite sesamoid with small fragments is present.[57]

The wound left by the removal of the sesamoid may be reinforced by an absorbable suture prior to closure. It must be emphasized that careful dissection is imperitive and that haphazard dissection can result in a complete laceration of the flexor hallucis longus tendon, which has its course just inferior to the sesamoids. Transection of the flexor hallucis longus could result in a flexion deformity of the hallux post-surgically.[20] Closure of the wound is routine although repair of the extensor wing[18] should be attempted if the tibial sesamoid has not been removed since this will help stabilize the pull of the tibial insertion of the flexor hallucis brevis.

The two technical complications affecting this approach to lateral sesamoidectomy are post-operative neuralgia, resulting from involvement of nerve trunks (the proper plantar and dorsal digital nerves) in the resulting scar tissue, and haematoma. The reader is referred to Chapters 8 and 10 for a discussion of these problems.

Post-operative results and complications

The complex biomechanical influences affecting these procedures have already been discussed, and it is hardly surprising that they may give rise to post-operative complications, the most common of which are defined by McGlamry[15] as 'weakening of the flexor hallucis brevis muscle and tendon by removing the fulcrum for the tendon' and 'leaving a somewhat loose tendon' which in turn may lead to the plantar tendons and capsule being overwhelmed by the dorsal structures, resulting in a trigger toe deformity of the hallux and/or hallux valgus.[8,15,20] Other complications include hallux varus, intractable plantar keratosis,[15] forefoot instability, keloid scars, impaired motion, and bursitis.[8] Only Inge and Ferguson have published a comprehensive analysis of their post-operative results (**Table 5.6**).

In reviewing these results, Inge and Ferguson conclude that since some 81% of patients having only one sesamoid removed fell within the two most successful groups of patients, as opposed to only 64% of those patients having both sesamoids removed, the results would tend to disprove the contention that when sesamoidectomy is performed both bones should be removed.[8] Inge and Ferguson also draw attention to the increased risk of post-operative complications that involve the dorsiflexion of the hallux and to pre-operative deformity not appearing to affect the outcome of surgery. Complications affect removal of both sesamoids.

Consensus lies against the removal of both sesamoids unless specifically indicated by the pathology, as removal will significantly weaken the effects of flexor hallucis brevis, resulting in a trigger deformity of the hallux.[5,8,15] It must be remembered that sesamoidectomy weakens the flexor hallucis brevis muscle and tendon by removing the fulcrum for the tendon and by leaving a somewhat loose tendon. Consequently, some provision must be made to prevent the dorsal structures from overwhelming the plantar tendons and capsule and resulting in a 'cock up' hallux or a hallux valgus, either or both of which may occur.[15]

Should the removal of both sesamoids become necessary, then it should be accompanied by an inverted-V capsulotomy, a Z-plasty lengthening of the extensor hallucis longus tendon, and tendonectomy of the extensor hallucis brevis.[15] The additional pressure that will develop on the flexor hallucis longus tendon, despite its protection from the fibro-fatty plantar pad, should also be anticipated, and the plantar surface of the first metatarsal should be smoothed before closure of the capsule. This latter procedure can not offer complete protection to the flexor hallucis longus, which in time must undergo degenerative changes and calcification—which, in any case, may precede surgery. Cartilagenous changes, ossification, and calcification can be found readily in dissected material; the latter two changes can be seen on radiographs, when pain or loss of movement has led to such as investigation being carried out.[12]

Table 5.6 Post-operative results (percentage breakdown in parentheses) of sesamoidectomy in 41 patients[8]

	Number of patients	Pre-operative condition of feet Normal	Deformed	Sesamoids removed Both	Single
Complete relief of symptoms and restoration of normal function	17 (41.5)	10 (24.4)	7 (17.0)	11 (26.8)	6 (14.6)
Persistence of mild pain and/or impaired joint motion	12 (29.3)	8 (19.5)	4 (9.8)	5 (12.2)	7 (17.0)
Division of plantar structures, with resultant hammer toe deformity requiring corrective surgery	7 (17.0)	6 (14.6)	1 (2.5)	6 (14.6)	1 (2.5)
Unimproved	5 (12.2)	2 (4.9)	3 (7.4)	3 (7.4)	2 (4.9)
Total	41 (100.0)	26 (63.4)	15 (36.6)	25 (61.0)	16 (39.0)

Complications of tibial sesamoidectomy

Removal of the tibial sesamoid in isolation of other procedures is the most common sesamoidectomy and has been reviewed by Kaiman and Piccora.[3] Again, the hammer deformity of the hallux is the most likely post-operative deformity to develop, but it is also likely to be accompanied by hallux abducto valgus. According to McGlamry,[15] the first obvious means of preventing these complications is to perform a tenoplasty (preferably a Z-plasty lengthening) of the extensor hallucis longus and a tendonectomy of the extensor hallucis brevis. The tendonectomy of the extensor brevis is particularly important since it is inserted almost directly opposite to the insertion of the flexor hallucis brevis tendon from which the tibial sesamoid has been removed. (This procedure may also be extended to ensure that the 'extensor wing'[18] is not also pulling the hallux into valgus.) Frequently, if there is a moderately severe dorsal contracture, it is wise to perform a dorsal capsulotomy of the metatarsophalangeal joint and to manipulate the great toe to assure that there will be no dorsal riding of the toe when released.[15] In practice, an inverted V- or Washington monument-type capsulotomy at the time of the sesamoidectomy is preferable to dorsal capsulotomy, especially if carried out in association with the tenoplasty/tendonectomy of the dorsal extensors. Dorsal capsulotomy is better retained as a post-operative procedure, since its completion at the time of the initial sesamoidectomy can destabilize the joint, which may then luxate.

In reviewing eight cases of tibial sesamoidectomy, Kaiman and Piccora[3] report that in 50% of the patients studied no change was noted in the lateral deviation of the hallux. Two patients exhibited a lateral deviation of the fibular sesamoid, whereas the others in the group demonstrated a medial excursion. Seventy-five per cent of the patients in the group who displayed consistent values of hallux abductus angles pre- and post-operatively, possessed round metatarsal heads. This phenomenon may be explained by either the low metatarsus adductus angle present amongst the group or may be the result of good capsular reapproximation.[3]

Structural modifications and complications affecting fibular sesamoidectomy

The relatively low incidence of fibular sesamoidectomy, in isolation of hallux abducto valgus surgery, tends to disguise the intrinsic benefits of this procedure to the structural integrity of the foot. The two main complications associated with the operation are (1) the (inevitable) trigger deformity of the hallux and (2) hallux varus. In practice, however, hallux varus is, fortunately, an uncommon complication that results from 'overcorrection' in the realignment of the hallux valgus. A significant benefit deriving from fibular sesamoidectomy is the derotation of the first metatarsal. When the fibular sesamoid is removed and the tibial sesamoid is returned to its rightful position, it exercises a constant force in the direction of derotation of the first metatarsal.[15] The restitution of the tibial sesamoid tendon is accompanied by that of the abductor hallucis, a very powerful muscle,[15] the combined effect being to move the hallux in a varus direction. This is conventionally facilitated in hallux abducto valgus surgery by tendonectomy of the adductor hallucis. However, in the absence of marked abducto valgus the attachment of the adductor hallucis should be retained as exercising a stabilizing influence on the hallux post-operatively, and mitigating against the development of hallux varus. Fibular sesamoidectomy from a dorsomedial incision makes an inverted-V capsulotomy impossible, nor is it really necessary, since the pull of the extensors can be mitigated by a Z-plasty lengthening of the extensor hallucis longus and tendonectomy of the extensor hallucis brevis.

In the event of hallux varus developing, correction usually requires the removal of the remaining sesamoid, arthrodesis of the interphalangeal joint, and, probably, tenoplasty of the extensor hallucis longus to an appropriate length and the flattening of the plantar surface of the first metatarsal head.[15] Severing the abductor hallucis may also be indicated.

In the few instances in which a second surgical intervention is required, the part can be treated as though a hallux extensus were present, i.e., so that the structures plantar to the joint predominate in strength after sesamoidectomy. Unless this approach is made, there is a good possibility that such a condition will occur shortly after removal of the remaining sesamoid. It is important that the predominating strength be plantar to the joint.[15] McGlamry's argument for ensuring that a predominantly flexory force is applied to the joint post-operatively is readily appreciated; the dorsiflexory influences of gait will serve to ensure that a balance is obtained.

On paper, the debate on balancing the influences of those forces acting on the first metatarsophalangeal joint appears straightforward. In practice, it devolves into a question of professional discretion and experience, which may be why so many procedures carried out on the first metatarsophalangeal joint appear compromised.

Post-operative care

Apart from routine post-operative dressings, post-operative care is especially important to the successful outcome of first metatarsal joint surgery, and carries both short-term and long-term implications. Even where a plantar incision has been avoided, weight-bearing should be modified with the use of a flexible orthotic for the first few months, not only to give the wound time to heal—healing of these tissues usually requires from two–three months[15]—but also to control weight distribution over the forefoot during gait. Rarely can a surgical procedure improve on nature, and any procedure on the first metatarsal joint is going to permanently compromise the joint. It is therefore imperative that the foot be permanently stabilized with flexible or semi-flexible orthotics, even in the absence of pronation. Such orthotics afford the additional benefit of providing a vehicle for medial forefoot posting to compensate for the functional shortening of the first metatarsal once the sesamoids have been removed, and for palliation of the plantar surface of the joint to obviate against the formation of plantar keratosis. In most instances, when keratosis begins to develop, the process can be reversed using simple mechanical padding or an inlay of appropriate construction.[15]

Helal,[2] in a very practical manner, implemented the assertion of Silver[24] that the replacement of displaced sesamoids was essential to the efficient functioning of the forefoot. Replacement of the sesamoids in a cross country runner, who had to have both sesamoids removed after injury to both in the right foot, was carried out as a prophylactic measure to avoid a plantar displacement of the first metatarsal head. The artificial bones were created out of a silicone rubber block. The patient is now completely free of symptoms.[3]

One final, if obvious, post-operative step, is to ensure that the principles of non-invasive sesamoid care are implemented post-operatively. In particular, the patient must be warned of the long-term consequences of wearing high-heeled footwear and of taking part in activities that produce excessive pressure at the site of the operation.

Interphalangeal and other inconstant sesamoids

The incidence of sesamoids associated with the other metatarsophalangeal joints is very low. Burman and Lapidus[51] give an incidence of 16.3% and Hubay[14] quotes Kassatkin as recording an incidence of 12.2% for tibial sesamoids of the fifth metatarsophalangeal joint, while Bizzaro[4] gives an incidence of 10%. Recorded incidences of other metatarsal sesamoids do not exceed 6.2% (see **Table 5.1**). Should these sesamoids become troublesome, and in reality this is unlikely, they can be treated as described for the counterparts underlying the first metatarsal.[13]

The incidence of interphalangeal sesamoids of the hallux, however, is somewhat higher, for while Bizzaro[4] records an incidence of only 5%, Pfitzner (as quoted by Hubay[14]) and Jahss[5] give incidences of 13.1% and 13%, respectively, while Pfitzner and Kassatkin give an average incidence of 55.6% (see **Table 5.1**). Where such sesamoids occur they are unlikely to develop problems unless there is an associated pathology of the first metatarsophalangeal joint, in which case the problem will be disguised by overlying callus and characterized by increasing discomfort,[6] which can only be satisfactorily treated by excision. Rarely, excision of the sesamoid may be necessary through a longitudinal approach.[5] The incision is placed directly over the sesamoid, and the flexor hallucis longus tendon carefully divided to remove the bone. The tendon is then sutured to restore its integrity and the wound closed.

The important characteristic of this lesion is not so much the lesion itself, or its treatment, as the condition of the first metatarsophalangeal joint pathology, which presents as hallux limitus or hallux rigidus. Evidence,[58] suggests that in some cases the first metatarsophalangeal joint functions like the knee joint in that it moves around a double axis and is dependent upon the plantar flexion of the first metatarsal head as the foot moves into the propulsive phase of gait, to enable the joint to extend fully. If this extension is prevented by a reduced angle of declination of the first metatarsal (as happens in pronation), dorsiflexion of the first metatarsophalangeal joint will be impaired, the dorsal edges of the joint will impinge against each other, and excessive pressure will devolve on the interphalangeal joint and its sesamoid, if present.

There can be little benefit therefore in operating for an interphalangeal sesamoid of the hallux unless the procedure is accompanied by surgery on the metatarsophalangeal joint or the patient is provided with orthotics to control the rearfoot instability and to palliate the joint post-operatively.

References

[1] Garrison, F.D. The bone called 'luz'. *New York Med. J.*, **92**: 149, 1910.
[2] Helal, B. The great toe sesamoid bones, *Clin. Orthopaed. Rel. Res.*, **157**: 82–87, 1981.
[3] Kaiman, M.E. and Piccora, R. Tibial sesamoidectomy: a review of the literature and retrospective study. *J. Foot Surg.*, **22**: 286–289, 1983.
[4] Bizzaro, A.H. On sesamoid and supernumerary bones of the limbs. *J. Anat.*, **55**: 256–268, 1920.
[5] Jahss, M.H. The sesamoids of the hallux. *Clin. Orthopaed. Rel. Res.*, **157**: 88–97, 1981.
[6] DuVries, H.L. *Surgery of the Foot.* St. Louis, C.V. Mosby, 1959, p.270.
[7] Kewenter, Y. Sesambeine des I. Metatarsophalangealgelenks des Menschen. *Acta Orthopaed. Scand.*, **2**, 1–113, 1936.
[8] Inge, G.E.L. and Ferguson, A.B. Surgery of the sesamoid bones of the great toe. *Arch. Surg.*, **27**: 466–489, 1933.
[9] Freiberg, E. Injuries of the sesamoid bones of the great toe. *Orthopaed. Surg.*, **2**: 453, 1920.
[10] Francis, C.C. Appearance of centers of ossification from 6 to 15 years. *Am. J. Phys. Anthropol.*, **27**: 127–138, 1940.
[11] Scranton, P.E. and Rutkowski, R. Anatomic variations in the first ray: Part II. Disorders of the sesamoids. *Clin. Orthopaed. Rel. Res.*, **151**: 256–264, 1980.
[12] Gallocher, J. A study of the sesamoid bones and related structures in the first metatarso-phalangeal joint of the foot. *The Chiropodist*, **XXI**: 419–435, 1967.
[13] Lapidus, P.W. Lesions of the inconstant sesamoids of the foot, *Radiology*, **40**: 581–585, 1943.
[14] Hubay, C.A. Sesamoid bones of the hands and feet. *Am. J. Roentgenol.*, **61**, 493–505, 1949.
[15] McGlamry, E.D. Hallucal sesamoids. *J. Am. Podiatry Assoc.*, **55**: 693–699, 1965.
[16] Lapidus, P.W. Operative correction of metatarsus varus primus in hallux valgus. *Surgery, Gynecology and Obstetrics*, **58**: 183–189, 1934.
[17] Haines, R.W. and McDougall, A. The anatomy of hallux valgus. *J. Bone Joint Surg.*, **36B**: 272–293, 1954.
[18] Sarrafian, S.K. and Topouzian, L.K. Anatomy and physiology of the extensor apparatus of the toes. *J. Bone Joint Surg.*, **51A**. 669–679, 1969.
[19] McMinn, R.M.H., Hutchings, R.T. and Logan, B.M. *Foot and Ankle Anatomy.* London, Wolfe Medical Publications, 1982.
[20] Lipsman, S. and Frankel, J.P. Criteria for fibular sesamoidectomy in hallux abducto valgus correction. *J. Foot Surg.*, **16**: 43–48, 1977.
[21] Jahss, M.H. LeLievre bunion operation. *AAOS Instructional Course Lectures, 21.* St. Louis, C.V. Mosby, 1972, p.295.
[22] D'Amico, J.C. and Schuster, R.O. Motion of the first ray. *J. Am. Podiatry Assoc.*, **69**: 71–73, 1979.
[23] Butterworth, R.F. Correspondence. 'Metatarsal and Sesamoids' *Br. J. Chirop.*, **29**(2), 1977.
[24] Silver, D. The operative treatment of hallux valgus. *J. Bone Joint Surg.*, **5**: 225, 1923.
[25] Colwill, M. Osteomyelitis of the metatarsal sesamoids. *J. Bone Joint Surg.*, **51B**: 464–468, 1969.
[26] Hawkins, F.B. Acquired hallux varus: cause, prevention and correction. *Clin. Orthopaed. Rel. Res.*, **76**: 169–176, 1971.
[27] Kelikian, H. *Hallux Valgus, Allied Deformities of the Forefoot and Metatarsalgia.* Philadelphia, W.B. Saunders, 1965, p.80.
[28] Hass, M. *In* Gerbert, J. and Sokoloff, T.H. (eds), *Textbook of Bunion Surgery.* New York, Futura, 1981, p.41.
[29] Jones, F. Wood. *Structure and Function as Seen in the Foot,* 2nd edn, London, Balliere, Tindall & Cox, 1949, p.99.
[30] Helal, B. Surgery of the forefoot. *Br. Med. J.*, 29th January, pp.276–280, 1977.
[31] Downey, M.A. and Dorothy, W.L. A radiographic technique to demonstrate the plantar aspects of the forefoot in stance. *J. Am. Podiatry Assoc.*, **59**: 140–143, 1969.
[32] Gamble, F.O. and Yale, I. *Clinical Foot Roentgenology,* 1st edn. Baltimore, Williams & Wilkins, 1966.
[33] Fuson, S.M., Blau, K. and Beilman, B.A. A new sponge axial poser. *J. Am. Podiatry Assoc.*, **69**: 681–682, 1979.
[34] Gerbert, J. and Sokoloff, T.H. *Textbook of Bunion Surgery.* New York, Futura, 1981.
[35] Mercado, O.A. *An Atlas of Foot Surgery. Vol. 1: Forefoot Surgery.* Illinois, Colorado Press, 1979.
[36] Schuster, R.O. Course lecture. Bushmills International Sports Academy, University of Ulster, 1986.
[37] Fielding, M.D. (Ed.) *The Surgical Treatment of Hallux-Abducto-Valgus and Allied Deformities.* New York, Futura, 1973, p.31.
[38] Bizzaro, A.H. On the traumatology of the sesamoid structures. *Ann. Surg.*, **74**: 783–791, 1921.
[39] Apley, G. Open Sesamoid! A re-appraisal of the medial sesamoid of the hallux. *Proc. Roy. Soc. Med.*, **59**: 120–121, 1966.
[40] Gordon, S.L., Evans, C. and Greer, R.B. Pseudomonas osteomyelitis of the metatarsal sesamoid of the great toe. *Clin. Orthopaed. Rel. Res.*, **99**: 188–189, 1974.
[41] Helfet, A.J. A neurological cause of pain under the head of the metatarsal bone of the big toe. *Lancet,* 23 October, p.846, 1954.
[42] Ilfeld, F.W. and Rosen, V. Osteochondritis of the first metatarsal sesamoid. *Clin. Orthopaed. Rel. Res.*, **85**: 38–41, 1972.
[43] Rowe, M. Osteomyelitis of the metatarsal sesamoid. *Br. Med. J.*, 20 April, 1071–1072, 1963.
[44] Smith, R. Osteitis of the metatarsal sesamoid including a case report of acute pyogenic osteomyelitis. *Br. J. Surg.*, **29**: 19, 1941.
[45] Speed, K. Injuries of the great toe sesamoids. *Ann. Surg.*, **60**: 478–480, 1914.
[46] Seder, J.I. Sesamoiditis. *J. Am. Podiatry Assoc.*, **64**: 444–446, 1974.
[47] Doury, P., Pattin, S., Delahaye, R.P., Metges, P.J., Milne. J. and Casanova, C. Sesamoidite du gros orteil au cours d'un syndrome de Fiessinger–Leroy–Reiter. *Rev. Rhum. Mal. Osteoartic*, **46**: 133, 1979.

[48] Resnick, D., Niwayama, G. and Feingold, M.L. The sesamoid bones of the hands and feet. Participators in arthritis. *Radiol.*, **57**: 123, 1977.
[49] Geschichter, C.F. and Copeland, M.M. Giant xanthomatous tumours of the sesamoids. *In* Tumours of Bone. New York, *American Journal of Cancer,* p.370, 1931.
[50] DeLuca, F.N. and Kenmore, P.I. Bilateral dorsal dislocations of the metatarsophalangeal joints of the great toes with a loose body in one of the metatarsophalangeal joints.
[51] Burman, M.S.M. and Lapidus, P.W. Functional disturbances caused by the inconstant sesamoids of the foot. *Arch. Surg.,* **22**: 936–975, 1931.
[52] Para, G. Stress fractures of the sesamoids of the foot. *Clin. Orthopaed. Rel. Res.,* **18**: 281–285, 1960.
[53] Mann, R.A. and DuVries, H.L. Keratotic disorders of the plantar skin. *In* Mann, R.A. (ed.), *DuVries' Surgery of the Foot,* 4th edn. St. Louis, C.V. Mosby, 1978.
[54] Jahss, M.H. Surgical principles and the plantigrade foot. *In* Jahss, M.H. (ed.), *Disorders of the Foot.* Philadelphia, W.B. Saunders, 1982.
[55] Viladot, A. The metatarsals. *In* Jahss, M.H. (ed.), *Disorders of the Foot.* Philadelphia, W.B. Saunders, 1982.
[56] Ferris, D.L., Thomas, J.C. and Owens, J.H. Extirpation of the fibular sesamoid simplified. *J. Foot Surg.,* **24**: 255–257, 1985.
[57] Cavolo, D.J. Extirpation of the fibular sesamoid simplified. *In Yearbook of Podiatric Medicine and Surgery.* Chicago, Year Book Medical Publishers, 1987, pp.75–76.
[58] Urry, S.R. Course lecture notes. Northern Ireland School of Chiropody, 1983.

Further reading

Gerbert, J. (Ed.) *Textbook of Bunion Surgery,* 2nd edn. New York, Futura, 1991.

6 Lesser metatarsal surgery

BYRON L. HUTCHINSON

Introduction

Lesser metatarsal surgery is a challenging area for the foot surgeon. Deformities of the lesser metatarsals are extremely complex, involving the interphalangeal joint, metatarsophalangeal joints, metatarsals, and the related soft tissue structures. Failure of the surgeon to fully understand the biomechanics, pathomechanics, and interrelations of these deformities can lead to dismal surgical failures.

It is important to emphasize that procedural choice is often less important than sound clinical assessment and determination of the level of the deformity. Many procedures have been described for lesser metatarsal surgery and it will not be the intent of this chapter to review them in their entirety. Rather, the purpose will be to give the surgeon a sound overview of the specific deformities, their pathomechanics, and a rational approach to treatment.

Surgical anatomy

One cannot discuss lesser metatarsal surgery without first looking at the surgical anatomy of the forefoot, including the digits. Central to this is the extensor complex of the lesser toes, which will be discussed shortly. We will review the various anatomical systems as they pertain to the lower extremity and concentrate on pertinent functional anatomy. Additionally, emphasis will be placed on clinical and surgical correlation.

Proximally, the lesser metatarsal bases form a transverse arch that is high medially and low laterally. Distally, the lesser metatarsal heads are located in the same horizontal plane and no transverse arch is present at this level. This is extremely important structurally and functionally when one considers aberrant friction patterns plantarly against ground reactive force. The metatarsal length formula, $2 > 3 > 1 > 4 > 5$, is accepted by most anatomists and surgeons.[1-5] Variations of this formula create deformities with specific clinical patterns.

The bases of the second and third metatarsals are cuneiform and help to create the high medial portion of the transverse arch. The medial surface of the second metatarsal provides attachment for the powerful Lisfranc's ligament, which plays an important role in the pathogenesis of Lisfranc's fracture dislocations.[6]

The base of the fourth metatarsal is quadrilateral and that of the fifth is flat, in a dorsoplantar direction, with a large styloid process laterally (**6.1**). This process gives rise to the insertion of the peroneus brevis tendon and plays an important role in the pathogenesis of fractures of the fifth metatarsal base.[7] The architecture of the fifth metatarsal base is important to consider when planning an osteotomy in this region. In order to close the osteotomy in a transverse plane, the hinge must be oriented dorsolaterally (**6.2**).

The shafts of the lesser metatarsals have a variable plantar concavity and are prismatic, with dorsal, medial, and lateral surfaces (**6.3**). The lesser metatarsal heads are flattened transversely and are quadrilateral (**6.4**). Surgical approaches to the lesser metatarsals are by far more effective dorsally than plantarly because of the numerous layers of vital structures plantarly.

Abnormal muscle function is a common cause of digital and subsequent metatarsal deformities. Many

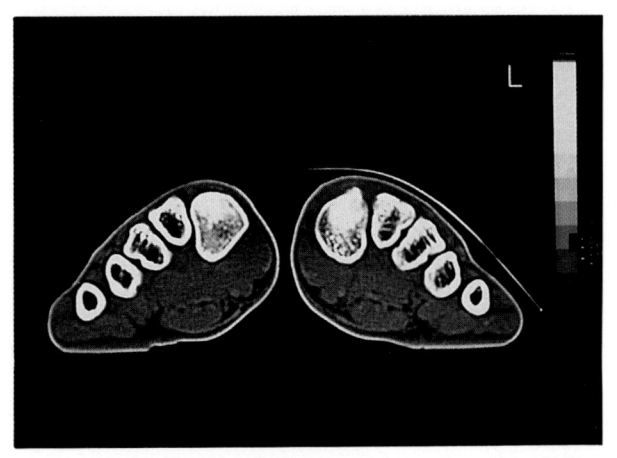

6.1 Computerized axial tomogram (CAT) scan cross-section of the foot, showing metatarsal shape and position.

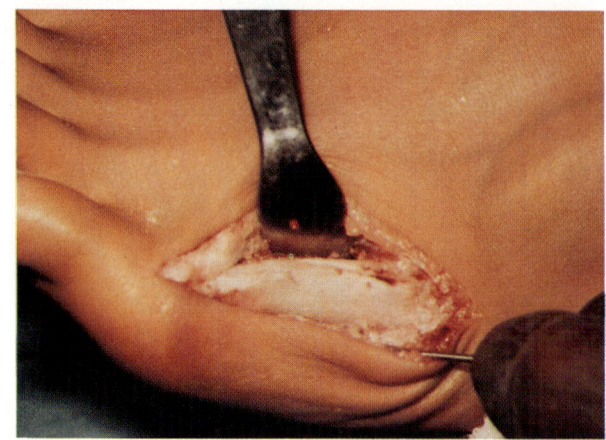

6.2 Surgical osteotomy of the fifth metatarsal, with hinge oriented in the dorsolateral position.

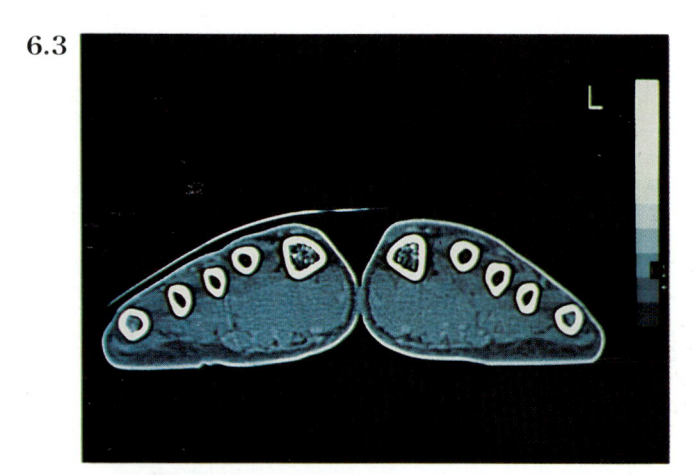

6.3 CAT scan cross-section of lesser metatarsal shafts, indicating prismatic variables.

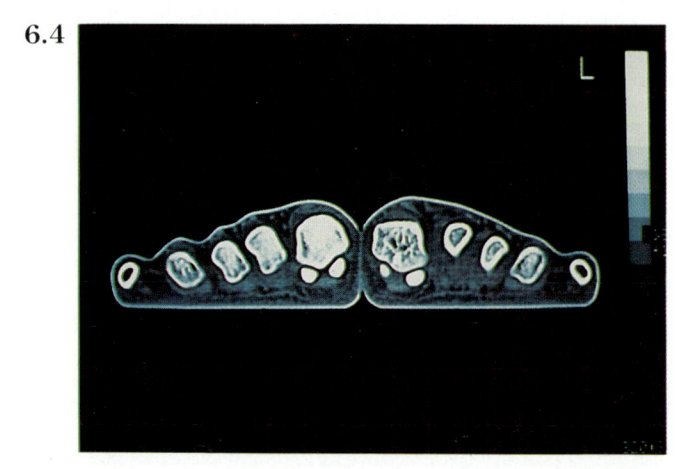

6.4 CAT scan cross-section of lesser metatarsal heads, showing transverse flattening.

myotendinous structures cross the metatarsophalangeal joints. Extrinsic and intrinsic muscles play major roles in the stability and function of the lesser rays. The extrinsic muscles will be considered in greater detail in the section on functional anatomy and biomechanics within this chapter.

The intrinsic muscles of the internal metatarsals (2–4) include four dorsal interossei, three plantar interossei, and four lumbricals. The functional axis of the foot passes through the second ray, with the relative motions of abduction and adduction occurring about this axis.[8] The dorsal interossei are the abductors of the toes and are easily remembered by the acronym, DAB, and the plantar interossei are the adductors PAD.

The dorsal interossei originate from adjacent sides of the metatarsals. The first dorsal interosseus occupies the interspace between the first and second metatarsals, the second is situated between the second and third metatarsals, the third between the third and fourth metatarsals, and the fourth between the fourth and fifth metatarsals.

The plantar interossei originate from the tibial (medial) aspects of the third, fourth, and fifth metatarsals and are named first, second, and third plantar interossei, from medial to lateral. The tendons of the interossei pass dorsal to the deep transverse metatarsal ligament. Their origins and insertions are depicted in **6.5**.

The lumbricals function to flex the lesser toes at the metatarsophalangeal joints and extend the phalanges at the interphalangeal joints. One simple way to remember this is that they allow us to 'wave goodbye'. They arise from the flexor digitorum longus tendon and also have a 'functional insertion' into the corresponding digits (**6.6**). The lumbricals pass plantar to the deep transverse metatarsal ligament. There are numerous variations of the intrinsic muscles to the internal metatarsals reported.[9] The blood supply to the lesser metatarsals comes from the terminal branches of the popliteal anterior and posterior tibial arteries. The anterior tibial artery in turn becomes the dorsalis pedis artery, and the posterior tibial artery gives rise to the medial and lateral plantar arteries. There is great variability in the distribution and anatomical location of the arteries of the lesser metatarsals.[3] One should be familiar with the arterial anatomy of the foot before performing any lesser metatarsal surgery.

Perforating arteries connecting the dorsal and plantar systems are located at the base of the metatarsals. The dorsal and plantar metatarsal arteries are also located near the metatarsal shafts. Careful elevation of subcutaneous tissues and sufficient retraction during surgery will help to avoid unwanted laceration of an artery.

The important motor nerves involved in the lesser metatarsus are the deep peroneal and tibial nerves.

The deep peroneal nerve innervates the extensor digitorum brevis and extensor hallucis brevis before it becomes a sensory terminal branch supplying sensation to the first interspace dorsally. All other intrinsic muscles to the foot are supplied by the tibial nerve as it courses through the tarsal tunnel. The medial plantar nerve terminal branch supplies the abductor hallucis, first lumbrical, flexor digitorum brevis, and flexor hallucis brevis. The lateral plantar nerve terminal branch supplies all the rest.

The sensory innervation to the dorsum of the foot is derived from the saphenous, sural, superficial, and deep peroneal nerves. The tibial nerve supplies all the sensation to the plantar pedis. Sensory nerve patterns are extremely variable, and meticulous soft tissue dissection should be employed during metatarsal surgery.

A significant functional and anatomical concept in lesser metatarsal surgery is the extensor complex of the lesser toes. This forms a 'functional insertion' for the extensor digitorum longus, extensor digitorum brevis, interossei, and lumbricals. The extensor complex affects digital function primarily, but through retrograde forces, it can also affect the lesser metatarsals.

The tendons of the extensor system are anchored at the level of the metatarsophalangeal joint and proximal phalanx by a fibroaponeurotic structure. The transverse fibres of this structure extend around the capsule of the metatarsophalangeal joint and blend on the plantar side with the plantar plate, deep transverse metatarsal ligament, and the flexor tendon sheath. This is termed the 'extensor sling'. Obliquely oriented fibres of this same structure are found more distally and are termed the 'extensor hood' (**6.7**).[10] The interossei, lumbricals, flexor, and extensor tendons all have attachments to this extensor complex and are interrelated to each other around the lesser metatarsophalangeal joints (**6.8**). Because of this close association, digital deformities often lead to metatarsal abnormalities. Loss of stability of the extensor complex leads to significant retrograde forces against the metatarsals and faulty biomechanics.

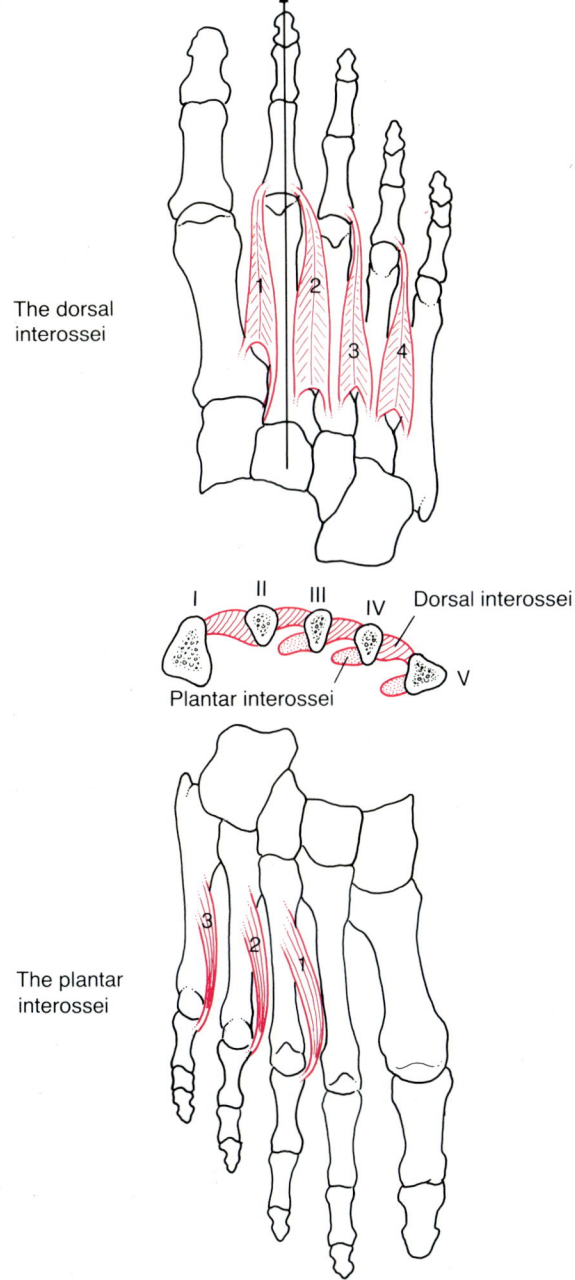

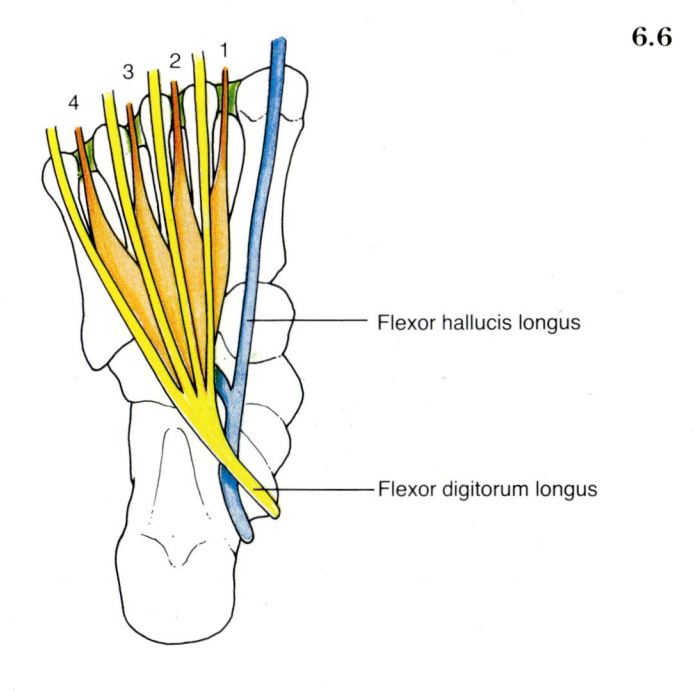

6.5 Dorsal and plantar interossei muscles.

6.6 The lumbrical muscles.

6.7

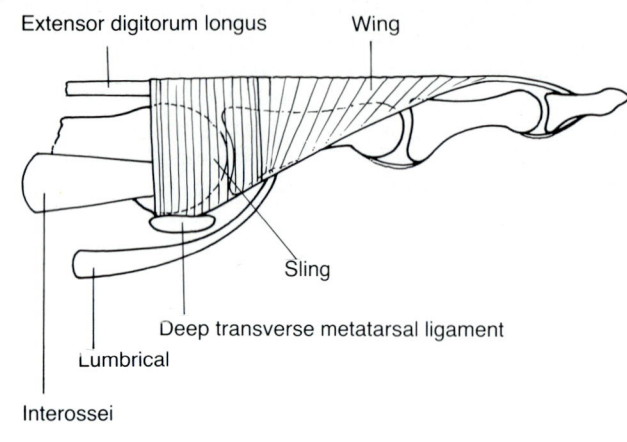

Extensor digitorum longus — Wing — Sling — Deep transverse metatarsal ligament — Lumbrical — Interossei

6.7 The extensor hood complex, lateral view.

6.8

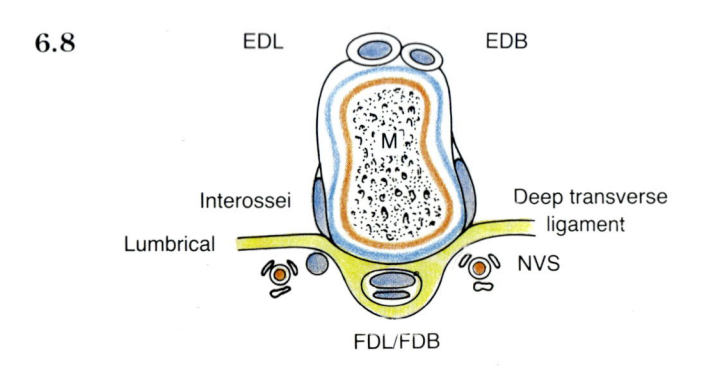

EDL, EDB, Interossei, Lumbrical, Deep transverse ligament, NVS, FDL/FDB, M

6.8 Cross-section of the metatarsophalangeal joint apparatus.

6.9

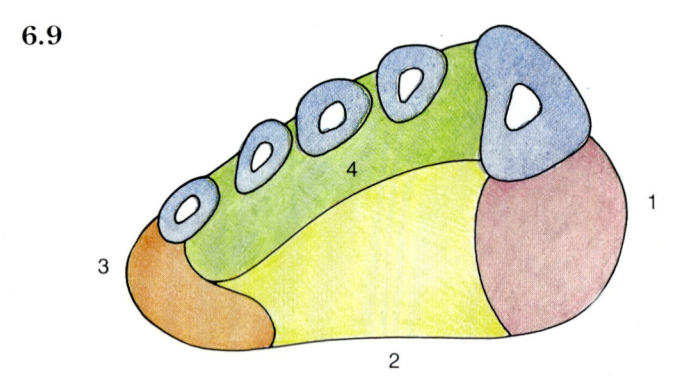

6.9 The functional layers (1–4) of the forefoot plantar muscles. See the text for a detailed explanation of the four layers.

Often, surgical procedures involve different compartments and layers in the plantar aspect of the foot. The foot surgeon should be knowledgeable of these compartments and layers.

The plantar muscles which effect forefoot function can be divided into four functional layers (**6.9**). The first layer contains the abductor hallucis, flexor digitorum brevis, and abductor digiti minimi. The second layer is occupied by the quadratus plantae, lumbricals, and the tendons of the flexor hallucis longus and flexor digitorum longus. The third layer contains the flexor digiti quinti, adductor hallucis, and flexor hallucis brevis. Finally, the fourth layer contains the interossei and the tendons of the peroneus longus and tibialis posterior muscles.

There are four plantar compartments of the sole of the foot (**6.10**). The central compartment contains the flexor digitorum brevis, flexor digitorum longus tendons with the lumbricals, the quadratus plantae, the adductor hallucis, peroneal longus tendon, and portions of the posterior tibial tendon. It is bounded medially and superficially by the medial segment of the plantar aponeurosis, laterally by the intermuscular septum, and dorsally by the first metatarsal.

The lateral compartment is bounded by the lateral segment of the plantar fascia, limiting it superficially and laterally. It is limited medially by the intermuscular septum and dorsally by the fifth metatarsal. This compartment contains the abductor digiti minimi, flexor digiti minimi, and opponens digiti minimi. The medial compartment is a potential closed space and is occupied by the abductor hallucis and its investing fascia.

Finally, the interosseous compartment contains all the interossei and is limited by the muscles, fascia, and the metatarsals themselves.

Biomechanics of forefoot deformities

Although isolated metatarsal deformities are sometimes seen, many forefoot deformities develop as a result of abnormal pronation. Metatarsal problems, callus patterns, 'tailor's bunions', and contracted digits are intimately related to faulty biomechanics. For the surgeon to effectively evaluate and treat these forefoot deformities, he should understand the pathomechanics of pronation. Digital deformities and first ray function are discussed in more detail in other chapters.

Pronation may result from a host of structural problems in the lower extremity: most commonly these include equinus, frontal, and transverse plane deformities, as well as torsional abnormalities. Ligamentous laxity and limb length discrepancies can also predispose patients to abnormal pronation and related forefoot deformities.

At heel strike, during the contact phase of gait, the normal subtalar joint pronates to aid in shock absorption and allows the midtarsal joint to 'unlock', so that the forefoot can adapt to the specific terrain.[11] As the foot continues through the contact phase and into the midstance phase of gait, the subtalar joint resupinates, 'locking' the midtarsal joint, so that the forefoot becomes rigid and stable for the propulsive phase of gait.

Abnormal subtalar joint pronation does not allow the midtarsal joint the opportunity of stabilizing the forefoot; this leads to certain pathological changes in the forefoot, depending on what structural deformities are present. The inability of the midtarsal joint to stabilize the forefoot puts the peroneus longus muscle at a mechanical disadvantage, which results in first ray hypermobility and sequelae associated with hallux abductovalgus. With hypermobility of the first ray, more ground reactive force is applied to the second and third metatarsal heads, leading to subsequent forefoot derangements.

In a closed kinetic chain, there continues to be medial displacement of the subtalar joint and apparent abduction of the forefoot on the rearfoot. This changes the relationship between the intrinsic muscles, long flexors, and extensors, creating digital deformities.[12,13] Retrograde forces against the metatarsophalangeal joints are created by the unstable digits forcing the metatarsal heads to bear excess weight. In the right circumstances, this abnormal pronation will also lead to pathological changes around the fifth ray.

Successful lesser metatarsal surgery is based on the ability of the surgeon to assess the biomechanical forces at work and to understand the local symptomatic deformities, such as an intractable plantar keratoma. Specific callus patterns can be a clue to the type of structural deformities that are present. For example, the presence of a callus under the fifth metatarsal head, in combination with a medial pinch callus on the hallux, might be a result of an uncompensated forefoot valgus.

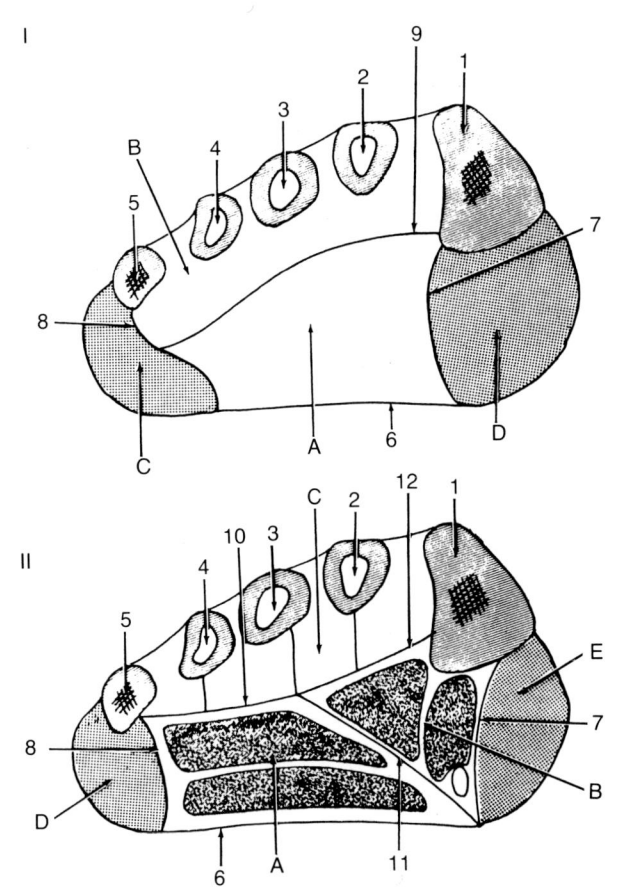

Plantar compartments of the sole of the foot. (I) Classical interpretation: *A*, central compartment; *B*, interosseous compartment; *C*, lateral or peroneal compartment; *D*, medial or tibial compartment; 1–5, metatarsals 1 to 5; 6, central segment of plantar aponeurosis; 7, medial intermuscular septum; 8, lateral intermuscular septum; 9, interosseous fascia. (II) Modified interpretation: *A*, superficial part of central or intermediary compartment; *B*, middle part of central or intermediary compartment; *C*, deep part of central or intermediary compartment; *D*, lateral compartment; *E*, medial compartment; 10, horizontal stem of Y septum; 11, inferomedial limb of Y septum; 12, superomedial limb of Y septum.

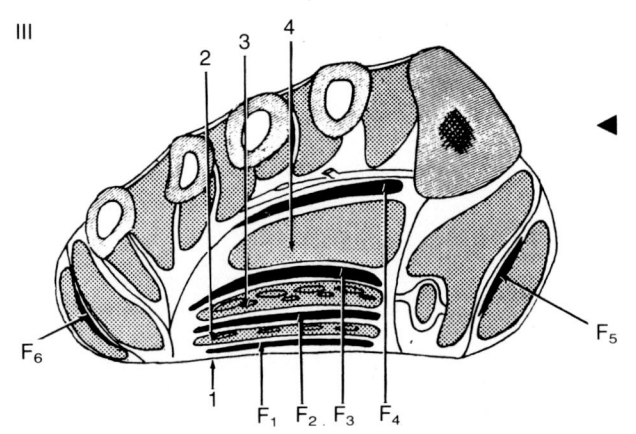

Fascial spaces of the sole of the foot: cross-section of foot at the level of the middle of the fifth metatarsal bone (proximal surface). *Central compartment:* F_1, fascial space between central plantar aponeurosis (1) and flexor digitorum brevis (2); F_2, fascial space between flexor digitorum brevis (2) and quadratus plantae (3); F_3, fascial space between quadratus plantae (3) and oblique head of adductor hallucis (4); F_4, fascial space between adductor hallucis (4) and interosseous fascia. *Medial compartment:* F_5, fascial space located between investing fascia of abductor hallucis and deep surface of muscle. *Lateral compartment:* F_6, fascial space located between investing fascia of abductor digiti quinti and deep surface of muscle.

6.10 Plantar compartments and fascial spaces of the sole of the foot.

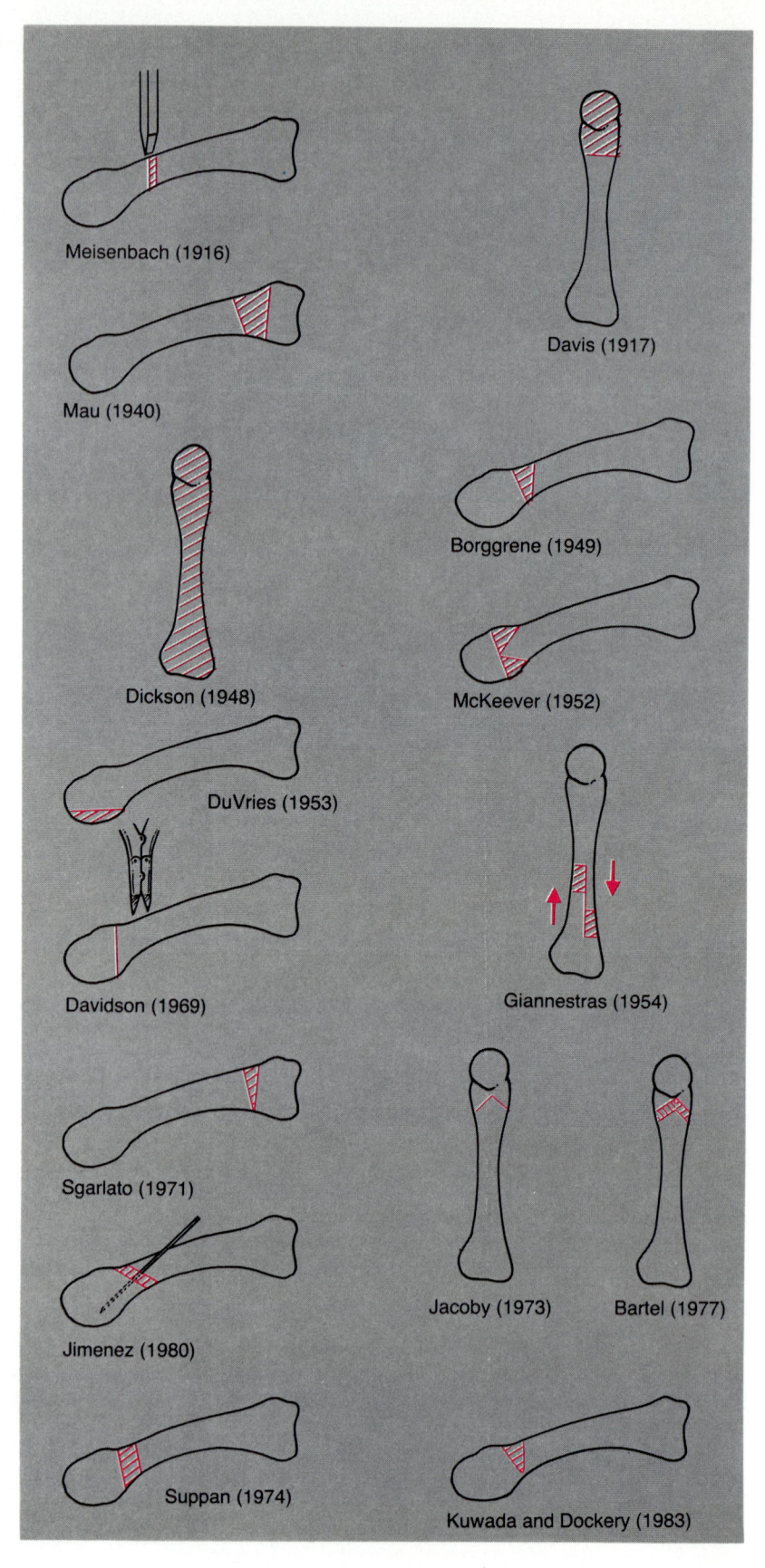

6.11 The major metatarsal osteotomy procedures; the osteotomy area is marked in red.

Meisenbach (1916)
Mau (1940)
Dickson (1948)
DuVries (1953)
Davidson (1969)
Sgarlato (1971)
Jimenez (1980)
Suppan (1974)
Davis (1917)
Borggrene (1949)
McKeever (1952)
Giannestras (1954)
Jacoby (1973)
Bartel (1977)
Kuwada and Dockery (1983)

If the forefoot varus is fully compensated, the callus pattern will be entirely different, with the plantar keratoma under the second metatarsal head.

Lesser metatarsal surgery: an historical review

Lesser metatarsal surgery has a fascinating history beginning in the early 1900s. Numerous procedures have been described, some with good design and others that are no longer performed because of poor clinical results. We will briefly review the pertinent history, with respect to lesser metatarsal surgery, and discuss the current procedures in greater detail in the section on specific lesser metatarsal deformities that is found later in this chapter. The major historical lesser metatarsal osteotomies are described in **6.11**.

Meisenbach is credited with performing the first lesser metatarsal surgery in 1916.[14] He used an osteotome, 3 cm from the metatarsophalangeal joint in diaphyseal bone, for deep-seated calluses. Metatarsal head resections were quite common at the time and he considered his procedure to be 'conservative' by comparison.

In 1917, Davis suggested removal of the metatarsal head, with excision of the plantar callus.[15] Mau, in 1940, removed a dorsiflexory trapezoidal piece of bone at the base of the lesser metatarsal and fixated this osteotomy with a wire suture.[16] This was done primarily for cavus feet; a considerable amount of bone was usually removed, resulting in excessive shortening.

In 1948, Dickson advocated ray resection and digital amputation for intractable verrucae.[17] Many of the original researchers did not distinguish between plantar verrucae and intractable plantar keratomas. Borggrene in 1949 performed the same procedure as Mau, but at the metaphyseal region of the metatarsal head.[18] In 1952, McKeever suggested a subcapital osteotomy of the involved metatarsal and telescoped the spiked end of the shaft into the capital fragment.[19] A year later, DuVries described the plantar condylectomy procedure, which was popular up until the late seventies.[20] This particular procedure has been abandoned at the Waldo Podiatric Residency Program because the corresponding digit was found to float dorsally due to loss of the flexor plate function.

Giannestras, in 1954 described his classic 'step down osteotomy', which was popular in the orthopaedic literature for many years,[21] reporting success in 17 of 21 patients. Then, in 1958, he reported on 40 procedures, with excellent results in 82.5%, good in 10%, and failure in 7.5%.[22]

Davidson, in 1969, performed an osteoclasis similar to Meisenbach, but at the surgical neck instead of in the diaphyseal region of the metatarsal.[23] He popularized

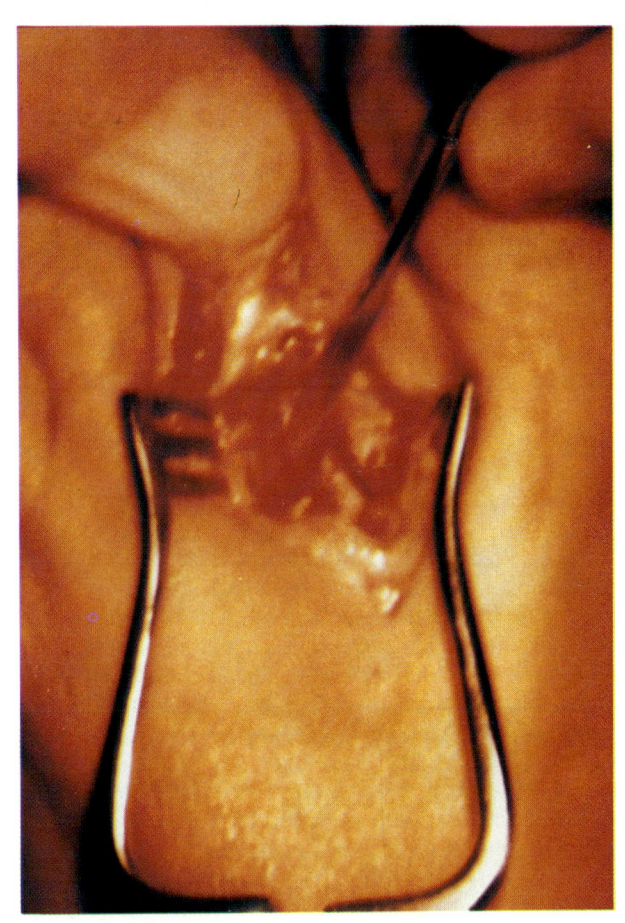

6.12 The second metatarsal shows a distal metaphyseal Jacoby V-osteotomy procedure.

weight-bearing, with no fixation post-operatively to allow the capital fragment to 'seek its own level'. This concept was adopted in 1973, when Jacoby described his 'V' osteotomy.[24] Jacoby found that, with other metatarsal osteotomies at the surgical neck, there was too much lateral shifting of the capital fragment; his procedure prevented this by virtue of the osteotomy design.

In 1971, Sgarlato reported on his E.O. technique, which was essentially a dorsiflexory wedge osteotomy at the base of the metatarsal.[25] Bartel, in 1977, described the shortening chevron osteotomy at the distal head region of the metatarsal.[26] Finally, in 1980 Jimenez reported on the double oblique osteotomy at the surgical neck of the metatarsal.[27] This procedure was fixated with a Kirschner wire.

From the multiplicity of procedures described in this overview, it is apparent that no one procedure produces consistent, satisfactory results. With a greater understanding of biomechanics and pathomechanics of various forefoot deformities, lesser metatarsal surgery for intractable plantar keratoma has evolved in the United States into the selection of a few time-tested procedures that are currently in use.

At the Waldo Podiatric Residency Program, the 'V' osteotomy, shortening chevron, and Jimenez osteotomies are generally accepted as the standard distal metatarsal osteotomies for isolated intractable plantar keratomas that are unresponsive to biomechanical control (**6.12**). Additional procedures, such as the Suppan cartilaginous articulation preservation (CAP) procedure[28] and the modified CAP procedure of Kuwada et al.,[29] are also still performed. The dorsiflexory base wedge osteotomy and modifications of this technique are the preferred proximal osteotomies in lesser metatarsal surgery. These base osteotomies are often carried out in conjunction with a distal metatarsal osteotomy, particularly when adjacent metatarsals are being performed. This helps prevent potential complications, such as bony coalition between metatarsal heads or the devitalizing of the corresponding digit because of increased soft tissue dissection. Whether or not osteotomies are fixated is still widely a matter of surgeon preference. The plantar keratoma is often removed at the time of the osseous procedure. Suturing techniques to evert skin margins and alleviate tension on the plantar skin are extremely important, as is non-weight-bearing for three to four weeks to help prevent painful plantar scars.

Clinical assessment

The personal history of the patient is always the cornerstone to diagnosis, with emphasis being placed on previous trauma or surgery and the onset and severity of symptoms. One should determine the disability that the deformity imposes and obtain a detailed family history of any similar conditions. One should also ask the appropriate questions necessary to rule out systemic involvement, such as rheumatoid arthritis, neuromuscular disease, or diabetes. Since many of the lesser metatarsal deformities respond so well to conservative care, it is extremely important to know what previous professional treatment has been rendered.

During the physical examination, the surgeon should be thinking of planal dominance of the deformity. Changes should be noted with the foot weight-bearing and non-weight-bearing.[30] Location as well as type of calluses are helpful in determining the structural and/or biomechanical deformities present. They may also give one clues as to the type of compensation present. Associated deformities should be noted and joint function assessed. The Jack test can be useful to determine if there are any retrograde forces from the digits on the lesser metatarsals.[31] Finally, no examination is complete unless an analysis of the patient's gait has been performed.

Radiographs of the lesser metatarsals are particularly helpful when evaluating obvious deformities such as tailor's bunions, Freiberg's, brachymetatarsia, and rheumatoid arthritis. When the problem is both structural and biomechanical, lesion markers can be useful in locating calluses with respect to underlying osseous structures. These X-ray films should be taken with the central beam perpendicular to the film, so as not to distort or displace the actual position of the callus. Axial films of the forefoot are used frequently to assess the position of the metatarsal heads relative to the transverse plane, but one should not rely on this particular view for assessment because of the supinated position of the foot with this technique. It is not a true representation of what is happening to the metatarsal heads during the midstance phase of gait when the foot is pronated and the metatarsal heads are subjected to ground reactive force. Taking X-ray films in both the weight-bearing and non-weight-bearing condition can help in the evaluation of compensation for certain deformities. Special radiographic techniques and bone scans can be useful in specific circumstances: for example, computerized axial tomography (CAT) scans can assist evaluation of bone tumours or fractures. Bone scans, on the other hand, can be essential in determining the presence or absence of a stress fracture, particularly during the initial phases when plain X-ray films may be negative. Magnetic resonance imaging (MRI) is an emerging technology that may also prove to be an excellent diagnostic aid in certain lesser metatarsal conditions[32] (**6.13**).

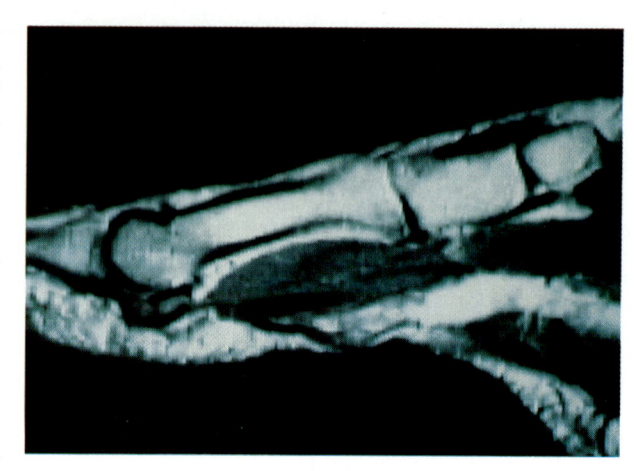

6.13 Magnetic resonance imaging (MRI) cross-section of the foot, showing anatomical structures clearly.

Ancillary diagnostic tests include diagnostic injections and laboratory arthritis profiles. Often it is difficult to distinguish between periarticular and intra-articular symptoms on examination. Diagnostic injections with local anaesthetic agents can be quite useful in such circumstances. Arthritis profiles can be obtained to rule out or document a systemic aetiology for the lesser metatarsal pathology.

Lesser metatarsal deformities

Traumatic

Technology has changed considerably in the past 10 years in regard to conservative as well as surgical treatment of lesser metatarsal fractures.[33,34] The diagnosis and management of metatarsal fractures has also become much more sophisticated, leading to better functional results with these fractures.

Metatarsal fractures are fairly common and result from either direct or indirect trauma. Direct trauma fractures, which are mainly the result of crush injuries or motor vehicle accidents where sudden impact forces are delivered, are generally more serious than indirect injuries, which are usually the result of torque or twisting applied to the foot in a closed kinetic chain.

Metatarsal neck fractures are the least common and are usually transverse (**6.14**); the force occurs perpendicular to the long axis of the bone, creating the fracture. These fractures are often displaced, and intrinsic muscular contracture usually prevents satisfactory reduction.[35]

Midshaft fractures of the lesser metatarsals are usually oblique and result in considerable shortening of the metatarsal (**6.15**); displacement may be significant, causing loss of the metatarsal parabola, or minimal.

Metatarsal base fractures, for the most part, are transverse and fairly rare for the internal metatarsals. When base fractures are present, the surgeon should have a high index of suspicion that a Lisfranc fracture–dislocation may be present (**6.16**).

Fractures of the fifth metatarsal are very common and can pose many problems because of the fifth metatarsal's independent range of motion as an external metatarsal. The head and midshaft fractures are similar to those already discussed. Fractures of the fifth metatarsal base are considered one of the most common foot fractures.[36,37]

The Jones fracture is a transverse diaphyseal fracture 1.5 cm distal to the tuberosity[38] (**6.17**). The insertion of the peroneus brevis tendon is proximal to the fracture line and plays an important role in the pathomechanics of this fracture. The mechanism is a supination external rotation force applied to the rearfoot and ankle with the foot supinated. The musculotendinous attachments at the metatarsal base stabilize the fifth metatarsal against the cuboid and fourth metatarsal. A powerful ground reactive force occurs at the head and neck of the metatarsal against the stable base and

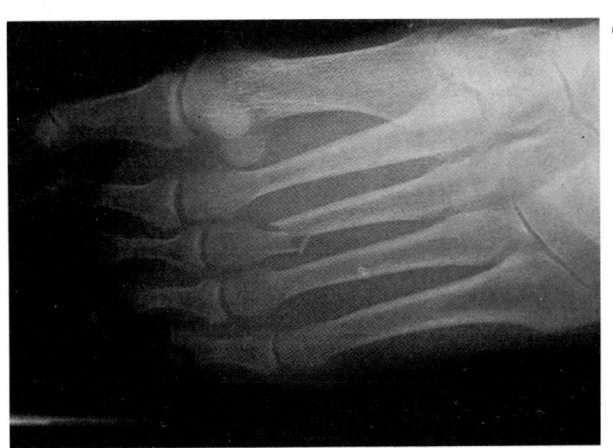

6.14 Third metatarsal neck fracture.

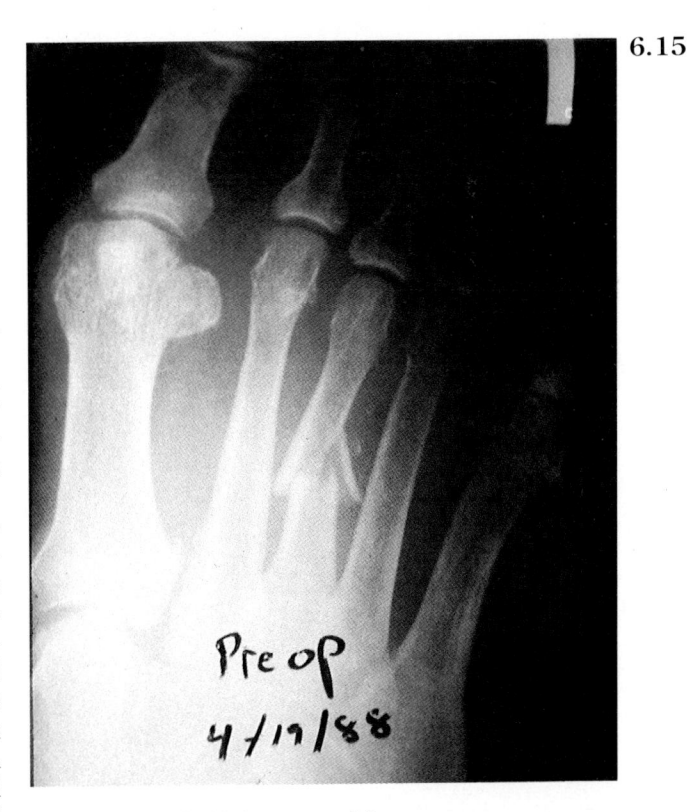

6.15 Midshaft third metatarsal fracture.

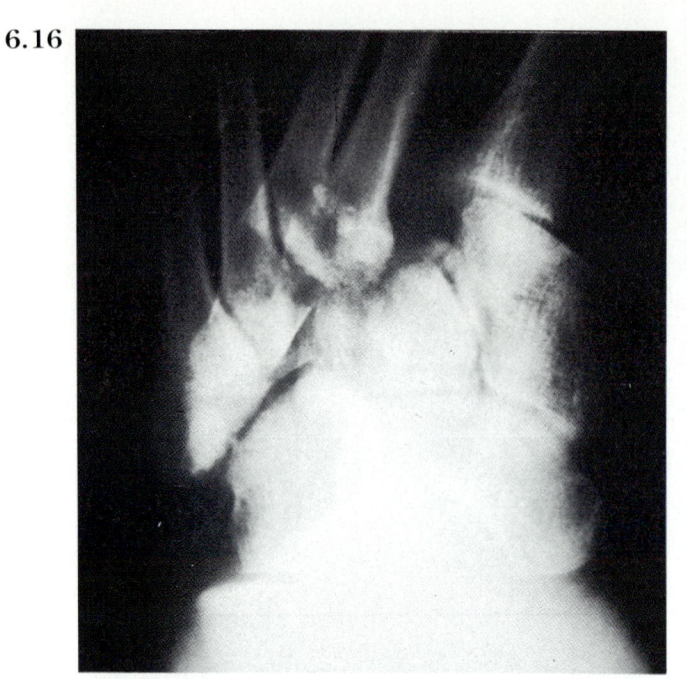

6.16 Lisfranc fracture–dislocation.

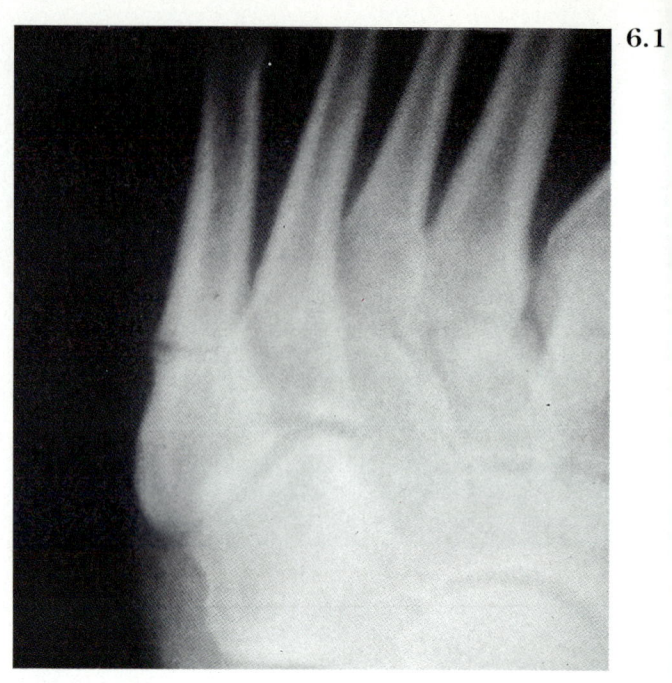

6.17 Jones fracture of the base of the fifth metatarsal bone.

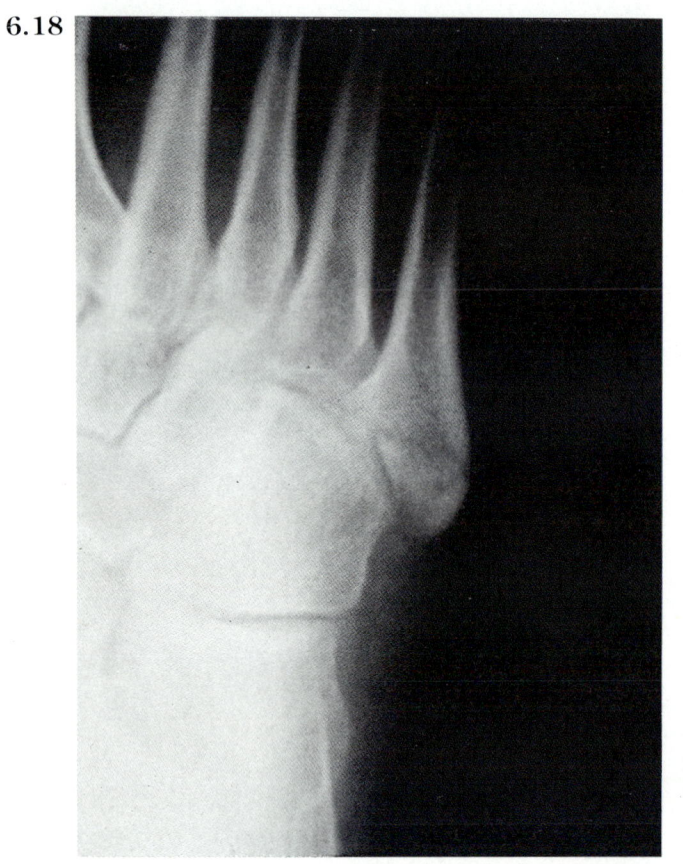

6.18 Avulsion fracture at the styloid process of the fifth metatarsal bone.

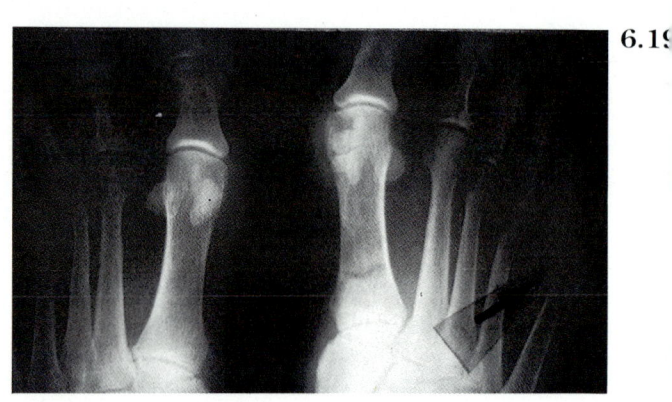

6.19 Fifth metatarsal fracture, with phalangeal dislocation.

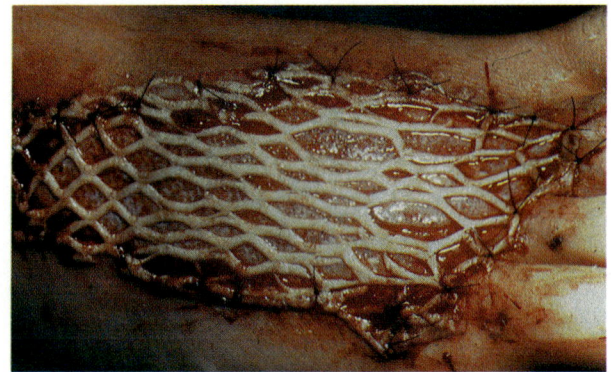

6.20 Meshed split-thickness skin graft covering an area of extensive tissue damage on top of the foot.

120

causes the transverse fracture.

Avulsion fractures of the styloid process of the fifth metatarsal base are caused by forced inversion of the foot (**6.18**). They rarely displace, because of the tension of the peroneus brevis on the fragment. Avulsion fractures respond well to conservative care unless they are displaced or intra-articular.

Lesser metatarsal fractures that involve joints carry a worse prognosis if not treated appropriately: many of them cannot be adequately reduced with closed reduction, such as the metatarsal neck fracture with dislocation (**6.19**). The mechanism is one of hyperextension of the proximal phalanx over the metatarsal head.[39] This drives the head through the plantar plate and it becomes trapped, making closed restoration of joint alignment impossible.

The major goal of fracture management is to return the injured part to full function. Of paramount importance is restoration of the normal weight-bearing alignment of the metatarsal heads. Axial radiographs should be a matter of routine to assess the sagittal plane. Small displacements in the frontal and transverse planes are acceptable, but sagittal plane displacement is not. With unstable fractures, strict anatomical reduction with rigid internal fixation is the key. Inferior methods of treatment lack an understanding of the pathomechanics, and as a result often lead to long-term complications.

If the fractures are the result of a crush injury, marked oedema may be present, compartment syndromes can develop, and open lacerations may also be a complication. All these problems deserve attention before evaluating the metatarsal fractures for treatment. Open injuries should be managed with meticulous debridement and lavage. Appropriate antibiotic coverage and tetanus prophylaxis must be administered. If significant soft tissue damage is present, resulting in necrosis, osseous stabilization may be necessary in conjunction with soft tissue coverage procedures (**6.20**).

Metatarsal neck fractures may require closed reduction with percutaneous wire fixation if displaced (**6.21**). Finger traps are often useful for reducing metatarsal fractures. If adequate reduction cannot be accomplished by closed methods, then open reduction may be necessary. Distal metatarsal fractures that are in good apposition and alignment can be treated conservatively. Metatarsophalangeal joint dislocations or intra-articular fractures require open reduction and internal fixation in most cases.

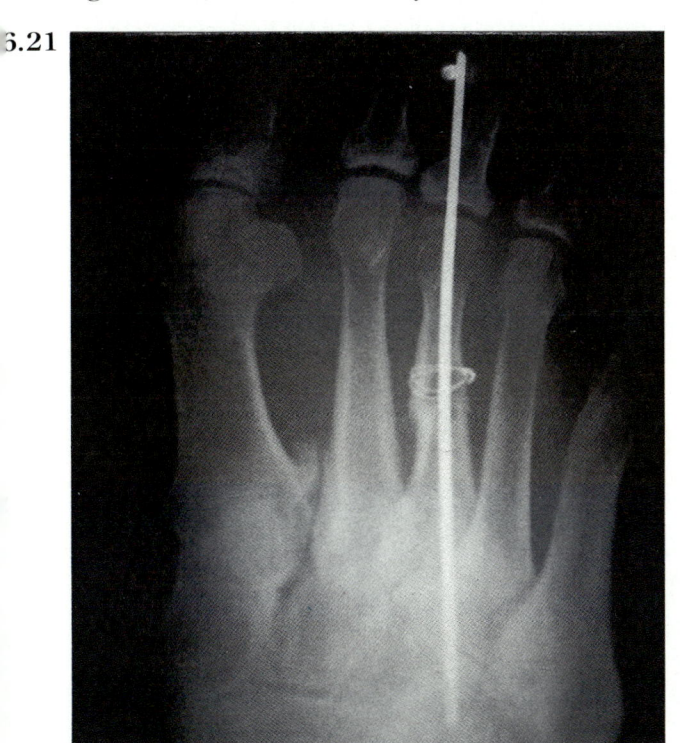

6.21 Midshaft metatarsal fractures may also require K-wire fixation for stability.

6.22 Internal fixation screws placed in an oblique fifth metatarsal fracture for rigid internal fixation.

6.23 Jones fifth metatarsal fracture with soft tissue damage.

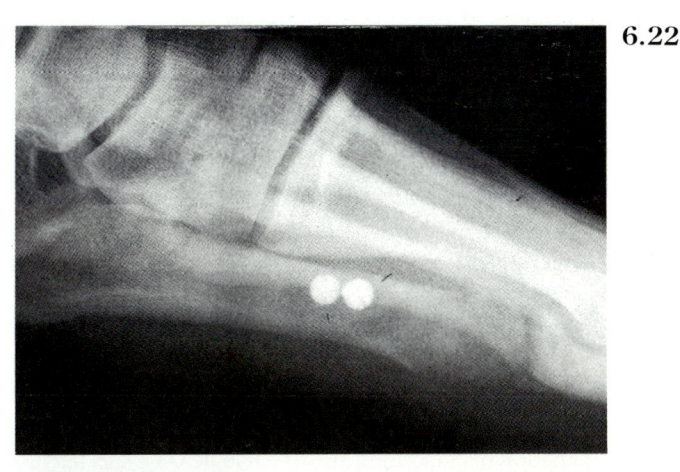

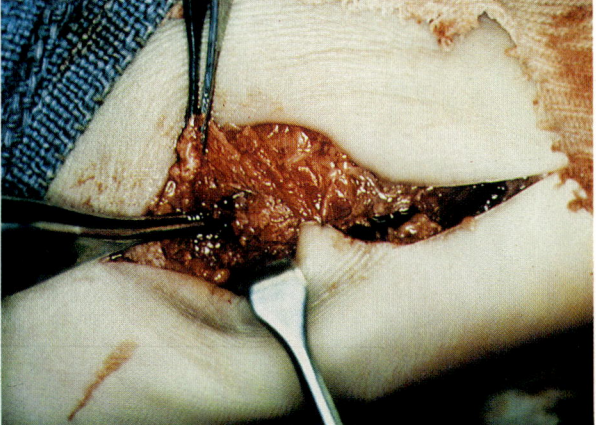

Isolated midshaft fractures with minimal displacement can usually be managed conservatively.[32,34] If there is considerable shortening or displacement, then open reduction and internal fixation is the treatment of choice (**6.22**).

Jones fractures are notorious for complications,[7,38,40] and, until recently, open reduction techniques with internal fixation were the standard method of treatment (**6.23**). Torg et al.,[41] who conducted a prospective study on Jones fractures in 1984, found that the non-union rate was considerably lower than had previously been reported.[41] They found that treating patients in a below-knee non-weight-bearing cast for six to eight weeks was the key to success.

Styloid process fractures are usually stable and have minimal displacement because of the strong ligamentous and tendinous attachments to the base. These fractures heal well in a below-knee walking cast for four to six weeks. Occasionally, displaced intra-articular fractures of the styloid process occur. Displacement and rotation of the fragment is maintained by the distal articular surface of the cuboid, which acts as a fulcrum to rotate the fragment.[42] These fractures need to be opened and reduced surgically.

Non-traumatic

Brachymetatarsia

Brachymetatarsia is a congenital shortening of one or more of the metatarsals and is not uncommon. A result of premature closure of the growth centre of the metatarsal,[43,44] brachymetatarsia appears to be primarily hereditary, but can also occur due to premature epiphyseal closure secondary to trauma.

The most common metatarsals involved are the first and fourth, respectively.[45] Morton, in 1935, first described a syndrome causing pain under the second and third metatarsal heads due to a short first metatarsal. He attributed this shortening to an 'atavistic regression of the human foot to a more primitive form'.[46] Many authors commonly believed that this syndrome was the cause of symptomatic flat feet. Harris and Beath, in 1947, determined that this was not the cause and that a short first metatarsal seldom caused foot disability.[47] It is important to consider the metatarsal protrusion distance during planning for first-ray surgery, but a short first metatarsal itself does not constitute a pathological foot.

When the lesser metatarsals are involved, typically there is overloading of adjacent metatarsals, with the formation of plantar keratoses. The flexor plate fails to load on weight bearing and this results in an unstable, floating digit (**6.24**). The instability of the digit usually results in migration of adjacent digits.

Brachymetatarsia may not result in symptoms at an early age. As the adjacent metatarsals grow and retraction of the toe occurs, the patient may become more symptomatic, with signs of metatarsalgia or pain along the corresponding digit secondary to shoe pressure.

Radiographs will demonstrate the short metatarsal and usually osteopenia of the metatarsal head. The toe is usually not deviated in the transverse or frontal planes, but will be retracted.

Usually no treatment is required and surgical treatment is primarily aimed at either functional correction of the short metatarsal or cosmetic improvement. Surgeons at the Waldo Podiatric Residency Program direct treatment at lengthening the metatarsal with a tricortical bone graft in conjunction with various soft tissue procedures about the involved metatarsophalangeal joint (**6.25**) or hinged implant to the metatarsophalangeal joint to help cosmetically lengthen the shortened toe.[48]

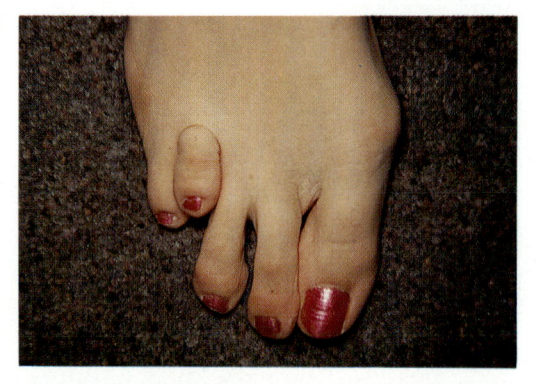

6.24 An unstable floating digit may result from failure of the flexor plate apparatus. (Courtesy of Dr G. Dockery, Seattle, Washington, USA.)

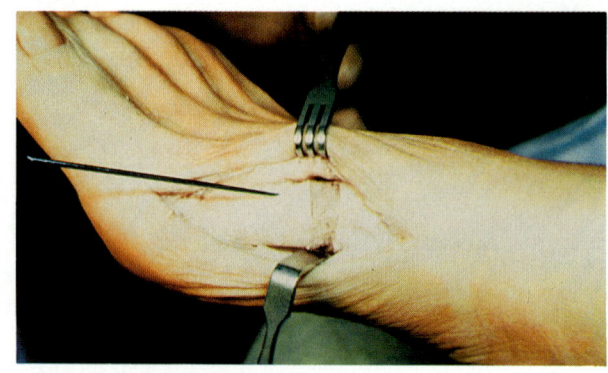

6.25 Lengthening of the first metatarsal bone with a tricortical bone graft and wire stabilization.

Osteochondrosis

In 1914, Freiberg described osteochondrosis of the second metatarsal head and coined the term 'Freiberg's infraction', meaning incomplete fracture.[49] It has also been described as Koehler's second disease and Panner's disease, especially in the European literature.[5]

The disease is seen in adolescents, usually after 13 years of age, and most commonly involves the second metatarsal. Females are affected more often than males and it can be bilateral.[45] The aetiology of osteochondrosis is unknown. It is generally regarded as an avascular necrosis of the epiphyseal plate of the involved bone.[50] Some authors feel that excessive loading of a long second metatarsal compromises the circulation to the subchondral bone, resulting in aseptic necrosis and collapse of the head.[51,52]

Clinically, one sees localized tenderness around the involved metatarsophalangeal joint. There may be local swelling or effusion and limitation of motion of the involved metatarsophalangeal joint. Radiographs usually reveal flattening of the articular end of the metatarsal, with periarticular osteophytes (**6.26**). Subchondral eburnation may also be present or complete collapse of the articular cartilage may be seen.

Treatment should be conservative in the adolescent. Some authors have taken a more aggressive approach in the acute phase by performing bone graft procedures to prevent collapse of the metatarsal head.[53] This author still prefers to put patients in a below-knee walking cast for three to four weeks, followed by nonsteroidal anti-inflammatory drug (NSAID) therapy, and orthotic foot devices.[21] If symptoms continue, surgery may be indicated. Consideration must be given to age, activity level, and condition of the joint at the time of surgery. Arthrotomy of the metatarsophalangeal joint, with removal of osteophytes and subchondral drilling in areas of erosion, is an excellent procedure for young, active patients who have minimal radiographic changes. In advanced stages, arthroplasty or implant arthroplasty may be necessary (**6.27**). Alignment of the digit and the prevention of collapse should be of paramount importance, regardless of the surgery performed.

Elongated metatarsals

This condition is hereditary and considered to be rare. Elongated metatarsals are usually symptomatic, especially when both elongated and plantar flexed. This is often associated with a long digit, which will increase the retrograde force against the long metatarsal, causing it to be prominent in a plantigrade direction. The second and/or third metatarsals are most often involved. Radiographs are usually diagnostic for this con-

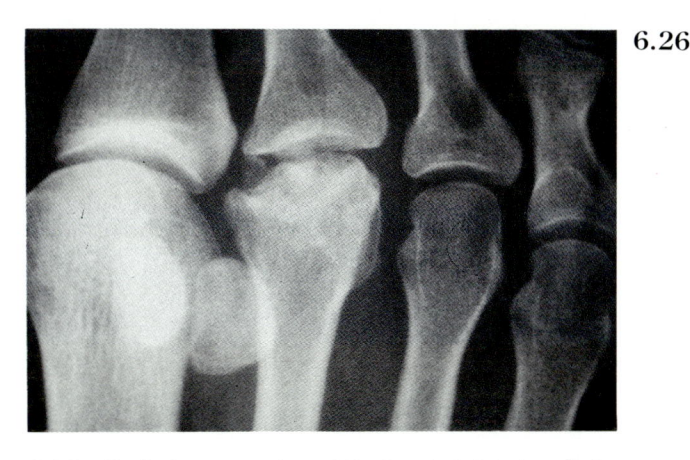

6.26 Typical presentation of Freiberg's infraction of the second metatarsal head with periarticular osteophytes.

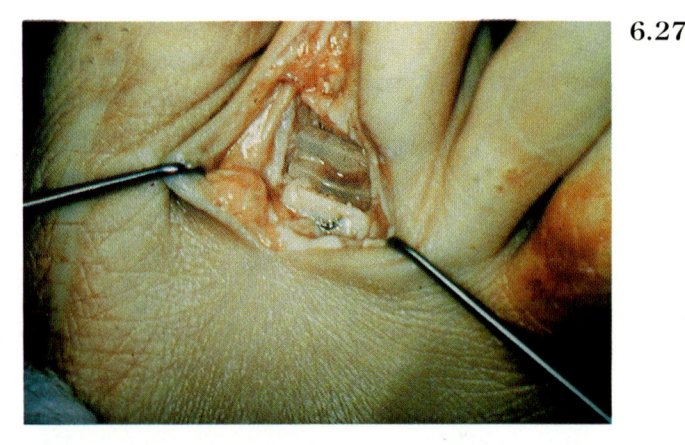

6.27 Total joint hinged implant arthroplasty performed for painful advanced Freiberg's infraction.

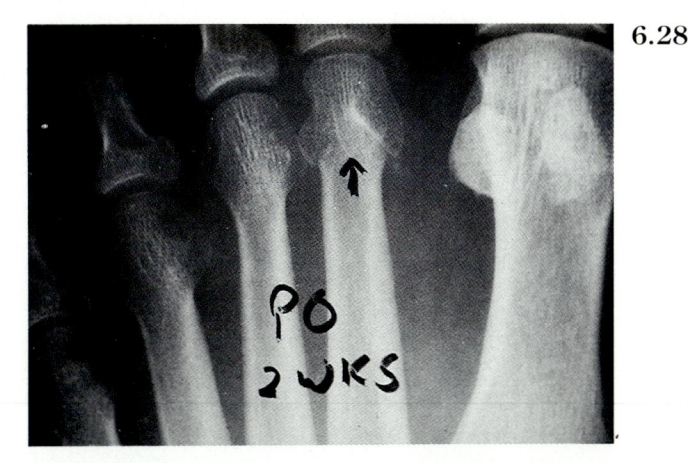

6.28 Post-operative double-shortening V-osteotomy of the second metatarsal metaphyseal region.

dition; one sees an abnormality in the metatarsal parabola, indicating an elongated metatarsal. Surgical treatment is aimed at shortening the metatarsal to re-establish a normal parabola. Many procedures have been devised for this purpose.[21,27,54,55,56] A shortening double-chevron osteotomy at the metaphyseal region of the metatarsal head is the most common technique used by surgeons in our programme (**6.28**).

Metatarsus adductus

Metatarsus adductus is a positional and/or structural deformity whereby the metatarsals are deviated medially in the transverse plane in relation to the longitudinal axis of the lesser tarsus. The apex of the deformity is at Lisfranc's joint[57] (**6.29**).

To briefly summarize, metatarsus adductus is one of the most frequent aetiologies of an 'intoed' gait. Historically, this condition has had numerous descriptions and treatments associated with it. In general, children that are under two years of age will often respond to manipulation and serial casting techniques (**6.30**). Once a child is over two years of age, the success of conservative measures becomes less optimal, and specific surgical procedures become beneficial.

Pre-operative planning with the child's family, establishing realistic goals, and evaluating specific clinical and radiographic criteria are essential to the success of these procedures. Children from two to six years of age respond to certain soft tissue procedures.[58–60] Osseous procedures become the procedures of choice in children over six years of age and into adult life.[61–65] Currently, the Lepird procedure is being performed when osseous correction is indicated (**6.31**).[57] The procedure allows for accurate correction of the deformity and utilizes the principles and techniques of internal fixation developed by AO/ASIF.

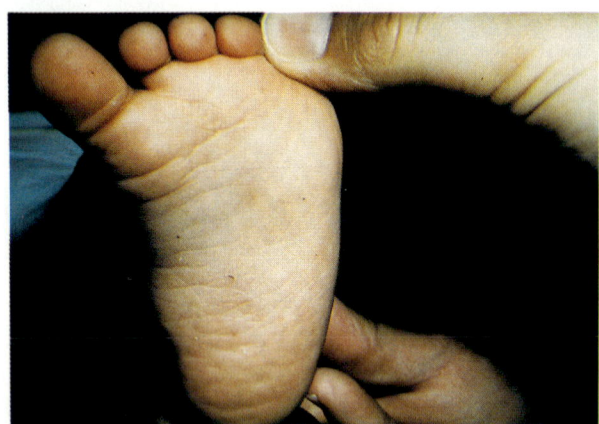

6.29 Metatarsus adductus in infant, showing C border presentation.

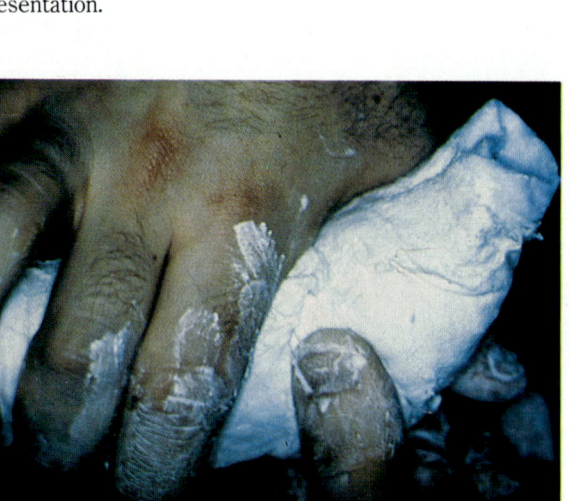

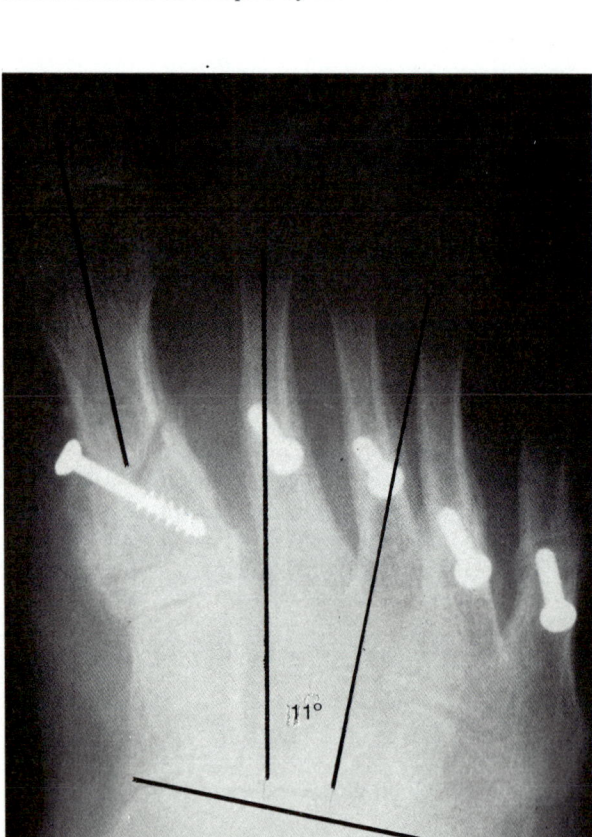

6.30 Serial casting performed to manipulate and hold correction of the metatarsus adductus condition in the infant.

6.31 Radiographic presentation of the post-operative Lepird procedure for the correction of metatarsus adductus in the older child.

Metatarsalgia

Metatarsalgia, by definition, is generalized pain in the region of the distal aspect of the metatarsals. Rarely seen in children, except when trauma or osteochondritis are present,[66] this generalized pain usually has a specific cause that should be determined. Some of the more common specific aetiologies include arthritis, capsulitis, osteochondrosis, stress fractures, neuromas and/or neuropathy, pronation, and faulty biomechanics, as well as iatrogenic causes. Treatment regimens are extremely variable and depend on the specific aetiology, which makes appropriate diagnosis essential.

Dependent upon historical and clinical findings, certain diagnostic tests may be helpful. Standard radiographs may give clues as to metatarsal deformities or malalignments that may be contributing to the metatarsalgia. They may also be helpful in determining specific arthritic patterns, stress fractures, or bone tumours. As mentioned earlier, diagnostic local anaesthetic injections are useful in localizing pathology in this situation. Electromyographic and nerve conduction studies can help to differentiate peripheral neuropathy or tarsal tunnel syndrome from generalized metatarsalgia.

Metatarsal equinus

The so-called plantarflexed lesser metatarsus or metatarsal equinus does occur, but is extremely rare. Usually the patient has a metatarsal equinus as a result of the retrograde force applied to the forefoot from a hammered digit syndrome, as discussed previously. Failure to recognize this will result in a compromised surgical result. Usually under these circumstances, surgical procedures that are devised to relieve the hammered digit syndrome (such as the Hibbs' tenosuspension procedure) are employed and will ultimately resolve the metatarsal equinus (**6.32**).

The retrograde force applied to all the metatarsals can be quite variable, but usually falls into one of four categories: flexor substitution, flexor stabilization, extensor substitution, or rheumatoid arthritis.

Flexor substitution. Flexor substitution occurs in the late stance phase of gait in a supinated foot. At this point, the flexors have gained mechanical advantage over the interossei. A hallmark of this kind of substitution is that the contracture of the digits is straight, with no adductovarus component. This occurs in the presence of a weak triceps surae, resulting in a calcaneus gait. The deep posterior and lateral compartment muscles in the leg try to substitute for the weak triceps surae by firing earlier and longer than usual; this causes severe contraction of the digits and results in metatarsal equinus.

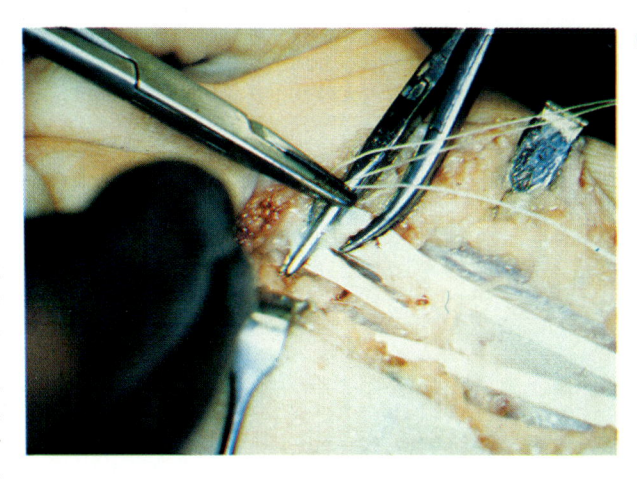

6.32 Extensor digitorum longus transfer into the midfoot (modified Hibbs' tenosuspension) used for control of extensor tendon substitution and flexible contracted lesser digits.

Flexor stabilization. Flexor stabilization occurs in the late stance phase of gait in a pronated foot. During late stance, the flexor digitorum longus and brevis have gained mechanical advantage over the interossei. There is usually an adductovarus component to the contracture. The pronated foot in a closed kinetic chain is an unstable foot at the subtalar and midtarsal joints.[4] The flexors fire earlier and longer during the gait cycle in an attempt to 'stabilize' the osseous structures of the forefoot.[67] Ultimately, these muscles overpower the small interossei, leading to hammered digit syndrome. The metatarsal equinus is not apparent in this type of abnormal digital function.

Extensor substitution. Extensor substitution occurs during the swing phase of gait in a pronated and/or supinated foot. The extensor digitorum longus gains a mechanical advantage over the lumbricals. An adductovarus contracture usually only occurs in the pronated foot type.[68] The hallmark of this type of hammered digit syndrome is that when the deformity is still flexible, it will reduce completely in a closed kinetic chain.

In an open kinetic chain, a passive pull of the extensor digitorum longus tendons creates an excessive metatarsal equinus or forefoot equinus. In the swing phase of gait, the extensor digitorum longus must move the joint of least resistance (MPJ) to their end range of motion before effecting ankle dorsiflexion without the stabilizing effects of the lumbricals. The metatarsophalangeal joints become excessively dorsiflexed, putting a retrograde force on the metatarsals and, at heel contact, one sees the extensor substitution graphically.[69]

Rheumatoid arthritis and hammered digit syndrome. It has been well documented that in the rheumatoid foot, one loses the plantar fat pad or has it displaced distally with digital contractures. The metatarsal heads ultimately become prominent and, over time, can lead to significant disability for these patients. The aetiology is unknown at this time but there is speculation that the periarticular chronic inflammatory process weakens the integrity of the soft tissue structures and muscles around the metatarsophalangeal joint.[70]

Splay foot

By definition, splay foot is a pathologically increased width of the forefoot in the transverse plane.[11] This is a progressive and acquired deformity. The author has also observed a high correlation between splay foot and benign hypermobile joint syndrome. There is usually radiographic evidence of increased intermetatarsal angles between the first and second metatarsals, and the fourth and fifth metatarsals, and occasionally between all metatarsals. Some authors believe splay foot involves the five metatarsals as well as the cuneiforms.[71,72]

The aetiology of splay foot seems to be related to abnormal subtalar joint pronation and subluxation of the rays at their basal joints. This is translated pathomechanically into loss of function of the transverse pedis muscle and excessive eversion of the foot because of abnormal subtalar joint pronation at a time when resupination is necessary for a propulsive gait. The ability of the transverse pedis muscle to stabilize the metatarsals during propulsion is the primary factor.

When the central three metatarsals do not spread during propulsion in a foot that is abnormally pronated, then a rearfoot varus is probably present. When all the metatarsals splay, then there are probably many components involved, including benign hypermobile joint syndrome.[73] Clinically, this type of foot will typically show a wide forefoot with weight bearing. There are marked signs of excessive pronation, with very little resupination present during gait. Intractable plantar keratomas may be seen under the second and fourth metatarsal heads, depending on the range of motion of the first and fifth rays.

The management of splay foot has not received much attention, and literature is sparse. In an effort to establish a normal anatomical alignment, osseous procedures should be chosen and directed at the structural abnormality.[74] In cases where there is significant increase in the intermetatarsal angle between the first and second as well as the fourth and fifth metatarsals, oblique osteotomies at the respective bases should be performed. The use of AO/ASIF internal fixation techniques is preferred for these types of osteotomies. Arthrodesis procedures of the first and fifth basal joints may be indicated if there is significant splaying in conjunction with benign hypermobile joint syndrome, to prevent reoccurrence (**6.33**).

Tailor's bunion

Tailor's bunion or 'bunionette' was popularized in the nineteenth century when tailors sat with their legs crossed as they sewed clothes. The bunion developed as a result of this sartorial position. Current thought is that this enlargement at the lateral aspect of the fifth metatarsal head occurs because of shearing of soft tissue between an unstable metatarsal and the shoe, creating an inflamed adventitious bursa.[5]

The aetiology of tailor's bunion remains elusive. Many theories have been suggested;[75–78] other authors have suggested a correlation with splay foot.[4,72,75,79,80] It becomes clear when reviewing the literature that the aetiology of tailor's bunion is multifaceted, including congenital, developmental, and biomechanical factors.[4,5,30,72,75–81]

Root *et al.*[4] provide probably the best, most detailed discussion of the pathomechanics of the tailor's bunion deformity. They summarize the pertinent aetiologies as (a) abnormal subtalar joint pronation of the foot; (b) any uncompensated varus position of the forefoot or rearfoot in a fully pronated foot; (c) congenital plantarflexed fifth-ray deformity; (d) dorsiflexed fifth ray deformity; and (e) idiopathic. They also correlate these aetiologies with the pathomechanics of the deformity.

Abnormal subtalar joint pronation alone will not cause the development of a tailor's bunion, except in a congenitally dorsiflexed fifth ray. Usually, abnormal subtalar joint pronation is seen in conjunction with one of the other aetiological factors, resulting in hypermobility of the fifth metatarsal during the midstance and propulsive phases of gait and in the development of a tailor's bunion. Any uncompensated or compensated varus deformity will produce a subluxed fifth ray in a fully pronated foot, when subjected to ground reactive force. In the presence of a congenitally plantarflexed

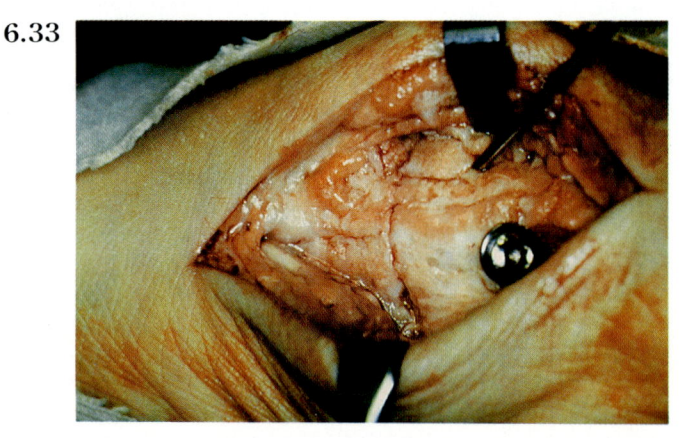

6.33 Fusion of the first metatarsal–cuneiform joint (modified Lapidus procedure) to control hypermobility and splaying of metatarsal.

fifth-ray deformity, a tailor's bunion will develop if the fifth metatarsal head will not reach the transverse plane of the other metatarsal heads when the fifth ray is in its maximally dorsiflexed position (**6.34**).

Clinical examination is particularly helpful in assessing the functional aspects of the deformity. The majority of patients have plantar or lateral pain, but this can also be dorsolateral over the fifth metatarsal head. There will be prominence of the fifth metatarsal, especially with the foot loaded. An adventitious bursa with erythema may also be present. Hyperkeratotic lesions, especially plantarly, are often present. The fifth digit is usually contracted in an adductovarus attitude and associated heloma dura or heloma molle may accompany this digital deformity. Range of motion of the fifth ray, as well as a good biomechanical examination, including stance and gait evaluation, should be performed. The examination should also include non-weight-bearing and weight-bearing assessment. All of these aspects of clinical assessment are important in preparing the patient for the appropriate treatment options.

Radiographic evaluation is important to confirm osseous and structural malalignments and to help plan definitive treatment. Standard X-ray films should be taken in the weight-bearing condition and should consist of anterior–posterior, lateral, and oblique views.[6,7]

The normal intermetatarsal angle between the fourth and fifth metatarsals is traditionally 0–8°,[77] but this measurement fails to take into account any lateral bowing of the metatarsal. Recently, criteria were established by Fallat and Buckholz to evaluate the anatomical and radiographic characteristics of a tailor's bunion deformity:[82] they established six pathomechanical types of tailor's bunions (**6.35**). From this work, it is clear that it is important to measure not only the intermetatarsal angle but also the amount of lateral bowing. This is done by drawing a line adjacent and parallel to the medial proximal surface of the fifth metatarsal shaft and a line bisecting the fourth metatarsal (**6.36**). The angle formed (A), is the intermetatarsal angle and should be, on the average, 6.47°. In the presence of a tailor's bunion, this angle can average 8.71°. Lateral bowing is determined by the lateral deviation angle.[82] A bisection of the head and neck of the fifth metatarsal and the angle (B) formed between that bisection and the line parallel to the fifth metatarsal forms the lateral deviation angle. This angle is 2.64° on the average and can increase to 8.05° in a tailor's bunion deformity (**6.37**).

Selection of the appropriate surgical procedure for a tailor's bunion deformity depends largely on the clinical and radiographic appearance of the fifth ray. Generally, if a purely plantar callus is present under the fifth metatarsal head and the fifth ray is not hypermobile, the Sponsel procedure with fixation is preferred[83] (**6.38**). If the callus is lateral or the dorsolateral aspect of the

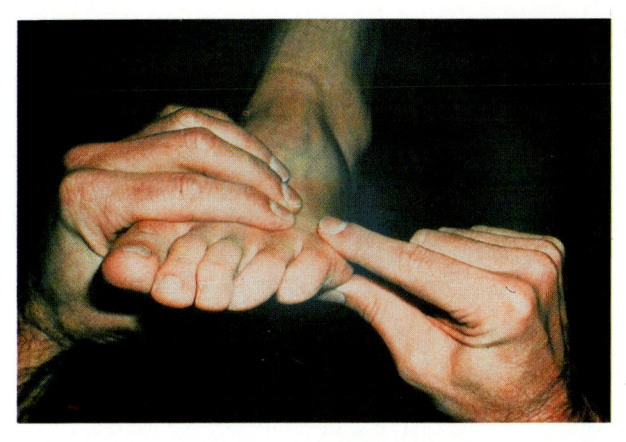

6.34 Proper technique for evaluation of fifth metatarsal range-of-motion in dorsiflexion and plantarflexion.

1. Rotation of the lateral plantar tubercle into a lateral position.
2. Increased intermetatarsal angle.
3. Increased lateral deviation angle.
4. A large dumbell-shaped fifth metatarsal head.
5. Arthritic changes resulting in exostosis formation at the fifth metatarsophalangeal joint.
6. Any combination of the above conditions with the first three being the most common.

6.35 Fallat and Buckholz[82] criteria for the evaluation of the anatomical and radiographic characteristics of a tailor's bunion formation.

6.36 Intermetatarsal and lateral deviation angles used to determine lateral bowing.

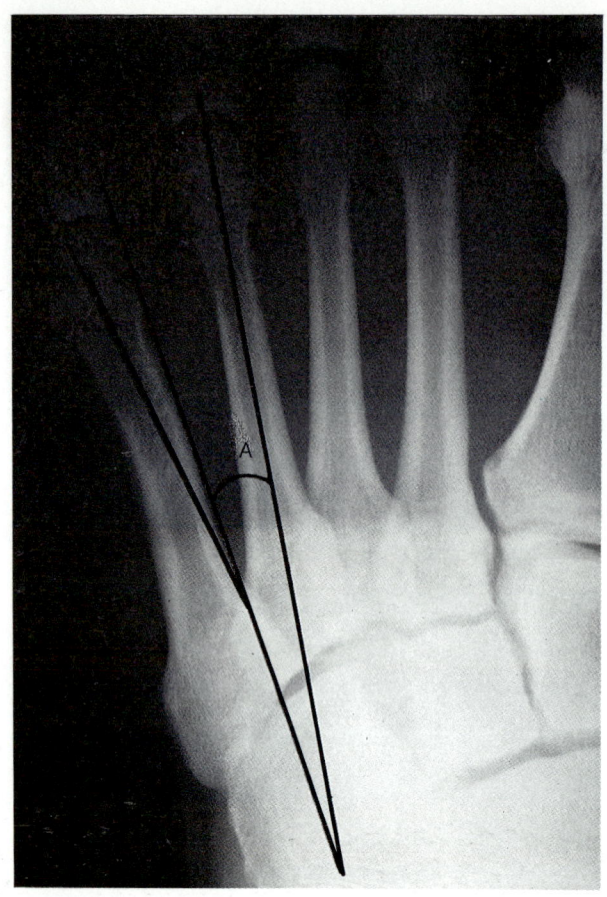

6.37 Clinical presentation on radiographs of measurements used to determine the intermetatarsal angle showing the presence of lateral metatarsal bowing.

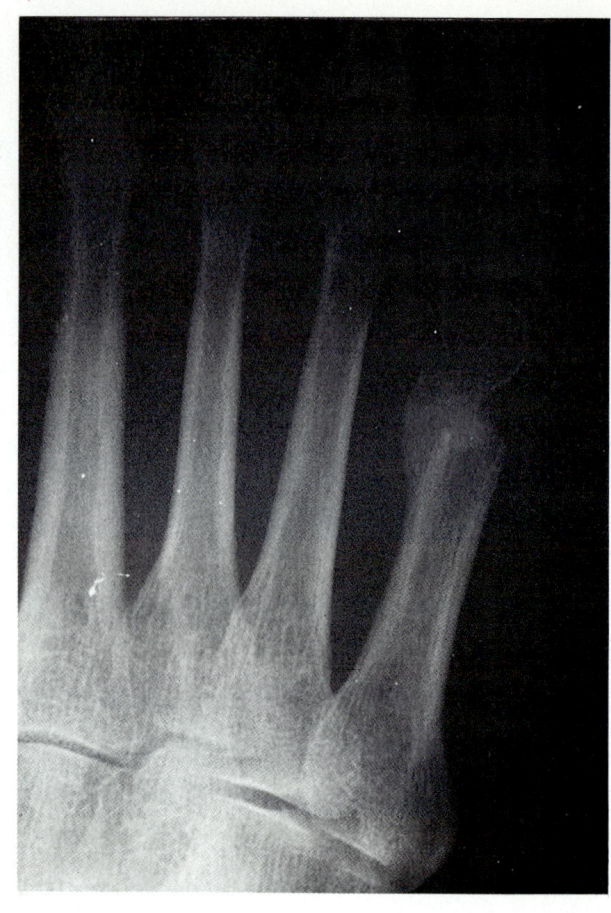

6.38 Post-operative radiographic presentation of a healed Sponsel osteotomy of the fifth metatarsal bone.

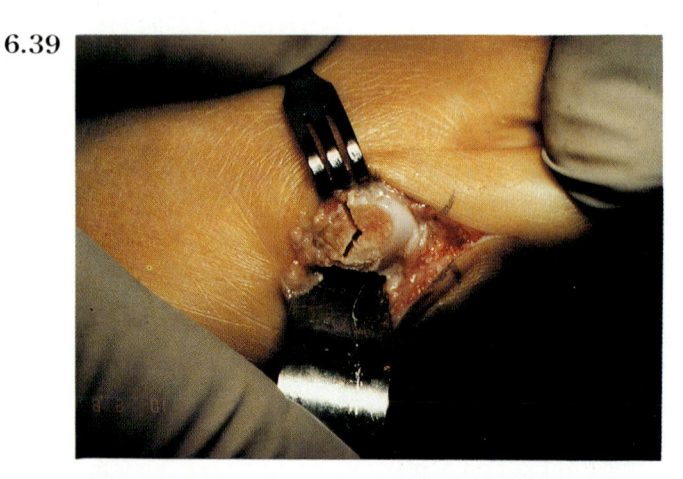

6.39 A distal transverse plane chevron-type of distal fifth metatarsal osteotomy for the correction of prominent metatarsal head.

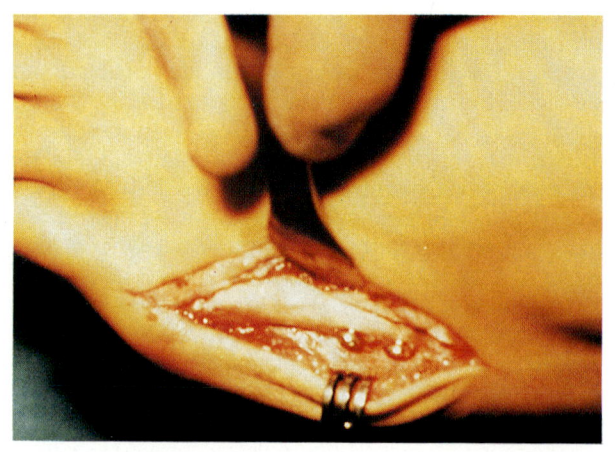

6.40 An oblique closing wedge osteotomy with internal screw fixation of the fifth metatarsal bone performed to reduce the intermetatarsal angle.

fifth metatarsal head is prominent, a distal transverse plane osteotomy is performed[84] (**6.39**). Finally, if there is significant hypermobility of the fifth ray and an increased intermetatarsal angle, the oblique base wedge osteotomy using AO/ASIF techniques is performed (**6.40**). Rarely is there a need to perform a fifth metatarsal head resection or total implant procedure for tailor's bunions. It has been our experience that fifth metatarsal head resections tend to leave patients with significant retraction of the fifth digit, and transfer lesions to the fourth metatarsal are commonplace.

Metatarsal tumours

Increasing attention has been paid in recent years to tumours of the foot, and references, usually in the form of case studies, have increased significantly. Fortunately, bone malignancies of the foot still remain rare by all accounts. In Berlin's study of 67,000 tumorous lesions of the foot, exostoses were the most common lesion found.[85] Just under 150 total bone lesions were reported and none of these was malignant. Usually, these lesions are picked up secondarily on radiographs taken for other probable conditions, such as stress fractures (**6.41**).

Early recognition and appropriate management of bone tumours generally increases survival rates among afflicted individuals. The surgeon should be aware of the clinical and radiographic characteristics of bone tumours as well as appropriate diagnostic aids and therapeutic regimens. All too often, diagnostic tests and treatment plans are thought of retrospectively, i.e. after the lesion has been removed surgically and identified.

Obtaining a good history, with emphasis on duration, onset, progression of symptoms, family history, and previous trauma, is essential. Differentiating a malignant process from a benign process should be accomplished on standard radiographs.

Lodwick has created an excellent grading system to establish bone tumour characteristics to aid in presumptive diagnosis.[86] The system looks at eight general characteristics. The first is the type of bone destruction present. Geographical, moth-eaten, or permeative forms of bone destruction can occur. The margin of the tumour is determined by growth rate and host response. Margins can be sharp or sclerotic, and cortical break may or may not be noted. The rate of growth and the matrix of the lesion itself are important to assess. Usually, solitary bone tumours have a lytic appearance, whereas osteogenic sarcoma will have calcified deposits within the matrix.

Periosteal reaction is another important characteristic. One should note if the periosteum is lamellated, solid, spiculated, or expanded. Is there reactive bone formation present and is there extension of the bone tumour into the soft tissues? Finally, the location of the lesion is important to know: certain tumours are purely diaphyseal and other are metaphyseal by nature.

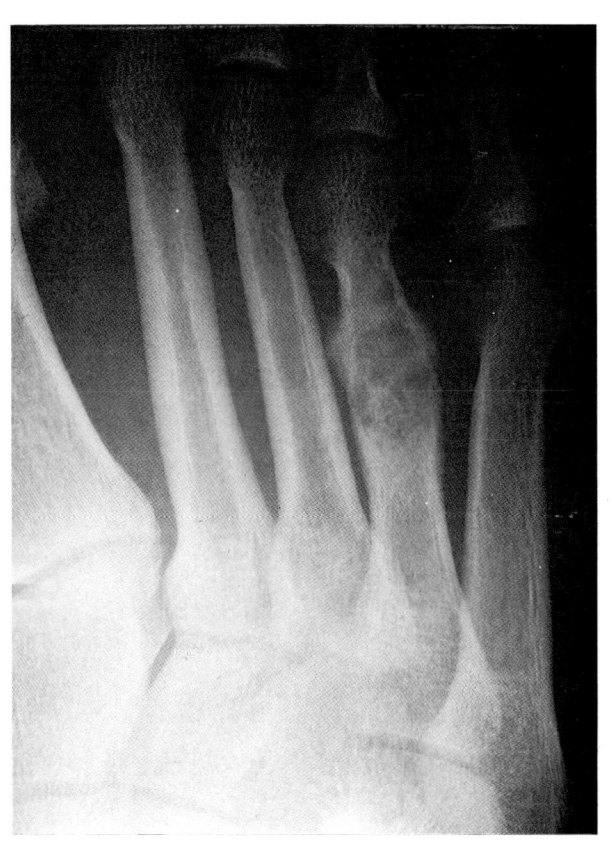

6.41 Typical presentation of a benign solitary bone cyst in the shaft of the fourth metatarsal bone.

After tumour characteristics have been identified on standard radiographs, the surgeon should be able to determine if a malignant process is present or if this is indeed a solitary benign bone tumour. If a malignant process has been diagnosed, then the patient should be referred to a tumour institute for proper staging and definitive treatment. If a benign bone tumour is suspected, it is prudent for the surgeon to obtain a complete bone scan to determine if the lesion is indeed solitary and not a metastatic process or occult malignancy.

If the benign bone tumour is diaphyseal and is less than 1 cm in diameter, the tumour should be curetted and packed with autogenous bone. If the lesion is over

1 cm and the cortical wall is fractured or weak, then an en bloc excision with a tricortical bone graft and rigid internal fixation is the procedure of choice. Another alternative might be the use of a cortical cancellous strut, such as rib strip.

Benign tumours of the metaphyseal region of the metatarsal can usually be curetted and packed with autogenous bone. Care must be taken to maintain strength to the subchondral bone to preserve the articular cartilage.

The rheumatoid foot

Rheumatoid arthritis affecting the human foot is a chronic systemic inflammatory process characterized by proliferative synovitis, joint pain, stiffness, and specific structural deformities (**6.42**). Sixty per cent of those afflicted with the disease will have involvement of the metatarsophalangeal and interphalangeal joints[87] (**6.43**).

The management of the rheumatoid foot is best accomplished through an organized team approach under the direction of the patient's rheumatologist. A good understanding of the roles played by other team members is essential. Now that remitative therapy is available, it should be the cornerstone of treatment in the rheumatoid foot.

In early and moderately severe involvement, efforts should be made at joint protection and maintaining function. Once the rheumatoid foot has progressed to the point of unremitting pain and severe deformity, panmetatarsal head resection is indicated. The primary goal of this surgery is to alleviate pain and to keep the patient ambulatory.

Hoffman, in 1911, first described panmetatarsal head resection in the rheumatoid foot.[88] This was performed through a single transverse curved plantar incision, with removal of the metatarsal heads. The procedure was gratifying because it essentially allowed end-stage rheumatoid patients to continue to be ambulatory without significant pain. One of the problems with this technique was that many patients developed similar plantar foot calluses and pain post-operatively.

Clayton, in 1963, felt that this reoccurrence of the calluses was a result of prominent bases of the proximal phalanges, which assumed a weight-bearing position because of shortening of the forefoot.[89] He advocated a dorsal transverse approach, with resection of the metatarsal heads as well as the bases. Since that time, other modifications have been described, but the purpose for the procedure has not changed and the procedure has withstood the test of time.[90–94]

Regardless of the procedural choice, maintenance of the metatarsal parabola is essential. The metatarsal heads should be resected obliquely to prevent any osseous prominence plantarly (**6.44**). The author prefers to utilize a three-incision dorsal approach unless contractures are so severe dorsally that exposure is too difficult. In those circumstances, a plantar transverse approach is performed (**6.45**). Kirschner wires are used in all lesser rays for three to four weeks to allow for optimum alignment during fibrosis[95] (**6.46**).

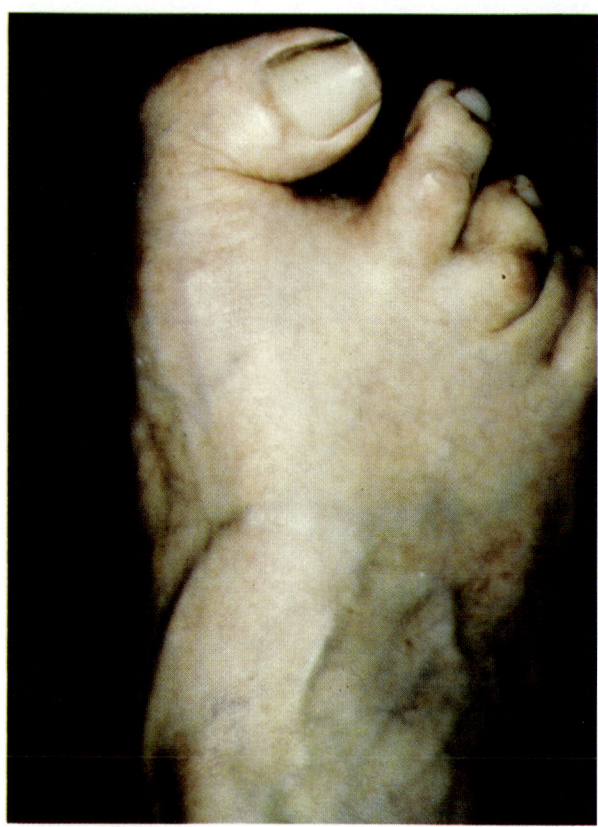

6.42 Severe presentation of rheumatoid foot in an adult.

A total implant or arthrodesis is usually performed on the first metatarsophalangeal joint, depending on the bone stock. We have found that with significant soft tissue adaptation in severe deformities this helps maintain alignment of the forefoot and provides additional stability to the foot.

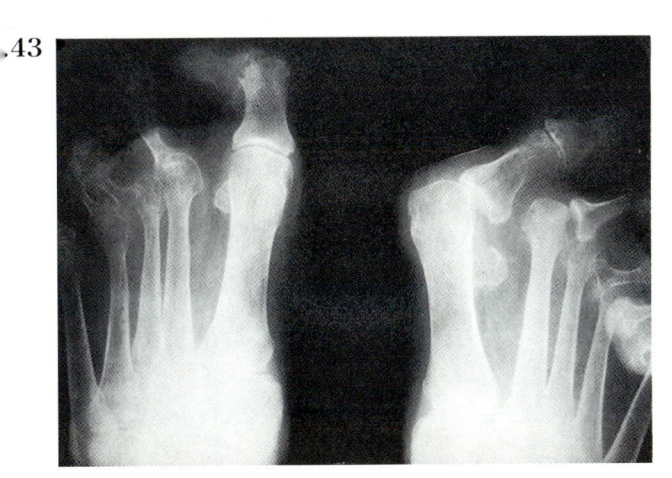

6.43 Radiographic presentation of severe dislocating rheumatoid arthritis in the feet.

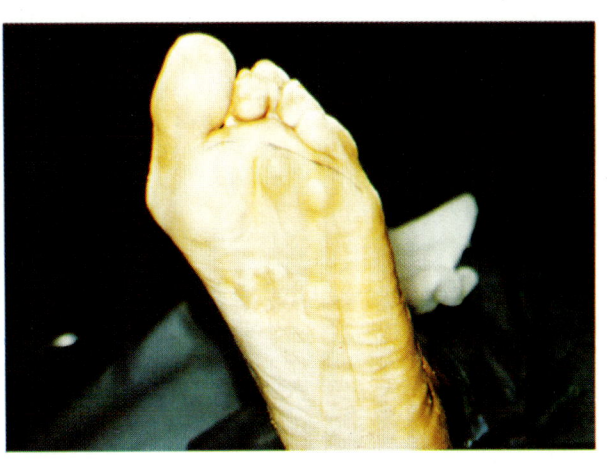

6.45 In selected cases, an arched plantar foot incision may be performed to provide access to the metatarsal heads for resection shaft.

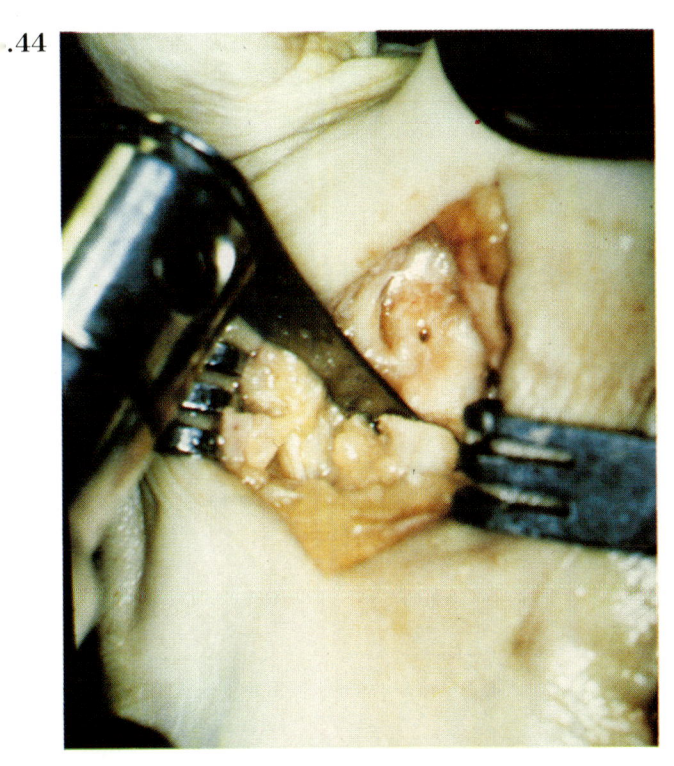

6.44 Resection of the metatarsal head is performed in such a manner as to decrease plantar pressure from the remaining metatarsal shaft.

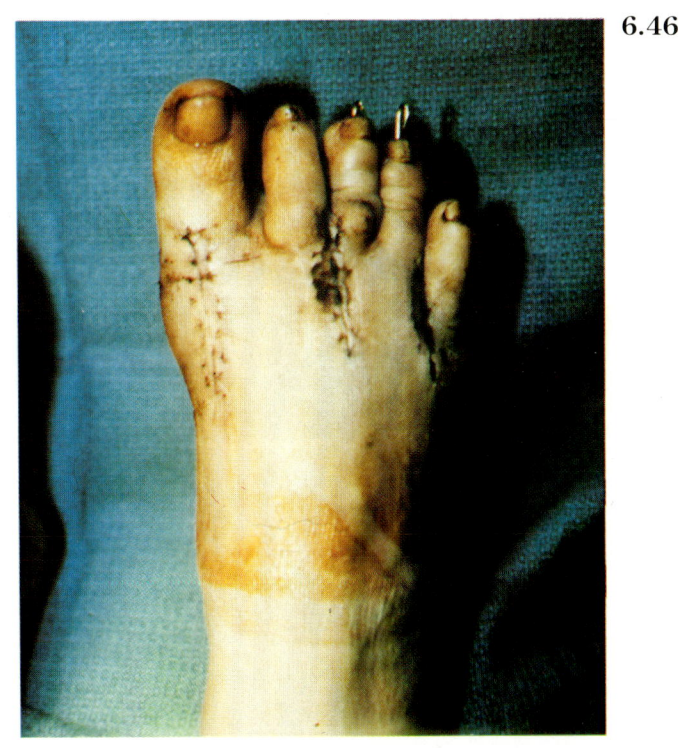

6.46 Post-operative status following three-incision approach panmetatarsal head resection procedure.

Lesser metatarsal implants

Implant arthroplasty of the lesser metatarsophalangeal joint prior to 1970 was being done to alleviate symptoms associated with plantar keratomas. Osseous procedures devised at that time had specific undesirable complications and many surgeons felt that implant arthroplasty was a good alternative.[96,97]

Most reports in the sixties were isolated uses of the duralumin implant devised by Seeburger.[96,98–100] The procedure lost popularity because of technical difficulties in implant design, lack of understanding of biomechanical function, and host response.

By the early seventies, it became apparent to most researchers that implant arthroplasty of the lesser metatarsals for plantar keratoma should be abandoned in favour of their use in joint arthrosis.[101] They regained popularity in the eighties with a better understanding of implant design, biomechanical function, and improved biomaterials.[102–104]

Currently, the role of implant arthroplasty of the lesser metatarsals is still not fully appreciated. Overutilization is common and no definitive criteria have been established. In isolated cases of flail toes or degenerative arthritis such as Freiberg's infraction, these implants can serve a useful purpose (**6.47**). Good, sound clinical judgement must be exercised to determine the benefit of using these implants rather than performing joint reconstruction.

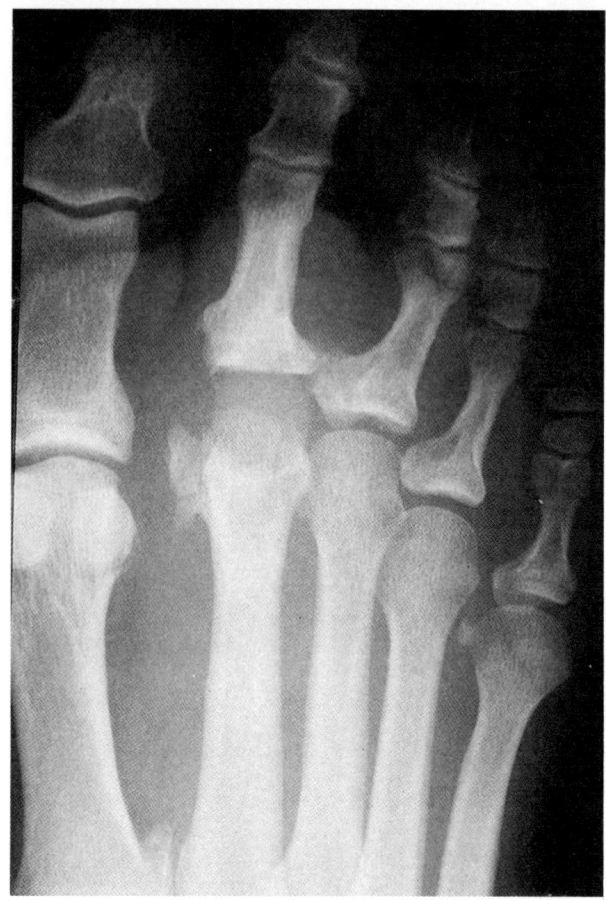

6.47 Post-operative status following condylar joint implant in second metatarsal head for treatment of Freiberg's infraction.

References

[1] McCarthy, D.J. Anatomy. *In* McGlamry, E.D. (ed.). *Fundamentals of Foot Surgery*. Baltimore, Williams & Wilkins, 1987, p.3.
[2] Sarrafian, S.K. *Anatomy of the Foot & Ankle*. Philadelphia, Lippincott, 1983, p.73.
[3] Anderson, J.E. *In* Chapt. 4: The lower limb. *Grant's Atlas of Anatomy*, 7th edn, Baltimore, Williams & Wilkins, 1978.
[4] Root, M.L., et al. *Clinical Biomechanics, Vol. II: Normal and Abnormal Function of the Foot*, 1st edn. Los Angeles, Clinical Biomechanics Corp., 1977, pp.367–371.
[5] Mann, R.A. (ed.). *DuVries' Surgery of the Foot*, 4th edn. St. Louis, C.V. Mosby, 1978, pp.251–252.
[6] Hardcastle, P.H., Reschauer, R., Kutcha-Lissberg, E. and Schoffman, W. Injuries to the tarsometatarsal joint, incident, classification, and treatment. *J. Bone Joint Surg.*, **64B**: 349, 1982.
[7] Devas, M. *Stress Fractures*. London, Churchill-Livingstone, 1975.
[8] McGlamry, E.D. (ed.) *Fundamentals of Foot Surgery*. Baltimore, Williams & Wilkins, 1987, p.71.
[9] Sarrafian, S.K. *Anatomy of the Foot and Ankle*. Philadelphia, Lippincott, 1983, p.247.
[10] Sarrafian, S.K., and Topouzian, L.K. Anatomy and physiology of the extensor apparatus of the toes. *J. Bone Joint Surg.*, **51**: 669, 1969.
[11] Root, M.L. *Clinical Biomechanics, Vol. II: Normal and Abnormal Function of the Foot*, 1st edn. Los Angeles, Clinical Biomechanics Corp., 1977, pp.46, 80.
[12] Basmajian, J.V. and Stecko, P. Role of muscles in arch support of the foot. *J. Bone Joint Surg.*, **45A**: 1184–1190, 1963.
[13] Jarrett, B.A., Manz, J.A. and Green, D.R. Interossei and lumbrical muscles of the foot, anatomical and functional study. *J. Am. Podiatry Assoc.*, **70**: 1–13, 1980.
[14] Meisenbach, R.O. Painful anterior arch of the foot and operation for its relief by means of raising the arch. *Am. J. Orthop. Surg.*, **14**: 206, 1916.
[15] Davis, G.F. Cure for hallux valgus: The interdigital incision. *Surg. Clin. North Am.*, **1**: 651, 1917.
[16] Mau, C. Eine operation des kontrakten spreizfusses. *Zbl. Chir.*, **67**: 667, 1940.
[17] Dickson, J.A. Surgical treatment of intractable plantar warts. *J. Bone Joint Surg.*, **30**: 757, 1948.
[18] Borggrene, J. Sur operation behandling dis kontraken spreizfusses zeitsch. *Orthop. Grenzzb.*, **78**: 581, 1949.
[19] McKeever, D.C. Arthrodesis of the first metatarsal phalangeal joint for hallux valgus, hallux rigidus, and metatarsus primus adductus. *J. Bone Joint Surg.*, **34A**: 129, 1952.
[20] DuVries, H.L. New approach to treatment of intractable verrucae plantaris. *J. Am. Med. Assoc.*, **152**: 1202, 1953.
[21] Giannestras, N.J. Shortening of the metatarsal shaft for the correction of plantar keratosis. *Clin. Orthop.*, **4**: 225–231, 1954.
[22] Giannestras, N.J. Shortening of the metatarsal shaft in the treatment of plantar keratosis. *J. Bone Joint Surg.*, **40**: 61–71, 1958.
[23] Davidson, M.R. A simple method for correcting second, third, and fourth plantar metatarsal head pathology—especially intractable keratomas. *J. Foot Surg.*, **8**: 23–26, 1969.
[24] Jacoby, R.P. V-osteotomy for correction of intractable plantar keratosis. *J. Foot Surg.*, **12**: 8, 1973.
[25] Sgarlato, T.E. *A Compendium of Podiatric Biomechanics*. San Francisco, California College of Podiatric Medicine, 1971.
[26] Bartel, P.F. Lesser metatarsal osteotomy. *J. Am. Podiatry Assoc.*, **67**: 358–360, 1977.
[27] Jimenez, A.L. Oblique 'V' lesser metatarsal osteotomy. *In* Schlefman, B.S. (ed.), Doctors Hospital Podiatric Education and Research Institute, Twelfth Surgical Seminar Syllabus, Tucker, O.A., Doctors Hospital Podiatry Institute, 1983, p.82.
[28] Suppan, R. The cartilagenous articulation preservation principle and its surgical implication for hallux abducto valgus. *J. Am. Podiatry Assoc.*, **64**: 635–656, 1974.
[29] Kuwada, G.T., Dockery, G.L. and Schuberth, J.M. The resistant, painful plantar lesion: a surgical approach. *J. Foot Surg.*, **1**: 29–32, 1983.
[30] McGlamry, E.D., Mahan, K.T. and Green, D.R. Pes valgo planus deformity. *In* McGlamry, E.D. (ed.), *Comprehensive Textbook of Foot Surgery, Vol. I*. Baltimore, Williams & Wilkins, 1987, pp.412–418.
[31] Jack, E.A. Naviculocuneiform fusion in the treatment of flatfoot. *J. Bone Surg.*, **57B**: 279, 1975.
[32] Forrester, D.M. *Imaging of the Foot and Ankle*. A. Aspen Publication, 1988, pp.283–313.
[33] Dorfman, G.R. Determination of treatment in fractures of the fifth metatarsal shaft. *J. Foot Surg.*, **17**: 16–21, 1978.
[34] Muller, M.E., Allgower, M., Schneider, R. and Willenegger, H. *Manual of Internal Fixation*, 2nd edn. Berlin, Springer-Verlag, 1979.
[35] Maxwell, J.R. Open or closed treatment of metatarsal fractures, indications and techniques. *J. Am. Podiatry Assoc.*, **73**: 100–106, 1983.
[36] Laurich, L.J., Witt, C.S. and Zielsdorf, L.M. Treatment of fractures of the fifth metatarsal bone. *J. Foot Surg.*, **22**: 207–211, 1983.
[37] Giannestras, N.J. and Sammarco, G.J. Fractures and dislocations in the foot. *In* Rockwood, C.A., Jr. and Green, D.P. (eds), *Fracture*. Philadelphia, J.B. Lippincott, 1975.
[38] Jones, R. Fractures of the base of the fifth metatarsal bone by indirect violence. *Am. Surg.*, **35**: 697–702, 1902.
[39] Rao, J.P. and Banzon, M.T. Irreducible dislocation of the metatarsal phalangeal joints of the foot. *Clin. Orthop.*, **145**: 224–226, 1979.

[40] Kavanaugh, J.H., Brower, T.O. and Mann, R.V. The Jones fracture revisited. *J. Bone Joint Surg.*, **60A**: 776–782, 1978.
[41] Torg, J.S., *et al.* Fractures of the base of the fifth metatarsal distal to the tuberosity. *J. Bone Joint Surg.*, **66-A**: 209–214, 1984.
[42] Pritsch, M., Heim, M., Tauber, H. and Horoszowski, H. An unusual fracture of the base of the fifth metatarsal bone. *J. Trauma*, **20**: 530–531, 1980.
[43] McGlamry, E.D. and Cooper, C.T. Brachymetatarsia: a surgical treatment. *J. Am. Podiatry Assoc.*, **59**: 259–264, 1969.
[44] McGlamry, E.D. and Fenton, C.F. Brachymetatarsia: a case report. *J. Am. Podiatry Assoc.*, **73**: 75–78, 1983.
[45] Tachdijian, M.O. *The Child's Foot.* Philadelphia, W.B. Saunders, 1985, pp. 314–317.
[46] Morton, D. *The Human Foot.* New York, Columbia University Press, 1935.
[47] Harris, R.I. and Beath, T. *Report 1574, Army Foot Survey.* Ottawa, National Research Council of Canada, 1947.
[48] Page, J.C., Dockery, G.L. and Vance, C.E. Brachymetatarsia with brachymesodactyly. *J. Foot Surg.*, **22**: 104–107, 1983.
[49] Freiberg, A.H. Infraction of the second metatarsal bone, a typical injury. *Surg. Gynec. Obstet.*, **19**: 191, 1914.
[50] Braddock, G.T.F. Experimental epiphyseal injury and Freiberg's disease. *J. Bone Joint Surg.*, **41**: 154, 1959.
[51] Jimenez, A.L., McGlamry, E.D. and Green, D.R. Lesser ray deformities. *In* McGlamry, E.D. (ed.), *Comprehensive Textbook of Foot Surgery*, Vol. I. Baltimore, Williams & Wilkins, 1987, pp. 75–76.
[52] Smillie, I.S. Freiberg's infraction (Koehler's second disease). *J. Bone Joint Surg.*, **37**: 580, 1955.
[53] Smillie, I.S. Treatment of Freiberg's infraction. *Proc. Roy. Soc., Lond. (Biol.)*, **60**: 29–31, 1967.
[54] Schwartz, N., Williams, J.E. and Marcinko, D.E. Double oblique lesser metatarsal osteotomy: A photographic essay. *J. Am. Podiatry Assoc.*, **73**: 218–220, 1983.
[55] Addante, J.B. Metatarsal osteotomy as an office procedure to eradicate intractable plantar keratosis. *J. Am. Podiatry Assoc.*, **60**: 397–399, 1970.
[56] Jacoby, R.P. V-osteoplasty for correction of intractable plantar keratosis. *J. Foot Surg.*, **12**: 8–10, 1973.
[57] Yu, G.V. Surgical management of metatarsus adductus deformity. *Clin. Podiatric Med. Surg.*, **4**: 207–232, 1987.
[58] Heyman, C.H., Herndon, C.H. and Strong, J.M. Mobilization of the tarsometatarsal and intermetatarsal joints for the correction of resistant adduction of the forepart of the foot in congenital clubfoot or congenital metatarsus varus. *J. Bone Joint Surg.*, **40A**: 299, 1958.
[59] Lichtblau, S. Section of the abductor hallucis tendon for correction of metatarsus varus deformity. *Clin. Orthop.*, 110–227, 1975.
[60] Thomson, S.A. Hallux varus and metatarsus varus. *Clin. Orthop.*, **16**: 109, 1960.
[61] Bankart, B. Metatarsus varus. *Br. Med. J.*, **2**: 685, 1921.
[62] Peabody, C.W. and Muro, F. Congenital metatarsus varus. *J. Bone Joint Surg.*, **15**: 171, 1933.
[63] McCormick, D. and Blount, W.P. Metatarsus adducto varus. *JAMA*, **141**: 449, 1949.
[64] Steytler, J.C.S. and VanDerWalt, I.D. Correction of resistant adduction of the forefoot in congenital club foot and congenital metatarsus varus by metatarsal osteotomy. *Br. J. Surg.*, **53**: 558, 1966.
[65] Berman, A. and Gartland, J.J. Metatarsal osteotomy for the correction of adduction of the fore part of the foot in children. *J. Bone Joint Surg.*, **53A**: 498, 1971.
[66] Giannestras, N.J. *Foot Disorders: Medical and Surgical Management.* 2nd edn. Philadelphia, Lea & Febiger, 1976.
[67] Mann, R. and Inman, V. Phasic activity of intrinsic muscles of the foot. *J. Bone Joint Surg.*, **46A**: 469–481, 1964.
[68] Dockery, G.L. Surgical treatment of the symptomatic juvenile flexible flatfoot condition. *Clin. Podiatric Med. Surg.*, **4**: 99–117, 1987.
[69] Green, D.R., Ruch, J.A. and McGlamry, E.D. Correction of equinus related forefoot deformities. *J. Am. Podiatry Assoc.*, **66**: 768–779, 1976.
[70] Schwartzmann, J.R. The surgical management of foot deformities in rheumatoid arthritis. *Clin. Orthop.*, **36**: 86, 1964.
[71] Sim-Fook, L. and Hodgson, A.R. A comparison of foot forms among the non-shoe and shoe wearing Chinese population. *J. Bone Joint Surg.*, **40A**: 1058–1062, 1958.
[72] Kilikian, H. *Hallux Valgus and Allied Deformities of the Forefoot and Metatarsalgia.* Philadelphia, W.B. Saunders, 1965.
[73] Wynne-Davies, R. Family studies and the cause of congenital clubfoot, talipes equinovarus, talipes calcaneo valgus and metatarsus varus. *J. Bone Joint Surg.*, **46B**: 445, 1964.
[74] Bishop, J., Kahan, A. and Turba, J.E. Surgical correction of the splay-foot: the Giannestras procedure. *Clin. Orthop.*, **146**: 234–238, 1980.
[75] Davies, H. Metatarsus quintus valgus. *Br. Med. J.*, **1**: 664–665, 1949.
[76] Lilievre, J. L'exostose de le 5 tete metatarsiene. *Le Concours Medical*, **78**: 4815–4816, 1956.
[77] Yancey, H.A. Congenital lateral bowing of the fifth metatarsal. *Clin. Orthop.*, **62**: 203–205, 1969.
[78] Leach, R.E. and Iyou, R. Metatarsal osteotomy for bunionette deformity. *Clin. Orthop.*, **100**: 171–175, 1974.
[79] Silverskiold, N. Metatarsus latus and hallux valgus. *Acta Chir. Scand.*, **61**: 543–560, 1927.
[80] Haines, R.W. The mechanics of the metatarsus in spread foot. *Chir.*, **2**: 197–209, 1947.
[81] Shoenhaus, I.T., Rotman, S. and Meshon, A.L. A review of normal intermetatarsal angle. *J. Am. Podiatry Assoc.*, **63**: 88–95, 1973.
[82] Fallat, L.M. and Buckholz, J.L. An analysis of the tailor's bunion by radiographic and anatomic display. *J. Am. Podiatry Assoc.*, **70**: 597–603, 1980.
[83] Sponsel, K.H. Bunionette correction by metatarsal osteotomy. *Orthop. Clin. N. Am.*, **7**: 809–819, 1976.

[84] Throckmorton, J.K. and Bradlee, N. Transverse V sliding osteotomy: a new surgical procedure for the correction of tailor's bunion deformity. *J. Foot Surg.*, **18**: 117–121, 1978.

[85] Berlin, S.J. A laboratory review of 67,000 foot tumors and lesions. *J. Am. Podiatry Assoc.*, **74**: 341–347, 1984.

[86] Lodwick, G.S. The bones and joints. *In* Hodes, P.J. (ed.), *Atlas of Tumor Radiology*. Chicago, Year Book Medical Publ., 1971.

[87] Yale, I. *The Arthritic Foot and Related Connective Tissue Disorders*. Baltimore, Williams & Wilkins, 1984, pp. 212–257.

[88] Hoffman, P. An operation for severe grades of contracted or clawed toes. *Am. J. Orthop. Surg.*, **9**: 441, 1911.

[89] Clayton, M.L. Surgery of the lower extremity in rheumatoid arthritis. *J. Bone Joint Surg.*, **45A**: 1517–1536, 1963.

[90] Cracchiolo, A. Management of the arthritic forefoot. *Foot Ankle*, **3**: 17–23, 1982.

[91] Freed, J.B. Alternative approaches to replacement of lesser metatarsal heads. *J. Foot Surg.*, **18**: 26–30, 1979.

[92] Gould, N. Surgery of the forepart of the foot in rheumatoid arthritis. *Foot Ankle*, **3**: 173–180, 1982.

[93] MacClean, C.R. and Silver, W.A. Dwyer's operation for the rheumatoid forefoot. *Foot Ankle*, **1**: 343, 1981.

[94] Hodor, L. and Dobbs, B. Pan metatarsal head resection. *J. Am. Podiatry Assoc.*, **73**: 287, 1983.

[95] Lipscomb, P.R., Benson, G.M. and Jones, D.A. Resection of the proximal phalanges and metatarsal condyles for deformities of the forefoot due to rheumatoid arthritis. *Clin. Orthop.*, **82**: 24, 1972.

[96] Seeburger, R. Surgical implants of alloyed metal in joints of the feet. *J. Am. Podiatry Assoc.*, **54**: 391–396, 1964.

[97] Kaplan, B.R. and Cohen, S.J. The use of the Calnan–Nicolle prosthesis for metatarsophalangeal joint replacement: a preliminary study. *J. Am. Podiatry Assoc.*, **66**: 165–172, 1976.

[98] Downey, M.A. A ball and socket metal prosthetic joint replacement as applied to the foot. *J. Am. Podiatry Assoc.*, **55**: 343–346, 1965.

[99] Myers, M.M. A four year observation of Freiberg's infraction. *J. Foot Surg.*, **6**: 185–188, 1967.

[100] Scioli, E.R. Metal prosthetic implantation for deformed lesser metatarsophalangeal joint. *J. Foot Surg.*, **6**: 105–106, 1967.

[101] McGlamry, E.D. and Ruch, J.A. Status of implant arthroplasty of the lesser metatarso phalangeal joints. *J. Am. Podiatry Assoc.*, **66**: 155–164, 1976.

[102] Swanson, A.B. Evolution and testing of flexible implants. *In* Swanson, A.B. (ed.), *Flexible Implant Resection Arthroplasty in the Hand and Extremities*. St. Louis, C.V. Mosby, 1973, p. 32.

[103] Sgarlato, T. A new implant for the metatarsophalangeal joint. *Clinics Podiatric Med. Surg.*, **1**: 69–77, 1984.

[104] Lawrence, B.R. and Papier, M.J. Implant arthroplasty of the lesser metatarsophalangeal joint—a modified technique. *J. Foot Surg.*, **19**: 16–19, 1980.

7 Surgery of the lesser digits

GERALD T. KUWADA

Surgical principles

Prior to any surgical considerations, it is necessary and prudent to obtain a complete history and physical from the patient, which includes determination of the neurovascular status of the lesser digits. If there is questionable vascular patency, circulatory assessment in the form of digital plethysmography or Doppler ankle–arm indices is indicated. If the neurovascular status is within normal limits and no other serious disease afflicts the patient (i.e. diabetes mellitus, arteriosclerosis obliterans, vasospastic disease), the surgeon can proceed to plan the digital correction.

Part of the plan should include performing surgical principles such as atraumatic technique, maintaining asepsis during the operation, using proper instrumentation, and ligating all bleeders. Keeping the digital tissues well hydrated by repeatedly flushing the exposed tissue with saline or lactated Ringer's solution is also important. Additionally, reducing tissue exposure by keeping the operation time as short as possible, and proper suture closure of tissue planes and skin will help establish a good end result.

Atraumatic technique

Atraumatic technique is an attitude of utmost respect towards tissue handling. Rough and careless handling of tissue adds to the unnecessary destruction of cells, requiring replacement and resulting in longer healing time. Proper use of instrumentation is an integral part of atraumatic technique. Furthermore, intimate familiarity with surgical anatomy is foremost in the application of atraumatic principles of surgery. Unnecessary injury or irreversible damage to neurovascular structures due to careless pre-operative surgical planning and technique is a prime example of violating atraumatic principles. It is therefore necessary to review the surgical anatomy of the lesser digits before presenting an in-depth discussion of the surgical procedures.

Surgical anatomy

The largest organ of the human body is the skin. Prior to surgery it is important to note the overall condition of the skin, including its texture, turgor, warmth, and sensitivity. Although the presence of hair on the digits is usually indicative of good or normal circulatory status, the absence of digital hair, especially in females, does not automatically imply poor circulation. In many Western cultures, hair removal is common to enhance the appearance of the feet. The condition of the nail may also reflect the overall general health of the patient.

Certainly any history of injury or fungal infections of the toes needs to be noted in the patient's history and physical examination. The nail plate, which is roughly accumulated keratin, is attached to the vascular nail bed inferiorly. The nail matrix is found laterally and proximally to the nail itself. This is where the nail plate

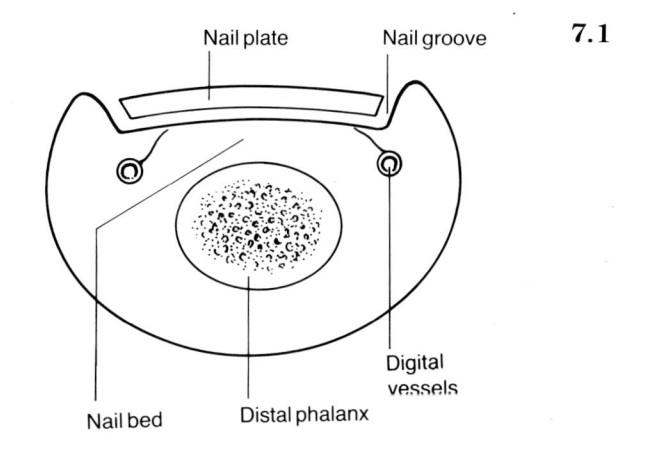

7.1 Cross-section of nail plate and bed area with nutrient blood supply.

grows from, and the lunula, a portion of the matrix, proximally attaches to the portion of the nail called the eponychium. The distal aspect of the nail plate is called the hyponychium. The nail bed receives its circulation from branches of the digital arteries (**7.1**).

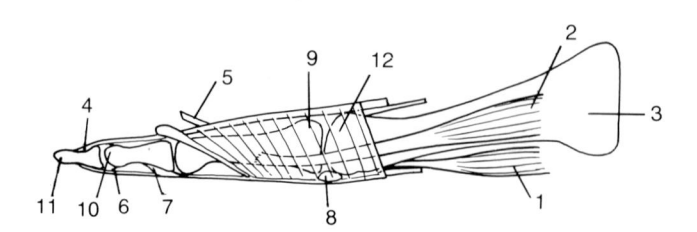

7.2

1 Lumbricale	7 Flexor digitorum brevis
2 Interossei	8 Transverse metatarsal ligament
3 Metatarsal	9 Proximal phalanx
4 Extensor digitorum longus	10 Intermediate phalanx
5 Extensor digitorum brevis	11 Distal phalanx
6 Flexor digitorum longus	12 Extensor hood apparatus

7.2 Side view of the digital intrinsic muscular structures of the extensor hood.

As we proceed proximally and dorsally, the tissue layers are skin, subcutaneous tissue, superficial fascia, extensor longus and brevis, and the extensor hood mechanism. The extensor hood is located over the proximal phalangeal joint, which includes capsule, medial and collateral ligaments, all of which contribute to the extensor hood function. The osseous structures are also noted, including the distal, intermediate, and proximal phalanges. Plantarly, there are the flexor longus and brevis tendons, the plantar capsule, and the plantar flexor tendon plate. Other anatomical structures, such as the dorsal and plantar interossei and the lumbricals, are also found. A side view of the digital intrinsic musculature structures of the extensor hood is shown in **7.2**.

Nail anatomy

The nail plate is primarily keratogenous material derived from the nail matrix, where there are essentially three germinal sites. The dorsal plate is formed from the upper nail root matrix, the intermediate nail is formed from the lower matrix, and a relatively thin ventral plate is derived from the nail bed. At the base of the nail, there is a region called the lunula, which is primarily less vascular and not as firmly adherent to the nail plate. Proximally, where the nail plate attaches to the matrix, is an area called the eponychium. Distally, where the nail plate adheres to the nail bed, is an area called the hyponychium. The deepest portion of the epidermis fuses with the periosteum of the distal phalanx.

The hyponychium, a thickened portion of the epidermis, that is primarily under the free edge of the nail plate, becomes continuous with the germinal layer of the nail bed. The nail groove is a furrow between the nail bed and the nail wall. At the bottom of the groove the epidermis loses all of its germinative layer and continues on to the undersurface of the nail plate (**7.3**).

There are many indications for the use of matrixectomy procedures to eliminate the matrix and nail plate. The primary indications include onychocryptosis, more commonly known as ingrown toenails; onychomycosis, or fungal nails; onychauxis, or thickened toenails; onychogryphosis and onychodystrophic toenails, or deformed toenails; and onycholysis, or separated toenail. Matrixectomy procedures can essentially be classified into three categories. Chemocautery techniques, of which there are several, cauterize the matrix and allow for permanent resolution of nail problems. The author prefers to use 89% carbolic acid or phenol. The goal of the technique is to expose and destroy the matrix tissue by using a cauterizing agent, thus eliminating nail plate growth. Another successful technique is the use of negative galvanism, in which an electrical current is applied to the matrix until the matrix is liquefied and sodium hydroxide is produced. It is the sodium hydroxide that cauterizes the matrix cells.

Other surgeons have modified these techniques by curetting the matrix after the chemocautery procedure to ensure that all matrix cells have been successfully eliminated. The second category is osteotripsy. In this technique, a high-speed burr is applied directly to the matrix, destroying it. The area is then curetted with a rasp to ensure all matrix cells have been eliminated. The third category is surgical ablation.

Surgical ablation

In this very common technique, employed in the permanent resolution of nail conditions, the matrix is exposed after an incision is made through the skin layer. The matrix is then completely dissected from the periosteum and, using a rasp, the area is smoothed. There are many surgical ablative techniques: laser matrixectomy is a recent technique that uses a laser to eliminate the nail matrix. Regardless of the type of laser used, the principle is essentially the same: burning or vaporizing the matrix cells. A burn is created and must be treated, as with other chemocautery techniques, post-operatively.

The overall efficacy of this procedure, however, is questionable; at this time, it does not appear to be superior to any of the more traditional techniques. The cost of the laser apparatus is exorbitant compared with that of instruments used in other matrixectomy techniques. There are also hazards in using the laser apparatus: training and extreme care are required. For these reasons, laser surgery is not currently being utilized by members of the surgical teaching staff of the Waldo Podiatric Residency Training Program in Seattle, Washington.

Phenol matrixectomy

After the digit has been anaesthetized and prepped and draped in the usual sterile manner, the offending nail—whether the procedure is a partial or total matrixectomy—is removed by nail avulsion. Either 89% carbolic acid or phenol is placed on a cotton tip applicator and applied directly to the matrix tissues for a total of 4 min. The total chemical exposure varies from surgeon to surgeon and ranges from three separate 15-second exposures to two exposures of 2 min each (which is the author's preference).

The phenol area is flushed with alcohol, and depending on surgeon preference, curettage may also be performed at this time. The wound is packed with either an antibiotic ointment or a hydrocortisone cream to treat the burn created by the chemical. The toe is then dressed in the usual sterile manner, and the patient is given post-operative instructions, including foot-soak instructions (primarily, using a solution of sodium chloride or of magnesium sulphate). The patient is instructed to soak once or twice a day post-operatively to ensure that there are no complications and that the area is healing properly. Patients are seen regularly, until at least six months post-operatively, to rule out any recurrence of the onychocryptosis or complications.

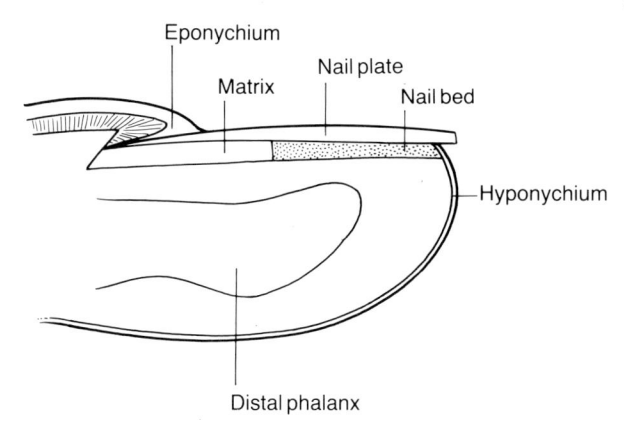

7.3 Side view cross-section of distal phalanx, showing nail anatomy.

Negative galvanism

The patient is prepared in the same manner as described for phenol matrixectomy. Once the anaesthetic status of the digit has been established, the negative galvanism probe or sabre is placed directly onto the matrix to be destroyed. The grounding pad and connecting cables must also be checked to ensure proper connection and application of the grounding pad.

Typically, the electrogalvanic generator has a time unit that allows the current to be administered for several minutes. The length of time depends on the procedure being employed: for example, with partial matrixectomies, the electric current should be applied to the matrix cells for approximately 2 min. With total matrixectomies, the probe should be applied for approximately 3–4 min. Next, the nail groove is irrigated with acetic acid, followed by saline. The toe is then painted with either a povidone-iodine solution or benzalkonium chloride and then dressed in the usual sterile manner.

Surgical ablation for matrixectomies

Operative technique

The following is an operative description for a partial matrixectomy of the lesser toenails. After the toe has been anaesthetized with a local anaesthetic and prepped and draped in the usual sterile manner, a partial nail avulsion is performed on the affected nail border (**7.4**). An incision is made approximately at the eponychium and extended lateral–proximal. The matrix is exposed, proximal and lateral, and excised totally. The bone is rasped smooth of any remaining matrix cells and then copiously flushed with a sterile saline-type solution. The incision is then closed with a 4-0 or 5-0 nonabsorbable suture of choice (**7.5**), and the wound is placed in a sterile dressing.

If an infection is suspected or there is a previous history of infection, an antibiotic flush may be used. The patient is seen post-operatively, where the dressings are removed. The sutures are removed in approximately 7–14 days. The patient is then allowed to bathe the foot and apply lotion to the incision site. Patients are seen at six months to one year post-operatively to ensure there is no recurrence of the nail plate or nail border.

Several other types of partial surgical matrixectomies have been described and are still popular with foot surgeons (**7.6–7.8**).

With regard to total matrixectomy, numerous operative techniques are employed to remove the entire nail plate permanently (**7.9–7.12**). The author utilizes a modified Zadik or Suppan technique in which the toenail has been avulsed from the lunula, proximally to the end of the matrix, and extending laterally and medially. The entire matrix is excised and the area rasped smooth of any remaining matrix and copiously flushed with a saline or antibiotic solution. The skin is then re-approximated to the remaining nail bed with a combination of a horizontal mattress and simple interrupted sutures, using a 4-0 or 5-0 nonabsorbable suture. The toe is then sterilely dressed and, at about 10–14 days post-operatively, the sutures may be removed.

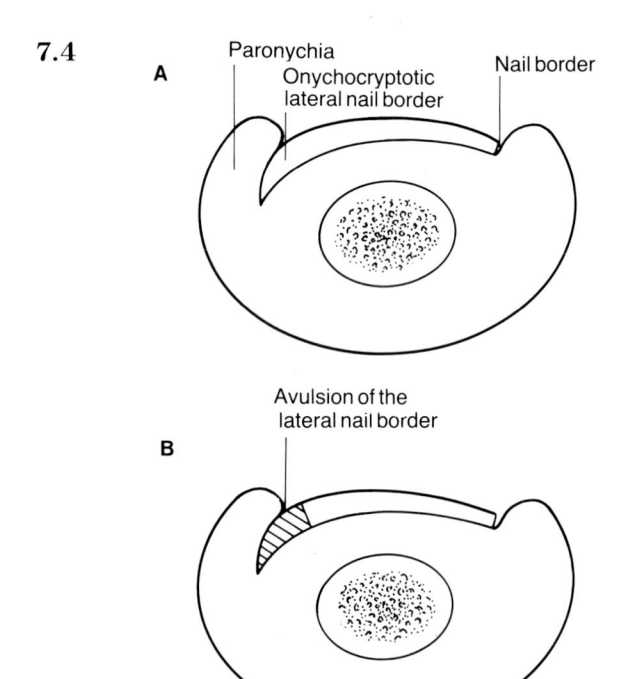

7.4 Cross-section of ingrown toenail (A) and area of nail avulsion (B).

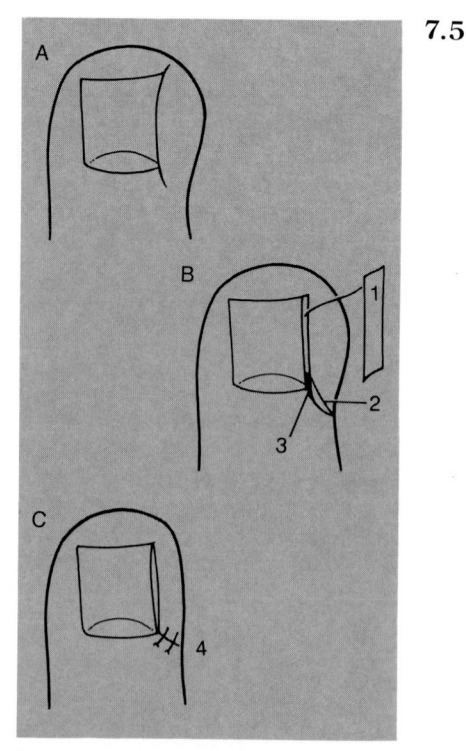

7.5 Partial nail avulsion with the partial matrixectomy procedure. A, Paronychia with onychocryptosis. B, Nail avulsion performed (1), incision exposes matrix (2), and excision of matrix (3). C, Non-absorbable suture used to reapproximate wound edges (4).

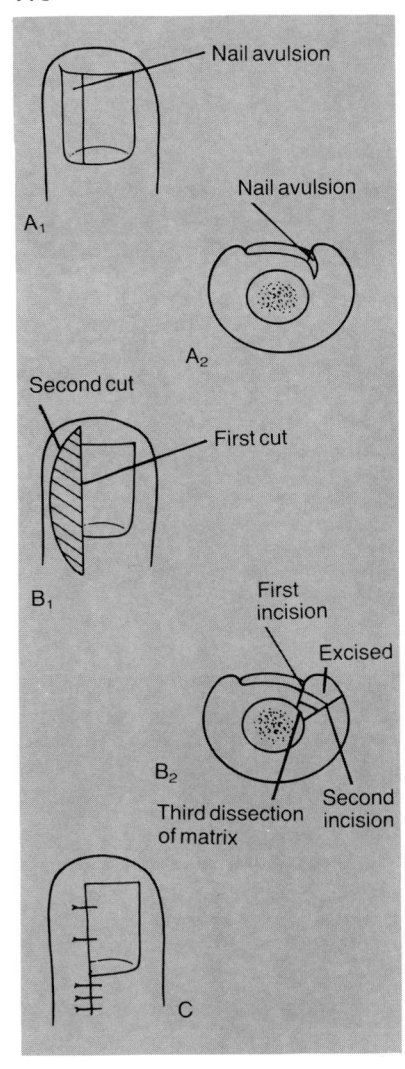

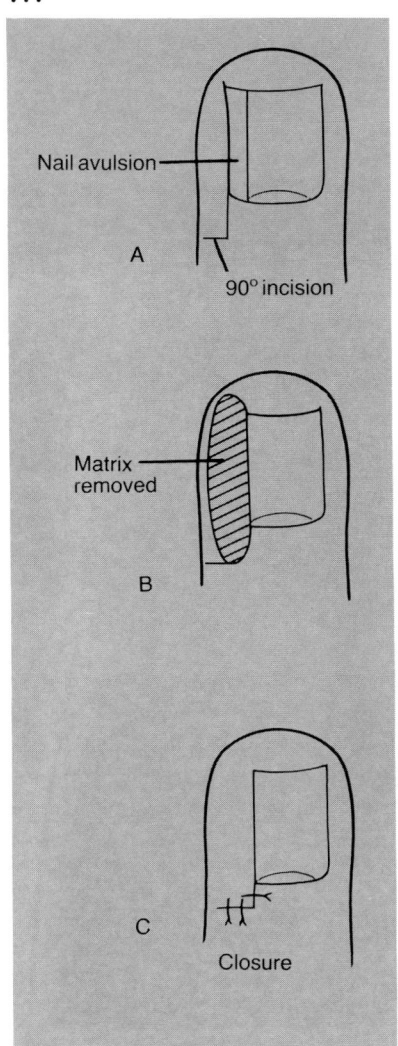

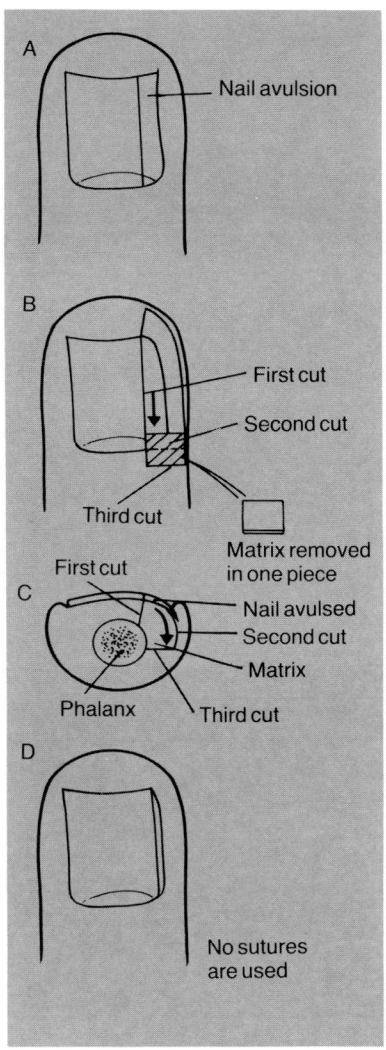

7.6 Winograd technique. A₁, Dorsal view—partial nail avulsion procedure. A₂, Cross-section of partial nail avulsion. B₁, Wedge resection of skin, nail bed, and nail groove down to phalanx, followed by dissection of matrix material. B₂, Cross-section of wedge resection. C, Dorsal view, with final suture closure of wedge resection incision.

7.7 Frost technique. A, Nail avulsion procedure with proximal nail skin incision made at 90°. B, Incision opened and matrixectomy performed. C, Flap suture closure.

7.8 Suppan nail technique 1. A, Nail avulsion procedure. B, First incision through the nail bed and under the proximal nail fold (no skin incision is made); second incision is carried out along the medial or lateral nail border; the third incision is placed behind (proximal to) the matrix material; the matrix is then excised as a unit. C, Cross-section showing angle of incisions. D, Final appearance without skin incisions prior to sterile dressings.

Results of matrixectomy procedures

In a 10-year follow-up study of 511 Steindler procedures the author found a 1% recurrence rate, a 4% infection rate, and a 3% scar rate. With the phenol–alcohol technique in 94 procedures, there was a 4% recurrence rate, a 3% infection rate, and a 2% scar rate. In 128 total matrixectomies, there was a 4% recurrence rate, a 5% infection rate, and a 2% scar rate. To be included in this retrospective study, the patient had to be seen at least one year postoperatively. No other complications were noted in these three techniques.

In summary, the overall results indicate that certain

procedures are more effective in eliminating the nail condition than others. Certainly, the overall success rate mainly depends upon the surgeon's skill and thoroughness in eliminating the matrix cells and in avoiding complications by using the correct techniques.

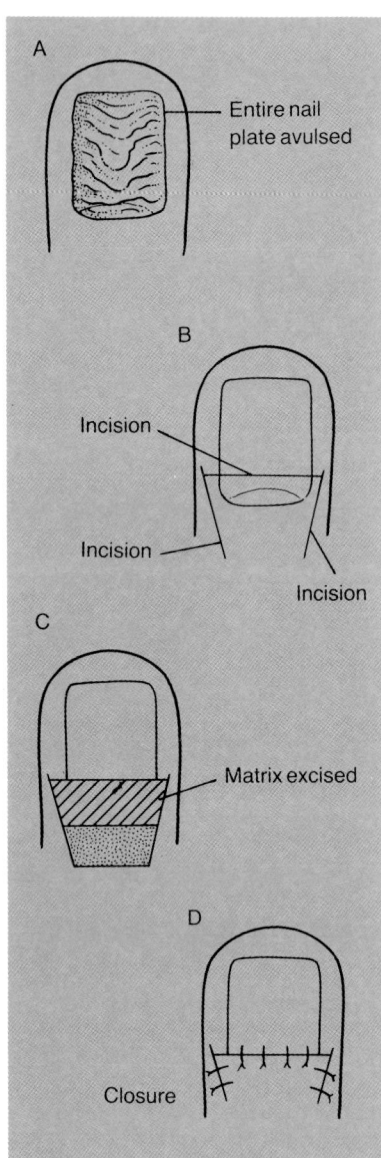

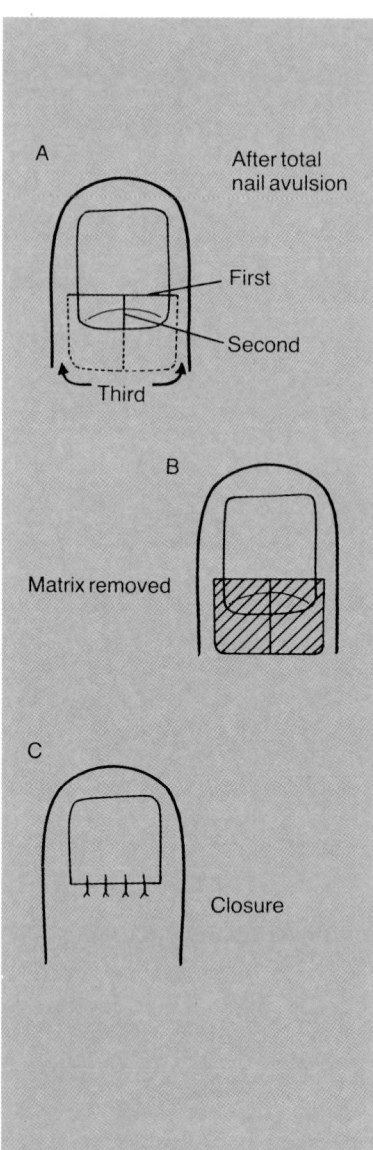

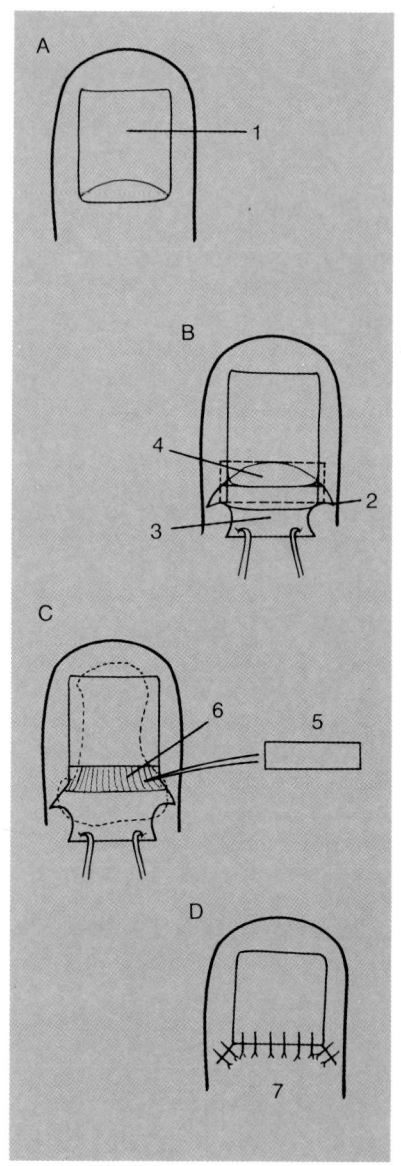

7.9 Zadik total nail technique. A, Thickened nail is totally avulsed. B, Three incisions are placed, as illustrated. C, Proximal portion of the incision flap is retracted to expose the underlying matrix, which is removed. D, Final suture closure.

7.10 Suppan nail technique 2. A, Incisions placed in the nail bed after the nail has been totally avulsed; dotted lines represent incisions placed under the skin. B, Total matrixectomy is performed. C, Final suture closure.

7.11 Kuwada technique for total matrixectomy. A, Total nail avulsion is perfomed (1). B, Skin and nail bed incisions are placed and the matrix is incised: two 1-cm incisions are made (2), skin is retracted proximally with skin hooks (3), and matrix is excised completely (4). C, Total matrixectomy is performed and the phalanx is rasped: matrix is removed (5) and bone is rasped to eliminate matrix (6). D, Final closure of incisions: suture with nonabsorbable sutures (7).

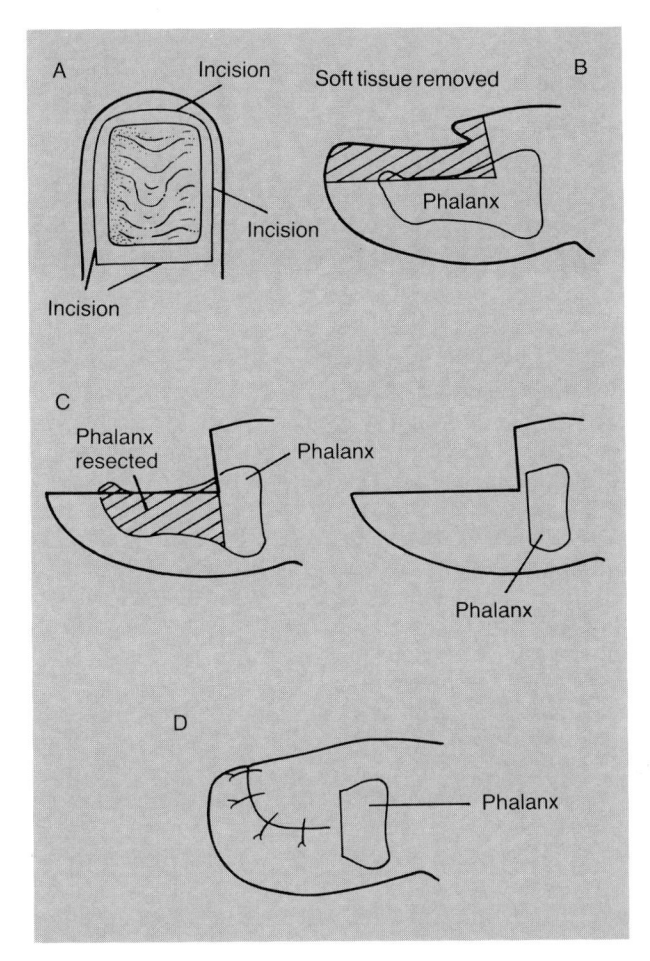

7.12 Lapidus technique. A, The entire periphery of the nail is incised deep to the bone. B, Side cross-section showing depth of incisions with tissue to be excised. C, Resection of the exposed distal phalanx. D, Post-resection of nail matrix and distal phalanx and final suture closure.

Laser matrixectomy

Types of laser

There are essentially three types of lasers suitable for primary coagulative therapy: carbon dioxide, argon, and Nd : YAG (neodymium: yttrium–aluminium–garnet) lasers. The CO_2 laser is one of the more commonly used instruments for laser surgery. Absorption of its middle-infrared output of 10 600 nm in the biological tissues is independent of tissue colour, unlike the argon laser, and its minimization of tissue damage, with virtually no scattering, differentiates it from the Nd : YAG laser. The high degree of absorption in soft tissue, with limited lateral damage, makes the CO_2 laser a more precise instrument for vaporizing tissues.

The CO_2 laser has also been utilized for coagulation techniques because of its precision and its ability to control excess bleeding. It has been used to weld arteries for microsurgery and to anastomose small vessels and nerves. The apparatus has also been used in dermatological surgery and, as previously mentioned, in foot surgery. The CO_2 laser beam can be used for cutting, evaporation, and coagulation. When the laser is used for cutting, the spot is focused directly on the tissues. The laser beam is then placed in the focused mode, so that when applied, the effect is precise and the damage is localized. The depth of the cut is determined by the power, density, and duration of the exposure. The surgeon must develop a certain feel for this technique through practice, to determine the density and duration of exposure required to eliminate the matrix.

The CO_2 laser can also evaporate tissues when used in the defocused-mode. Small areas can be evaporated with a focus spot, but larger areas tend to get ridges or furrows when they evaporate in this manner. Evaporation is useful in tumour removal or in removing tissue from delicate structures precisely, such as one cell layer at a time. Ablative-type lesions may also be produced with the defocused beam.

The argon laser was the first major application of laser technology; it was used in the treatment of diabetic retinopathy in 1965. Since that time, and with extensive experience, the argon laser photocoagulator has become the treatment of choice for retinal disorders. Dermatological disorders are the other major application of argon laser therapy. The argon laser produces a visible blue-green light, of wavelengths ranging from 488 to 515 nm, which is easily transmitted through transparent and aqueous tissues. Certain types of tissues, such as pigments and haemoglobin, absorb the argon laser light very easily. Dermatological deformities that have been used with the argon laser include the port wine-type haemangiomas and telangiectasias. The argon beam passes through the overlying skin without substantial absorption and reaches the pigmented layer of the lesion, causing protein coagulation in this layer.

As stated earlier, the Nd : YAG laser is best suited primarily for coagulative therapy. It will coagulate vessels up to 4 mm in diameter and larger, with manipulation. The argon laser has also been used to coagulate tissue, but its effects are primarily on haemoglobin and not on the vessel walls. The Nd : YAG laser is a solid crystal that is stimulated to emit laser light in the near-infrared region, at wavelengths of 1 060 nm. Nd : YAG laser units are capable of power levels of 15–100 W. The larger beam is transmitted to the target tissue through a fibreoptic system. What is interesting is that the Nd : YAG beam can be transmitted through transparent tissues and can be used in the eye or other water-filled cavities such as the bladder. Its absorption by tissue is not as colour-dependent as the argon laser and, thus, it can be absorbed by almost any tissue that is not transparent. Obviously, the darker the tissue, the greater the absorption.

The primary difference between the Nd : YAG laser and other types of laser is that it has a high degree of scattering on impacting tissues. Therefore, when focusing on very small lesions, the Nd : YAG laser may not be the instrument of choice. The zone of damage produced by the impact of this laser is not as precise as for the CO_2 laser and often the necrosis can be quite severe, including full thickness-type injuries to vessels, nerves, and even cortices of the bone.

Finally, there are combination laser units in which CO_2 and Nd : YAG lasers are applied together. Combined units provide increased flexibility and greater range in terms of treatment applications. Outside of ophthalmic surgery, the most common application for Nd : YAG lasers at the present time is tumour-ablation treatment of acute gastrointestinal tract haemorrhage. In foot surgery, the CO_2 laser is probably the apparatus of choice.

Laser operative technique

After carrying out the same preparatory technique as for anaesthesia and sterile prepping and draping of the digit(s), the laser apparatus is prepared; and the laser beam is directed at the matrix, which immediately emits a vapour that indicates the destruction of the matrix cells. The area is often curetted and then flushed copiously with a saline solution after the laser has been used. During this time, goggles are worn by the surgeon and any other personnel.

The wound is then dressed in the usual sterile manner. The patient may be given a post-operative antibiotic and an oral analgesic, and instructed to return for periodic post-operative examinations.

Pathomechanics of hammertoe

The pathomechanics of hammertoe deformity occur as a result of excess pronation of the foot, causing the musculotendinous structures to contract abnormally. Gradual weakening of the intrinsic musculature occurs, followed by contracture of the extensor sling mechanism and the flexor tendons. Once joint adaptation occurs, limitation or rigidity may follow. Other aetiologic factors might also contribute to the development of hammertoe deformity, including a plantar flexion deformity of the respective metatarsal of the adjacent toe. There may be loss of function of the lumbrical muscle or imbalance between the medial and lateral interosseous muscle.

Flaccid paralysis of both the extensor digitorum brevis and longus tendons may also contribute to overpowering of the flexor longus and brevis tendons, producing a hammertoe deformity. Often associated with hammertoes of the fourth and fifth toes is a forefoot valgus deformity. Abduction pressure from hallux abductovalgus deformity will also contribute to dorsal subluxation of the second toe, which may also affect the lesser digits. A fifth metatarsal, which is subluxed during pronation, may also cause hammertoe deformity of the fifth toe, primarily with the fifth toe in a varus position.

Certainly any trauma that occurs to the articular structures of the metatarsophalangeal joints or to the lesser toe joints may also cause hammertoe deformity. Other conditions, such as gastrocnemius equinus and gastrocnemius-soleus (triceps surae) equinus may also contribute to the abnormal pathomechanics of the subtalar joint and mid-tarsal joint, which may lead to hammertoe deformity in the form of extensor substitution or, if the triceps muscle group is weakened, digital flexor tendon substitution.

Hammertoe procedures

Arthroplasties

Painful heloma dura located over the proximal phalanx as a result of hammer digit syndrome is one of the more common digital problems encountered on the foot. The painful heloma dura may also occur over the distal interphalangeal joint and distal tip of the toe.

If the fifth digit is underriding the fourth, a heloma molle between the digits may also be seen, especially if the shoes are pointed or narrow-toed. If the hammertoe is semi-flexible or not totally manually reducible to a straight alignment, often an arthroplasty is indicated. This is a commonly performed digital procedure, and in most instances is very successful and reliable. The arthroplasty is indicated for correction of painful heloma dura or heloma molle, either dorsally or laterally. The toe is in a contracted state and is either flexible or semi-rigid. The toe is not displaced at the metatarsophalangeal joint and no neuromuscular defect is present. The digital circulation must also be patent and viable.

Operative procedure

There are several incisional approaches that are commonly used. The most common incision is the dorsal linear incision along the mid-line of the lesser digit. The incision is centred, and extends across the interphalangeal joint to totally expose the joint involved. The proximal phalanx head is then removed at the surgical neck.

Another approach is the two semi-elliptical incision (also known as the fusiform incision) to excise the heloma dura over the proximal interphalangeal joint. The surgeon must make use of the 3 : 1 rule (the length of the incision is approximately three times the width of the incision), in order to adequately close the wound. This technique continues with the performance of a transverse tenotomy and capsulotomy, exposing the head of the proximal phalanx. The collateral ligaments are released, allowing the entire head to be resected at the surgical neck. The remaining shaft of the proximal phalanx is rasped smooth and flushed with sterile saline or lactated Ringer's solution (**7.13**).

The two semi-elliptical excision of the heloma dura is preferred, since it allows for the re-approximation of the capsule and tendon, eliminates the excess soft tissue, and usually prevents a floppy or weak toe after resection of the proximal phalanx. Deep closure of the tissues (tendon and capsule) is carried through by using a 4-0 absorbable suture. The skin is sutured with a 4-0 or 5-0 nonabsorbable suture in a simple interrupted

7.13

A — Heloma dura / Phalanx / Metatarsal

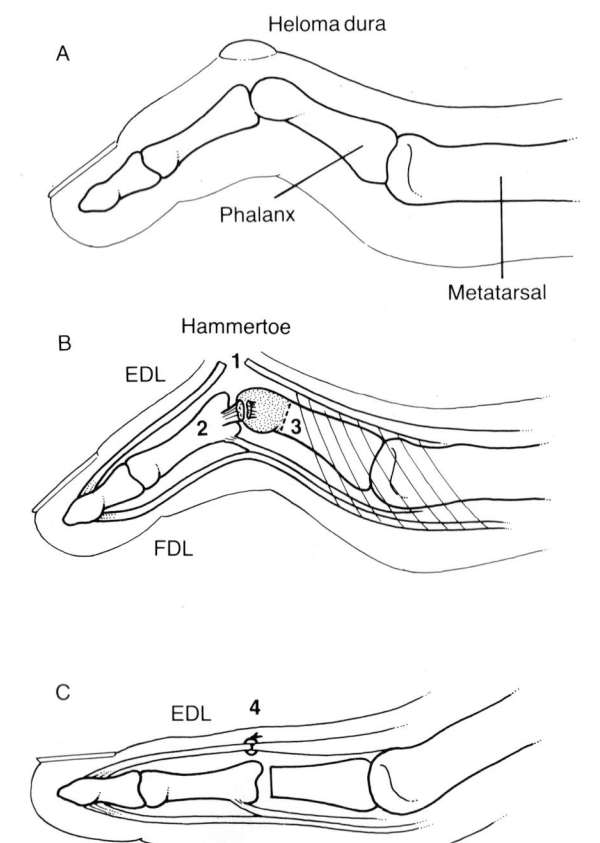

B — Hammertoe / EDL / FDL

C — EDL / FDL

7.13 Post-arthroplasty hammertoe operation. A, Typical side view presentation of hammertoe condition. B, Dorsal transverse incision with tenotomy and capsulotomy (1), the collateral ligaments are severed (2), and a partial phalanx head resection is performed (3). C, The dorsal extensor digitorum longus tendon is repaired: the tendon and capsule are sutured with an absorbable suture and tightened to decrease the laxity of the toe (4).

manner. Sterile dressings are carefully applied, splinting the toe in a straight attitude without compromising the digital circulation. The surgeon must be aware of post-operative oedema with tight dressings, which results in severe pain unless the dressings are removed or loosened.

If the heloma dura occurs at the distal aspect of the toe and the contracture occurs at the distal interphalangeal joint, the resection is performed at the neck of the intermediate digital phalanx. In this case, the transverse semi-elliptical skin incision approach is recommended because of a more secure and superior closure, with concomitant correction of the contracture.

The heloma molle (soft corn) of the fourth or fifth toes can also be approached with arthroplasties. If the heloma molle is on the inner medial aspect of the fifth toe web space, an arthroplasty of the fifth toe is usually effective in eliminating the soft corn.

If the fifth toe underrides and is irritated by the fourth toe, an arthroplasty is performed with an incision that helps de-rotate the fifth toe out of the varus position. If the fourth proximal phalanx is enlarged, an arthroplasty of the fourth toe may also be necessary to ensure elimination of the painful heloma molle. This requires good judgement and experience in determining what procedures will adequately correct the digital problem. The patient is seen 2–3 days post-operatively, to examine the wound and to ensure that no complication has occurred. The sutures are removed, typically, after 7 to 10 days, depending upon how well the incision heals.

Should a complication occur, the foot surgeon should be well aware of this, and provide immediate and proper treatment. Once the sutures have been removed, the patient is allowed to bathe and to apply skin lotion and moisturizers over the incision. Furthermore, the patient is instructed to massage the toe two to three times a day for 10 min and also to visualize the toe healing.

Swelling may occur during this time, and may preclude the use of certain styles of shoes. Usually, a flat, post-operative shoe or sandal or laced-up wide shoe can be worn comfortably. Post-operative oedema may last up to 3 months from the physiological point of view. Physiotherapy is frequently necessary to reduce the oedema and to regain strength in the digit as well as to treat any potential scar formation or adhesions.

In compromised patients with extensive medical problems but with good neurovascular status, prophylactic antibiotics should be administered peri-operatively to reduce the risk of infection. Other complications include continuous oedema or sausage toe, flail or weak toe, hypertrophic scar formation, and recurrence of the heloma dura or heloma molle. The results following the use of the arthroplasty, based on a retrospective analysis by the author over a 14-year period have shown a 98% success rate. The most common complication encountered was hypertrophic scar (1%), superficial infection (less than 1%), and recurrence of the heloma durum or heloma molle (less than 1%). From this analysis, it appears that this procedure is a reliable and dependable technique for the indications discussed previously. Using the procedure beyond these indications may lead to poor results and a higher complication rate. The treatment of the complications should be done pre-operatively and intra-operatively.

As for the treatment of the oedematous or sausage toe, let me remind you that at least a 3-month period is frequently necessary before pronouncing that the toe is a sausage or swollen toe. However, if the oedema exceeds a 3-month period and the patient is expressing great concern, treatment should be initiated to decrease the swelling and a discussion to alleviate the emotional and psychological anxiety should be addressed.

The simplest treatment plan should be used first, before moving on to more technical treatments. In this case, ice, elevation, and compression may be all that is needed (if this is done on a daily basis or more). If this is unsuccessful, physical therapy and anti-inflammatory measures may be implemented to stimulate movement of the excess oedema from the toe. When these conservative methods appear not to be helpful, injection therapy may be beneficial. Chronic swollen toes may be injected with a local anaesthetic agent and a corticosteroid.

In severe cases, if the entire lower extremity is oedematous, excess fluid retention requires short-term use of diuretic medications. Usually with time and patience, the excess swelling will subside. In some cases, a permanent swollen toe may remain, one that the patient can live with and still continue their previous levels of physical activities.

Treatment of hypertrophic scar or cicatrix should be implemented by the surgeon as early as possible. Even then, a few patients will have resultant cicatrix formation, despite the best treatment efforts and surgical technique. Pre-operative planning to screen these patients is highly important.

Using incisions that alleviate excess tension across the incision during the healing phase and also reduce stress during the walking phase is also important. An S-shaped or curvilinear-type incision is helpful in reduction of stress and tension across the incision site. Using less-reactive suture material will also help reduce scar formation. Physical therapy modalities, such as ultrasound therapy and massage, may also be effective. The use of enzymatic agents, via injection therapy into the hypertrophic scars has been reported to be of some success. Finally, excision of the cicatrix or hypertrophic scar may be performed if the discomfort and pain continue and all conservative treatment modalities have failed to alleviate the suffering.

Recurrence of the external excrescence may indicate an insufficient amount of bone has been removed or an inadequate shoe, which continues to aggravate and apply pressure to the digit. Certainly, any type of injury to the toe, or neuromuscular and arthritic disease processes, will also contribute to recurrence post-operatively. If the latter conditions have occurred and another procedure is contemplated, arthrodesis of the digital phalanges may be recommended. Finally, should severe vascular compromise to the digit occur from a traumatic episode or from other causes, partial or complete amputation of the digit may be necessary to alleviate this problem.

Arthrodesis of the lesser digits

As described earlier, rigid hammertoes from severe arthritis, recurrent hammertoes, and hammertoes associated with moderate to severe pes cavus, and neuromuscular disorders are indications for arthrodesis. Contracture of the proximal phalangeal joint requires arthrodesis at this level. Furthermore, rigid contracture of the distal interphalangeal joint, proximal interphalangeal joint, and contracture of the metatarsophalangeal joint often respond well to arthrodesis at the distal interphalangeal joint and proximal interphalangeal joint. Capsulotomy and release of contracted structures at the metatarsophalangeal joint is performed simultaneously to achieve a corrected position. Fixation can be achieved by using a Kirschner wire (K-wire), as shown in **7.14**.

The use of K-wire fixation for arthrodesis of digits is very common: this technique provides some stability while allowing the toe to rotate around the K-wire. Utilizing AO bone screw fixation of the arthrodesis site has also been performed by the author with some success: this technique provides rigid internal fixation and superior osseous union and stability. The drawback with the AO technique in digits is one of application, which has to be precise and correct. Several failed attempts to get the bone screw through the toe will result in the lack of adequate bone stock to hold the

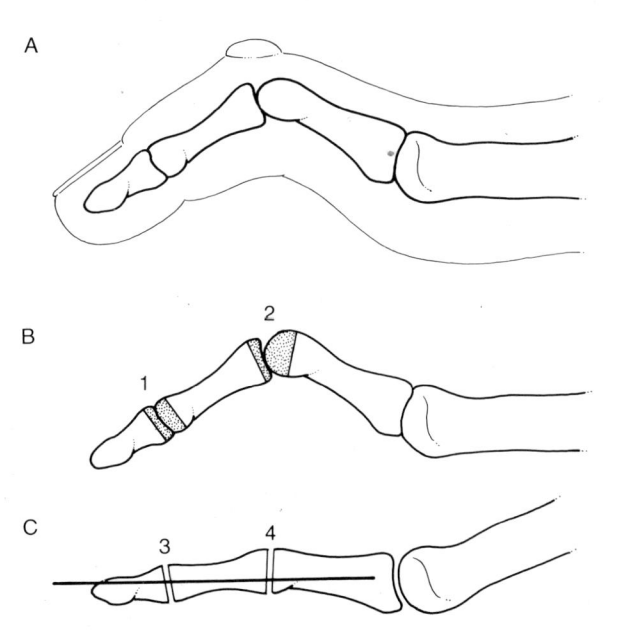

7.14 Digital arthrodesis with K-wire fixation. A, Side view of hammertoe condition. B, Marked areas to be resected (in some cases it may be advisable to resect only the proximal interphalangeal joint): resect joint surfaces at distal interphalangeal joint (1); reset joint surfaces at proximal interphalangeal joint (2). C, K-wire fixation of realigned digit for total arthrodesis: insertion of K-wire through the digit (3, 4).

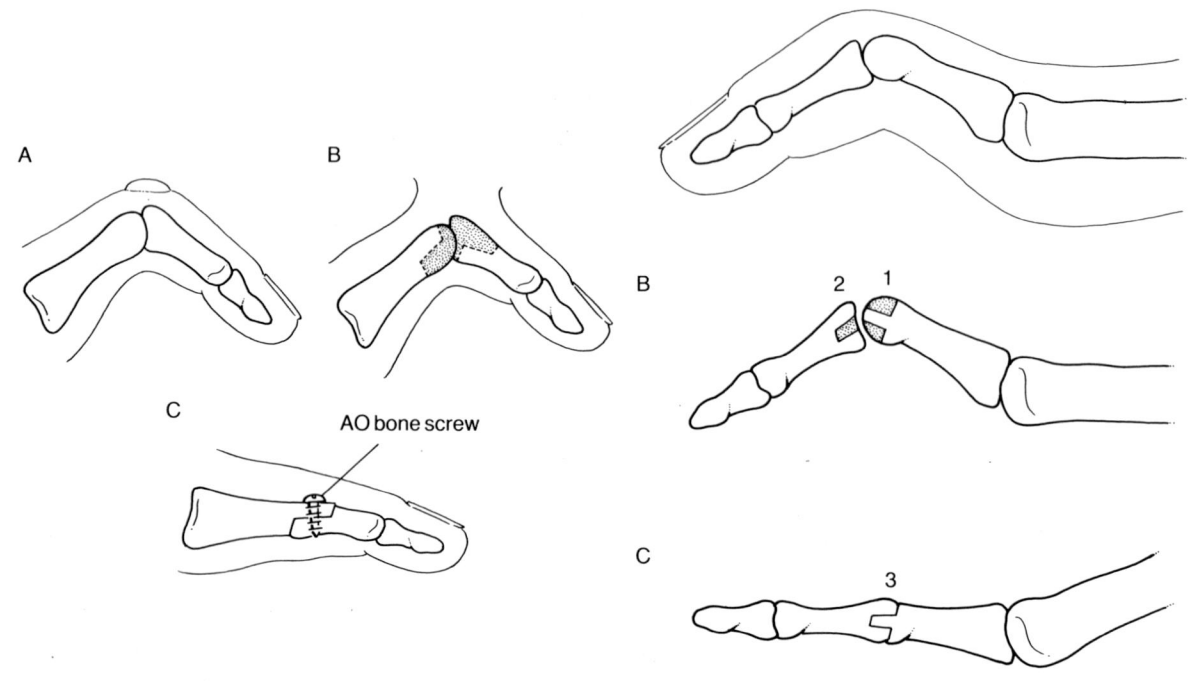

7.15 Digital arthrodesis with AO bone screw fixation. A, Side view of hammertoe condition. B, Dorsal capsulotomy and tenotomy is performed (shaded areas of bone are resected) C, Cut bone ends are placed together and fixed with the screw.

7.16 Peg-in-hole arthrodesis procedure. A, Side view of hammertoe condition. B, Shaded areas of bone at the proximal phalanx are resected to form the peg (1) and intermediate phalanx is resected to allow the peg to fit snugly in the shaft of the phalanx (2). C, The peg portion of the proximal phalanx is then inserted into the hole portion of the intermediate phalanx and arthrodesis of the digit is achieved (3). (A K-wire may be inserted for added security if necessary.)

screw in place (**7.15**).

Other techniques, such as a peg-in-hole procedure, have been devised for arthrodesis of the proximal phalangeal joint (**7.16**). This technique seems to allow for early fusion and stability of the arthrodesis site; the only difficulty is in performing the partial ostectomies accurately, to allow the end of the bones to fit correctly.

Operative techniques–proximal interphalangeal joint arthrodesis

After the digit has been anaesthetized and prepped and draped in the usual sterile manner, either a transverse semi-elliptical incision or a dorsal linear incision may be utilized. The incision is then carefully dissected through the subcutaneous and superficial fascial layers, exposing the extensor tendon, where a transverse tenotomy and capsulotomy is performed at the proximal interphalangeal joint. The collateral ligaments are also released and the extensor tendon is then reflected proximally, exposing the proximal phalanx and the base of the intermediate phalanx.

Using a bone saw or bone-cutting forceps, the base of the intermediate phalanx and the head of the proximal phalanx are resected. Care must be taken to ensure proper fitting of these two osseous structures. Using K-wire fixation, the K-wire is drilled first through the intermediate phalanx distally and then, reversing the direction, through the proximal phalanx until it is stable.

If there continues to be contracture of the metatarsophalangeal joint, a capsulotomy and release of tight collateral structures with lengthening of contracted tendons is performed. In some cases, the K-wire will be passed across the metatarsophalangeal joint to maintain the corrected position. X-rays are taken intraoperatively to ensure proper placement of the K-wire through the digit. The digit is then sutured and dressed in the usual sterile manner.

A Jones-type splint (a post-operative bandage utilizing multiply layers of sterile dressings with cotton wrap, plaster posterior splints, and elastic bandages) is utilized to protect the pins and the toes in order to maintain correction. Approximately 3 or 4 days postoperatively, the patient is instructed to return to the office for the first follow-up visit. Post-operative X-rays are taken at this time, the incisions are inspected, and the toe is then redressed using sterile dressings. A Jones-type splint is re-applied for another 1–2 weeks.

At approximately 3–4 weeks post-operatively, X-rays are taken to assess the osseous healing across the arthrodesis site. If there appears to be adequate osseous union, the pin is removed. Post-operative care entails the use of a Jones-type splint or a cast boot to protect the pins, at least for 3–4 weeks. This avoids distracting or breaking of the K-wire pin, which can occur with normal weight-bearing. Similarly, if AO fixation screws are used, the same precautions must be administered post-operatively.

At 10–14 days, the sutures are removed from the digit. The K-wire is often removed at 3–4 weeks, depending on the osseous healing (based on post-operative radiographs and clinical findings). AO bone screws are typically removed at 6 months or more post-operatively: removal of the hardware can be performed in the surgery under local anaesthesia.

Once healing has occurred and the oedema subsided, the patient is instructed to wear loose-fitting shoes initially; eventually, they may return to their usual footwear. Loose-fitting shoes are generally recommended, to reduce irritation to the lesser digits during the healing phase. Furthermore, daily massage and application of skin lotions and softeners assists in the healing process and also has a very soothing effect.

In terms of the results, the arthrodesis procedure in lesser digits has been very successful in achieving the goals of the surgical plan. However, the patient must be thoroughly informed that the toe will be rigid and lose flexibility and some function.

The most common early complication is distraction of the K-wire pin from the digit. In correcting severe contraction and dislocated hammertoes, the K-wire is placed through the metatarsophalangeal joint for greater stability after arthrodesis of the toes. In this case, it may be wise to keep the patient non-weight-bearing to avoid distraction or pin breakage. However, in most instances, pin distraction has been minimal, with little or no displacement of the digits. If the displacement has been severe and the correction has been compromised, the pin must be sterilely replaced through the digit. Re-insertion of a displaced K-wire pin may lead to pin-tract infection. The same complications noted with arthroplasty are possible with arthrodesis: the reader is referred to the section on arthrodesis for more details.

Tendon lengthening and transfers

The flexible contracted digit that may be totally corrected by manipulation may need only a simple tendon-lengthening procedure. Generally, it must be determined if the contracture is secondary to extensor or flexor pull. When the long extensor tendon to the digit is the primary problem, a slide or Z-plasty tendon lengthening is recommended. When the long digital flexor is involved, a flexor set (tenotomy of the long flexor tendon) is performed.

For flexible or semi-flexible hammertoes, a flexor tendon transfer is often an alternative to arthroplasty or arthrodesis. Girdlestone described a procedure where the long flexor tendon was transferred through the base of the proximal phalanx where it was attached directly to the long extensor of the toe. The idea was to decrease the contracted state and utilize the contracted nature of the flexor tendon to pull plantarly on the extensor with the hope of effectively pulling the toe down and straight. However, this author argued that the drill hole was too proximal and needed to be placed more distal and at the level of the deformity where the full fulcrum effect would occur. Thus, the modification of the Girdlestone technique was performed in which the drill hole was relocated from the base of the proximal phalanx to the surgical neck of the proximal phalanx, which provided immediate and reliable reduction of the contracted toe (Kuwada–Dockery flexor transfer) (**7.17**).

Sgarlato split the long digital flexor tendon in half, brought it over the dorsum of the proximal phalanx, and sutured it to itself and into the periosteum. He reported that this also reduced the contracted status, and this procedure is still recommended in patients who have had arthroplasty procedures or in digits that have poor bone stock.

Sorto argued that flexor transfers were effective in reducing the contracted toe but also caused severe stiffness in the lesser interphalangeal joints to the extent that the toes were functioning arthrodesed. This assessment is correct and in most cases joint mobility is eliminated primarily at the proximal interphalangeal joint. The advantage, however, with flexor tendon transfer is that recurrence of dorsal contracture is rare, there are few floating toe problems, no arthrodesis hardware is required, and it yields excellent results, with the elimination of the hammertoe and subsequent external excrescence.

As with any surgical procedure, there are drawbacks to each of the flexor transfer techniques. With Sgarlato's technique, periosteal irritation and cortical bone erosion occur as a result of the apparent contracture and friction from the flexor tendons. With the Girdlestone technique, unreliable correction of the hammertoe contracture has been noted, with medial and lateral drift of the digits. With the Kuwada–Dockery flexor tendon transfer, the flexor

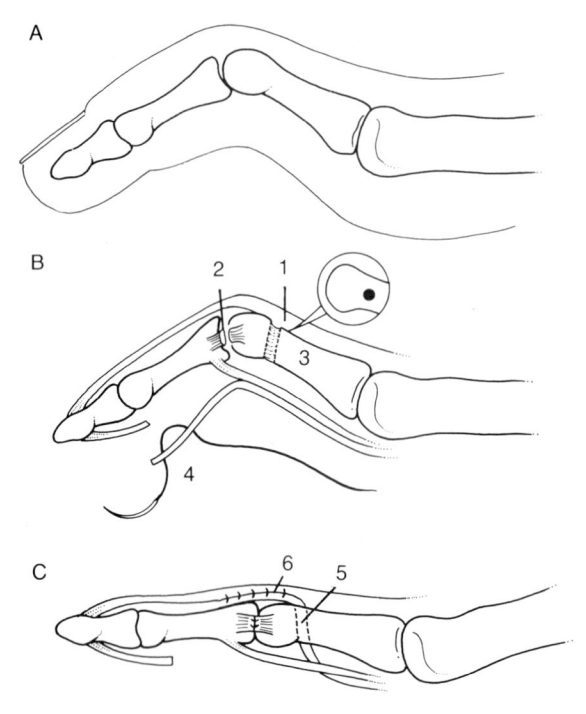

7.17 Kuwada–Dockery flexor tendon transfer procedure. A, Side view of hammertoe condition. B, Drill hole placed in the diaphyseal neck region of the proximal phalanx extensor longus and extensor hood retracted laterally (1); collateral ligament severed (2); drill hole is made (3); flexor longus tendon is severed and the end is sutured to pass plantar–dorsal through the drill hole (4). C, Final passing of the flexor digitorum longus tendon through the drill hole with the toe plantarflexed (5) and the flexor tendon is sutured directly to the extensor tendon medial, central, and lateral, with the toe plantarflexed (6). (From Kuwada, G.T. and Dockery, G.L. Modified flexor tendon transfer for the correction of flexible hammertoes. *J. Foot Surg.*, **19**(1): 30–40, 1980; with permission.)

was sutured to the dorsal aspect of the phalanx of the toe, allowing a small knot to form in some instances. Swelling for up to 3 months post-operatively was usual and common with this flexor tendon transfer, because of the bone drill hole. However, the external excrescence was gone within 1 month, and the pain and discomfort level, as well as the cosmesic appearance, was found to be very satisfying for the patients. Furthermore, no immobilization was necessary with this procedure.

With regard to arthrodesis, as stated earlier, some form of immobilization is required to protect the hardware and also to maintain the correction.

The benefits of flexor tendon transfer outweigh any negative aspect. The procedure may be used with young patients or patients concerned with the cosmetic appearance of their digits: since the incision is made on the dorsolateral aspect of the toe, it is not usually visible, which makes this procedure very attractive to female patients. Physiotherapy is usually not necessary with flexor tendon transfers. Typically, returning to ambulation is possible immediately, and after about 2–3 weeks, physical exercise is recommended to increase the range of motion and the strength of the lesser digits.

Some surgeons perform a digital arthroplasty at the head of the proximal phalanx and then perform a flexor tendon transfer. Inevitably, the distal segment of the toe is hyperextended dorsally due to pull from the long extensor tendon, sometimes causing pain and discomfort plantarly. This is not recommended.

Obviously, if the intrinsic musculature is weak, as a result of a neurological dysfunction, this should be recognized and considered before performing a flexor tendon transfer. In this case, an arthrodesis of the digit would be more beneficial for this patient long term than a flexor tendon transfer.

Operative procedures—flexor tendon transfer procedure

A dorsolateral incision is made from the distal interphalangeal joint, extending into the web along the lateral aspect of the toe. The incision is carefully dissected through the tissues, avoiding all vital structures. The bleeders are clamped, coagulated, or ligated. The flexor plate and the flexor longus tendon are identified and carefully severed distally. Using the same incision, an incision is made along the extensor tendon through the hood mechanism. The extensor tendon is then retracted medially, exposing the proximal phalanx head and neck. A lateral capsulotomy is performed and the collateral ligament is severed.

Using a small rotary burr, a drill hole is made from dorsal to plantar through the surgical neck region. The drill hole is carefully made in order to avoid thinning of the phalanx cortices, which might lead to fracture of the digit. The long flexor is then passed through the drill hole plantarly and brought up dorsally with a nonabsorbable suture. The tendon is then sutured medially, laterally, and centrally, into the extensor tendon, while the toe is placed in the corrected and slightly plantarflexed position to the adjacent digits using absorbable sutures. The collateral ligament is repaired and the subcutaneous layer is closed with an absorbable suture. The skin is then re-approximated using a subcuticular closure. The toe is dressed in the usual sterile manner and a 4-inch Ace wrap is applied.

Post-operatively, the patient may experience moderate-to-severe oedema in the lesser digits following this procedure. This can be of concern; however, for the most part, all patients have some degree of swelling that usually resolves.

The toe is dressed in a splint-type manner, using sterile gauze and elastic wrap to hold the toe straight, for at least 2 weeks and the patient is allowed to wear an open-toed shoe or sandal. If the patient has an extra-depth shoe, this will also avoid irritation to the lesser digits. As stated previously, ambulation and physical exercise will eventually strengthen the digit and, usually at 2 weeks, patients are able to resume some of their physical activities. High-heeled shoes are not recommended during this period and should be strongly avoided for maximum correction.

Results of the flexor tendon transfer

The results of most flexor tendon transfer procedures are, in general, anecdotal and not available at this time in the medical literature. The author, however, has provided a preliminary report on the procedure, as well as a five-year retrospective analysis of flexor tendon transfer in 81 digits (in 29 patients) that were surgically corrected using the Kuwada–Dockery flexor tendon transfer procedure. There was a 100% success rate (81 toes) for elimination of the heloma dura over the proximal phalanx or distal aspect of the digit and a 98% success rate (79 toes) for elimination of the contracture state of the digit. Three digits were deviated laterally.

No infections were reported in this series. Most of the digits were swollen to some extent for up to 3 months, until complete healing occurred. There were no sausage or swollen toes thereafter. Scarring along the incision, a problem reported by one patient, was eventually resolved by ultrasound therapy and massage. All of the digits in this study had some degree of stiffness at the proximal interphalangeal joint. Twenty-eight of the patients on whom this procedure was performed were very happy with their surgical result. One patient was pleased that the painful corn was gone, but was not happy with the deviation of the toe. However, she elected not to have any corrective measures performed, since her main concern, the elimination of a painful corn, had been achieved.

Complications

Subluxation or deviation of the digit, either dorsal medial or dorsal lateral, indicates either surgeon error or post-operative injury. If the surgeon is not careful suturing the flexor tendon medially or laterally, deviation of the toe will result. Infection, scarring, periosteal irritation, phalangeal fracture, lack of correction, and sausage toe are also possible complications. Patients should be informed pre-operatively that complications with flexor tendon transfer can and do occur; furthermore, they should be reassured that the surgeon can correct any of these complications should they occur. The advantage to flexor tendon transfer is that if a failure does occur or if there is a complication, more commonly performed digital surgery, such as arthroplasty or arthrodesis, can be easily performed.

Joint prosthesis of the lesser digits

Several endoprosthetic devices can be implanted into the lesser digits to restore joint function and maintain digital length and normal cosmetic appearance (**7.18**). In arthritic conditions, where joint motion is painful and contracture is severe, joint replacement is indicated. In conditions where cosmetic appearance is important, this procedure is an alternative to straight arthroplasty or arthrodesis. The earlier prosthetic implants were described as the ulnar caps over the ends of the proximal phalanx after arthroplasty procedures. Prosthetic implant deterioration with normal use is reported and, certainly, allergic reaction to the prosthetic device and detritic synovitis can also occur.

Prosthetic implants for lesser digits may have limited use overall. The author's experience also supports the general premise that more commonly performed procedures yield similar or more beneficial results long term, with fewer potential post-operative complications. Implants may dislodge, become displaced and fracture. In these cases, it is best to remove the implant and perform a standard surgical procedure. Fortunately, these patients do well and are usually satisfied with the surgical result. No great advantage over the more commonly performed procedures for digital problems was observed by using the implants in digits other than digital length may be preserved. The newer design implants (Zang:Sutter, Sgarlato:Sgarlato Labs, Weil:Dow-Corning Wright) offer less complications and problems and may become more popular in time.

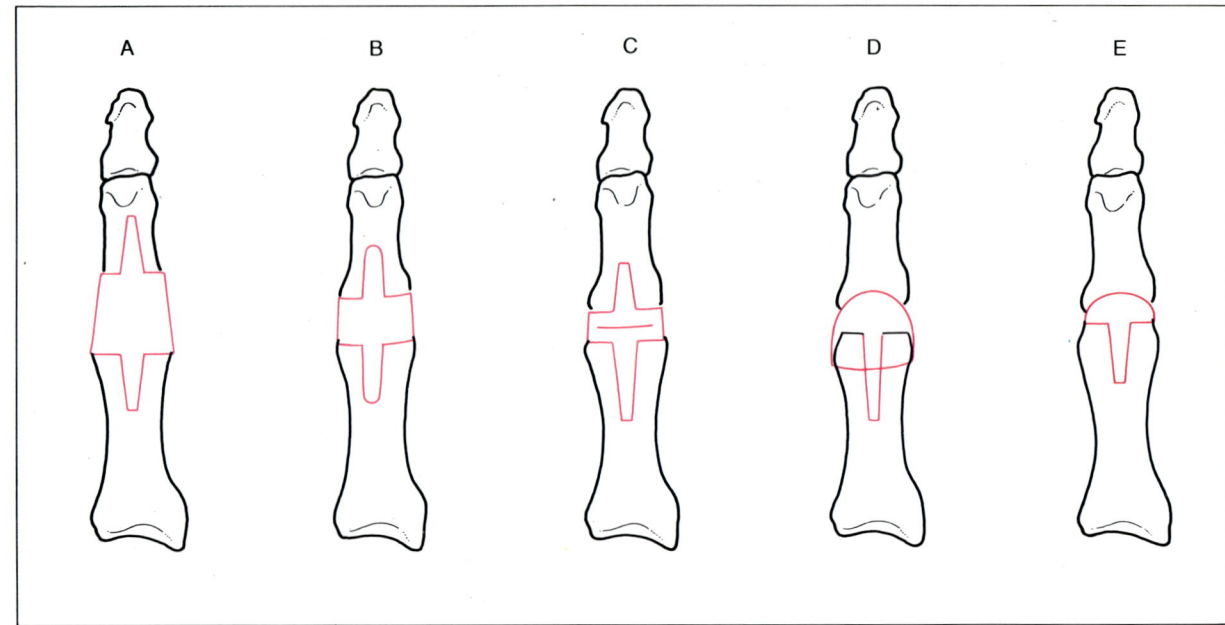

7.18 Digital arthroplasties with joint implants. A, Total joint digital implant (Sgarlato design). B, Total joint digital implant (Weil design). C, Total joint digital implant (Swanson design). D, Ulnar cap implant (Zang design). E, Hemi-digital implant (condylar).

Operative procedure

After the digit has been anaesthetized and prepped and draped in the usual sterile manner, a dorsally entered incision is made over the proximal interphalangeal joint. The incision is deepened through the tissues, avoiding all vital structures. A dorsal linear tenotomy and capsulotomy is performed, exposing the proximal interphalangeal joint, which is then resected in total using a power saw. A total digital joint implant, Dow–Corning Wright (Weil design), is described here. The intermediate phalanx is then centrally reamed to allow the distal stem to fit into the intermediate phalanx properly. This is also performed on the proximal phalanx to allow for the proximal stem of the prosthesis to fit securely.

Sizers are then placed into the lesser digit. When the correct size has been identified, the endoprosthetic device is implanted into the lesser digit. The soft tissue structures, such as the extensor tendon and capsule, are re-approximated using an absorbable suture. The skin may be closed with either an absorbable or a non-absorbable suture. The toe is then dressed in the usual sterile manner and a 4-inch Ace wrap is applied to the foot and ankle to prevent excessive swelling. A post-operative shoe is also used to facilitate ambulation.

Post-operative care

The toes are usually splinted with sterile 4 × 4s and gauze for a period of 3–4 days. After the initial post-operative visit, the patient is instructed to begin a more active range of movement of the lesser digit. The dressings are then changed after the toe has been inspected. After 2 weeks, the sutures are removed if they are nonabsorbable. Once again, the patient is instructed to begin range-of-motion exercises to tolerance: full weight-bearing is allowed at this time, unless pain and discomfort are being experienced. The patient is allowed to wear shoes between 2–4 weeks post-operatively, depending on the degree of swelling in the lesser digits. The patient is seen at various intervals, such as at 3 months, 6 months, and 12 months post-operatively.

Results

The overall results of lesser digital implant surgery have been, at best, satisfactory. As stated earlier, it is felt that the results of digital implant surgery are no better than those of more commonly performed digital procedures; in addition, they certainly have greater potential for complications. For these reasons, the use of the digital implant, in the author's view, is limited, and the overall benefit is questionable. Long-term follow-up of the newer implants for digital surgery is indicated as with all commonly performed surgical procedures.

Syndactylism

Certain conditions require syndactylism of the digits in order to correct a chronic problem: for example, a chronic and painful heloma molle between the toes is sometimes unresponsive to conservative or previous surgical care. To permanently alleviate this condition, the toes may be syndactylized. This is often necessary when one or both of the toes are flail or weak and thus non-functioning.

This procedure can be performed when the lesser metatarsal head is resected or when the digit is elevated and unstable. This avoids severe shortening of the digit and further distraction or displacement of the digit. By digital syndactylism, a degree of positioning is achieved and avoids the above-mentioned complications. Other surgical indications for the use of surgical syndactylization of the digits include chronic hammertoe deformities, flail or weak toes, overlapping fifth toes, following metatarsal head resection, and macrodactyly correction of the second digit. One of the other purposes of surgical syndactylism is to stabilize the adjacent digits when an excessive amount of bone has been resected during a surgical procedure.

Syndactylization of the digit to one or more of the adjoining digits adds to the stability of that digit and prevents subluxation of the toe or retraction of the digit.

Operative technique

The digits that are to be syndactylized together are prepared in the usual sterile technique. They are prepped and draped and the anaesthesia is also checked. The web space, where the skin will be removed, is marked off using a sterile marking pen. Primarily, the apex is slightly distal to the proximal phalanx of both lesser digits in the web space. The two toes are then brought together to see if enough of the skin has been removed. Once again, there has to be enough skin available to suture the two toes together and not leave any gaps or openings along the incision line. Using simple interrupted sutures, the skin edges are then re-approximated (**7.19**).

Various techniques can be employed in the actual suturing of the web space. The sutures are placed across the dorsal aspect, one in the middle of the web space and one plantarly, and then sutures are further placed equidistant from each other in between, until the incision line is completely closed. Another technique, taught by Dr Dockery, is to simply begin a running continuous suture from the superior towards the inferior portion of the incision. After completion, the running suture is tightened and tied plantarly. Once the syndactylism has been performed, the toe is then dressed in the usual sterile manner.

Following the surgical procedure, approximately 3 or 4 ml of 0.25–0.5% bupivacaine is injected about the operative site for post-operative analgesia. The patient is placed in a flat wooden shoe or standard post-operative shoe (to be worn for the first several weeks after surgery) and is discharged from the office or surgery centre with post-operative instructions and medications.

The initial post-operative visit is scheduled usually 3–4 days later. At that time, the incision is carefully examined and the patient's vital signs are taken and recorded. The wound is dressed in the usual sterile manner, an elastic wrap is re-applied, and the foot is placed back into the post-operative shoe. At approximately 10–14 days, the sutures are removed. The

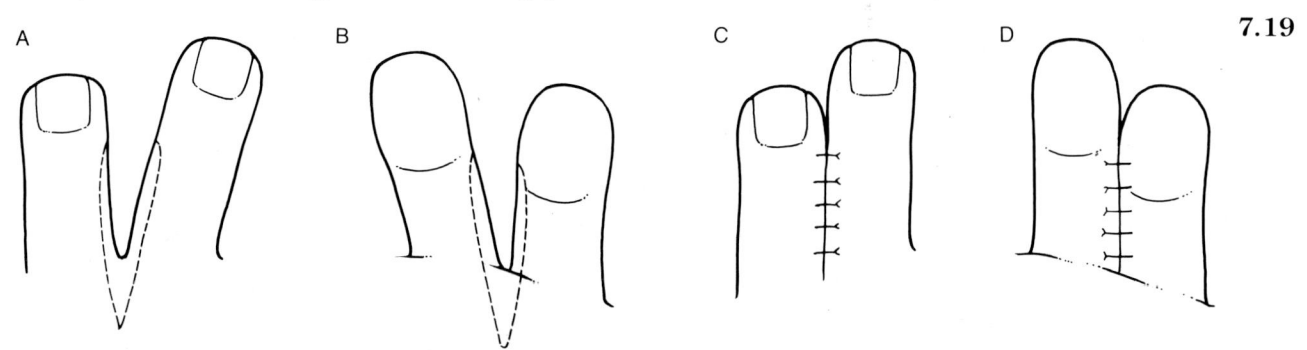

7.19 Digital syndactylism procedure. A, Dorsal view. B, Plantar view. C, Dorsal closure. D, Plantar closure.

patient is then allowed to wear a loose-fitting shoe; once the post-operative oedema and discomfort has subsided, the patient is allowed to get into regular footwear.

The overall results of syndactylism are good. The important element is ensuring that there is thorough patient education pre-operatively, so that expectations are reasonable. Especially important is the utilization of pictures and illustrations that inform the patient as to what to expect. When we find the patient's expectations are reasonable, the long-term results and acceptance rates are extremely high. Syndactylism is an effective procedure when performed with the above indications.

The primary complications are failure of the procedure, infection, scarification, and wound dehiscence. Some patients do not like the post-operative effects of surgical syndactylism because of the cosmetic appearance; good pre-operative illustration will prevent this complaint. If it done meticulously and correctly, the syndactylism will heal uneventfully.

Desyndactylization

Patients may report with a complaint of an extra digit or webbing of adjacent digits. This condition is often challenging to correct surgically. Phalangeal syndactyly is usually asymptomatic and surgical correction is frequently requested by the patient or the parent, primarily for cosmetic reasons. There have been many surgical procedures described in the medical literature to eliminate syndactylization. There are multiple choices, including a straight line-type incision, a zigzag-type incision, a Z-type incision, a wavy S-line-type incision, and rectangular flap-type incisions. This has caused some confusion as to the efficacy of each of the different skin incision approaches.

An S- or a Z-type incision to eliminate syndactyly has been used with some success. The important point here is that the surgery must be performed delicately and atraumatically; surgical principles must be closely adhered to in order to avoid complications with devitalization of any of the skin flaps or compromise of the neurovascular structure. Hypertrophic scar formation and post-operative haematoma and infection may result in wound dehiscence and skin slough, which can be devastating to the final results.

Operative technique

Using a lazy S- or a Z-type incision on the dorsal and plantar aspect of the web syndactyly, the incision is carefully dissected to the subcutaneous tissue. The skin incisions are cut precisely, so that the flaps match up to the dorsal and plantar aspect of each of the digits. This is to ensure adequate closure and also to eliminate any large gaping in the skin incision. Care must be taken not to restrict blood flow to the digits.

Neurovascular structures must be identified and preserved as much as possible. Using 5-0 or 6-0 non-absorbable monofilament suture material, the incisions are carefully sutured with a simple interrupted technique. Avoidance of post-operative haematoma is accomplished by maintaining a constant and even pressure on the newly created graft toe web space area without strangulating the tissues (by improper suture handling) and by post-operative dressings. The procedure discussed for desyndactylization has produced successful and acceptable cosmetic and functional results. Once again, the importance of following atraumatic surgical principles and techniques cannot be overemphasized.

Varus toe

Varus fifth-toe correction can usually be performed by using a derotation procedure of the digit by simple arthroplasty of a proximal phalanx and utilization of a teardrop skin incision to satisfactorily derotate the varus toe (**7.20**). The teardrop incision is placed with the apex distal lateral and proximal medial. If the flexor tendon is also found to be contracted, it is released by tenotomy. If the digit still has a tendency to stay in the varus position, a K-wire pin is placed through the digit to maintain correction.

Correction of an overlapping fifth toe may be accomplished by a V–Y Wilson skinplasty (see Chapter 1), as well as by simple arthroplasty. If the toe still tends to ride dorsally over the fourth digit, a pinch skinplasty of the fifth digit plantarly may also be performed simultaneously with extensor tendon lengthening, capsulotomy, and arthrotomy at the metatarsophalangeal joint. A K-wire may also be employed to maintain the corrected position of the digit once accomplished.

Other techniques that have been employed to correct an overlapping fifth toe include resection of a large amount of bone of the proximal phalanx and syndactylization of the fifth toe to the fourth toe.

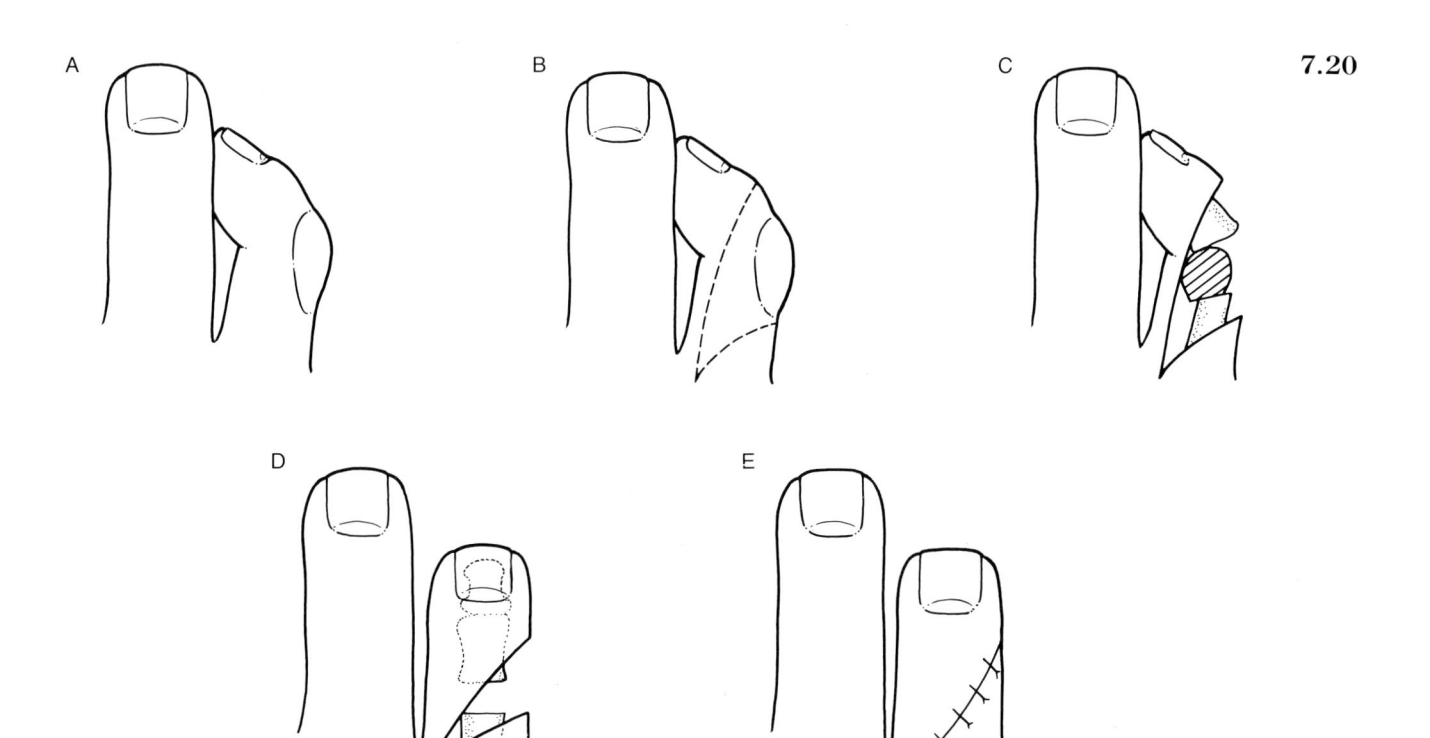

7.20 Derotational arthroplasty technique for varus toe (A). The incision is placed over the heloma in such a manner as to provide exposure to the underlying soft tissue (B). The head of the proximal phalanx is removed (C) and the toe is derotated (D) and sutured in the corrected position (E).

Elongated toes

Patients may complain of the cosmetic appearance of their elongated toes and may be quite embarrassed by this deformity: there may have been a congenital shortening deformity of the hallux or the lesser digits may be truly elongated. A technique reported by Kuwada and Dockery may be performed for this condition. Diaphysectomies in the proximal phalanx and in the intermediate phalanx are performed. K-wires are placed through the phalanges to re-approximate and maintain the corrected position of the toes. The K-wires are kept in place for approximately 3–4 weeks and then removed in the office under sterile conditions. At times, the K-wires can be easily rotated inside the toes and carefully removed without anaesthesia (**7.21**).

Surgical correction for floating toe syndrome

The floating toe syndrome is a pathological condition in which the toe fails to bear weight during stance or ambulation. In this condition, the long and short flexor and flexor plate are not functioning properly and thus allow the digit to float dorsally (**7.22**). The cause may be congenital or post-surgically shortened metatarsals, excessively elevated metatarsals after metatarsal osteotomies, or congenital or surgical toe problems. There may be dislocation of the flexor plate, which includes the long and short flexors, medially or laterally. In the case with brachymetatarsia, the metatarsal is congenitally short, even though muscle and tendon function are normal. The digit floats as a result of lack of plantar fascial tension on the involved proximal phalanx. Correction of this entails lengthening of the metatarsal by a bone graft and K-wire, Steinmann pin, or an AO plate. The proximal or distal phalangeal joint may also be fused to maintain the corrected position of the digit on the metatarsal (see Chapter 6).

The concern here is increasing the length severely,

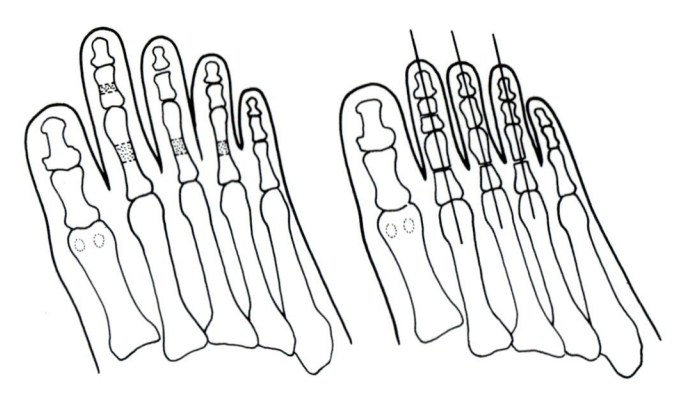

7.21 Correction of elongated toes. Marked areas of bone are resected and K-wire fixation stabilizes the digits in the corrected position. (From Kuwada, G. and Dockery, G.L. Cosmetic surgical correction for forefoot anomaly secondary to congenital short hallux. *J. Foot Surg*, **20**(2): 84–87, 1981; with permission.)

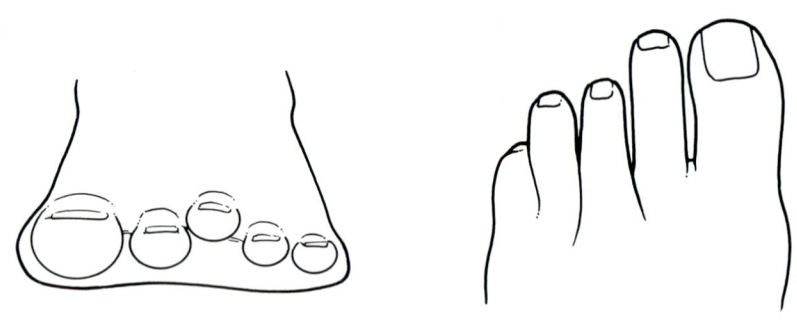

7.22 Floating toe syndrome. This condition may be due to a short metatarsal or to dislocation of the flexor plate apparatus, or if may be secondary to muscle–tendon imbalance.

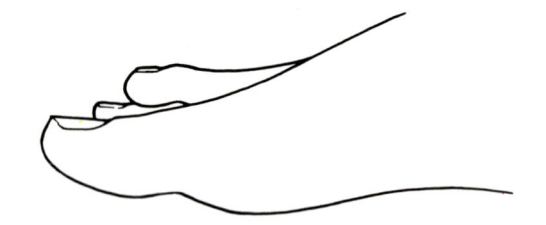

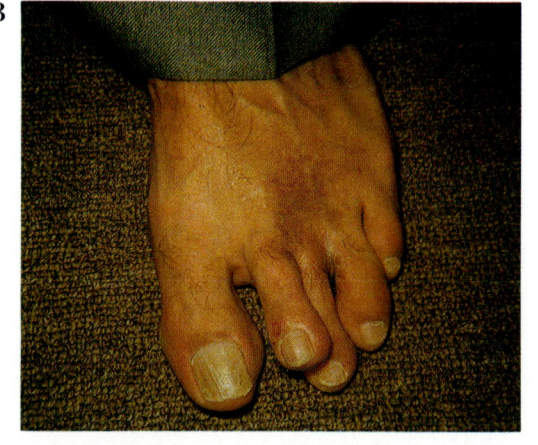

7.23 Floating second toe caused by previous surgery to elevate the metatarsal. (Courtesy of Dr G. Dockery, Seattle, Washington, USA.)

which will cause contracture of all the neurovascular structures, thus compromising the circulatory status of the digit. When the floating toe is iatrogenically created as a result of an elevated metatarsal or dislocation of the flexor plate, this is corrected surgically by re-establishing the metatarsal at a proper position, thus allowing the digit to retain its normal anatomical position and function (**7.23**). For example, in a situation where there has been a delayed or non-union after distal osteotomy, a plantar flexor-type osteotomy may be necessary to correct a floating toe situation. Furthermore, K-wire fixation through the digit, with arthrodesis of the proximal interphalangeal joint, may also be necessary to maintain the corrected anatomical position of the digit. Extreme shortening as a result of non-union or cheilectomy can be corrected by bone grafting and interphalangeal joint stabilization, capsulotomy, and tendon lengthening. The surgeon must be concerned about vascular embarrassment, which has been reported in the medical literature with these types of lengthening procedures using bone graft.

In the post-operative treatment of these conditions, where internal fixation devices or a K-wire is used, the patient is placed in a non-walking-type foot splint or cast in order to prevent other complications. Typically, the K-wire or Steinmann pins are removed approximately 4–6 weeks post-operatively. If AO bone screws or plates have been utilized, the hardware is removed approximately 6 months post-operatively.

Summary

In summary, the overall results indicate that certain procedures are more effective in eliminating digital conditions than others. Procedures that have stood the test of time are still favoured. Newer, and potentially better, procedures still need documentation of results before they can be placed into the same categories of standard procedures. Certainly, the overall success rate of digital procedures depends principally on the surgeon's knowledge, skill, and thoroughness in avoiding complications by using proper, aseptic, and atraumatic techniques.

Further reading

Apfelberg, D.B., Rothermel, E., Widtfeldt, A. *et al.* Progress report on use of carbon dioxide laser for nail disorders. *Curr. Podiatry*, **32**: 29, 1983.
Baden, H.P. *Diseases of the Hair and Nails.* Chicago, Year Book Medical Publishers, 1987.
Bernbach, E.H. and Bernbach, M.R. A box joint arthrodesis for the proximal interphalangeal joint in a clawtoe deformity. *J. Am. Podiatric Med. Assoc.*, **75**: 575–580, 1985.
Borovoy, M., Fuller, T.A., Holtz, P. and Kaczander, B.L. Laser surgery in podiatric medicine present and future. *J. Foot Surg.*, **22**: 353, 1983.
Bouche, R.T. Matrixectomy utilizing negative galvanic current. *Clin. Podiatric Med. Surg.*, **3**: 449, 1986.
Bouche, R.T. and Kuwada, G.T. Equinus deformity in the athlete. *Physicians and Sports Med.*, **12**(1), 1984.
Coleman, W.B., Kissell, C.G. and Sterling, H.D., Jr. Sydactylism and its surgical repair. *J. Am. Podiatry Assoc.*, **71**: 545–550, 1981.
David, L. (ed.) *Christopher's Textbook of Surgery,* 6th ed. Philadelphia, W.B. Saunders, 1956.
Dockery, G.L. Nails: fundamental conditions and procedures. *In* McGlamry, E.D. (ed.), *Comprehensive Textbook of Foot Surgery.* Baltimore, Williams & Wilkins, 1987, pp.3–37.
Dockery, G.L. and Nilson, R.Z. Intralesional injections. *Clin. Podiatric Med. Surg.*, **3**: 463–472, 1986.
DuVries, H.L. Hypertrophy of unguilabia. *Chiropody Rec.*, **16**: 13, 1933.
DuVries, H.L. *Surgery of the Foot*, 3rd edn. St. Louis, C.V. Mosby, 1973.
Dyer, A.M. and Cohen, M.F. A report on the use of negative galvanic current for the correction of incurvated nails. *J. Nat. Assoc. Chiropodists*, **45**: 21–22, 1955.
Feller, S.R. and Dockery, G.L. Vasospastic diseases, diagnosis and management, *Clin. Podiatric Med. Surg.*, **3**: 463–472, 1986.
Frost, L.A. Root resection for incurvated nail. *J. Am. Podiatry Assoc.*, **40**: 19, 1950.
Frost, L.A. A definite surgical treatment for sore lateral nail problems. *J. Nat. Assoc. Chiropodists,* **47**: 493, 1957.
Gardner, P. Negative galvanic current in surgical correction of onychocryptotic nails. *J. Am. Podiatry Assoc.*, **48**: 555–560, 1958.
Gastwirth, B.W., Anton, V. and Martin, R.A. The terminal Syme procedure. *J. Foot Surg.*, **20**: 95, 1981.
Giannestras, N.J. *Foot Disorders, Medical and Surgical Management,* 2nd edn. Philadelphia, Lea & Febiger, 1976.
Girdlestone, G.R. *Chartered Soc. Physiother.*, **32**: 167, 1947.
Heim, V. and Pfeiffer, K.M. *Small Fragment Set Manual Technique Recommended by the ASIF Group.* Berlin, Springer-Verlag, 1974.
Jay, R. *Current Therapy in Podiatric Surgery.* Philadelphia, D.C. Decker, 1989.
Jones, R. Clawfoot. *Br. Med. J.*, **1**: 749–751, 1916.
Kaplan, E.G. Elimination of onychauxis by surgery. *J. Am. Podiatry Assoc.*, **50**: 111, 1960.
Kelikian, H. *Hallux Valgus, Allied Deformities of the Forefoot and Metatarsalgia.* Philadelphia, W.B. Saunders, 1965.
Kufdakis, A.D. Ingrown toenail surgery: a new procedure. *Int. Surg.*, **6** 339, 1981.
Kuwada, G.T. A retrospective analysis of modification of the flexor tendon transfer for correction of hammertoes. *J. Foot Surg.*, **27**(1): 57–59, 1988.

Kuwada, G.T. and Dockery, G.L. Modified flexor tendon transfer for the correction of flexible hammertoes. *J. Foot Surg.,* **19**(1): 30–40, 1980.

Kuwada, G.T. and Dockery, G.L. Cosmetic surgical correction for forefoot anomaly secondary to congenital short hallux. *J. Foot Surg.,* **20**(2): 84–87, 1981.

Lapidus, P.W. Complete and permanent removal of toenail in onychogryphosis and subungual osteoma. *Am. J. Surg.,* **19**: 92, 1933.

Levy, L.A. and Hetherington, V.J. *Principles and Practice of Podiatric Medicine.* London, Churchill Livingstone, 1989.

Losch, G.M. and Duncker, H.R. Anatomy and surgical treatment of syndactylism. *Plast. Reconstr. Surg.,* **50**: 167–173, 1972.

Marcus, S.A. and Block, B.H. *American College of Foot Surgeons, Complications in Foot Surgery Prevention and Management,* 2nd edn. Baltimore, Williams and Wilkins, 1984.

McGlamry, E.D. Approaches to digital surgery. *J. Am. Podiatry Assoc.,* **68**: 358, 1978.

McGlamry, E.D. Indications for arthrodesis in the toes including clinical reports. *J. Foot Surg.,* **22**: 370–371, 1983.

McGlamry, E.D. *Fundamentals of Foot Surgery,* Baltimore, Williams & Wilkins, 1987.

McGlamry, E.D. *Comprehensive Textbook of Foot Surgery,* Vol. 1. Baltimore, Williams and Wilkins, 1987.

Mercado, D.A. *An Atlas of Foot Surgery. Vol. 1: Forefoot Surgery.* Oak Park, Illinois, Carolando Press, 1979.

Miller, M.E., Allogower, M. and Schnieder, R. *Manual of Internal Fixation.* Berlin, Springer-Verlag, 1979.

Murray, W.R. and Bedi, B.S. The surgical management of ingrowing toenail. *Br. J. Surg.,* **62**: 409, 1975.

Palmer, B.V. and Jones, A. Ingrowing toenails: The results of treatment. *Br. J. Surg.,* **66**: 575, 1979.

Page, J.C., Dockery, G.L. and Vance, C.E. Brachymetatarsia with brachymesodactyly. *J. Foot Surg.,* **22**: 104–107, 1983.

Perrone, M.A. Nail matrixectomy by onychotripsy with airmotor. *J. Am. Podiatry Assoc.,* **60**: 92–93, 1970.

Polokoff, M. Ingrown toenail and hypertrophied nail lip surgery by electrolysis. *J. Am. Podiatry Assoc.,* **51**: 805–808, 1961.

Pyper, J.B. The flexor extensor transplant operation for clawtoes. *J. Bone Joint Surg.,* **40B**: 548, 1958.

Raty, J.L. *Lasers in Cutaneous Medicine and Surgery.* Chicago, Year Book Medical Publishers, 1986.

Robb, J.E. and Murray, W.R. Phenol cauterization in the management of ingrowing toenails. *Scot. Med. J.,* **27**: 236, 1982.

Root, M.L. et al. *Clinical Biomechanics, Vol. II: Normal and Abnormal Function of the Foot.* Los Angeles, Clinical Biomechanics Corp., 1977.

Rubin, L.M. and Weiss, S.G. Complete nail eradication utilizing galvanic current: A preliminary report. *J. Am. Podiatry Assoc.,* **54**: 401–403, 1964.

Sarrafian, S.K. *Anatomy of the Foot and Ankle.* Philadelphia, J.B. Lippincott, 1983.

Sgarlato, T.E. Transplantation of flexor digitorum longus muscle tendon in hammertoes. *J. Am. Podiatry Assoc.,* **60**: 383, 1970.

Sgarlato, T.E. *A Compendium of Podiatric Biomechanics.* San Francisco, California College of Podiatric Medicine, March 1971.

Silverman, S.H. Cryosurgery for ingrowing toenail. *J. Roy. Coll. Surg. Edin.,* **20**: 289, 1984.

Sorto, L.A. Surgical correction of hammertoes: A five-year post-operative study. *J. Am. Podiatry Assoc.,* **64**: 940, 1974.

Suppan, R.J. and Ritchlin, J.D. A non-disabilitating surgical procedure for ingrown toenail. *J. Am. Podiatry Assoc.,* **42**: 900, 1962.

Taylor, R.G. The treatment of clawtoes by multiple transfers of flexor into the extensor tendons. *J. Bone Joint Surg.,* **33**: 539, 1951.

Thompson, T.C. and Terwilliger, C. The terminal Syme operation for ingrown toenail. *Surg. Clin. North Am.,* **31**: 575–584, 1951.

Trethowen, W.H. The treatment of hammertoe. *Lancet,* 1925.

Vanore, J., O'Keefe, R. and Pikscher, I. Complications of silicone implants in foot surgery. *Clin. Podiatry,* **31**: 175–198, 1984.

Whitney, A.K. Total matrixectomy procedure. *J. Am. Podiatry Assoc.,* **58**: 157, 1968.

Winograd, A.M. A modification in the technique of operation of ingrown toenail. *JAMA,* 91: 229, 1929.

Winograd, A.M. Results in operation for ingrown toenail. *Illinois Med. J.,* **70**: 197, 1936.

Yale, J.F. (ed.) *Podiatric Medicine,* 3rd edn. Baltimore, Williams & Wilkins, 1987.

Zadik, F.R. Obliteration of the nailbed of the great toe without shortening of the terminal phalanx. *J. Bone Joint Surg.,* **32**: 66, 1950.

8 Intermetatarsal neuromas and associated nerve problems

STEPHEN J. MILLER

Introduction and anatomy

The aetiology of a number of syndromes that cause neuralgic pain in the forefoot can be traced to the peripheral nerves. When the presenting symptoms sound as though there is nerve involvement—burning, tingling, numbness, and other paraesthesias—it is important to exclude proximal and systemic causes of neuropathy. Examples include radiculopathy, compression syndromes, entrapment neuropathies, autonomic dysfunction, diabetes mellitus, ischaemia, pernicious anaemia, polycythaemia vera, hypothyroidism, erythromelalgia, alcoholism, and other systemic diseases.

To further isolate the problem within the nerves of the forefoot, a thorough understanding of neuroanatomy and cord innervation is essential. There are six nerves that cross the ankle joint into the foot: the posterior tibial nerve, saphenous nerve, medial dorsal cutaneous nerve, intermediate dorsal cutaneous nerve, deep peroneal nerve, and the lateral dorsal cutaneous or sural nerve (**8.1, 8.2**).

After piercing the crural fascia at the lower one-third of the leg, passing from deep to superficial, the superficial peroneal nerve divides into two branches. The medial dorsal cutaneous nerve branches to supply the medial aspect of the great toe, the lateral aspect of the second toe, and the medial aspect of the third toe. In addition, it sends a small twig to the first web space dorsally, which may reinforce the deep peroneal nerve branches or supply part of the area by itself.

The intermediate dorsal cutaneous nerve innervates the lateral aspect of the third toe, the medial and lateral aspects of the fourth toe, and the medial aspect of the fifth toe. In rare instances, it sends a twig to augment the sural nerve.

In as many as 22% of the population, there is an accessory deep peroneal nerve, a branch of the superficial peroneal nerve. It passes through the peroneus muscle belly and supplies branches to all three lateral ankle ligaments plus the portions of the extensor digitorum brevis muscle controlling the third and fourth toes.[1]

Just above the ankle joint the deep peroneal nerve divides into a medial and a lateral branch. The lateral branch innervates the extensor digitorum brevis muscle and sends small branches to lie on the second, third, and fourth interosseous muscles. These nerve fibres supply the tarsometatarsal, metatarsophalangeal, and interphalangeal joints of the lesser toes. The medial branch courses distally to the dorsomedial surface of the second toe and the dorsolateral surface of the great toe. The deep peroneal nerve also has a muscular function, supplying the tibialis anterior, the extensor digitorum longus, the extensor hallucis longus, and the peroneus tertius (**Table 8.1**).

The sural nerve, arising from the tibial nerve,

Table 8.1 Motor innervation to the leg and foot

Muscle	Peripheral nerve	Spinal level
Tibialis anterior	Deep peroneal	$L_{4,5}$
Extensor digitorum longus	Deep peroneal	$L_{4,5}$
Extensor hallucis longus	Deep peroneal	$L_{4,5}$
Peroneus tertius	Deep peroneal	$L_{4,5}$
Gastrocnemius	Tibial	$S_{1,2}$
Soleus	Tibial	$S_{1,2}$
Plantaris	Tibial	$S_{1,2}$
Popliteus	Tibial	$L_{4,5}S_1$
Flexor hallucis longus	Tibial	$S_{2,3}$
Flexor digitorum longus	Tibial	$S_{2,3}$
Tibialis posterior	Tibial	$L_{4,5}$
Peroneus longus	Superficial peroneal	$L_5 S_{1,2}$
Peroneus brevis	Superficial peroneal	$L_5 S_{1,2}$
Extensor digitorum brevis	Deep peroneal	$S_{1,2}$
Abductor hallucis	Medial plantar	$S_{2,3}$
Flexor digitorum brevis	Medial plantar	$S_{2,3}$
First lumbricalis	Medial plantar	$S_{2,3}$
Flexor hallucis brevis	Medial plantar	$S_{2,3}$
Abductor digiti quinti brevis	Lateral plantar	$S_{2,3}$
Quadratus plantae	Lateral plantar	$S_{2,3}$
Second, third, fourth, lumbricales	Lateral plantar	$S_{2,3}$
Adductor hallucis	Lateral plantar	$S_{2,3}$
Flexor digiti quinti brevis	Lateral plantar	$S_{2,3}$
Plantar interossei	Lateral plantar	$S_{2,3}$
Dorsal interossei	Deep peroneal, lateral plantar	
First, second		$S_{1,2,3}$
Third, fourth	Lateral plantar	$S_{2,3}$

8.1

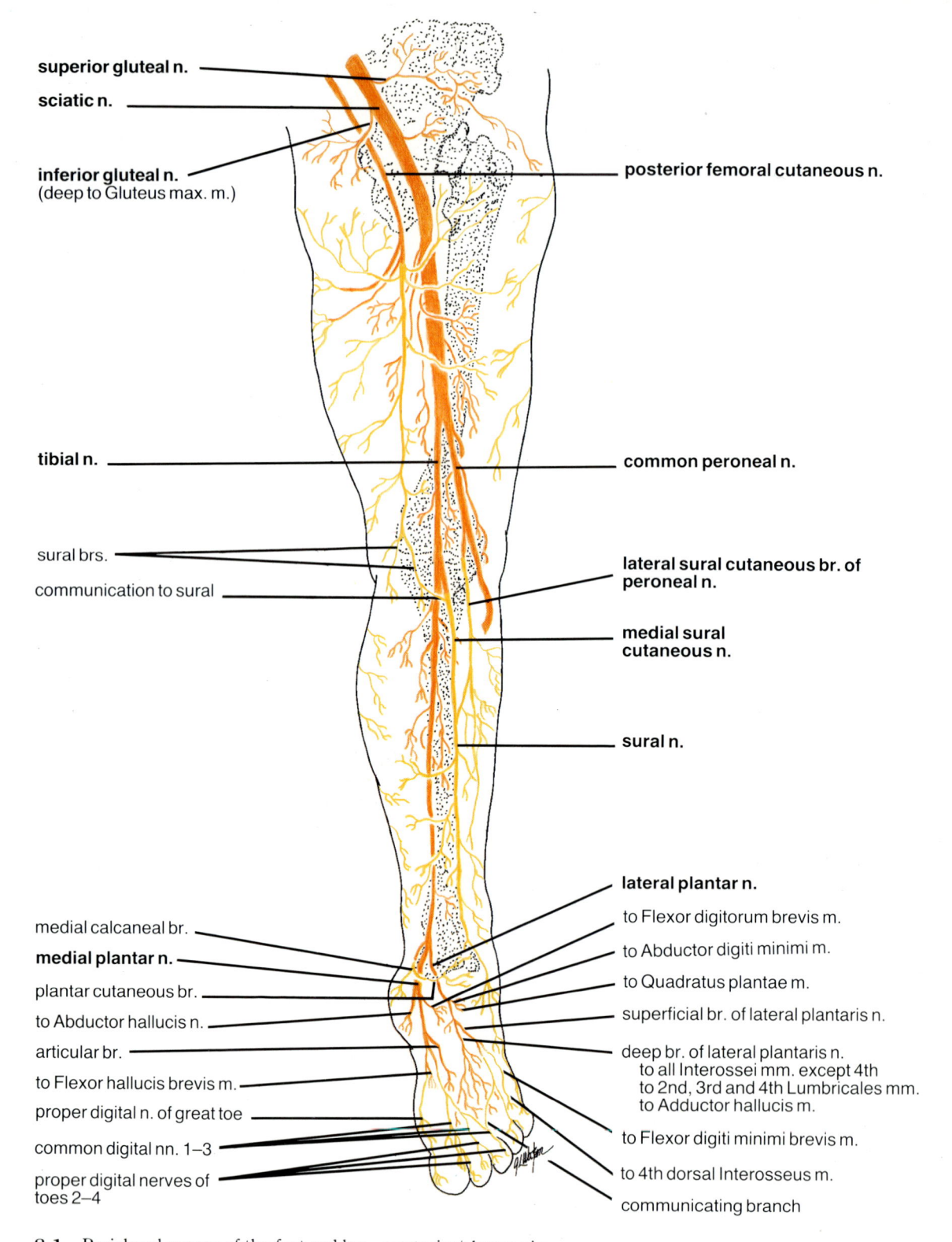

- superior gluteal n.
- sciatic n.
- inferior gluteal n. (deep to Gluteus max. m.)
- posterior femoral cutaneous n.
- tibial n.
- common peroneal n.
- sural brs.
- communication to sural
- lateral sural cutaneous br. of peroneal n.
- medial sural cutaneous n.
- sural n.
- lateral plantar n.
- to Flexor digitorum brevis m.
- medial calcaneal br.
- **medial plantar n.**
- to Abductor digiti minimi m.
- to Quadratus plantae m.
- plantar cutaneous br.
- superficial br. of lateral plantaris n.
- to Abductor hallucis n.
- articular br.
- deep br. of lateral plantaris n.
  - to all Interossei mm. except 4th
  - to 2nd, 3rd and 4th Lumbricales mm.
  - to Adductor hallucis m.
- to Flexor hallucis brevis m.
- proper digital n. of great toe
- to Flexor digiti minimi brevis m.
- common digital nn. 1–3
- to 4th dorsal Interosseus m.
- proper digital nerves of toes 2–4
- communicating branch

8.1 Peripheral nerves of the foot and leg— posterior/plantar view.

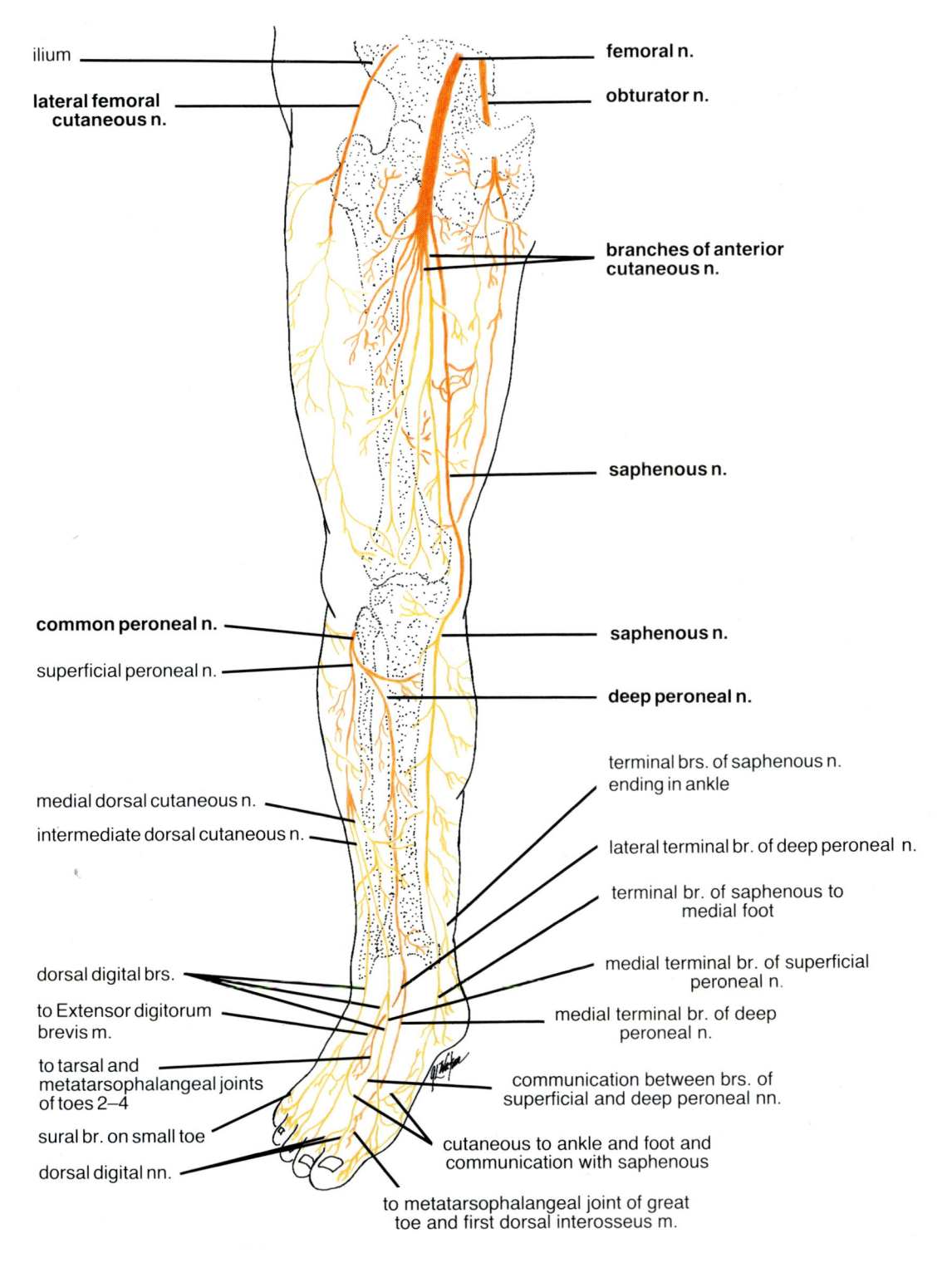

8.2 Peripheral nerves of the foot and leg— anterior/dorsal view.

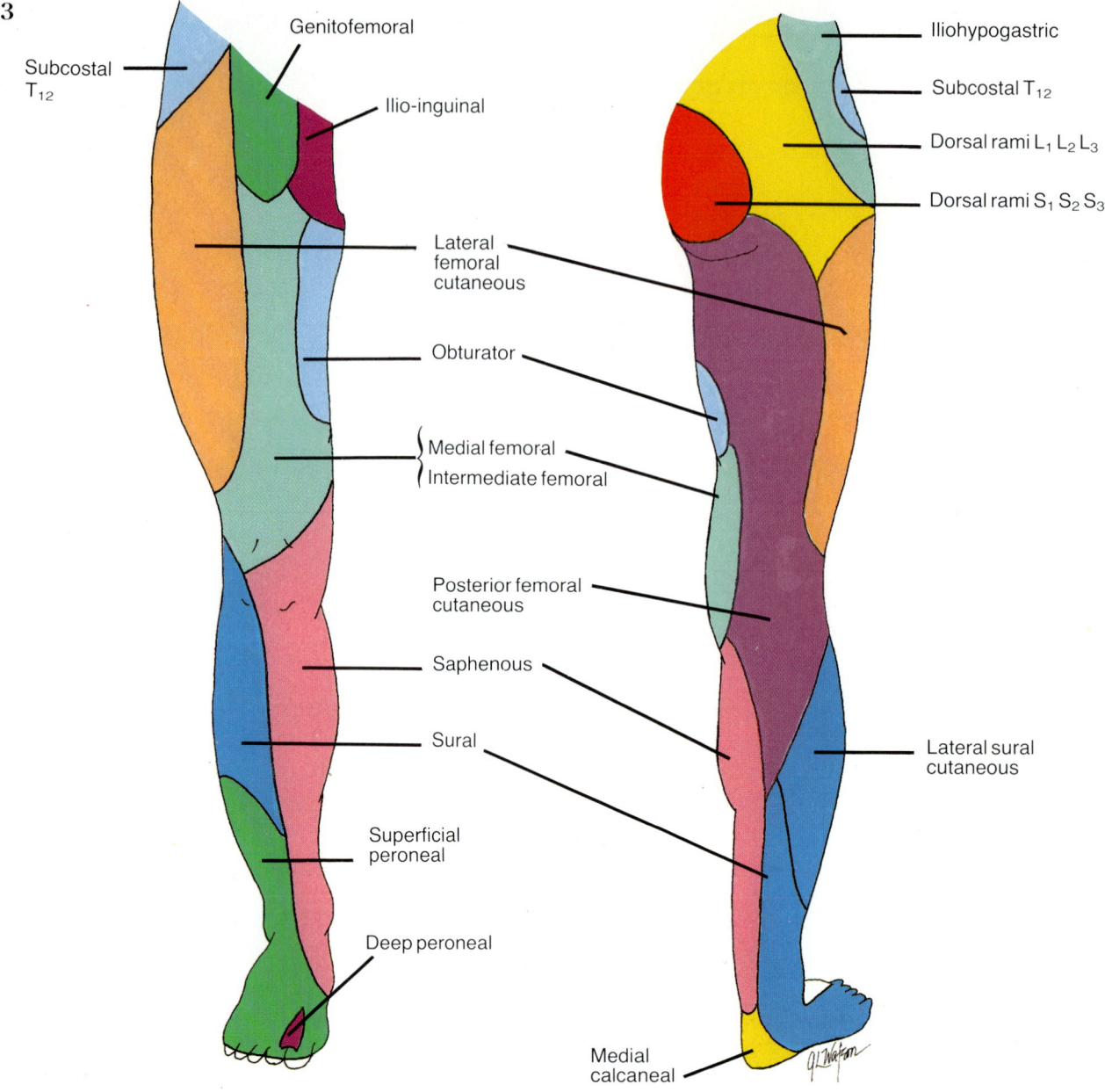

8.3 Anteromedial dermatomes.

8.4 Posterolateral dermatomes.

courses around the posterior and inferior lateral malleolus, splitting into two branches. The lateral branch supplies the lateral heel, including the Achilles tendon, plus the lateral forefoot and fifth toe. The medial branch usually supplies or augments innervation to the lateral fourth toe and medial fifth toe. There are also articular branches to the ankle and subtalar joints.

The saphenous nerve is the cutaneous terminal branch of the femoral nerve. It passes into the dorsomedial foot adjacent to the greater saphenous vein, terminating in the skin just before reaching the medial surface of the great toe.

After supplying all muscles in the posterior crural compartment, the posterior tibial nerve gives off the medial calcaneal nerve just before entering the third compartment beneath the laciniate ligament. Within this canal, it divides into two terminal branches: the medial and lateral plantar nerves. These enter the plantar foot via the porta pedis deep to the abductor hallucis muscle belly. The posterior tibial nerve also sends an articular branch into the medial ankle joint.

The medial calcaneal nerve pierces the aponeurosis

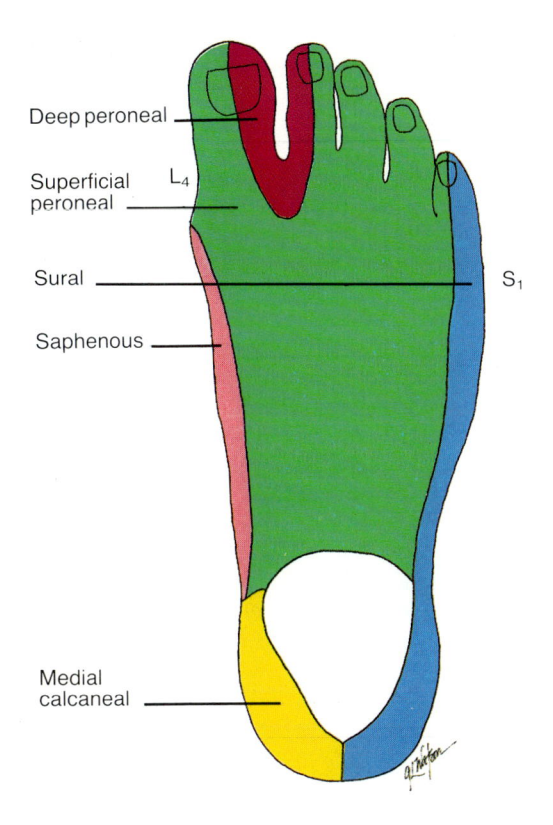

8.5 Dorsal foot dermatomes.

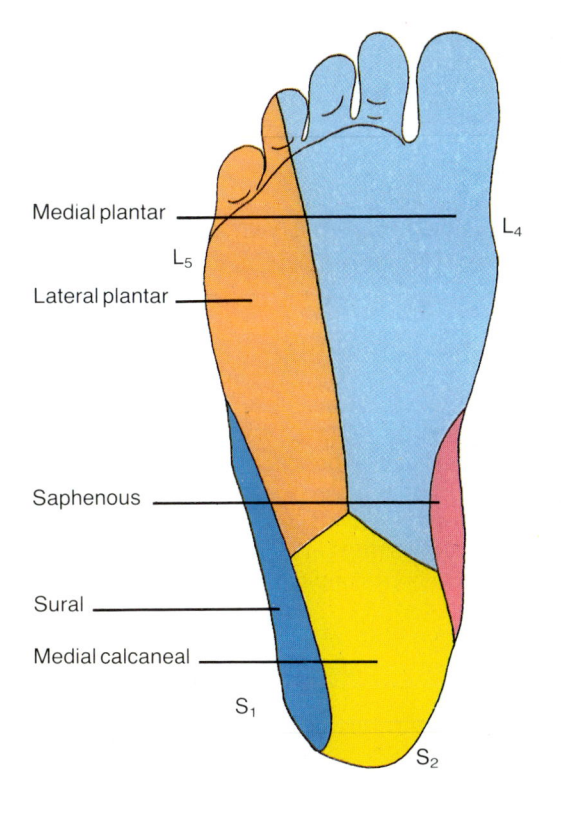

8.6 Plantar foot dermatomes.

and divides into two branches. The posterior branch supplies the skin covering the medial aspect of the Achilles tendon plus the medial and posterior heel. The anterior branch passes forward to supply the skin of the proximal one-third of the medial plantar foot.

Usually larger than its lateral division, the medial plantar nerve lies anteriorly as it passes into the plantar foot. It is plantar to the Master Knot of Henry, then passes within the septum between the abductor hallucis and flexor digitorum brevis, innervating both of these muscles. Distal branches also innervate the flexor hallucis brevis as well as the first and second lumbrical.

Finally, there are two terminal branches, the medial of which becomes the medial plantar nerve of the great toe. The lateral terminal branch divides into three common digital branches, each passing plantar to a deep transverse intermetatarsal ligament. At about this level, the first common digital nerve bifurcates to supply the lateral plantar surface of the great toe and the medial plantar surface of the second toe. The second common digital nerve divides to supply the lateral plantar surface of the second toe and the medial plantar surface of the third toe. Lastly, the third common digital nerve branches to supply the plantar lateral surface of the third toe and the medial plantar surface of the fourth toe. This third common digital nerve often receives an anastomotic branch from the lateral plantar nerve.

The lateral plantar nerve passes into the plantar foot posterior to its medial counterpart, along with the posterior tibial artery. After passing between the quadratus plantae and flexor digitorum brevis muscles, sending branches to each, it then pierces into and passes along the lateral intermusclar septum. It sends a rather larger motor branch transversely into the abductor digiti quinti, passing just anterior to the tuberosities of the calcaneus, and then dividing into two terminal branches.

The superficial branch divides into the fourth common digital nerve, supplying the lateral plantar surface of the fourth toe and the medial plantar surface of the fifth toe, and the lateral plantar cutaneous nerve to the fifth toe. The deep branch of the lateral plantar nerve courses laterally, then medially, generally following the lateral plantar artery arc as it gives off branches to the adductor hallucis heads, the lateral two or three lumbricales, and all four interossi, and then ends in a motor anastomosis to the flexor hallucis brevis.

There can be anatomical variations of all the nerves that deviate somewhat from the above descriptions. The basic pattern, however, must be understood and applied in the clinical setting. Also required is a

163

thorough knowledge of the neurodermatomes (8.3–8.6) and muscle innervation by peripheral nerve and spinal cord level. This battery of information is essential for the clinician to isolate and locate peripheral nerve pathology in the foot.

Peripheral nerve anatomy

The central unit of a peripheral nerve is the nerve fibre, which may vary in length from 0.5 mm to 1 m or more.[2,3] A nerve fibre comprises the axon, with its thin outer layer or axolemma surrounding the viscous axoplasm, the Schwann cell, and the Schwann cell sheath, with or without myelin (8.7). Myelinated nerves have one axon per Schwann cell, while unmyelinated fibres have several axons enveloped by a single Schwann cell (8.8). It should be noted that, since conduction rates are directly related to fibre size, myelinated fibres conduct at a more rapid rate than unmyelinated axons.

Each nerve fibre is surrounded by an endoneurial sheath which includes the basal membrane of the Schwann cell outside the myelin sheath as well as the reticular and collagen fibres that provide the supporting framework.

A fascicle is a unit within a peripheral nerve (8.9),[4] consisting of a group of nerve fibres surrounded by the perineurium. This perineurial sheath is composed of epithelial-like cells as an inner layer and collagen connective tissue as an outer layer.

Finally, a single fascicle or group of fascicles make up the peripheral nerve itself while the collagenous connective support tissue surrounding these fascicles is known as the epineurium, which may be external or interfascicular.

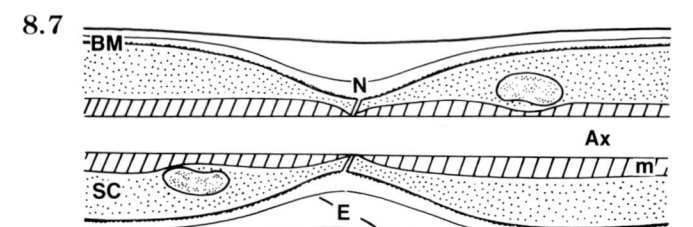

8.7 Microanatomy of a nerve fibre. Longitudinal section of a myelinated nerve fibre (axon). E, endoneurium (inner and outer layers); SC, Schwann cell; m, myelin; Ax, axon; BM, basement membrane; N, node of Ranvier. (Redrawn from Battista and Lusskin.[2])

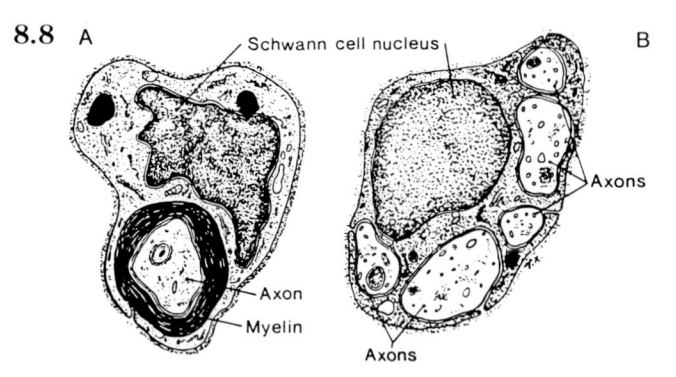

8.8 Myelinated axon: note the Schwann cell nucleus and its relation to the myelin sheath; the basal lamina surrounds the plasma membrane of this satellite cell (A). An unmyelinated fibre consisting of several unmyelinated axons enveloped by a single Schwann cell (B). (From Millesi and Terzis.[3])

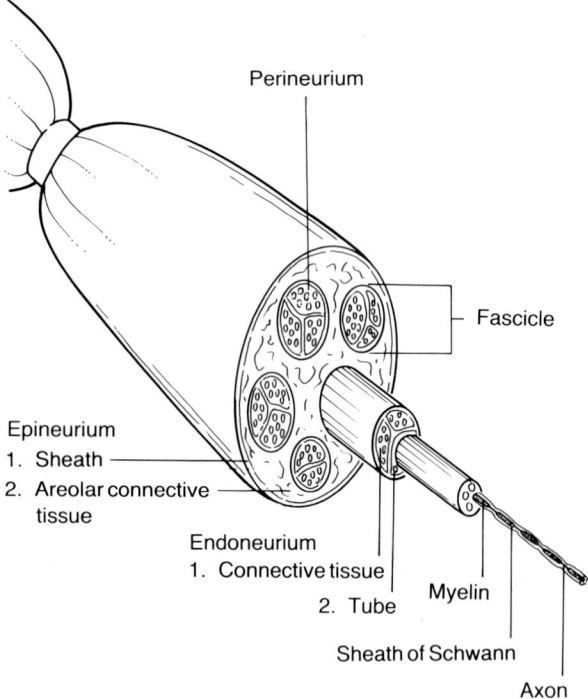

8.9 Microanatomy of a peripheral nerve. (Redrawn from Malay et al.[4])

Definitions

Nerve disorders fall under the general category known as 'peripheral neuropathies'. Peripheral neuropathy is defined as deranged function and structures of peripheral, motor, sensory, and autonomic neurons, involving either the entire neuron or selected levels.[5,6] The major categories of peripheral neuropathies are seen in **Table 8.2**. Since this chapter deals with nerve problems seen in the foot that are most amenable to local treatment, only the last four categories will be considered.

A true neuroma consists of an unorganized mass of ensheathed nerve fibres embedded in scar tissue which originates from the proximal end of a transected peripheral nerve.[7] Neuromas are always the result of trauma. When the injury is incomplete (partial laceration, traction) or the result of blunt trauma, the lesion will form within the epineurium and produce a fusiform or eccentric nodular swelling, termed 'neuroma-incontinuity'.[8] In either case, the axonal elements are disrupted such that they are arranged in a rather haphazard fashion.

Morton's neuroma, the interdigital or intermetatarsal lesion accurately described initially by the English chiropodist Louis Durlacher,[9] is actually a misnomer. It is neither a true neuroma nor a neoplasm. Rather, it is best defined as a mechanical neuropathy, with compression, stretching, and entrapment components in its aetiology. Pathologically, this lesion is a progressive degenerative, and at times regenerative, process in which early and late changes may be found. Characteristic histological findings support the above aetiology (**Table 8.3**). As a result, Morton's neuroma might be more accurately termed a perineural fibroma.[10,11]

Mechanical peripheral neuropathies are those due to local or extrinsic compression phenomena or impingement by an anatomical neighbour that causes localized entrapment.[12] Entrapment may also be caused by scarring or fibrosis, which tends to bind the nerve down, thus restricting or preventing normal mobility within the tissues.

Traumatic neuropathies are the result of either closed or open injuries to peripheral nerves. Early treatment usually involves prophylaxis and repair, while later attention is directed towards the painful neuromas or nerve entrapments that result from the body's healing processes.

Finally, nerve sheath tumours fall under another general category known as parenchymatous disorders, since they can involve the specific neural elements: neuron or axon, Schwann cell, perineurial cell, and eponeurial fibroblast. This is in contrast to the lesions described above, which are termed interstitial disorders, where the derangement is mediated from without.[5,6] Nerve sheath tumours are named according to their structure derivation. They may be either benign or malignant.

Table 8.2 Peripheral neuropathies

Vascular–ischaemic
Metabolic
Nutritional
Infectious
Toxic
Hereditary
Inflammatory demyelinating
Mechanical
   Compression
   Entrapment
Traumatic
   Closed injuries
   Open injuries
Painful neuromas
Nerve sheath tumours

Table 8.3 Histopathology of Morton's neuroma (perineural fibroma)

Venous congestion (early stages)
Endoneural and neural oedema (early stages)
Perineural, epineural, and endoneural fibrosis and hypertrophy (late stages)
Renaut's body formation (evidence of local pressure damage)
Hyalinization of the walls of endoneurial blood vessels
Subintimal and perivascular fibrosis that may lead to occlusion of local blood vessels (resembling healed vasculitis)
Mucinous changes endoneurially and perineurally
Demyelination with axonal loss

Morton's neuroma—the syndrome of intermetatarsal neuroma

Definition and anatomy

Morton's neuroma is a misnomer used to describe a painful pedal neuropathy that most commonly appears as a benign enlargement of the third common digital branch of the medial plantar nerve located between and often distal to, the third and fourth metatarsal heads. In addition, the lesion is usually supplied by a communicating branch from the lateral plantar nerve (**8.10**).[10] In the subsequent discussion the lesion will generally be referred to as an intermetatarsal neuroma or perineural fibroma.

Classically, the involved nerve passes plantar to the deep transverse intermetatarsal ligament. The only additional structures traversing this immediate area are the third plantar metatarsal artery with its accompanying vein or veins, and the tendon slip from the third lumbrical muscle that inserts into the extensor hood apparatus on the medial aspect of the fourth toe. The perineural fibroma is separated from the sole by the subcutaneous fat pad, plantar fascial slips, and connective tissue compartments (**8.11**). Frequently, there is found, either alone or in close association with the perineural fibroma, an intermetatarsal bursa which is deep and usually distal to the deep transverse intermetatarsal ligament (**8.12, 8.13**).[13–16]

Interestingly, this is also the area in which pacinian corpuscles are normally found in the subcutaneous tissues[17] and it is common to find multiple sensory branches diving plantarly from the nerve trunk and/or neuroma at the time of dissection. As an observation, these usually are the patients with the greater neuralgic symptoms causing the metatarsalgia.

Aetiology and biomechanics

Recent published information leaves little doubt that the syndrome of intermetatarsal neuroma is indeed a mechanical entrapment neuropathy,[18–21] with degenerative changes largely the result of both stretch and compression forces. In reference to the development of fibrosis within nerve support structures, Goldman suggests that the epineurium responds to mechanical compression whereas the perineurium responds to stretch.[22]

The next question is what is the source of these mechanical forces? A common observation is that the majority of intermetatarsal neuromas occur in the pronated foot,[23–26] where there are not only excessive stretch forces imposed on the interdigital nerves but also compressive and shearing forces from adjacent hypermobile metatarsal heads.[27–29]

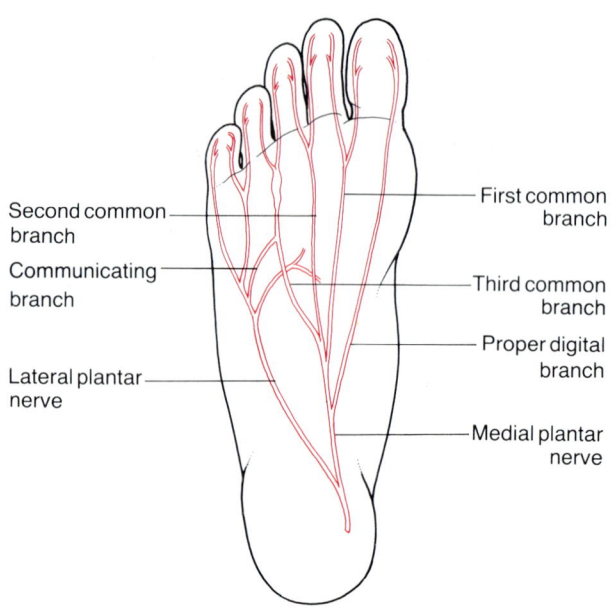

8.10 Classical site of Morton's neuroma in relation to the plantar nerves. (Redrawn from Miller,[10] with permission.)

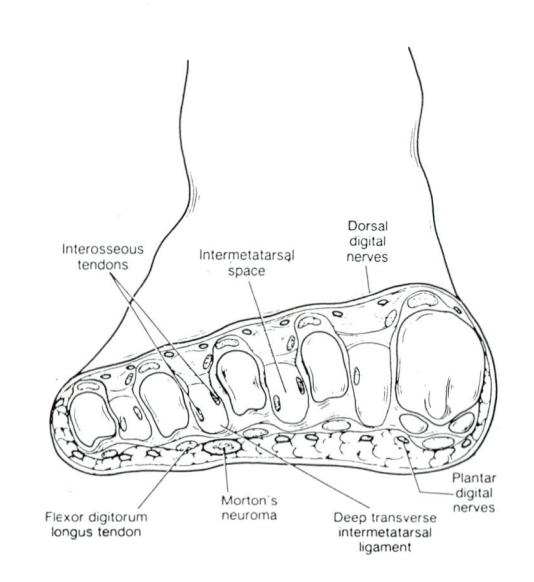

8.11 Cross-section through the forefoot at the level of the metatarsophalangeal joint. (Adapted from Miller.[10])

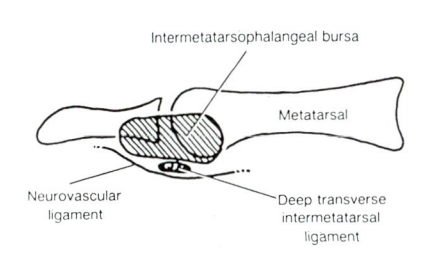

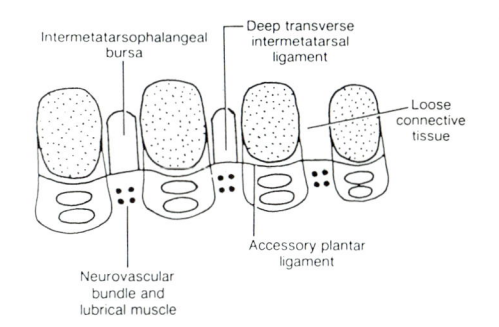

8.12, 8.13 Longitudinal section through third intermetatarsal space (**8.12**). Frontal section through bases of proximal phalanges (**8.13**). There is no bursa in the lateral web space. (Redrawn from Bossley and Cairney.[15])

Since the medial and lateral plantar nerves pass down the medial side of the foot and dive plantarly under the arch, it is easy to see the stretch placed on these nerves during prolonged mid-stance pronation as the foot is everted, abducted, and dorsiflexed. Tension is increased as the nerves pass around the flexor digitorum brevis 'sling'[30] and are drawn up tightly against the plantar and anterior edge of the unyielding deep transverse intermetatarsal ligament. Further tension and compression will occur at this ligament when the toes hyperextend or dorsiflex at the metatarsophalangeal joint.[12,20,30–35] Even occupations that require toe hyperextension can result in the development of an intermetatarsal neuroma, regardless of foot type.

Finally, pointed-toe or narrow shoes can definitely add compressive forces towards the development of intermetatarsal neuromas.[30,32] In addition, high heels will not only throw weight forward onto the ball of the foot, jamming it into the narrow front of the shoe, but will also force the toes into hyperextension and thus contribute to the aetiology.

Histopathology

The microscopic pathology of intermetatarsal neuroma is summarized in **Table 8.3**.[18,22,36–43] Although many of these findings are also found in 'normal' plantar nerves after years of wear and tear, endoneural oedema, exceptional fibrosis, and demyelination are diagnostic of intermetatarsal neuroma (**8.14**).[44] Serial section analysis has revealed that these degenerative nerve changes are usually found distal to the deep transverse intermetatarsal ligament.[20]

Interestingly, as a result of the findings of several investigators, a neuroma does not have to be particularly large or be present for a long time to undergo pathological changes and cause painful symptoms.[25,33,40] Also of interest is that, except for Reed and Bliss[13] and Hauser,[45] other researchers found no histological evidence of inflammation in a neuroma.[40,42,46]

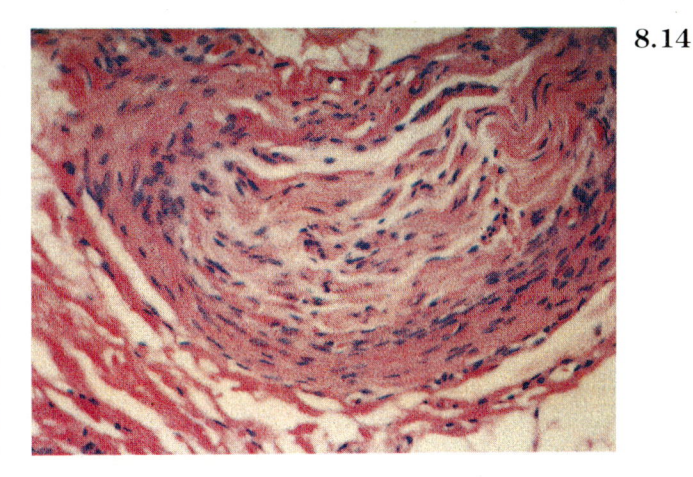

8.14 Photomicrograph of cross-section through a Morton's neuroma (H&E stain, × *100*).

Diagnosis

Intermetatarsal neuromas are classically and most commonly found in females in the third intermetatarsal space (**Table 8.4**); they are also seen frequently in the second but rarely in the first or fourth intermetatarsal space (**Table 8.5**). Although the lesion usually presents as a single entity, more than one intermetatarsal neuroma may develop in the same or both feet (**Table 8.6**).[35,47–52] The lesion is most commonly diagnosed in patients between 40 and 60 years old and the patient is likely to be overweight.[17,26] Symptoms may be present from a few weeks to several years.

Initially, the patient may describe a sensation as if walking on a wrinkle in her stocking or a lump in her toe. In more advanced cases, the pain may be sharp,

167

Table 8.4 Distribution of intermetatarsal neuromas by sex

Study	Male	Female	n
Bradley, et al.[47]	14 (16%)	71 (84%)	85
Gauthier[48]	19 (9%)	187 (91%)	206
Mann and Reynolds[49]	3 (5%)	53 (95%)	56
Wachter et al.[35]	7 (17%)	7 (83%)	7
Gudas and Mattana[50]	7 (16%)	36 (84%)	43
Addante et al.[51]	27 (20%)	109 (80%)	136
Johnson[52]	? (22%)	? (78%)	124
Average	15%	85%	

Table 8.5 Intermetatarsal space location of neuromas

Study	1st	2nd	3rd	4th	Other
Wachter, et al.[35]		43%	57%		
Gudas and Mattana[50]		5.1%	86.4%	8.5%	
Addante et al.[51]	3.9%	17.8%	66.4%	2.6%	9.2%
Johnson[52]		16%	84%		

Table 8.6 Post-operative symptoms of neuroma (from Mann and Reynolds[49])

Study	Single	Double	Bilateral	Repeat	(n)
Bradley et al.[47]	63%	4%	27%	6%	85
Gauthier[48]	42%	23%	35%	—	304
Mann and Reynolds[49]	61%	—	39%	15%	76
Gudas and Mattana[50]	63%	11%	26%	—	43
Johnson[52]	82%	2%	14%		149
Average	62%	10%	28%	11%	

Table 8.7 Pre-operative symptoms of neuroma (from Mann and Reynolds[49])

Symptoms	Neuromas N = 65	(%)	Recurrent neuromas N = 11	(%)
Pain radiating to toes	40	62	4	36
Burning pain	35	54	4	36
Aching or sharp pain	26	40	7	63
Pain up foot or leg	22	34	2	18
Relief by removing shoe	46	70	6	54
Relief by rest	58	89	11	100
Cramping sensation	22	34	0	0
Pain increased with walking	59	91	11	100
Plantar pain	50	77	11	100
History of associated injuries	10	15	1	9
Numbness into toes or foot	26	40	2	18

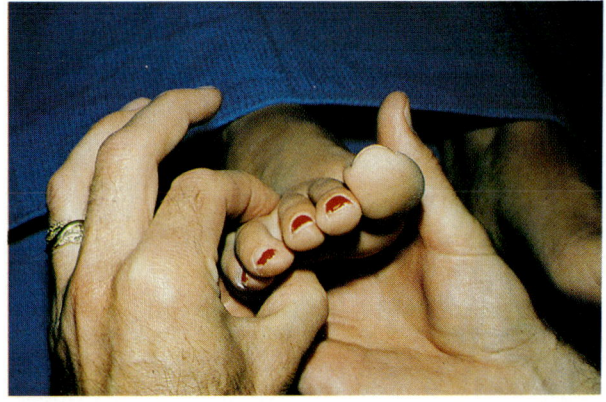

dull, or throbbing but classically presents as a paroxysmal burning sensation 'like walking on a hot pebble' or 'having a hot poker thrust between the toes'.

The pain is most often localized to the region of the third and fourth metatarsal heads and may radiate distally into adjacent toes, especially the fourth, or proximally up the leg to the knee and, in rare instances, as high as the hip. Numbness in the third and fourth toes may be the presenting symptom; however, there is seldom a sensory deficit. Patients sometimes describe a 'cramping' sensation in the arch of the toes but there is no physical evidence of cramping (**Table 8.7**).[49,53]

Normally, the pain is greatly aggravated by walking in shoes and is relieved somewhat by rest. Occasionally, the pain remains at rest, and at night the patient might even find that pressure from the bed sheets is intolerable. The overwhelming desire to remove the shoe, massage the forefoot, and flex the toes is pathognomonic, although relief is only transient.

In many cases, acute pain symptoms appear after an incidence of trauma of some sort. Examples include stepping on a rock, twisting an ankle, jamming the foot into the floorboard in a motor vehicle accident, or simply changing into a pair of new shoes and doing an extraordinary amount of walking. Narrow or tight-fitting shoes can both instigate and aggravate pain symptoms.

The intermetatarsal spaces are often tender to direct plantar palpation. A thickened nerve cord can

8.15 The 'lateral squeeze test' is positive when the manoeuvre reproduces pain symptoms.

frequently be rolled against a thumb over the distal metatarsal heads in the plantar sulcus when the toes are dorsiflexed. This may reproduce a varying amount of pain. Dorsoplantar palpation of the affected intermetatarsal space with simultaneous side-to-side compression of the metatarsal heads (the 'lateral squeeze test') can reproduce the pain by directly trapping the neuroma with pressure (**8.15**).

When lateral compression of the metatarsal heads elicits a silent, palpable, and sometimes painful 'click', Mulder's sign is said to be positive.[54] However, the intermetatarsal bursa can also be responsible for the click.[55]

Electrodiagnostic techniques for evaluating intermetatarsal neuroma are not that accurate because of the difficulty in isolating a single interdigital nerve with an electrode to measure sensory conduction velocity.[19] However, in one such study the diagnosis was confirmed by electrophysiological testing of five patients.[56] Positive results were characterized by an 'abnormal dip phenomenon', a relatively normal nerve conduction velocity, and normal duration of the sensory compound nerve action potential. These findings are the hallmarks of a neuropathy with predominantly axonal degeneration.

The differential diagnosis of intermetatarsal neuroma includes intermetatarsal bursitis, rheumatoid arthritis, osteochondritis dissecans of metatarsal heads, localized vasculitis, ischaemic pain, nerve root compression syndromes, metabolic peripheral neuropathy, tarsal tunnel syndrome, and metatarsal stress fractures. Weight-bearing radiographs should be taken to rule out other possible osseous pathology. However, the neuroma itself is not visible on X-ray films or xeroradiographs.

Conservative management

Initial measures for treatment should be directed towards reducing or preventing irritation of the neuroma. Wider shoes with good arch support and adequate toe room is the simplest approach. Avoiding high heels can be helpful, but most patients have already discovered this. Metatarsal pads set just at the proximal edges of metatarsal heads two, three, and four will help splay the bones and draw the weight proximally off the neuroma (**8.16**). Several padding techniques designed to relieve pressure have been described.[57-62] This can be combined with a Lo–Dye strapping to add more support (**8.17**). Toe crest pads sometimes provide relief.

If successful results occur with pads and strappings, then cast-fitting neutral position orthoses may be helpful. The goal is to limit pronation and hypermobility of the forefoot, both of which cause painful irritation of the neuroma.[63-66]

Injection therapy can provide a measure of relief using proper techniques.[67] Vitamin B_{12} or cyanocobalamin infiltration advocated by one author[59] resulted in some success, although the results may have been caused by the sclerosing effects of the preserving agent, 1% benzoyl alcohol.

Several writers have described injection therapy using various steroid preparations combined with a local anaesthetic.[67-71] Infiltration starting dorsally should be directed between the metatarsal head, injecting before and after penetration of the deep transverse intermetatarsal ligament, then distally into the

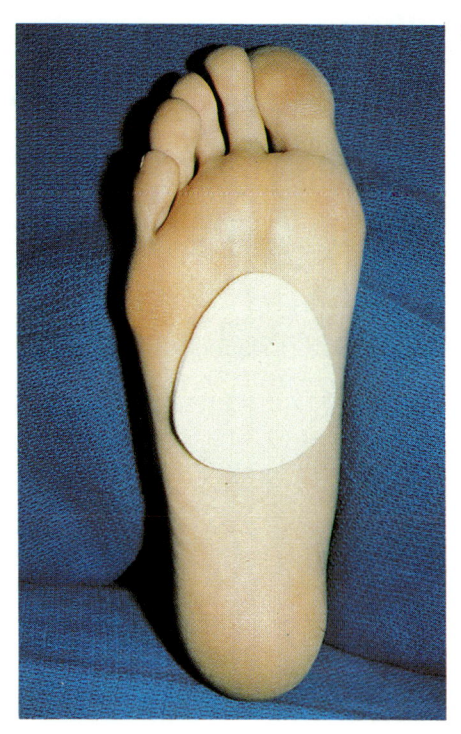

8.16 Placement of a metatarsal pad to treat Morton's neuroma.

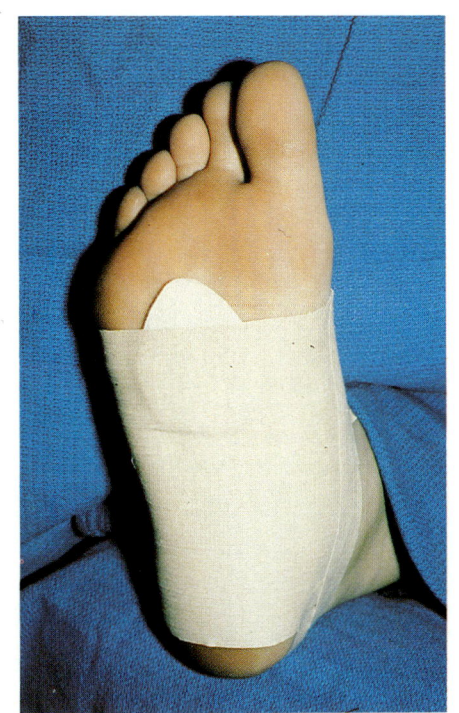

8.17 Lo–Dye strapping to relieve metatarsalgia.

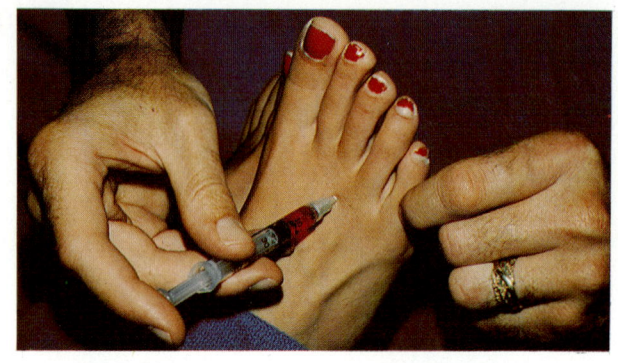

8.18 Injection therapy for treatment of intermetatarsal neuroma.

8.19 Incisional approaches for resection of Morton's neuroma. A, Longitudinal plantar incision;[30,31,54,76,79] B, transverse plantar incision;[37,76] C, web-splitting incision;[32,76] D, dorsal incision.[77,78] (Redrawn from Miller.[10])

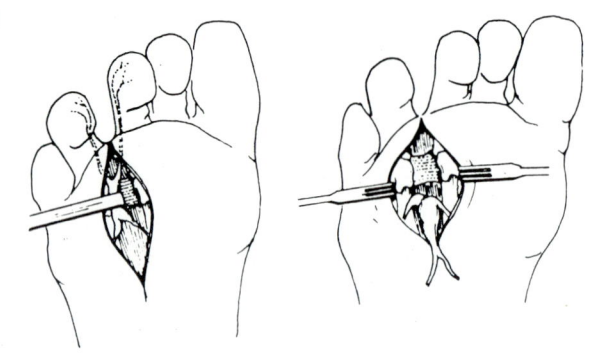

8.20 Plantar approach for resection of Morton's neuroma. (Redrawn from Miller.[10])

sulcus area (**8.18**). The patient should be cautioned that the symptoms may even get worse for 1 or 2 days before the desired effects are obtained. This so-called steroid flare is seen especially when less-soluble steroid salts are utilized. Pain may also be accentuated if there is direct injury to the nerve tissue by the needle.

The use of a local anaesthetic by itself, acting as a nerve block, is rarely therapeutic but may give helpful diagnostic information.

Finally, Dockery and Nilson[67] state that infiltration with a dilute (4%) ethanol solution can be effective when the neuroma has a chronic history; injection of approximately 1 ml at a time provides the necessary sclerosing effect. The solution is made by withdrawing 2 ml from a 50 ml vial of 2% Lidocaine (lignocaine) and replacing it with 2 ml of alcohol USP (ethanol). A minimum of three injections, at weekly intervals, is usually necessary to obtain complete and permanent results.[67] Care must be taken to inject only the diluted alcohol; infiltration of pure alcohol has led to disastrous results, including sloughing of the skin and intervening tissues.[72]

Surgical management

Indications
When conservative measures fail and painful symptoms persist, surgical excision becomes the treatment of choice.[10,11,14,16,31,32,42,53,54,61,66,73–75]

Although no well-controlled studies have been reported that analyse and compare the conservative approaches to intermetatarsal neuromas, except for mixed results from injection therapy, it is the general experience that only 29–30% of symptomatic patients respond to non-operative measures. Patients should be made aware of this early in their management programme, since the majority will go on to surgical resection for relief of their painful symptoms. However, even with surgical intervention, 8–13% of the patients will have unsatisfactory results.[47–50]

Surgery is usually performed in an out-patient setting under general, regional, or local anaesthesia. When excised under local anaesthesia, field infiltration should be augmented with a posterior tibial nerve block to prevent the lancinating pain that can occur when the proximal nerve trunk is sharply severed.

Four approaches have been described for access to the intermetatarsal neuroma: plantar longitudinal,[30,31,54,76] plantar transverse,[37,76] web-splitting,[32,74] and dorsal.[77,78] All have advantages and disadvantages (**8.19**). The two most frequently used techniques will be described.

Plantar approach
The second most common approach is via plantar longitudinal incision. This approach provides the best ex-

8.21 Dorsal approach A–E for resection of Morton's neuroma. (Redrawn from Miller.[10])

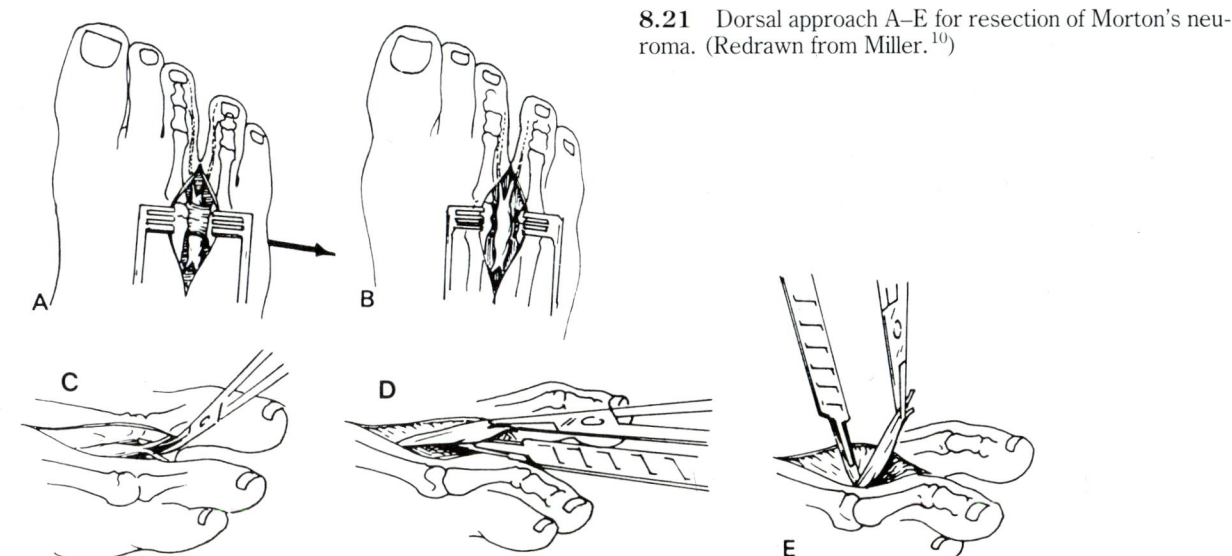

posure to the neuroma and leaves the deep transverse intermetatarsal ligament intact. The disadvantage is the potential for a painful plantar scar on the weight-bearing surface. Prophylaxis includes careful placement of the incision between the metatarsal heads and 3 weeks of absolutely no weight-bearing postoperatively.[11] Excision via the plantar approach has achieved a 93% success rate in one study.[80]

Once the plantar incision is made and haemostasis achieved, minimal dissection will expose the entire neuroma. Vascular structures are easily identified and preserved and the deep transverse intermetatarsal ligament is left undisturbed because the neuroma lies plantar to it. The digital branches are isolated and clearly transected, followed by the proximal nerve trunk and, if present, accessory branches. Using vertical mattress sutures, deep closure is made, with little or no dead space (**8.20**).

Dorsal approach

The more common dorsal approach has the advantage of allowing early ambulation, since the incision is on a non-weight-bearing surface (**8.21**). There is some disadvantage in the initial awkwardness of dissecting deep between the metatarsal heads as well as in having to sever the deep transverse intermetatarsal ligament. These tasks are facilitated with the use of the Schink Metatarsal Spreader (**8.22**). There is also greater potential for dead space[11] and damage to intrinsic neurovascular and muscular units.

After the initial dorsal incision over the intermetatarsal space, blunt dissection is carried down to the deep transverse intermetatarsal ligament, which is sharply incised. The metatarsal spreader is inserted for maximum exposure. Gentle finger pressure on the plantar sulcus will deliver the fusiform neuroma into the wound so the digital branches can be isolated, clamped, and cut distally (**8.23**). Vascular structures must be identified and divided for haemostasis only when necessary. The neuroma is then dissected as far proximal as possible, placed under tension, and cleanly transected along with any other communicating branches present. Routine closure should include a large over-and-over suture through adjacent capsules to bring the metatarsal heads close together and allow healing of the deep transverse intermetatarsal ligament. A closed suction drain can be inserted if necessary to prevent haematoma formation.

Deep transverse intermetatarsal ligament

The role of the deep transverse intermetatarsal ligament has raised some interesting issues. Gauthier[48] achieved an 83% overall success rate by simply transecting the ligament (which he identified as plantar fascia) and then performing microscopic epineural neurolysis. Bradley et al.[47] achieved better results when the neurectomy was combined with percutaneous fas-

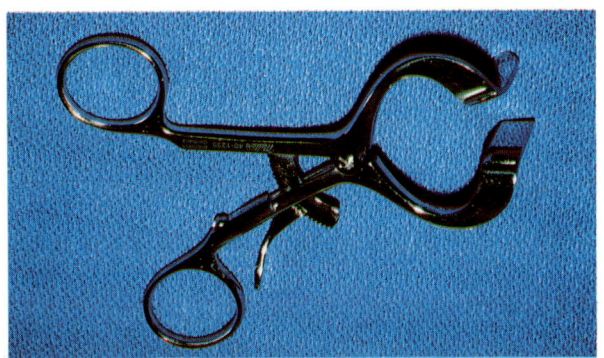

8.22 Schink Metatarsal Spreader. Strong, thin retractor blades allow ease of introduction into the surgical site to spread the metatarsals for less traumatic access to the proximal trunk of the neuromas. (Courtesy of Miltex Instrument Company, Inc., New York.)

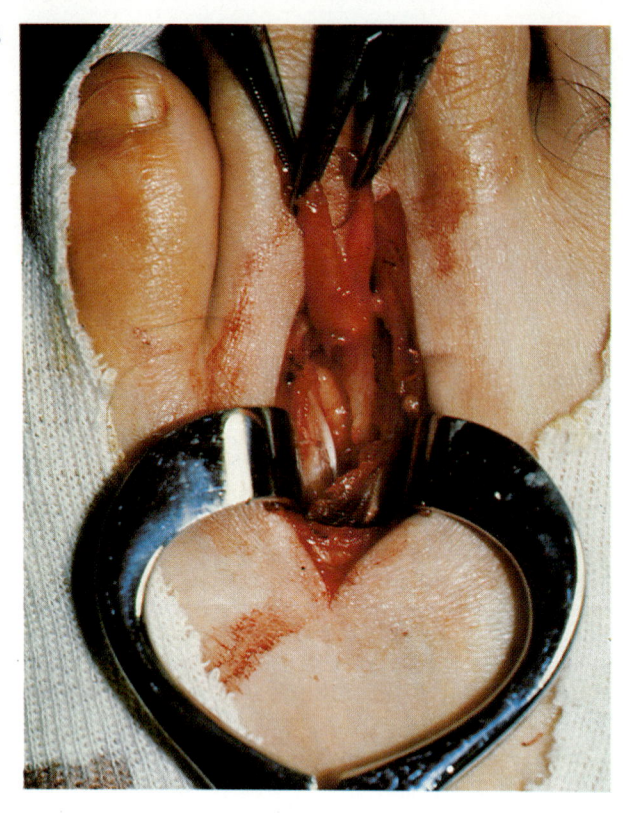

8.23 Dissection for dorsal excision of Morton's neuroma.

ciotomy, 83% as compared with 66% without. Gudas and Mattana reported good to excellent results in 79% of their series in which the neuromas were excised via the dorsal approach leaving the said ligament intact.

It is important to preserve the function of the deep transverse ligament as it provides a fulcrum around which the lumbrical tendon stabilizes the lesser toes. When this tendon loses its functional ability, the affected lesser toe begins a dorsal contracture at the proximal phalanx, until the extensor tendon and hood apparatus take over; the result is a full hammertoe deformity. Suturing the adjacent capsules will bring the metatarsal heads close enough for the ligament to heal. In re-operating on recurrent neuromas, Mann and Reynolds noted complete reconstitution of the deep transverse intermetatarsal ligament that had been sectioned at initial surgery.

Adjacent interspaces

Since neuromas can occur in adjacent intermetatarsal spaces, excision of both neuromas simultaneously adds to the risk of vascular embarrassment. The use of magnifying glasses or surgical loupes will aid proper visualization of the micro-anatomy. Separate incisions should be kept as far apart as possible to avoid necrosis of the intervening skin. When using a single incision, the incorporation of curves will make allowance for scar contracture and help prevent digital deformities. When a single incision is utilized, make sure dissection is carried down to a level below the subcutaneous tissue that contains the vascular structures before undermining into either intermetatarsal space. When circulation is identified as marginal, the more painful neuroma should be excised first and the adjacent intermetatarsal neuroma resected 1–2 months after the primary incision has healed.[11]

Surgical complications

Whatever approach is made for intermetatarsal neuroma surgery, observance of several principles will minimize complications. These include:

1. Gentle handling of tissues at all times.
2. Meticulous haemostasis. A cuff or tourniquet is not necessary.
3. Identification of the digital branches before completing the resection.
4. Removal of the neuroma without damaging the intermetatarsal artery or the local tendon from the lumbrical muscle.
5. Clean transection of the nerve trunk far enough proximally to prevent irritation or adhesions to the stump.
6. Intraneural injection of the proximal nerve trunk prior to transection, with one or two drops of steroid solution to impede scar adhesions and sensitive axon sprouts at the nerve end.
7. Closure of dead space as necessary. When this is not possible, a closed suction drain should be inserted.
8. Use of a firm, even compression dressing, which is essential to help prevent post-operative haematoma formation.

Haematoma can form in the dead space, following a neuroma resection, as a result of blood and serum accumulation. This will not only intensely prolong the initial inflammatory phase of healing, with added pain and frustration, but will also provide excellent media for bacteria proliferation. Prophylactic antibiotics, expression of the haematoma, compression dressing, needle aspiration, and surgical removal of the clot are approaches to treatment.

Vascular ischaemia of the toes results from interruption of arterial supply, vasospasm, and congestion due to post-operative oedema. Early recognition should lead to prompt treatment, such as loosening of any tight dressing, removal of ice, reflex heat, sympathetic nerve blocks, reversal of epinephrine effects using local infiltration with phentolamine (Regitine), abstinence from caffeine and nicotine, and warming up the surrounding environment. In emergency situations, 5–10 mg of isoxuprine (Vasodilan), intramuscularly, or 10 mg of nifedipine (Procardia), orally, should stimulate effective vasodilation. Unchecked, a cyanotic toe

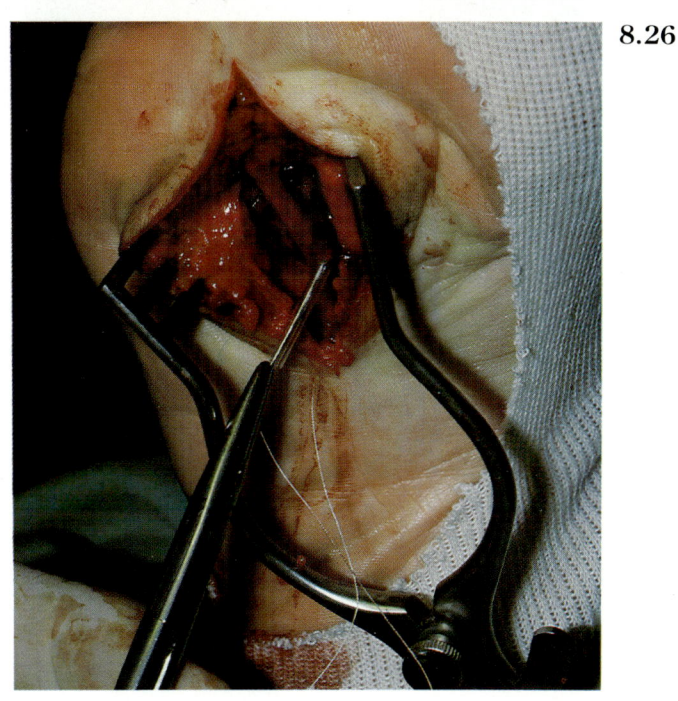

8.24 Usual point of maximum tenderness following excision of Morton's neuroma.

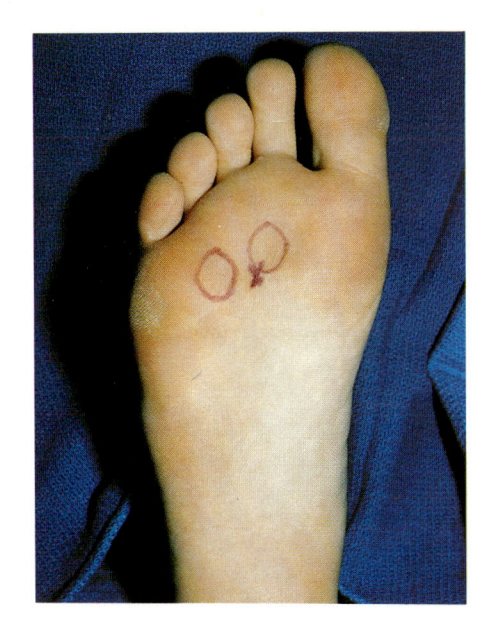

8.25 Adherence of nerve stump to adjacent metatarsal head capsular tissue as seen on re-entry (plantar approach).

8.26 Application of silicone plastic nerve cap to protect the transected end of the nerve.

can progress to frank gangrene with subsequent amputation.

Probably the most troublesome complication is the painful *stump neuroma* or *recurrent neuroma* formation. Actually, a true bulbous stump neuroma is a rare finding at secondary operation. In most instances, recurrent neuromas presented with adhesions to the plantar joint capsule of a metatarsal head; the pain appeared to be the result of traction/impingement forces causing mechanosensitivity at the transected nerve ending.[49,81] The same authors[49] identified in one-third of their re-operated cases an accessory nerve trunk passing under the deep transverse intermetatarsal ligament. It appeared to have developed into a 'recurrent neuroma', having been damaged at the time of the primary surgery.

The 'recurrent neuroma' is identified by sharp, often lancinating, or burning paraesthesias, aggravated by weight-bearing or point-pressure, and persisting well after local tissues have healed (**8.24**). Symptoms can even be similar to those experienced prior to the initial surgery. Treatment is initially conservative, using various padding and injection techniques. Triamcinalone acetonide infiltration is thought to soften the scar tissue adhering the nerve end to surrounding tissue, thus providing a measure of scar release.[82]

Surgical re-entry must be via a plantar incision to provide good visualization and access to the more proximal nerve trunks (**8.25**). The goal is neurolysis to free the nerve and a clean transection of the nerve more proximally with the nerve under tension. The nerve end should then withdraw into the intrinsic muscle bellies, away from weight-bearing areas, for protection. Implementation of several prophylactic measures will help minimize further adhesions or stump neuroma formations. The use of an interneural steroid injection, a 4% alcohol sclerosing solution,[67] and a metal ligation clamp help discourage neurite formation.[11] Containment of the axon sprouts and protection against adhesions is the goal of silicone caps, which can be applied to the end of the nerve in order to isolate it (**8.26**).[83–85] Unfortunately, there are no good controlled studies to examine the efficacy of such treatment.

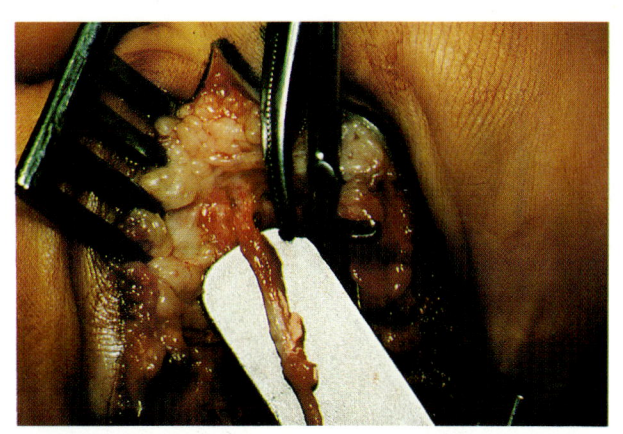

Results of re-operation for intermetatarsal neuromas vary widely. Bradley et al.[47] found unsatisfactory results in 4 out of 5 patients re-explored, while Mann and Reynolds[49] reported significant improvement in 9 of 11 patients (81%) and Beskin and Baxter[86] achieved 50% or more improvement in 33 out of 38 patients (87%). Nelms et al.[87] were able to obtain good to excellent results in 24 of 27 patients (89%) by tucking the nerve end into a drill hole in an adjacent metatarsal.

Results of Surgery

Several studies have shown that satisfactory results occur in an average of 84% of the patients who undergo neurectomy surgery (**Table 8.8**),[47–50,52] although a good number of these will still have some uncomfortable, yet tolerable, lingering sensations. Results are better when the third intermetarsal space alone is involved and decrease dramatically when the condition persists bilaterally or when the second or other spaces are also involved.[50,86]

Beskin and Baxter identified two clinical groups of patients who experienced pain following neurectomy: those that remain symptomatic after neurectomy and those that recur after a period of quiescence.[86] Identifying patients pre-operatively who are at risk for recurrent neuroma formation is virtually impossible, although it is a goal worthy of pursuit.

Actually, what remains after neurectomy is a severed nerve end, the same as when a limb is amputated. Spontaneous firing starts the day the nerve is cut and has two peaks of activity: the first occurs at about the third day and the second occurs within the third week.[88] For some people this is a much more sensitive phenomenon than for others, perhaps moderated or enhanced by neighbouring sympathetic fibres.[89,90]

As the end of the nerve degenerates, immature axon 'sprouts' form (**8.27**). These can be quite sensitive, especially to mechanical pressure. The axons will extrude with unlimited growth potential, seeking to connect with the distal axons. When blocked by local tissues or scar, the axons can convolute into a painful stump neuroma. Simultaneously, the fibroblasts within the supporting perineurium and epineurium are forming scar tissue that can bind down the end of the nerve and place it under traction tension or compression.

In conclusion, excision of the intermetatarsal neuroma is a procedure not to be undertaken without a thorough patient work-up and meticulous surgical technique. Honest patient rapport and responsible postoperative management will lead to a cooperative relationship when complications persist.

8.27 Formation of 'axon sprouts' through the proximal end of a cut nerve. (Redrawn from Millesi.[91])

Table 8.8 Unsatisfactory results of neuroma surgery

Study	Unsatisfactory rate (%)
Bradley et al.[47]	13 (34.3)
Gauthier[48]	17
Mann and Reynolds[49]	20
Gudas and Mattana[50]	21
Karges[80]	7
Johnson[52]	19
Average	16

Diagnosis of nerve injuries and entrapments

Patients afflicted with nerve injuries or compression problems tend to experience pain and paraesthesias typical of nerves. Sometimes, they are enhanced with bizarre symptoms, especially when the patient has an overly anxious or hysterical personality. The pain is characteristically of a sharp or burning nature, localized over the sensory distribution of the involved nerve. The extent of the area involved will depend on what portion of the nerve trunk is damaged or impinged.

Early in the entrapment process, the patient may experience muscle cramps or a feeling of tight, heavy, or swollen feet. Dysaesthesia, hypaesthesia, and hyperaesthesia can be extremely uncomfortable. It may then progress to altered sensations of tingling, burning, or numbness. The pain is often present at rest and may increase in severity at night, causing restlessness. It is aggravated by increased extremity movement and activity. Proximal radiation is common. Altogether, the symptoms can be very exasperating and debilitating, causing complete disability.

When a motor nerve is primarily involved, the symptoms are less well defined as to distribution. Motor nerve pain is characteristically dull and aching, affecting the muscle or muscles innervated by the affected nerve. Local joints will also hurt, especially proximally. As the neuropathy persists over time, muscle tenderness can be found, leading eventually to paresis and disuse atrophy.

Sensorimotor examination is central to objective evaluation. Decreased two-point tactile discrimination over 6 mm is an early sign. When the nerve is accessible, deep palpation may reveal enlargement and/or elicit tenderness and paraesthesias. Often it will reproduce the patient's symptoms.

Percussion of the nerve, causing distal radiation of paraesthesias, is a positive Tinel's sign, while proximal and distal radiation indicates a positive Valleix phenomenon. Both are indicative of traumatic or compression damage.

Diagnostic nerve blocks that selectively anaesthetize the suspected nerve with Lidocaine or Bupivacaine will result in dramatic relief when there is a nerve entrapment. This helps identify the nerve trunk and localize nerve branches to further isolate the problem. Perineural infiltration with steroid at the site of the entrapment can also decrease symptoms remarkably, by reducing inflammation and fibrosis, another good diagnostic aid.

Nerve condition velocity is decreased in most cases of nerve entrapment, although normal findings do not rule out impingement. Electromyographic studies are less helpful, unless there is virtually complete nerve conduction blockade.

Magnetic resonance imaging (MRI) has provided some rather striking visualizations of nerve entrapments, although diagnostic value relative to cost must be considered since it is currently an expensive test. MRI can give good contrasts in soft tissue density.

Entrapment neuropathy about the first metatarsophalangeal joint

The four nerve branches crossing this joint correspond roughly to the four corners of the hallux. The dorsolateral surface is supplied by the deep peroneal nerve and its pathology is described elsewhere.

Joplin described a perineural fibrosis of the proper digital nerve as it coursed along the plantomedial first metatarsal head. He reported the removal of 265 of these entities.[92] The nerve either displaces laterally from its usual anatomical position or, in the course of the development of hallux valgus deformity, the metatarsal head drifts medially to bear weight directly on top of the nerve. Pronatory forces that concentrate body weight through the medial foot provide further compressive forces that stimulate perineural oedema and fibrosis, axon degeneration, and Renaut body formation. The result is pain, paraesthesias, and numbness.

Treatment with pads and orthotic devices to redistribute weight will help relieve pressure on the nerve. Steroid injections can be helpful and anaesthetic infiltration may be diagnostic. Surgery is the curative treatment, by means of a neurectomy through a medial incisional approach at the junction of the dorsal and plantar skin. Clean transection of the proximal nerve trunk under tension will allow the nerve end to retract into the abductor hallucis muscle belly for protection (**8.28**).[93]

Another location for entrapment compression neuropathy is the dorsomedial first metatarsophalangeal joint.[94] The most medial branch of the medial dorsal cutaneous nerve becomes compressed between an enlarged medial eminence and the shoe, with very little enlargement necessary to develop the problem. Avoidance of shoe pressure, padding, injection therapy, and bunionectomy will all help alleviate the pressure. At times, nerve excision is necessary to relieve painful paraesthesias that are unresponsive to other forms of treatment. Similar neuromas can be found in association with tailor's bunions, where treatment is generally the same.[95]

Intermetatarsal plantar neuromas are rarely found between the first and second metatarsal heads, only 3.9% in one study.[96] Such a painful lesion can remain after corrective bunion surgery, having been over-

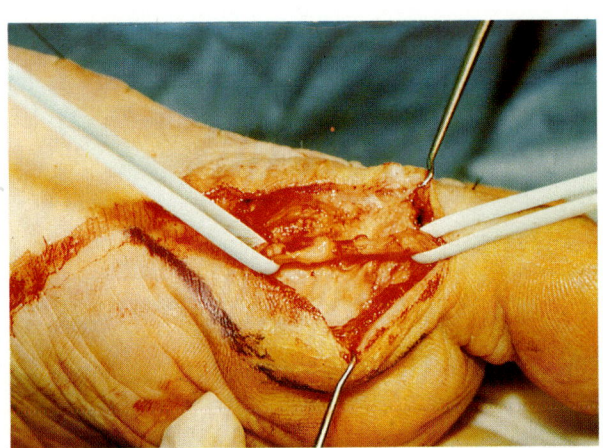

8.28 Example of Joplin's neuroma dissected from beneath the medial edge of a bunion.

Failure of conservative treatment requires surgical excision through a dorsal or plantar approach, or a fibular sesamoidectomy. Again, the nerve trunk must be sharply divided and allowed to retract into the intrinsic muscle bellies. The patient must be made aware of the areas of anaesthesia that will result.

looked as contributing to the patient's symptoms preoperatively. Hypermobility is part of the cause of intermittent nerve compression, but a contributing factor can be the laterally displaced fibular sesamoid impinging the nerve against the second metatarsal head. Neuralgic symptoms are usually the result.

Compression neuropathy of the deep peroneal nerve

Compression neuropathy involving the anterior tibial or deep peroneal nerve has been described as 'anterior tarsal tunnel syndrome.'[97] It may be an entrapment of the nerve at the inferior extensor retinaculum (**8.29**).[98,99] It can also be caused by traction, trauma, local exostoses, oedema, or shoe pressure. Altered sensation in the third web space is the hallmark diagnostic sign.[100]

EMG studies may reveal distal latency in the deep peroneal nerve and there may be signs of denervation in the extensor digitorum brevis muscle.

Treatment includes avoidance of shoe pressure, steroid injections, and pads to disburse direct pressure on the nerve. If conservative therapy fails, surgical intervention for relief of symptoms includes exostectomy, neurolysis, or retinacular release.

Sural nerve entrapment

Entrapment of the sural nerve will cause sensory alterations and pain locally at the site of entrapment or all the way along its course laterally to the fifth toe. Local trauma, surgical nerve injury, and long-term chronic tendonitis of the tendo Achilles are the leading aetiologies of this compression syndrome.[4]

If unresponsive to the usual conservative approaches, surgical intervention is frequently necessary. Neurolysis is the first choice for release, but since the sural nerve is totally sensory, sectioning and excising the nerve are commonly necessary to alleviate the pain. Care must be taken to allow the nerve end to retract into the shelter of soft tissues to prevent sensitive stump neuroma formation.

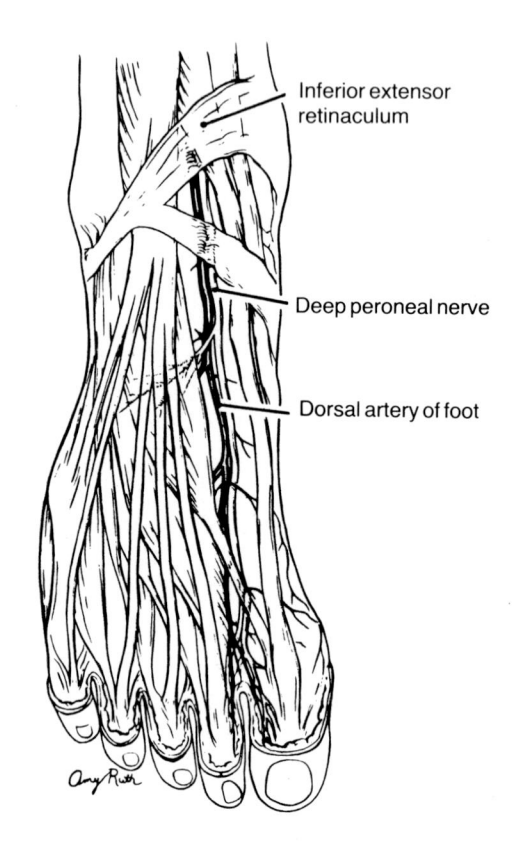

8.29 Deep peroneal nerve anatomy. (From Adelman et al.[100])

Dorsal forefoot nerve injury and entrapment

In addition to entrapment of the deep peroneal nerve on the dorsum of the foot, compression of the superficial peroneal nerve, as it exists the deep fascia in the lower leg, can cause painful symptoms. The peroneal nerve can also be trapped against dorsal exostoses along the course of its branches or can be injured by trauma.

Since many surgical approaches occur via the dorsal foot, surgical trauma can result in painful sensory neuromas in that area. In one study, 19 of 25, or 76% of the neuromas occurred within the medial two-thirds of the dorsal midfoot, an area termed the neuromatous or

N-zone (**8.30**). Although nerves are frequently damaged in bunion surgery, they are seldom symptomatic. In addition, toe surgery rarely results in painful neuromas or nerve injuries.[101]

Once identified, nerves trapped in scar tissue can be treated by injection therapy using enzyme mixtures, sclerosing solutions, steroid preparations, or volume injection adhesiotomy techniques.[67,102] If they remain painful, they are best treated by neurolysis and excision. This is a technically difficult and often painful approach that can yield up to 26% unsatisfactory results.[103] The conclusion is that it is much easier to prevent a sensory neuroma by careful surgical technique than to treat a highly symptomatic neuroma. This involves thoughtful planning for the location of the incision, gentle tissue separation and retraction, identification of peripheral nerves, and judicious suturing technique.

Symptoms can also occur on the dorsal foot when the superficial peroneal nerve suffers a traction injury or entrapment at the fibular neck[104,105] or where it exits the deep fascia in the anterior lower leg.[106] Local injury can occur from contusions, fractures, midfoot exostoses, or by compression from adjacent soft tissue masses such as ganglia.

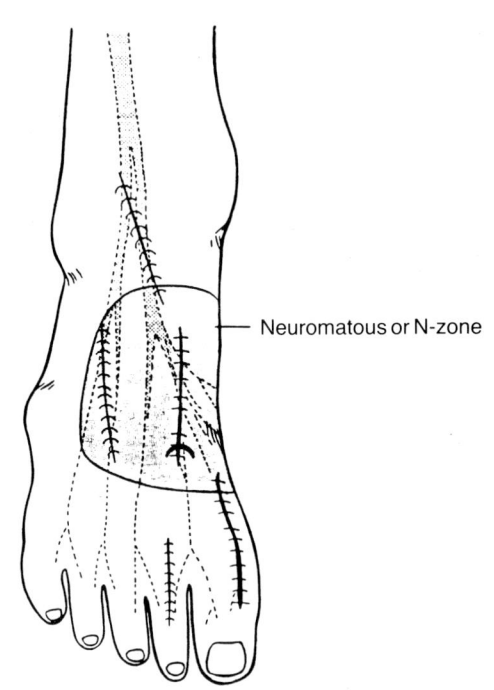

8.30 Neuromatous or N-zone where incisions are more likely to lead to symptomatic neuromas. (Redrawn from Kenzora.[101])

Tarsal tunnel syndrome

The symptom complex caused by entrapment of the posterior tibial nerve was first described by Pollock and Davis in 1933,[107] then named by Keck in 1962[108] and later the same year by Lam.[109] Entrapment may result from recent weight gain, post-traumatic fibrosis, chronic compression from fascial bands, restriction within the laciniate canal, and entrapment by the abductor hallucis muscle (**8.31, 8.32**).[111] It has also been postulated to occur in association with os trigonum syndrome.[112] Goodman and Kehr reported 27 cases of bilateral tarsal tunnel syndrome, suggesting that it is more common than previously believed.[113] The condition is also commonly seen in the chronically pronated foot and ankle.

Symptoms consist primarily of sharp or burning paraesthesias radiating into the plantar aspect of the foot, aggravated by activity and relieved somewhat by rest and removing shoes. Proximal radiation is common, although usually not past the knee. Pain may occur at night with the patient in bed. Patients may also relate a feeling of 'fullness' or 'tightness' in the arch, while others complain of a sensation of impending arch cramps.[114] The onset of the neuropathy is usually 'spontaneous' or slow and insidious and may be mistakenly diagnosed as intermetatarsal neuromas.[115] When symptoms of multiple intermetatarsal neuromas are present, it would be wise to carefully rule out tarsal tunnel syndrome before starting treatment.

There is rarely any motor weakness detectable, although EMG studies often demonstrate abnormal fibrillation potentials within the intrinsic muscles. Prolonged latency in the conduction of impulses along the medial and plantar nerves, greater than 6.1 ms and 6.7 ms, respectively, help confirm the presence of a compression neuropathy.[116]

In cases of tarsal tunnel syndrome, percussion of the posterior tibial nerve will almost always elicit a positive Tinel's sign as well as a positive Valleix phenomenon. Turk's test, performed by inflating a thigh cuff to just below the systolic blood pressure, can exacerbate symptoms as the venae comitantes become engorged within the tarsal tunnel.[117]

Conservative measures include control of excessive pronation, non-steroid anti-inflammatory drugs, massage, ultrasound, and the injection of steroid preparations or large volumes of local anaesthetic into the third canal of the tarsal tunnel. If symptoms persist, then surgical decompression is indicated. The laciniate ligament must be incised over the third canal followed by careful neurolysis, first proximally and then distally, where the porta pedis is dilated as the nerve passes beneath the abductor hallucis muscle belly into the plantar vault. Tortuous veins in the area are excised and ligated. Only the superficial fascia is sutured, leaving the laciniate ligament open. A compression dressing is applied and the patient kept non-weight-

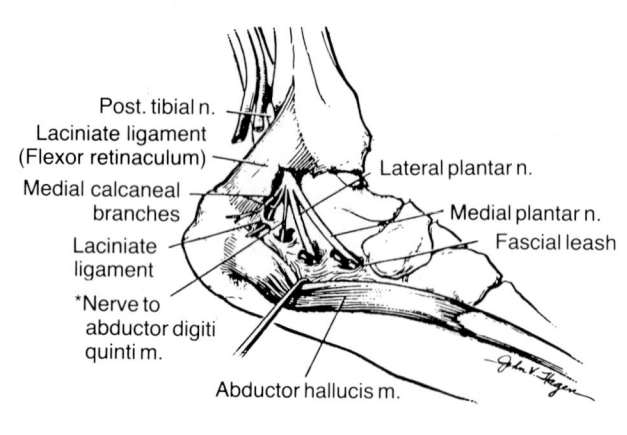

8.31, 8.32 Medial view of the foot showing branches of the posterior tibial nerve as they pass beneath the laciniate ligament through the third compartment of the tarsal canal. (Redrawn from Baxter and Thigpen.[110])

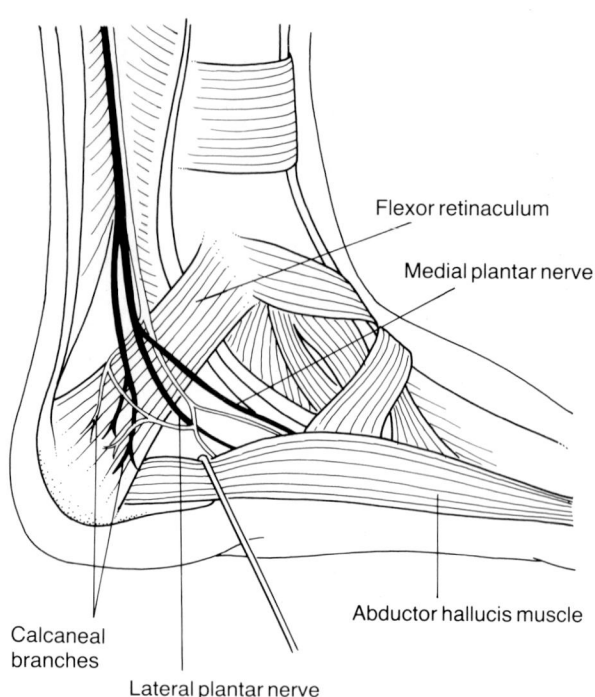

bearing for no longer than 2 weeks so as to mobilize the tissues early. The post-operative Tinel's sign will usually diminish with time.[4]

With symptoms generally the same, an extension of the tarsal tunnel syndrome involves entrapment or compression of the plantar nerves at the level of the abductor hallucis upon entering the foot or beneath the midtarsus in the severely collapsed flat foot. In the latter case, the nerve is placed under severe stretch when abduction is present and the patient may actually be placing full weight on the nerve through the bones of the tarsus. This is an extremely difficult condition to treat successfully. Conservative care involves using soft orthoses to distribute the weight away from the nerve. Surgery, when necessary, must not only free the nerve tissue but also create some form of arch architecture, through arthrodesing procedures, in order to get the weight-bearing pressure off the nerve.

Calcaneal nerve entrapment

Heel involvement has been reported as part of the tarsal tunnel syndrome,[111,118] but generally the area is spared. However, patients with recalcitrant heel pain—with or without calcaneal spurs—have been shown to experience good relief from decompression and neurolysis of the calcaneal nerve, usually the mixed sensorimotor branch to the proximal abductor digiti quinti muscle.[110,119,120]

The most common origins of the calcaneal nerve are from the posterior tibial or lateral plantar nerves. Origins from the posterior tibial nerve occur in equal frequencies within and proximal to the tunnel. Origins from the lateral plantar nerve occur almost always within the tunnel.[121]

Except when involved in tarsal tunnel syndrome, entrapment of the calcaneal nerve branch to the abductor digiti quinti muscle can cause severe and disabling heel pain. The nerve can be traumatized and compressed primarily at two sites: at the firm fascial edge of the abductor hallucis muscle;[122,123] and at the medial edge of the calcaneus, where the nerve traverses either beneath the medial tuberosity or along the origin of the flexor brevis muscle and plantar fascia (**8.33, 8.34**).[120]

The symptoms usually differ from those of plantar fasciitis in that they involve a sharp, burning pain that often radiates up the posteromedial leg. It can be reproduced by deep compression just medial or distal to the medial tuberosity. Patients frequently fail to experience the pain on weight-bearing after rest (post-static dyskinaesia) that is almost pathognomonic of the plantar fasciitis enthesopathy.

Pronation can be a great contributor to this entrapment, but the syndrome also occurs in feet with normal

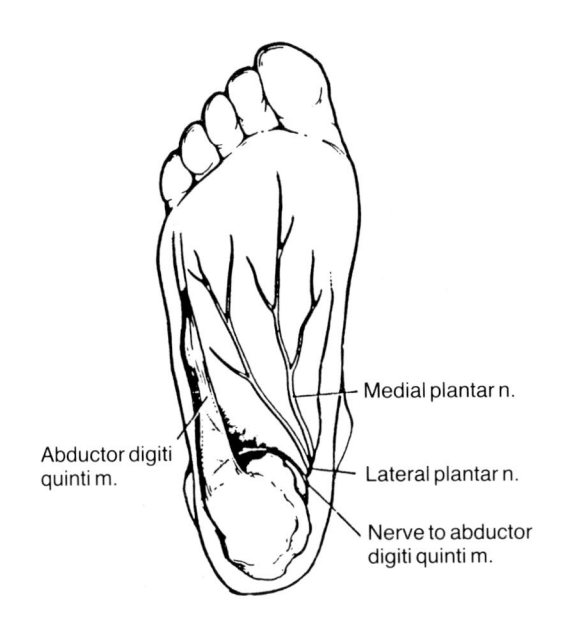

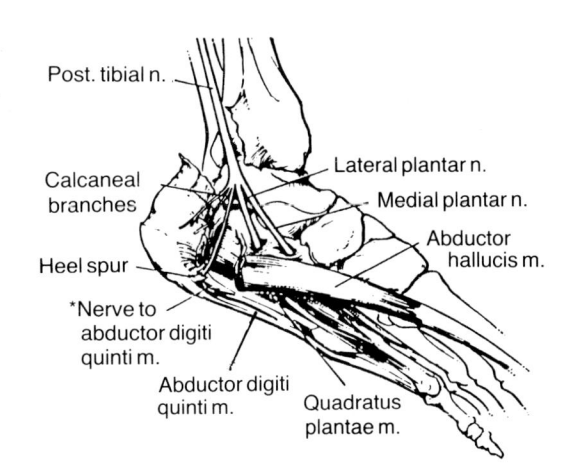

8.33, 8.34 Course of the calcaneal nerve branch to the abductor digiti quinti muscle. (Redrawn from Baxter and Thigpen.[110])

or supinated architecture. Affected patients are commonly athletes or people whose occupations require long hours on concrete or other unforgiving surfaces. They characteristically do not respond to the variety of conservative therapeutic measures used to treat heel pain, including rest, tape strappings, steroid injections, shoe adjustments, orthotic devices, ultrasound, and massage. In fact, many of these therapies tend only to aggravate the condition.

Surgery involves a medial incision to access the nerve at or distal to the medial tuberosity. The deep fascia of the abductor hallucis muscle is released. The nerve is then freed along its course distal and deep to the medial tuberosity as it approaches the abductor digiti quinti muscle. The medial plantar fascia should be incised and only a small portion of heel spur removed, when present, but only if it appears to be contributing to the entrapment. Results are often in the form of dramatic relief the next day. Patients should be kept non-weight-bearing for 2 weeks, with a gradual return to full activity.

References

[1] Sarrafian, S.K. *Anatomy of the Foot and Ankle: Descriptive, Topographic and Functional.* Philadelphia, J.B. Lippincott, 1983, p.317.

[2] Battista, A.F. and Lusskin, R. The anatomy and physiology of the peripheral nerve. *Foot Ankle,* **7**: 65–70, 1986.

[3] Millesi, H. and Terzis, J. Nomenclature in peripheral nerve surgery. Committee report of the International Society of Reconstructive Microsurgery. *Clin. Plast. Surg.,* **11**: 3–8, 1984.

[4] Malay, D.S., McGlamry, E.D. and Nava, C.A., Jr. Entrapment neuropathies of the lower extremities. *In* McGlamry, E.D. and McGlamry, R, (eds), *Textbook on Foot Surgery,* Vol. II. Baltimore, Williams & Wilkins, 1987, pp.668–684.

[5] Dyck, P.J. The causes, classifications and treatment of peripheral neuropathy. *New Eng. J. Med.,* **307**: 283–286.

[6] McQuarrie, I.G. Peripheral nerve surgery—today and looking ahead. *Clin. Plast. Surg.,* **13**: 255–268, 1986.

[7] Fisher, G.T. and Boswick, J.A. Neuroma formation following digital amputations. *J. Trauma,* **23**: 136–142, 1983.

[8] Mathews, G.J. and Osterholm, J.L. Painful traumatic neuromas. *Surg. Clin. N. Am.,* **51**: 1313–1324, 1972.

[9] Durlacher, L. *A Treatise on Corns, Bunions, the Disease of Nails and the General Management of the Feet.* London, Simkin, Marshall, 1845, p.52.

[10] Miller, S.J. Surgical technique for resection of Morton's neuroma. *J. Am. Podiatry Assoc.,* **71**: 181–188, 1981.

[11] Miller, S.J. Morton's neuroma: A Syndrome. *In* McGlamry E.D. and McGlamry, R. (eds), *Textbook on Foot Surgery,* Vol I. Baltimore, Williams & Wilkins, 1987, pp.38–56.

[12] Kravette, M.A. Peripheral nerve entrapment syndromes in the foot. *J. Am. Podiatry Assoc.,* **61**: 457–472, 1971.

[13] Reed, R.J. and Bliss, B.O. Morton's neuroma: regressive and productive intermetatarsal elastofibrositis. *Arch. Pathol.,* **95**: 123, 1973.

[14] Shepherd, E. Intermetatarsophalangeal bursitis in the causation of Morton's metatarsalgia. *J. Bone Joint Surg.,* **57B**: 115, 1975.

[15] Bossley, C.J. and Cairney, P.C. The metatarso-phalangeal bursa—its significance in Morton's metatarsalgia. *J. Bone Joint Surg.,* **62B**: 184–191, 1980.

[16] Burns, A.E. and Stewart, W.P. Morton's neuroma. *J. Am. Podiatry Assoc.,* **72**: 135–141, 1982.

[17] Goldman, F. and Gardner, R. Pacinian corpuscles as a cause for metatarsalgia. *J. Am. Podiatry Assoc.,* **70**: 561, 1980.

[18] Ochoa, J. The primary nerve fibropathology of plantar neuromas. *J. Neuropathol. Exp. Neurol.,* **35**: 370, 1976.

[19] Guiloff, R.J., Scadding, J.W. and Klenerman, L. Morton's metatarsalgia: clinical, electrophysiological, and histological observations. *J. Bone Joint Surg.,* **66B**(4): 586–591, 1984.

[20] Graham, C.E. and Graham, D.M. Morton's neuroma: A microscopic evaluation. *Foot Ankle,* **5**(2): 150–153, 1984.

[21] Alexander, I.J., Johnson, K.A. and Parr, J.W. Morton's neuroma: A review of recent concepts. *Orthopedics,* **10**(1): 102–106, 1987.

[22] Goldman, F. Intermetatarsal neuroma: Light microscopic observations. *J. Am. Podiatry Assoc.,* **69**: 317, 1979.

[23] Gilbey, V.P. The non-operative treatment of metatarsalgia. *J. New Ment. Health Dis.,* **19**: 589, 1894.

[24] Pincus, A. Intractable Morton's toe (neuroma). Review of the literature and report of cases. *J. Am. Podiatry Assoc.,* **40**: 19–35, 1950.

[25] Tate, R.O. and Rusin, J.J. Morton's neuroma: Its ultrastructural anatomy and biomechanical etiology. *J. Am. Podiatry Assoc.,* **68**: 797, 1978.

[26] Bartolomei, F.J. and Wertheimer, S.J. Intermetatarsal neuromas: distribution and etiologic factors. *J. Foot Surg.,* **22**: 279–282, 1983.

[27] Carrier, P.A., Janigan, J.D., Smith, S.D. and Weil, L.S. Morton's neuroma: a possible contributing etiology. *J. Am. Podiatry Assoc.,* **65**: 315, 1975.

[28] Sgarlato, T.E. *Compendium of Podiatric Biomechanics.* California College of Podiatric Medicine, San Francisco, 1971.

[29] Root, M.L., Orien, W.F. and Weed, J.M. Normal and abnormal function of the foot. *Clinical Biomechanics,* Vol. 2. Los Angeles, Clinical Biomechanics, 1977, pp.112, 296, 322–325.

[30] Bickel, V.H. and Dockerty, M.B. Plantar neuromas, Morton's toe. *Surg. Gynecol. Obstets.,* **84**: 111, 1947.

[31] Betts, L.O. Morton's metatarsalgia. *Med. J. Aust.,* **1**: 514, 1940.

[32] McElvenny, R.T. The etiology and surgical treatment of intractable pain about the fourth metatarsophalangeal joint (Morton's toe). *J. Bone Joint Surg.,* **25**: 675, 1943.

[33] Baker, L.D. and Kuhn, M.H. Morton's metatarsalgia: localized degenerative fibrosis with neuromatous proliferation of the fourth plantar nerve. *South. Med. J.,* **37**: 123, 1944.

[34] Denny-Brown, D. and Doherty, M.M. Effects of transient stretching of peripheral nerve. *Arch. Neurol. Psych.,* **54**: 116, 1945.

[35] Wachter, S., Nilson, R.Z. and Thul, J.R. The relationship between foot structure and intermetatarsal neuromas. *J. Foot Surg.,* **23**(6): 436–439, 1984.

[36] King, L.S. Note on the pathology of Morton's metatarsalgia. *Am. J. Clin. Pathol.,* **16**: 124, 1946.

[37] Nissen, K.I. Plantar digital neuritis. *J. Bone Joint Surg.,* **30B**: 84, 1948.

[38] Scott, T.M. The lesion of Morton's metatarsalgia (Morton's toe). *Arch. Pathol.,* **63**: 91, 1957.

[39] Lassmann, G. and Machacek, J. Clinical features and histology of Morton's metatarsalgia. *Wien Klin. Wochenschr.,* **81**: 55, 1969.

[40] Meachim, G. and Aberton, J.J. Histological findings in Morton's metatarsalgia. *J. Pathol.,* **103**: 209, 1971.

[41] Lassmann, G., Lassmann, H. and Stockinger, L. Morton's metatarsalgia. Light and electron microscopic observations and their relation to entrapment neuropathies. *Virchows Arch. Pathol. Anat.*, **370**: 307, 1976.
[42] Lassmann, G. Morton's toe: clinical, light, and electron microscopic investigations in 133 cases. *Clin. Orthop.*, 142–73, 1979.
[43] Goldman, F. Intermetatarsal neuromas—light and electron microscopic observations. *J. Am. Podiatry Assoc.*, **70**: 265–278, 1980.
[44] Ringertz, N. and Unander-Scharin, M.L. Morton's disease: a clinical and pathoanatomical study. *Acta Orthop. Scand.*, **19**: 327, 1950.
[45] Hauser, E.D.W. Neurofibroma of the foot. *J. Am. Med. Assoc.*, **121**: 1217, 1943.
[46] Viladot, A. and Moragas, A. Entermedad de Morton. *Podologic*, **5**: 233, 1966.
[47] Bradley, N., Miller, W.A. and Evans, J.P. Plantar neuromas: analysis of results following surgical excision in 145 patients. *South. Med. J.*, **69**: 853–854, 1976.
[48] Gauthier, G. Thomas Morton's disease: a nerve entrapment syndrome. A new surgical technique. *Clin. Orthop. Rel. Res.*, **142**: 90–92, 1979.
[49] Mann, R.A. and Reynolds, J.C. Interdigital neuroma—a critical analysis. *Foot Ankle*, **3**: 243–248, 1983.
[50] Gudas, C.J. and Mattana, G.M. Retrospective analysis of intermetatarsal neuroma excision with preservation of the transverse metatarsal ligament. *J. Am. Podiatric Med. Assoc.*, **76**: 459–463, 1986.
[51] Addante, J.B., Peicott, P.S., Wong, K.Y. and Brooks, D.L. Interdigital neuromas: results of surgical excision of 152 neuromas. *J. Am. Podiatric Med. Assoc.*, **76**: 493–495, 1986.
[52] Johnson, K.A. *Surgery of the Foot and Ankle*. New York, Raven Press, 1989, pp. 69–82.
[53] Pincus, A. The syndrome of plantar metatarsal neuritis. *J. Am. Podiatry Assoc.*, **52**: 746, 1962.
[54] Mulder, J.D. The causative mechanism in Morton's metatarsalgia. *J. Bone Joint Surg.*, **33B**: 94, 1951.
[55] Berlin, S.J., Domick, I., Block, L.D. and Costa, A.L. Nerve tumors of the foot: diagnosis and treatment. *J. Am. Podiatry Assoc.*, **65**: 157, 1975.
[56] Oh, S.J., Kim, H.S. and Ahmed, B.K. Electrophysiological diagnosis of interdigital neuropathy of the foot. *Muscle and Nerve*, **7**: 218–225, 1984.
[57] Schreiber, L.J. Method of padding for Morton's neuralgia. *J. Am. Podiatry Assoc.*, **29**: 5, 1939.
[58] Polokoff, M.M. The treatment of Morton's metatarsalgia. *J. Am. Podiatry Assoc.*, **38**: 27, 1948.
[59] Brohner, M.D. Morton's toe or Morton's neuralgia. *J. Am. Podiatry Assoc.*, **59**: 18, 1969.
[60] Silverman, L.J. Old principles and new ideas. *J. Am. Podiatry Assoc.*, **31**: 7, 1941.
[61] Milgram, J.E. Morton's neuritis and management of post-neurectomy pain. *In* Omer, G.E. and Spinner, M. (eds), *Management of Peripheral Nerve Problems*. Philadelphia, W.B. Saunders, 1980, pp. 203–215.
[62] Milgram, J.E. Office methods for relief of the painful foot. *J. Bone Joint Surg.*, **49A**: 1099, 1964.
[63] Whitman, R. Anterior metatarsalgia. *Trans. Am. Orthop. Assoc.*, **11**: 34–53, 1898.
[64] Hohmann, G. Uber die Mortonsche neuralgie am fuss Bietrage. *Orthopad*, **13**: 649, 1966.
[65] Silverman, L.J. Morton's toe or Morton's neuralgia. *J. Am. Podiatry Assoc.*, **66**: 749, 1976.
[66] Milgram, J.E. Design and use of pads and strappings for office relief of the painful foot. *In* Kiene, R.H. and Johnson, K.A. (eds), *Symposium on the Foot and Ankle*. St. Louis, C.V. Mosby, 1983, pp. 95–101.
[67] Dockery, G.L. and Nilson, R.Z. Intralesional injections. *Clin. Podiatric Med. Surg.*, **3**: 473–485, 1986.
[68] Steinberg, M.D. The use of vitamin B-12 in Morton's neuralgia. *J. Am. Podiatry Assoc.*, **45**: 41, 1955.
[69] Wright, E.W. Injection therapy in Morton's neuralgia. *J. Am. Podiatry Assoc.*, **45**: 566–567, 1955.
[70] Cozen, L. Neuroma of plantar digital nerve. *In Clinical Orthopedics*, Vol. 2. Philadelphia, J.B. Lippincott, 1958, pp. 224–226.
[71] Greenfield, J., Rea, J. and Ilfeld, F.W. Morton's interdigital neuroma: indications for treatment by local injections versus surgery. *Clin. Orthop. Rel. Res.*, **185**: 142–144, 1985.
[72] Lapidus, P.W., and Wilson, M.J. Morton's metatarsalgia. *Bull. NY Med. Coll.*, **12**: 34–46, 1969.
[71] Giannestras, N.J. *Foot Disorders, Medical and Surgical Management*. Philadelphia, Lea & Febiger, 1967, pp. 494–498.
[73] May, V.R., Jr. The enigma of Morton's neuroma. *In* Bateman, J.E. (ed.), *Foot Science*. Philadelphia, W.B. Saunders, 1976, pp. 222–234.
[74] Joplin, R.J. Some common foot disorders amenable to surgery. *AAOS Instructional Course Lectures*, **15**: 144, 1958.
[75] Kelikian, H. *Hallux Valgus, Allied Deformities of the Forefoot, Metatarsalgia*. Philadelphia, W.B. Saunders, 1965, pp. 359–368.
[76] Kaplan, E.B. Surgical approach to the plantar digital nerves. *Bull. Hosp. Joint Dis. Orthop. Inst.*, **1**(1): 96–97, 1950.
[77] KcKeever, D.C. Surgical approach for neuroma of plantar digital nerve (Morton's metatarsalgia). *J. Bone Joint Surg.*, **34A**: 490, 1952.
[78] Kitting, R.W. and McGlamry, E.D. Removal of an intermetatarsal neuroma. *J. Am. Podiatry Assoc.*, **63**: 274, 1973.
[79] Hoadley, A.E. Six cases of metatarsalgia. *Chicago Med. Rec.*, **5**: 32, 1893.
[80] Karges, D.E. Plantar excision of primary interdigital neuromas. *Foot Ankle*, **9**: 120–124, 1988.
[81] Nelms, B.A., Bishop, J.O. and Tullos, H.S. Surgical treatment of recurrent Morton's neuroma. *Orthopedics*, **7**(11): 1708–1711, 1984.
[82] Smith, J.R. and Gomez, N.H. Local injection therapy of neuromata of the hand with triamcinalone acetonide. *J. Bone Joint Surg.* **52**(1): 71–83, 1970.
[83] Swanson, A.B., Boeve, N.R. and Lumsden, R.M. The prevention and treatment of amputation neuromata by silicone capping. *J. Hand Surg.*, **2**: 70–78, 1977.

[84] Burke, B.R. A preliminary report in the use of silastic nerve caps in conjunction with neuroma surgery. *J. Foot Surg.*, **17**(2): 53–57, 1978.

[85] Midenberg, M.L. and Kirschebaum, S.E. Utilization of silastic nerve caps for the treatment of amputation neuromas. *J. Foot Surg.*, **25**(6): 489–494, 1986.

[86] Beskin, J.L. and Baxter, D.E. Recurrent pain following interdigital neurectomy—a plantar approach. *Foot Ankle*, **9**(1): 34–39, 1988.

[87] Nelms, B.A., Bishop, J.O. and Tullos, H.S. Surgical treatment of recurrent Morton's neuroma. *Orthopedics*, **7**(11): 1708–1711, 1984.

[88] Scadding, J.W. Development of ongoing activity, mechanosensitivity, and adrenaline sensitivity in severed peripheral nerve axons. *Exp. Neurol.*, **73**: 345–364, 1981.

[89] Devor, M. and Janig, W. Activation of myelinated afferents ending in a neuroma by stimulation of the sympathetic supply in the rat. *Neurosci. Lett.*, **24**: 43–47, 1981.

[90] Wall, P.D. and Gutnick, M. Ongoing activity in peripheral nerves: the physiology and pharmacology of impulses originating from a neuroma. *Exp. Neurol.*, **43**: 580–593, 1974.

[91] Millesi, H. Healing of nerves. *Clin. Plast. Surg.*, **4**: 459, 1977.

[92] Joplin, R.J. The proper digital nerve, vitallium stem arthroplasty, and some thoughts about foot surgery in general. *Clin. Orthop. Rel. Res.*, **76**: 199–212, 1971.

[93] Merritt, G.N. and Subotnick, S.I. Medial plantar digital proper nerve syndrome (Joplin's neuroma): typical presentation. *J. Foot Surg.*, **21**: 166, 1982.

[94] Lee, B. and Crowhurst, J.A. Entrapment neuropathy of the first metatarsophalangeal joint: two case reports. *J. Am. Podiatric Med. Assoc.*, **77**(12): 657–659, 1987.

[95] Thul, J.R. and Hoffman, S.J. Neuromas associated with tailor's bunion. *J. Foot Surg.*, **24**: 342, 1985.

[96] Addante, J.B., Peicott, P.S., Wong, K.Y. and Brooks, D.L. Interdigital neuromas: results of surgical excision of 152 neuromas. *J. Am. Podiatric Med. Assoc.*, **76**(9): 493–495, 1986.

[97] Krause, K.H., Witt, T. and Ross, A. Anterior tarsal tunnel syndrome. *J. Neurol.*, **217**: 67–74, 1977.

[98] Borges, L.F., Hallett, M., Selkoe, D.J. and Welch, K. The anterior tarsal tunnel syndrome. Report of two cases. *J. Neurosurg.*, **54**: 89–92, 1981.

[99] Gessini, L., Jandolo, B. and Pietrangeli, A. The anterior tarsal tunnel syndrome. Report of four cases. *J. Bone Joint Surg.*, **66A**: 786–787, 1984.

[100] Adelman, K.A., Wilson, G. and Wolf, J.A. Anterior tarsal tunnel syndrome. *J. Foot. Surg.*, **27**: 299–302, 1988.

[101] Kenzora, J.E. Symptomatic incisional neuromas on the dosum of the foot. *Foot Ankle*, **5**: 2–15, 1984.

[102] Edwards, W.G., Lincoln, C.R., Bassett, F.H. and Goldner, J.L. The tarsal tunnel syndrome: diagnosis and treatment. *J. Am. Med. Assoc.*, **207**(4): 716–720, 1969.

[103] Kenzora, J.E. Sensory nerve neuromas—leading to failed foot surgery. *Foot Ankle*, **7**: 110–117, 1986.

[104] Meals, R.A. Peroneal-nerve palsy complicating ankle sprain. *J. Bone Joint Surg.*, **59A**: 966–968, 1977.

[105] Vastamaki, M. Decompression for peroneal nerve entrapment. *Acta Orthop. Scand.*, **57**: 551–554, 1986.

[106] Lemont, H. and Hernandez, A. Recalcitrant pain syndromes of the foot and ankle: Evaluation of the lateral dorsal cutaneous nerve. *J. Am. Podiatry Assoc.*, **62**: 331–335, 1972.

[107] Pollock, L.J. and Davis, L. *Peripheral Nerve Injuries.* New York, Hoeber, 1933, pp. 484–493.

[108] Keck, C. The tarsal tunnel syndrome. *J. Bone Joint Surg.*, **44A**: 180–184, 1962.

[109] Lam, S.J.S. The tarsal tunnel syndrome. *J. Bone Joint Surg.*, **49B**: 87–92, 1967.

[110] Baxter, D.E. and Thigpen, C.M. Heel pain—operative results. *Foot Ankle*, **5**: 15–25, 1984.

[111] Edwards, W.G., Lincoln, C.R., Bassett, F.H. and Goldner, J.L. The tarsal tunnel syndrome: diagnosis and treatment. *J. Am. Med. Assoc.*, **207**(4): 716–720, 1969.

[112] Havens, R.T., Kaloogian, H., Thul, J.R. and Hoffman, S. A correlation between os trigonum syndrome and tarsal tunnel syndrome. *J. Am. Podiatric Med. Assoc.*, **76**: 450–454, 1986.

[113] Goodman, C.R. and Kehr, L.E. Bilateral tarsal tunnel syndrome: A correlative perspective. *J. Am. Podiatric Med. Assoc.*, **78**: 292–294, 1988.

[114] Radin, E.L. Tarsal tunnel syndrome. *Clin. Orthop. Rel. Res.*, **181**: 167–170, 1983.

[115] Mann, R.A. Tarsal tunnel syndrome. *Orthop. Clin. N. Am.*, **5**: 109–115, 1974.

[116] Johnson, E.W. and Ortiz, P.R. Electrodiagnosis of tarsal tunnel syndrome. *Arch. Phys. Med.*, **45**: 548–554, 1964.

[117] Gilliat, R.W. and Wilson, T.G. A pneumatic tourniquet test in carpal tunnel syndrome. *Lancet*, **2**: 595, 1953.

[118] Dellon, A.L. and MacKinnon, S.E. Tibial nerve branching in the tarsal tunnel. *Arch. Neurol.*, **41**: 645–646, 1984.

[119] Przylucki, H. and Jones, C.L. Entrapment neuropathy of muscle branch of lateral plantar nerve: a cause of heel pain. *J. Am. Podiatry Assoc.*, **71**: 119–124, 1981.

[120] Henricson, A.S. and Westlin, N.E. Chronic calcaneal pain in athletes: entrapment of the calcaneal nerve. *Am. J. Sports Med.*, **12**: 152–154, 1984.

[121] Havel, P.E., Ebraheim, N.A., Clark, S.E., Jackson, W.T. and DiDio, L. Tibial branching in the tarsal tunnel. *Foot Ankle*, **9**: 117–119, 1988.

[122] Kopel, H.P. and Thompson, A.L. Peripheral entrapment neuropathy of the lower extremity. *New Engl. J. Med.*, **262**: 56–60, 1960.

[123] Rask, M.E. Medial plantar neuropraxia (Jogger's foot): report of three cases. *Clin. Orthop.*, **154**: 193–195, 1978.

9 Soft tissue tumours: diagnosis and treatment

JEFFREY C. PAGE

Soft tissue tumours, which are encountered frequently in private practice, commonly pose diagnostic and therapeutic challenges. This chapter will discuss some of the more common soft tissue tumours that present in the foot and ankle. Clinical presentation, diagnostic aids, and therapeutic alternatives will be presented for each entity following a general discussion of soft tissue principles.

Diagnostic considerations

An accurate diagnosis of soft tissue tumours will seldom be arrived at without a thorough history-taking, careful physical examination, and appropriate testing. During the clinical presentation, one should obtain information regarding gradual or sudden onset of symptoms, duration of the mass and any changes in its shape, size or coloration, and the nature and location of any pain. A history of antecedent trauma and any previous therapeutic manipulation is important. A social history regarding employment and avocations should not be neglected. A review of systems will, in some cases, shed light on a systemic connection to pedal complaints.

Physical examination of the patient presenting with a soft tissue mass should be systematic and include neurological, vascular, dermatological, and musculoskeletal systems. Important diagnostic clues are derived from both inspection and palpation, such as the presence of oedema, colour of the lesion and surrounding tissues, induration, or fluctuation of the mass, mobility or adherence of the tumour to adjacent tissues, and proximity to bony prominences. Fluid-filled cysts are often capable of being transilluminated.

An often under-utilized diagnostic tool is the biopsy. Biopsies may be incisional or excisional. A surgical punch, a wedge resection, shaving of superficial lesions, or converging semi-elliptical incisions provide an adequate specimen for pathological analysis. Laboratory testing may require haematology, chemical analysis, sedimentation rate, arthritis screen, or culture to provide a complete assessment.

Radiographs allow assessment of soft tissue density, calcification, or bony erosion. Computerized tomography provides a three-dimensional evaluation and a comparison of tissue densities. Magnetic resonance imaging often provides the best contrast and clarity of soft tissue structures.

Therapeutic considerations

Soft tissue masses may be approached with a variety of methods, but emphasis must be given to patient symptomatology. In certain instances, no therapy at all is the prudent choice. For example, a benign lesion, such as a dermatofibroma on the lower leg, is rarely symptomatic and does not require excision; however, cosmetic concerns may justify surgical treatment in selected cases. Other tumours may respond to non-surgical care, such as aperture padding, accommodative orthoses, or changes in footwear. Intralesional injections with corticosteroids or sclerosing solutions will occasionally cause resolution of discrete lesions, including ganglion, bursitis, and rheumatoid nodules.[1] Another non-surgical tool that may be of value in patients who are poor surgical candidates is physical therapy. Ultrasound, phonophoresis, and iontophoresis can soften firm masses and reduce inflammation.

When conservative care has failed or when the operative approach is the initial treatment of choice, an understanding of the basic principles of soft tissue surgery is important. The placement of the incision is the first concern. A linear scar over a metatarsophalangeal joint or the ankle joint is susceptible to contracture or hypertrophy. Serpentine or curvilinear incisions will help to avoid these complications. Skin lines should be followed whenever possible and plantar incisions should be placed to avoid weight-bearing areas. In general, curved or S-shaped incisions should provide greater exposure (see Chapter 1).

Meticulous dissection and delicate tissue handling not only improve the rate and quality of healing, but contribute to less post-operative pain. If a dead space is created by excision of a mass, it should be closed. If this is not possible, the wound may be packed or a drain should be placed to allow fluid egress.

Proper closure will be accomplished with careful pre-operative planning. Tension on the wound margins must be avoided. With the use of converging semi-elliptical incisions, dehiscence may be avoided by making the length of the incision at least three times the width. In less mobile tissues, undermining or even adjacent parallel relaxing incisions may be required.

Retention sutures of a large diameter placed as vertical mattress or horizontal mattress sutures often serve to counteract tension across a wound. Plantar incisions are subject to considerable stress with weight bearing. Therefore, special measures should be taken to minimize tension on plantar wounds. The surgeon may utilize 3 weeks of non-weight-bearing, casting, a shortened post-operative shoe for forefoot wounds, or felt padding in the standard surgical shoe.

The size, shape, and location of some soft tissue tumours may not allow simple excision with primary closure. Consideration must then be given to the use of a split- or full-thickness graft, rotational, transpositional, or vascularized flaps, and the removal of underlying bone to improve closure. A complete discussion of flaps and grafts is given in Chapter 1.

Ganglion

Ganglia are soft, fluctuant, thin-walled, fluid-filled cysts that occur most often in the extremities. The fluid varies in viscosity and may be clear to amber-coloured (**9.1**). They may be transilluminated in many cases. Ganglion cysts are found in association with joints or tendon sheaths, but have also been described in bone.[2–6] They are very common in the feet, appearing on the ankle and the dorsum of the foot.[7] Their aetiology is unknown, but is presumed to be traumatic in nature.[8,9] A 'valve-theory' was proposed in 1970.[10] Ganglia have been described histologically as herniations of synovial tissue.[11] The cysts have also been postulated to be the result of mucinous degeneration of connective tissue. *De novo* development of cysts from multi-potent mesenchymal-like cells has been supported by histological analysis.[12]

Ganglia are not always symptomatic. Symptoms depend upon the size and location of the lesion and the degree of pressure against nerves, tendons, and joints.[13,14] Irritation from footwear is no small problem. Mucocutaneous cysts (digital mucous cysts) are very similar to ganglion cysts, but are generally quite small, superficial, and overlie the interphalangeal joints of the digits. The lesions are most often firm, but may fluctuate in size. Ganglia usually present as movable growths in the subcutaneous layer, 1–2 cm in diameter.[15,16] Symptoms are generally related to irritation from shoes. Onychodystrophy may result from distortion of the nail matrix.

Treatment of ganglia and mucocutaneous cysts can be frustrating due to the high recurrence rate. Aspiration of ganglionic fluid followed by the installation of corticosteroids is sometimes successful. However, if this method fails, then surgical excision should be considered. Meticulous dissection is required to avoid puncturing the cyst and to allow location of the 'stalk' or source (**9.2**). Injection of radiopaque dye and radiographic imaging can help determine the extent of the cyst and facilitate dissection. Cautery or ligation of the source may help prevent recurrence. Recurrence from simple excision of mucocutaneous cysts may be as high as 50%, so arthroplasty should also be performed at the underlying joint (which is most often the distal interphalangeal joint).[17]

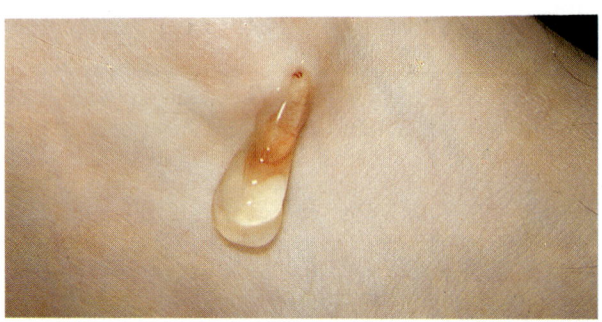

9.1 This ganglion, located near the ankle, was punctured during aspiration and reveals a clear, viscous fluid.

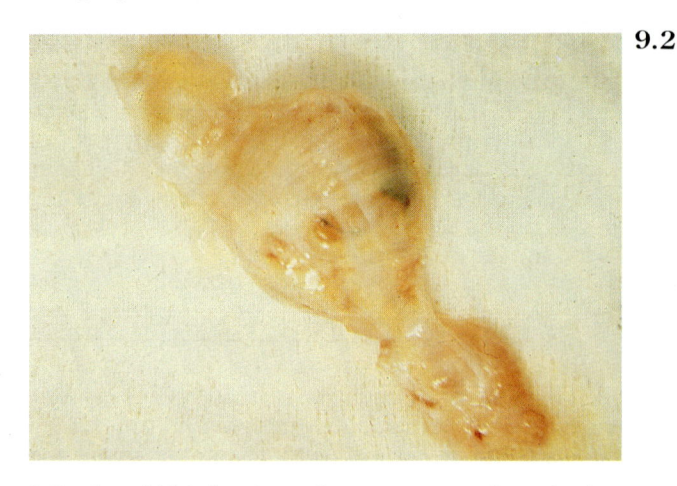

9.2 A multi-lobulated ganglion was excised from the foot intact by careful dissection.

Fibrous tumours

Fibrohistiocytic tumours that appear in the foot and leg include both benign and malignant varieties. Enzinger and Weiss suggested a classification of these lesions that describes tumours of the skin as cutaneous fibrous histiocytoma and tumours of deeper tissues as simply fibrous histiocytoma.[18] However, a precise histological differentiation of the two types is not always possible.[19]

Cutaneous fibrous histiocytoma (dermatofibroma) is not common in the foot but appears more frequently on the anterior surfaces of the lower legs. The lesions are circular, raised, firm, non-tender, and usually appear singly (**9.3**). Multiple tumours may be a manifestation of tuberous sclerosis. Cutaneous fibrous histiocytomas are generally more deeply pigmented than surrounding skin. These tumours may also appear periungually. Periungual fibromas presenting with tuberous sclerosis have been called Kernan's tumours.[20] The treatment of choice for cutaneous fibrous histiocytomas is surgical excision. Recurrence has been noted with low incidence in the foot and leg and with higher incidence in periungual lesions.[17,21]

Fibrous histiocytomas may occur in the adipose, fascial, synovial, or tendinous tissues of any part of the foot.[22–24] These tumours usually present as painless masses, except when occurring on the sole of the foot. The lesions are firm, nodular, often movable beneath the skin, and may appear with multiple lesions. The aetiology is unknown but trauma is a likely factor.

Fibrous histiocytomas appear most commonly as benign, reactive lesions of the plantar fascia, where they are labelled plantar fibromatosis (**9.4**). Plantar fibromatosis has been associated with Peyronie's disease and with Dupuytren's contracture of palmar fascial structures. Fibrous histiocytomas do not require surgical excision unless they are symptomatic or are rapidly growing. Recurrence rate following excision of plantar fibromatosis can be greater than 65%.[17] The surgeon must complete an *en bloc* resection and include 0.5 cm of normal fascia. Radical fasciectomy may rarely be necessary in cases of recurrent fibromatosis (**9.5**). Interposition of polyethylene woven mesh may reduce recurrence rates.[25]

Malignant fibrohistiocytic tumours are rare in the foot and ankle.[26–28] They are low-grade malignancies but have the potential for metastasis. They may involve fascia, subcutis, dermis, or epidermis and are also known as fibrosarcomas and dermatofibrosarcomas. These tumours vary widely histologically, making diagnosis more challenging and giving rise to such confusing names as pseudosarcomatous fibromatosis. When both mitotic activity and pleomorphism are present, malignancy must be considered.[18] Wide local excision or amputation is generally required. The presence of metastases at diagnosis significantly lowers survival rate.

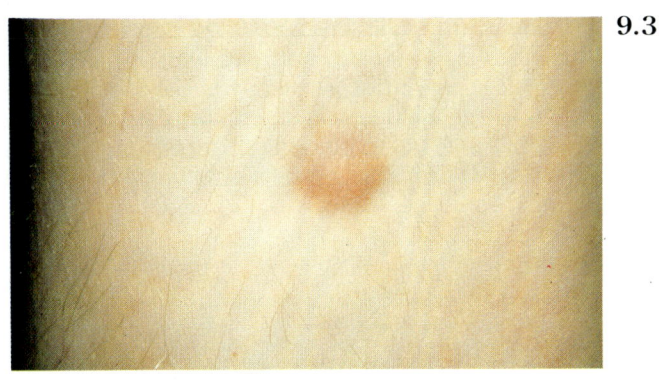

9.3 Fibrous histiocytomas (dermatofibromas) most often appear on the anterior shins and lower leg.

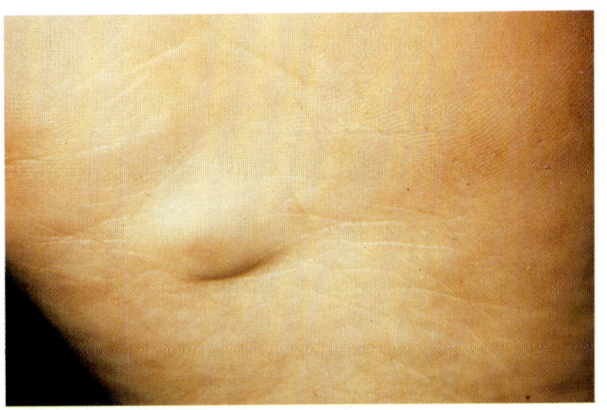

9.4 Typical presentation of plantar fibroma. The plantar fibroma shown became painful after insidious growth.

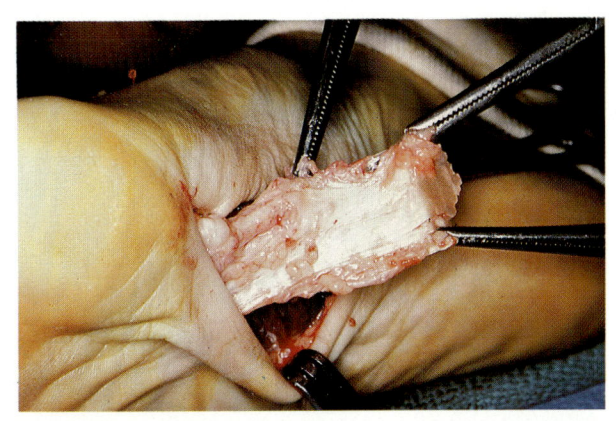

9.5 Radical fasciectomy was required to correct this recurrent plantar fibromatosis.

Lipoma

Lipomas are solid, benign, well-defined adipose tumours. They may occur anywhere that fat is deposited, but appear most frequently in the subcutaneous layer. These multi-lobulated, encapsulated lesions are generally not tender; however, increasing size and encroachment on nerves or other structures may lead to pain. Occasionally, they attain great size.[29] Tenderness or cosmetic disfigurement usually brings the patients to the clinic. A common location in the foot is adjacent to the malleoli.[30]

Lipomas are common in the torso but less common in the extremities. The diagnosis of lipoma applies to more than 50% of all soft tissue tumours in the extremities.[31] Lipomas are idiopathic, slow-growing masses found with increased frequency in patients with obesity, diabetes mellitus, and hypercholesterolaemia. They may present anywhere on the foot.[32,33] Radiographs may reveal a globular radiolucent mass outlined by the greater density of surrounding tissues.[34]

Lipomas appear microscopically very similar to ordinary adipose tissue. Increased fibrous tissue may be present. At surgery, the masses appear darker yellow and firmer than surrounding adipose tissue. The presence or size of lipomas is not related to the percentage of overall body fat.[35]

An uncommon morphological variant of lipoma is the angiofibrolipoma. It manifests a proliferation of fibrous and vascular tissue,[31] and is also benign.

Although malignant degeneration of lipomas is quite rare, liposarcoma is a known malignancy that can occur on the foot. The presence of vascular tissue in liposarcomas means that at times they are called angiolipomas. They may be metastatic and have a highly variable presentation.

The treatment of choice for lipoma or its variants is excision. Recurrence is uncommon.

Giant cell (pigmented villonodular synovitis)

Pigmented villonodular synovitis has been described in three different forms: an isolated, well-defined lesion that involves the tendon sheath; a solitary intra-articular nodule (nodular pigmented villonodular synovitis); and a diffuse, villous form (diffuse pigmented villonodular synovitis).[36] These lesions were originally thought to comprise a benign inflammatory condition rather than a true neoplasm. Newer research has demonstrated that the lesions rarely show inflammatory changes or progressive fibrosis.[37] Distinct borders and centrifugal growth patterns also mitigate for a true neoplastic process.[38] An assortment of synonyms for giant cell tumours of the tendon sheath has given rise to some confusion. These include benign synovioma, fibrous histiocytoma, pigmented nodular synovitis, xanthomas, giant cell haemangiofibroma, and benign polymorphocellular tumour. Differential diagnosis at clinical presentation should include lipoma, ganglion, rheumatoid nodule, synovial sarcoma, and various arthritides.[39]

The aetiology of pigmented villonodular synovitis is unknown but trauma has a close association.[39] It occurs most often in the thirties and forties in both sexes. Lesions appear almost exclusively in the extremities and a number of cases have been reported in the foot or ankle.[36,40–48] Most cases are benign, but malignant giant cell tumours have been reported.[49]

Clinical presentation of pigmented villonodular synovitis is highly variable with one or more areas of swelling, tenderness, limited motion, and occasional warmth. Some lesions are entirely asymptomatic until progressive enlargement causes impingement or shoe irritation. The tumour itself also has a variable appearance. Intra-articular nodules and isolated giant cell tumours of the tendon sheath are most often discrete, well-defined pigmented nodules.

The diffuse form is multi-lobulated with gross villi (**9.6**). Colour ranges from red-brown to grey-black. Histopathology reveals giant cells, fusiform fibroblasts, histiocytes, and areas of haemosiderin and fibrin deposition. Definitive diagnosis is based on cytological examination of the excised tumour. Radiographs

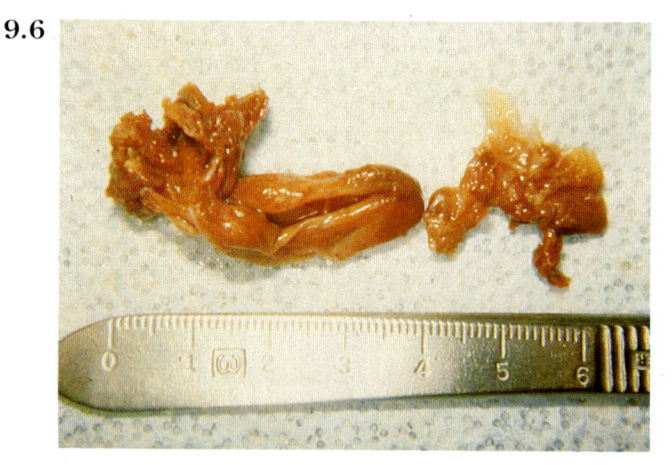

9.6 Diffuse pigmented villonodular synovitis often presents with multiple villi, as seen in this specimen removed from the anterior ankle.

may reveal increased soft tissue density, subchondral cystic changes, or bone erosion and sclerosis from pressure by the expanding tumour.

Excision is the treatment of choice but is accompanied by a high rate of recurrence. When the diffuse form presents in a large joint such as the ankle, more than one incision will be required. Prolonged post-operative re-evaluation and follow-up is recommended.

Neuroma

Morton's neuromas are probably the most common type of neural lesion to afflict the foot.[50] These lesions are not true tumours but consist of reactive, inflammatory tissue and degenerative intraneural fibrosis. The plantar interdigital nerve of the third web space is most frequently involved but more than one nerve may be involved at the same time.[51] The presenting complaint is usually lancinating pain that radiates into the digits and/or numbness and tingling of the involved toes.

Traumatic neuromas result from either blunt or sharp trauma and may occur in any part of the foot. These lesions can be quite painful and disabling.

Neuromas may respond to conservative care, including steroid injections, padding, orthoses, and wider shoes. However, surgical intervention is often required with long-standing lesions.[52,53] Both the diagnosis and treatment of neuromas is described extensively in Chapter 8.

Neurilemmoma

Neurilemmoma (schwannomas) are uncommon benign tumours of the nerve sheath. They are slow-growing, encapsulated, and usually solitary. Perforation of the cortical bone with soft tissue invasion by the tumour is common.[54,55] The histological appearance is that of Schwann's cells in a collagenous matrix. Size varies, but pressure on adjacent axons often causes pain or paraesthesia.[56] Small nerves may be obliterated by the expanding mass, while involvement of the major nerves of the lower extremity may lead to foot drop or other dysfunction. Differential diagnosis includes intraosseous neurilemmoma,[57,58] neurofibroma, aneurysmal schwannoma, and plexiform schwannoma.

Complete excision of the tumour and invaded tissues should effect a cure. When found in association with larger nerves, the tumour should be removed utilizing loupes or a microscope and meticulous dissection to avoid permanent loss of sensation or motor control (**9.7, 9.8**). Sacrifice of smaller nerves will sometimes be required.

9.7, 9.8 Three distinct neurilemmomae were discovered upon dissection of the tarsal canal and the posterior tibial nerve (**9.7**). The encapsulated neurilemmomae were removed from within the fibres of the posterior tibial nerve. One tumour is cross-sectioned to demonstrate the solid mass (**9.8**).

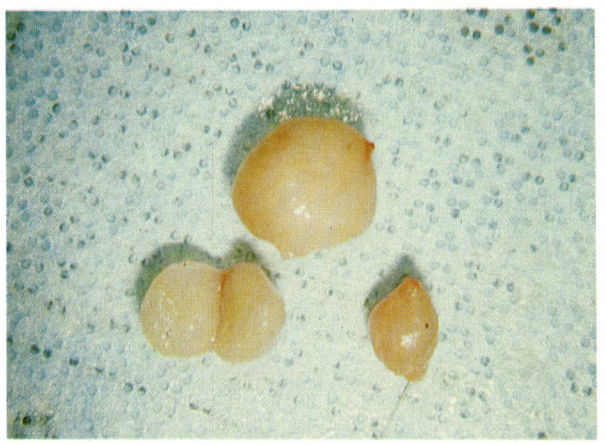

Leiomyoma

Leiomyomas are slow-growing, benign, usually asymptomatic smooth muscle tumours. They arise from smooth muscle in the walls of vessels (angioleiomyoma)[59–61] or from the erector pilorum muscles in the skin.[62,63] Leiomyomas are rare in the foot and their aetiology in unknown.[64] These lesions occur most commonly over the extensor surfaces of the extremities and the anterior surface of the trunk.[65] A benign variant, angiomyolipoma, has been reported in the foot.[66,67] Dockery and Wendel[61] presented a digital case in 1980 and Berlin *et al.*[63] presented a comprehensive review of leiomyomas in 1976.

The firm nodular appearance of leiomyomas makes it difficult to differentiate them from fibromas or ganglia. Most lesions range in size from a few millimetres to a few centimetres; long-standing lesions may become quite large. Leiomyomas are, generally, very painful tumours, giving a sharp, stabbing pain. Histological analysis reveals poorly defined proliferation of smooth muscle fibres that interlace with surrounding collagen. The encapsulated lesion will also show numerous thick-walled blood vessels in the vascular variant. Intraoperative presentation is well defined and ranges from white to grey in colour. Inasmuch as most leiomyomas are benign, surgical excision is generally successful.[61] However, leiomyomas were found to be malignant in 10% of reported cases.[68]

Leiomyosarcoma is fortunately a rare malignancy of smooth muscle: it is extremely rare in the foot.[69] If bone involvement is apparent, malignancy must be suspected. Leiomyosarcoma may arise in the smooth muscle of abdominal organs. Oncological consultation is necessary, due to the incidence of metastases. Wide surgical excision or amputation coupled with radiation or chemotherapy may improve the survival rate.

Neurofibroma (von Recklinghausen's disease)

Neurofibromatosis was first described nearly a century ago as a genetic disorder characterized by *café au lait* spots, neurofibromas of both the skin and internal organs, and lisch nodules.[70,71] In contrast to neurilemmomas, the neurofibromas of neurofibromatosis often appear as multiple lesions. The lesions are slow-growing, well-defined, benign neoplasms composed largely of Schwann's cells. Neurofibromas are not uncommonly found on the foot,[72–75] but are rarely seen on the plantar surface.[76]

The tumours of this disease are non-tender, firm nodules that may or may not be movable (**9.9**). Laboratory testing is not available, therefore, and only histological evaluation will give a definitive diagnosis. The disease is progressive with age as the number of lesions expands. Most lesions are small, but they can attain considerable size.[77]

The lesions of neurofibromatosis are usually easy to excise. The surgeon must be concerned about the potential for malignant transformation.[78] Malignant schwannomas are very rare in the foot but are associated with von Recklinghausen's disease 35% of the time.

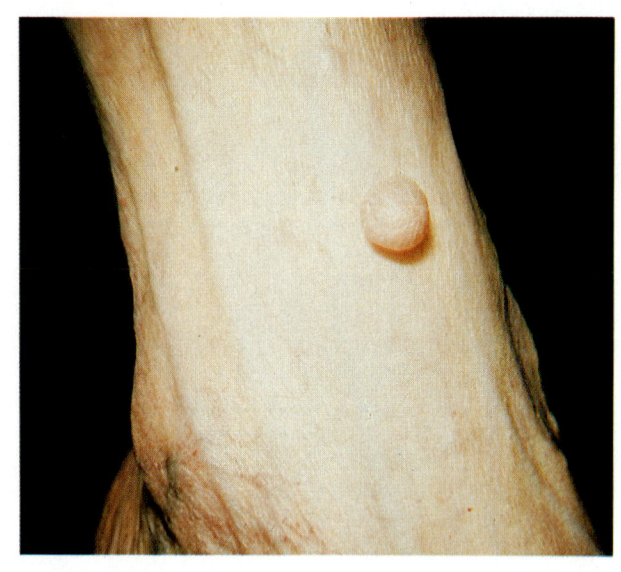

9.9 The tumours of neurofibromatosis may appear pedunculated, as this lesion on the anterior ankle demonstrates, but many lesions are sessile.

Kaposi's sarcoma

Kaposi's sarcoma was first described by a Hungarian physician, Moriez Kaposi, in 1872. It has previously been considered most common in mature Caucasian males of Jewish or Italian descent.[79,80] In recent years, the incidence has grown in other populations along with the prevalence of acquired immune deficiency syndrome (AIDS).[81] One-third of the patients with AIDS develop Kaposi's sarcoma lesions.[82] Diabetes mellitus is also associated with 32% of patients with Kaposi's sarcoma.[79] There is also an increased incidence of this tumour in iatrogenically immunosuppressed individuals.[83]

The characteristic lesions of Kaposi's sarcoma are brown, red, or bluish, well-circumscribed patches of nodules that most often appear on the lower extremities. It is considered to be among the most common malignant skin tumours of the foot.[84,85] This malignant, endothelial neoplasm may appear singly or as multinodular haemorrhagic placques. The lesions are usually non-tender, soft, somewhat mobile, and slow-growing. Itching, burning, and some pain may be present. Metastasis can occur to regional lymph nodes and internal organs. Ten per cent of cases appear first in the internal organs. Biopsy is imperative to the correct diagnosis, inasmuch as the differential diagnosis is long, including glomus tumour, pyogenic granuloma, lichen planus, haemangioma, melanoma, mycosis fungoides, and psoriasis.

The disease has been described with three different but sometimes overlapping presentations: locally aggressive, nodular, and generalized.[86] Generalized disease is rapidly fatal but is fortunately rare as is locally aggressive disease. Morbidity and mortality relate most often to gastrointestinal haemorrhage, widespread cutaneous ulceration, or concomitant infection.

Cryosurgery has proven to be a successful method of eradicating smaller cutaneous lesions, but lesions under 1.5 cm in diameter may be completely excised. Inasmuch as the tumours of Kaposi's sarcoma are radiosensitive, larger lesions should be irradiated. Widespread disease will require chemotherapy with cytotoxic drugs.

Pyogenic granuloma

Pyogenic granuloma is a benign vascular tumour that appears both on skin and mucous membranes. The aetiology has not been clearly established, but chronic inflammation, infection, and trauma are suspected.[87] An angiogenic factor may be released, causing a reactive proliferation of blood vessels. These tumours are not restricted by age, sex, or race and occur most often on the face and fingers.[88] They usually occur singly, but may develop numerous satellites.[89,90]

Also known as granuloma pyogenicum, these tumours present as soft, red papules which may be sessile or pedunculated (**9.10, 9.11**). An exudate is present and may be malodorous or purulent. With time, colour may change to brown or black and crusting is commonly seen. The friable nature of the lesion often leads to considerable haemorrhage with minor trauma.[91] The typical pyogenic granuloma is painless and about 1 cm in diameter, but size varies. The differential diagnosis list is very long and is well described by Hirsh *et al.*[92]

Histopathological analysis demonstrates a proliferating capillary haemangioma, with a larger central artery entering the lesion through the pedicle. Acanthosis, hyperkeratosis, atrophy, and changes in rete ridges are variably present.

Chemical cautery (for small lesions), electrocautery, cryocautery, surgical excision, or laser treatment are all successful alternatives for pyogenic granuloma. Sur-

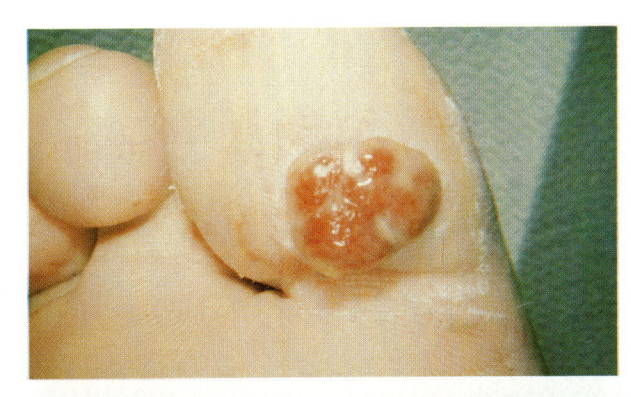

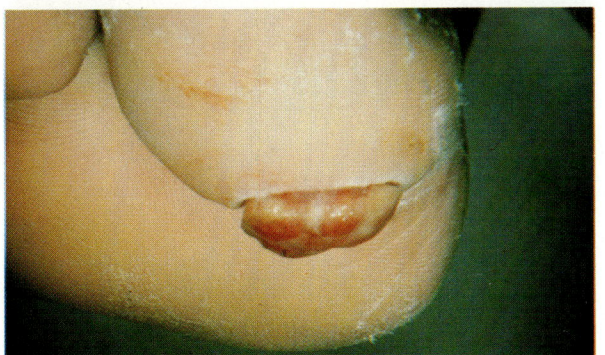

9.10 This pyogenic granuloma developed following minor trauma to the hallux.

9.11 Pyogenic granulomae are often raised and exudative.

gical excision coupled with electrocautery of the base may aid in preventing recurrence.[91] All excised lesions should be sent for pathological analysis.

Miscellaneous soft tissue tumours

Rheumatoid nodules are benign soft tissue masses commonly found in patients with both seropositive and seronegative rheumatoid arthritis.[93] These tumours are generally firm, subcutaneous, sometimes tender masses that appear most often on the plantar surface of the foot.[94] Trauma of the soft tissue overlying bony prominences is thought to be the common aetiology.[95] The masses are often bilateral and symmetrical. Though firm to palpation, rheumatoid nodules may be cystic, with central cavitation. Multiple loculations or channels are filled with fluid or gelatinous material and correspond to a multi-lobulated appearance.

Infiltration of fibrinoid necrosis and granulation tissue is commonly seen on histology. Rheumatoid nodules have also been reported in association with symptomatic neuromas.[96,97] The importance of conservative care should be emphasized. The use of aperture padding, accommodative insoles, shoes with extra depth, and intra-lesional steroids can give resolution of symptoms. In recalcitrant cases surgical excision will be needed.

Bursitis results in a soft tissue mass very similar to a rheumatoid nodule. Ovoid or multinodular, these lesions occur over bony enlargements as a result of shoe irritation (**9.12**). Adventitious tissue organizes between fascia and subcutaneous layers in response to chronic pressure. Bursae are often fluid-filled and may contain a grey caseous material (**9.13**). Bursitis responds to corticosteroid injection, oral anti-inflammatory agents, changes in footwear, and other protective measures. However, bursae are easily excised and can be removed at the time of correction of the causative bony deformity.

Glomus tumours are benign neuroarterial tumours often found in the subcutaneous tissue and the dermis. The presence of neural tissue with multiple vascular channels gives rise to an extremely painful lesion. These lesions may be red or blue, are typically of small size, and may present subungually.[98] Surgical excision gives prompt relief and recurrence is rare.

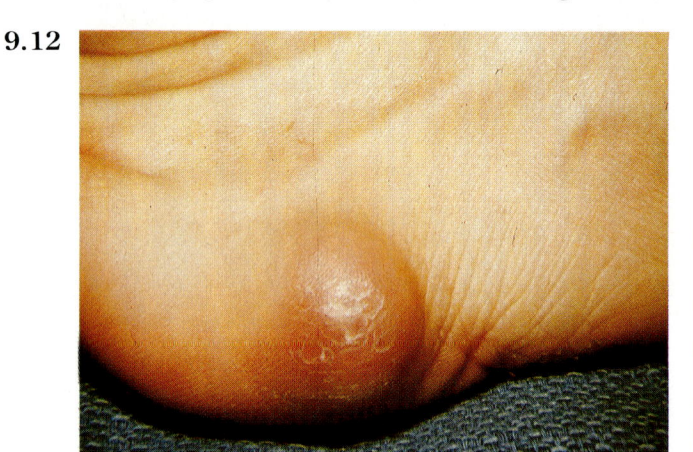

9.12 Bursitis commonly develops from shoe irritation over a bony prominence.

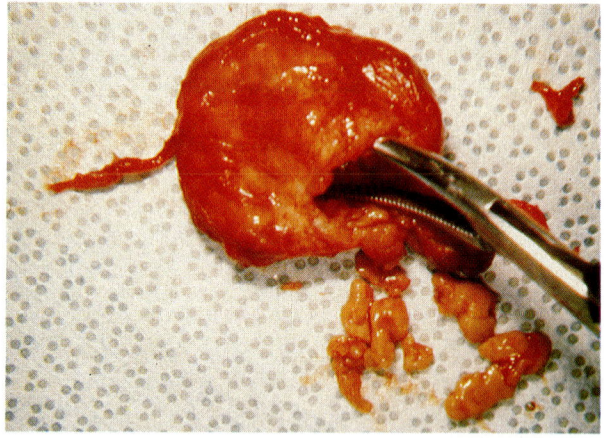

9.13 Bursae typically contain a cavity filled with fluid and a grey-brown caseous material.

Summary

Soft tissue tumours of the lower extremity present in a variety of ways and it is very important for the foot surgeon to understand the proper approach for diagnosis and treatment. The word 'tumour' is generally very frightening to the patient and must be used with discretion when describing most of the common lesions presenting on the legs and feet.

References

[1] Dockery, G.L. and Nilson, R.Z. Intralesional injections. *Clin. Podiatric Med. Surg,* **3**: 473–486; 1986.
[2] Schram, A.J. and Kirschenbaum, S.E. Presentation of a unique ganglionic cyst. *J. Foot Surg.,* **27**: 530, 1988.
[3] Rubenstein, S.A. and Bardfeld, L.A. Ganglia (synovial cysts) of bone. *J. Foot Surg.,* **27**: 71–75, 1988.
[4] Goldman, R.L. and Friedman, N.B. Ganglia (synovial cysts) arising in unusual locations. Report of three cases, one primary in bone. *Clin. Orthoped.,* **63**: 184, 1969.
[5] Crabbe, W.A. Intraosseous ganglia of bone. *Brit. J. Surg.,* **53**: 15, 1966.
[6] Newland, A. and Moore, R.M. Intraosseous ganglion of the ankle. *J. Foot Surg.,* **25**: 241, 1986.
[7] Berlin, S.J. A laboratory review of 67,000 foot tumors and lesions. *J. Am. Podiatric Assoc.,* **74**: 341, 1984.
[8] Carp, L. A discussion of ganglia. *J. Am. Podiatric Med. Assoc.,* **62**: 60, 1972.
[9] Berlin, S.J., Domick, I.I., Block, L.D. and Costa, A.J. Ganglion cysts and metatarsalgia. *J. Am. Podiatric Med. Assoc.,* **66**: 491, 1976.
[10] Jayson, M.I.V. and Dixon, A.S.J. Valvular mechanism in juxtaarticular cysts. *Ann. Rheum. Dis.,* **29**: 415, 1970.
[11] Kliman, E.K. and Friedberg, A. Ganglion of the foot and ankle. *Foot Ankle,* **3**: 45, 1982.
[12] Wenig, J.A. and McCarthy, D.J. Synovial cysts of the hallux: a case report. *J. Am. Podiatric Med. Assoc.,* **76**: 7, 1986.
[13] Brooks, D.M. Nerve compression by simple ganglia—a review of 13 collected cases. *J. Bone Joint Surg.,* **34B**: 391, 1952.
[14] Rinaldi, R.R. and Sabia, M.L. A large and unusual ganglion. *J. Am. Podiatric Med. Assoc.,* **65**: 580, 1975.
[15] Slavitt, J.A., Behesti, F., Lenet, M. and Sherman, M. Ganglions of the foot. A six-year retrospective study and review of the literature. *J. Am. Podiatric Med. Assoc.,* **70**: 459, 1980.
[16] Rosenberg, A. Dorsal tendosynovial cyst. *J. Am. Podiatric Med. Assoc.,* **76**: 455, 1986.
[17] Berlin, S.J. Tumours and tumorous conditions of the foot. *In* McGlamry, E.D. (ed.), *Comprehensive Textbook of Surgery.* Baltimore, Williams & Wilkins, 1987, pp. 618–624.
[18] Enzinger, F.M. and Weiss, S.W. *Soft Tissue Tumors,* St. Louis, C.V. Mosby, 1983.
[19] Freedman, D.J., Luzzi, A., Pellegrino, P. and Picciotti, J. Benign and malignant fibrohistiocytic tumors. *J. Am. Podiatric Med. Assoc.,* **77**: 544, 1987.
[20] Fielding, M. (ed.) *Skin Tumors of the Foot: Diagnosis and Treatment.* Mt. Kisco, Futura Publ., New York, 1984, pp. 79–87.
[21] Saeva, J.T., Lynch, D.M. and Guthrie, J.D. Bourneville's disease, a review and case report of tuberous sclerosis. *J. Am. Podiatric Med. Assoc.,* **78**: 590, 1988.
[22] Jacobs, A.M., Amarwek, D.L. and Oloff, L.M. Atypical fibrous histiocytoma of the great toe. *J. Foot Surg.,* **23**: 250, 1984.
[23] Novicki, D.C. and Anselmi, S.J. Fibrous histiocytoma. *J. Am. Podiatric Med. Assoc.,* **68**: 606, 1978.
[24] Gill, P.W., Rosenthal, L. and Wagreich, C.R. Tenosynovial fibroma, a case report. *J. Am. Podiatric Med. Assoc.,* **78**: 368, 1988.
[25] Oster, J.A. and Miller, A.E. Resection of plantar fibromatosis with interposition of Marlex surgical mesh. *J. Foot Surg.,* **25**: 217, 1986.
[26] Smith, L.S., Lenet, M. and Sherman, M. Malignant fibrous histiocytoma: a rare soft tissue tumor of the foot. *J. Am. Podiatric Med. Assoc.,* **66**: 459, 1976.
[27] Weiss, S.W. and Enzinger, F.M. Malignant fibrous histiocytoma: an analysis of 200 cases. *Cancer,* **41**: 2250, 1978.
[28] Nachlas, M. and Ketai, D. An unusual variation of malignant fibrous histiocytoma: a case report. *J. Foot Surg.,* **19**: 212, 1980.
[29] Bartis, J.R. Massive lipoma of the foot: a case report. *J. Am. Podiatric Med. Assoc.,* **64**: 874, 1974.
[30] Eibel, P. Juxtamalleolar lipomata. *Clin. Orthoped.,* **49**: 191, 1966.
[31] Kershisnik, W., McCarthy, D.J. and O'Donnell, E. Angiofibrolipoma, a histologic variant of the lipoma. *J. Am. Podiatric Med. Assoc.,* **76**: 67, 1986.
[32] Gilchrist, K. Fatty type tumors of the foot: a report of two cases. *J. Am. Podiatric Med. Assoc.,* **65**: 142, 1975.
[33] Greenberg, G.S. Lipomas: discussion and report of an unusual case. *J. Foot Surg.,* **19**: 68, 1980.
[34] Lisch, M., Mittleman, M. and Albin, R. Digital lipoma of the foot: an extraordinary case. *J. Am. Podiatric Med. Assoc.,* **67**: 330, 1977.
[35] Feldman, M., Healey, K., Nach, W., Kaplan, N. and Taylor, H. Plantar approach for excision of bilateral soft tissue masses in a child. *J. Foot Surg.,* **28**: 60, 1989.
[36] Jaffe, H.L., Lichtenstein, L. and Sutro, C.J. Pigmented villonodular synovitis bursitis, and tenosynovitis. *Arch. Pathol.,* **31**: 731, 1941.
[37] Rao, A.V. and Vigorita, V.J. Pigmented villonodular synovitis (giant cell tumor of the tendon sheath and synovial membrane). *J. Bone Joint Surg.,* **66A**: 76, 1984.
[38] Stout, A.P. and Lattes, R. *Atlas of Tumor Pathology: Tumors of Soft Tissue.* Washington, DC, Armed Forces Institute of Pathology, 1967.
[39] Goldberg, S., Feit, J. and McCarthy, D.J. The podiatric implications of giant cell tumors. *J. Foot Surg.,* **25**: 208, 1986.
[40] Frankel, S.L., Chioros, P.G. and Sidlow, C.J. Giant cell tumor of the plantar fascia: a case report. *J. Am. Podiatric Med. Assoc.,* **77**: 557, 1987.
[41] Gold, A.G., Bronfman, R.A., Clark, E.A. and Comerford, J.S. Giant cell tumor of the extensor tendon sheath of the foot: a case report. *J. Am. Podiatric Med. Assoc.,* **77**: 561, 1987.

[42] Roth, I., Frisch, D.R. and Mercado, O.A. Nodular pigmented villonodular synovitis. *J. Foot Surg.*, **24**: 51, 1985.

[43] McGinness, L.E., Schiffgen, S.T. and Mercado, O.A. Pigmented villonodular synovitis: a case report. *J. Am. Podiatric Med. Assoc.*, **70**: 335, 1980.

[44] Floyd, E.J., Cohen, R.S. and Daily, J.H. Giant cell tumor of the tendon sheath: a report of two cases. *J. Am. Podiatric Med. Assoc.*, **73**: 312, 1983.

[45] Steinberg, R.I. and Harant, W. Giant cell tumor of the foot: a case report. *J. Am. Podiatric Med. Assoc.*, **66**: 534, 1976.

[46] Galinski, A.W. and Vlahos, M. Giant cell tumor of the sheath in podiatric medicine: report of two cases. *J. Am. Podiatric Med. Assoc.*, **68**: 825, 1978.

[47] Coster, A.A. Giant cell tumor of tendon sheath: benign synovioma. *J. Am. Podiatric Med. Assoc.*, **66**: 538, 1976.

[48] Buggiani, F.P., Rutan, G.M. and Holt, W.P. Giant cell tumor of the tendon sheath: a case report. *J. Am. Podiatric Med. Assoc.*, **71**: 166, 1981.

[49] Carstens, H.B. and Howell, R.S. Malignant giant cell tumor of the tendon sheath. *Virchows Arch. (Pathologic Anatomy)* **382**: 237, 1979.

[50] Berlin, S.J., Domick, I.I., Block, L.D. and Costa, A.J. Nerve tumors of the foot: diagnosis and treatment. *J. Am. Podiatric Med. Assoc.*, **65**: 157, 1975.

[51] Silverman, E.J. Three neuromas of one foot. *J. Am. Podiatric Med. Assoc.*, **77**: 53, 1987.

[52] Gaynor, R., Hale, D., Spinner, S.M. and Tomczak, R.L. A comparative analysis of conservative *versus* surgical treatment of Morton's neuroma. *J. Am. Podiatric Med. Assoc.*, **79**: 27, 1989.

[53] Mann, R.A. and Reynolds, J.C. Interdigital neuroma: a critical clinical analysis. *Foot Ankle*, **3**: 238, 1983.

[54] Fawcett, K.J. and Dahlin, D.C. Neurilemmoma of bone. *Am. J. Clin. Pathol.*, **47**: 759, 1967.

[55] Wirth, W.A. and Bray, C.B. Intra-osseous neurilemmoma: case report and review of thirty-one cases from the literature. *J. Bone Joint Surg.*, **59A**: 252, 1977.

[56] Coulter, K.R., Gerbert, J. and Shea, T.P. Neurilemmoma of the lateral plantar nerve: a case report. *J. Am. Podiatric Med. Assoc.*, **68**: 721, 1978.

[57] Barley, S.W., Williams, J.T. and Baerg, R.H. Intraosseous neurilemmoma of the foot: a case report. *J. Am. Podiatric Med. Assoc.*, **77**: 294, 1987.

[58] Morton, K.S. and Vassar, P.S. Neurilemmoma in bone: report of a case. *Can. J. Surg.*, **7**: 187, 1964.

[59] Sweeny, J. and Keating, S.E. Angioleiomyoma. *J. Foot Surg.*, **22**: 21, 1983.

[60] Hosey, T.C., Jacob, T. and Kallet, H.A. Vascular leiomyoma. *J. Am. Podiatric Med. Assoc.*, **74**: 93, 1984.

[61] Dockery, G.L. and Wendel, R.E. Benign vascular leiomyoma angioma of the digit: a case report. *J. Am. Podiatric Med. Assoc.*, **69**: 438, 1979.

[62] Cullen, T.H. Solitary leiomyoma of the skin. *Brit. J. Surg.*, **43**: 178, 1955.

[63] Berlin, S.J., Binder, D.M., Emiley, T.J., Hatch, K.L., *et al.* Leiomyoma of the foot: a review of the literature and report of cases. *J. Am. Podiatric Med. Assoc.*, **66**: 450–458, 1976.

[64] Genakos, J.J., Wallace, J.A., Napoli, A.A., Pontarelli, A. and Terris, A. Angioleiomyoma. A case report and literature review. *J. Am. Podiatric Med. Assoc.*, **77**: 101, 1987.

[65] Fisher, W.C. and Helwig, E.B. Leiomyomas of the skin. *Arch. Dermatol.*, **88**: 510, 1963.

[66] Krolick, W.D. and Black, J.R. Angiomyolipoma in the foot. A case report. *J. Am. Podiatric Med. Assoc.*, **77**: 290, 1987.

[67] Moien, A.J. and Giltman, L.I. Angiomyolipoma of the foot: a case report. *J. Am. Podiatric Med. Assoc.*, **68**: 773, 1978.

[68] Sout, A.P. Solitary cutaneous and subcutaneous leiomyomas. Am. J. Cancer, **29**: 435, 1937.

[69] Wu, K.K. Leiomyosarcoma of the foot. *J. Foot Surg.*, **27**: 362, 1988.

[70] Riccardi, V.M. Von Recklinghausen neurofibromatosis. New Engl. J. Med., **305**: 1617, 1981.

[71] McCarroll, H.R. Clinical manifestations of congenital neurofibromatosis. *J. Bone Joint Surg.*, **32A**: 601, 1950.

[72] Cohen, M.D. Neurofibromatosis manifested in the foot. *J. Am. Podiatric Med. Assoc.*, **74**: 143, 1984.

[73] Bauder, T. and DiPrimio, R.R. Neurofibromatosis of the feet. *J. Am. Podiatric Med. Assoc.*, **70**: 372, 1980.

[74] Serdoz, L.L., Lepow, G.M. and Lepow, R.S. Neurofibromatosis: a case history. *J. Am. Podiatric Med. Assoc.*, **68**: 720, 1978.

[75] Taylor, P.M. Case report of neurofibromatosis. *J. Am. Podiatric Med. Assoc.*, **61**: 272, 1971.

[76] Gazivoda, P.L., Hart, T.J. and Wolf, J.A. Surgical management of plantar von Recklinghausen Neurofibroma. *J. Foot Surg.*, **27**: 52, 1988.

[77] Harris, W.C., Alpert, W.J. and Marcinko, D.E. Elephantiasis neuromatosa in von Recklinghausen's disease: a review and case report. *J. Am. Podiatric Med. Assoc.*, **72**: 70, 1982.

[78] Sands, M.J., McDonough, M.T., Cohen, A.M., *et al.* Fatal malignant degeneration in multiple neurofibromatosis. *JAMA*, **233**: 1381, 1975.

[79] Laor, Y. and Schwartz, R. Epidemiologic aspects of American Kaposi's sarcoma. *J. Surg. Oncol.*, **12**: 299, 1979.

[80] Hood, A.F., Fanner, E.R. and Weiss, R.A. Kaposi's sarcoma. *Johns Hopkins Med. J.*, **151**: 222, 1982.

[81] Jarvis, B.D., Lessenden, C.M., D'Amico, H.R. and Iyer, L.B. Kaposi's idiopathic hemorrhagic sarcoma. *J. Am. Podiatric Med. Assoc.*, **77**: 354, 1987.

[82] Shilling, G.A. and Black, J.R. Kaposi's sarcoma of the lower extremity. *J. Am. Podiatric Med. Assoc.*, **77**: 89, 1987.

[83] Klepp, C., Dahl, O. and Stenwig, J.T. Association of Kaposi's sarcoma and prior immunosuppressive therapy. *Cancer*, **42**: 2626, 1978.

[84] Stern, D. and Jacobs, C. Kaposi's sarcoma. *J. Am. Podiatric Med. Assoc.*, **71**: 694, 1981.

[85] Winston, L., DeWolf, A.R., Tarr, R.P. and Tarr, M.A. Kaposi's sarcoma. *J. Am. Podiatric Med. Assoc.*, **68**: 821, 1978.

[86] Templeton, A.C. and Bhana, D. Prognosis in Kaposi's sarcoma. *J. Nat. Cancer Inst.,* **55**: 1301, 1975.
[87] Wolf, J.E. and Hubler, W.R. Origin and evolution of pyogenic granuloma. *Arch. Dermatol.,* **110**: 958, 1974.
[88] Estersohn, H.S. and Stanoch, J.F. Pyogenic granuloma. *J. Am. Podiatric Med. Assoc.,* **73**: 297, 1983.
[89] Warner, J. and Jones, E.W. Pyogenic granuloma recurring with multiple satellites: a report of eleven cases. *Brit. J. Dermatol.,* **80**: 218, 1968.
[90] Amerigo, J., Gonzaliz-Campora, R., Galera, H., *et al.* Recurrent pyogenic granuloma with multiple satellites: clinicopathological and ultrastructural study. *Dermatologica,* **166**: 177, 1983.
[91] Berlin, S.J., Block, L.D. and Domick, I.I. Pyogenic granuloma of the foot. *J. Am. Podiatric Med. Assoc.,* **62**: 94, 1972.
[92] Hirsch, S.P., Cicero, J.R. and Feldman, M.R. Plantar pyogenic granuloma. *J. Am. Podiatric Med. Assoc.,* **78**: 469, 1988.
[93] Kaye, B.R., Kaye, R.L. and Bobrove, A. Rheumatoid nodules: review of the spectrum of associated conditions and proposal of a new classification, with a report of four seronegative cases. *Am. J. Med.,* **76**: 279, 1984.
[94] Taylor, P.M. A review of changes of the hands and feet in rheumatoid arthritis. *J. Am. Podiatric Med. Assoc.,* **68**: 817, 1978.
[95] Greenberg, A.J. Rheumatoid nodules. *J. Am. Podiatric Med. Assoc.,* **72**: 84, 1982.
[96] Higgins, K.R., Burnett, O.E., Krych, S.M. and Harkless, L.B. Seronegative rheumatoid arthritis and Morton's neuroma. *J. Foot Surg.,* **27**: 404, 1988.
[97] Miller, H.G., Abadesio, L. and Heaney J.P. Morton's neuroma symptoms from a rheumatoid nodule: a case report. *J. Am. Podiatric Med. Assoc.,* **73**: 311, 1983.
[98] Koushoubis, C.E. Subungual glomus tumor: a clinical–pathological study. *J. Dermatol. Surg. Oncol.,* **9**: 4, 1983.

10 Surgical procedures of the first ray

JOHN M. SCHUBERTH

Introduction

Surgical procedures performed on the first ray often have the combined goal of the improvement of function and the correction of deformity. In many cases, the achievement of one goal will attain the other. Conditions which afflict the first ray are among the most common presenting to the foot surgeon. The inherent nature of the biomechanical forces that are necessary for bipedal ambulation place the first ray under tremendous strain. With uncontrolled pronatory moments of force, the first metatarsophalangeal joint fails to maintain its integrity, and deformity ensues. It is these deformities that impede pain-free ambulation and provide the patient with an impetus to seek treatment.

Although many of these maladies can be managed on a conservative basis, the majority of problems are due to structural malalignments. The mere presence of these malalignments is clearly not an absolute indication for surgical treatment, but only a condition. The decision to operate will only come from a strict adherence to sound medical principles, honest evaluation of the patient's needs, and a critical assessment of the surgeon's abilities to achieve the goals of the patient.

This chapter will provide the reader with a discussion of the pertinent surgical anatomy of the region. Radiographic assessment of the foot as it relates to the first metatarsal and its functional and structural variances will also be discussed. The procedures discussed in this chapter are designed to reestablish a more normal and more functional position of the first metatarsal and thereby assure a more optimal function of the first metatarsophalangeal joint. The indications and the advantages and disadvantages for each procedure will be discussed. Actual technique of the surgical procedure is beyond the scope of this chapter; however, practical suggestions and tips on technique that the author has found useful will be presented.

Surgical anatomy

Effective surgical procedures on the first metatarsal are only possible if the surgeon has the ability to obtain access and exposure to the entire first ray complex. Versatility and innovation are often necessary for some special procedures that require seldom-used exposures. However, the vast majority of the procedures performed on the first metatarsal can be performed through standard surgical approaches. A thorough knowledge of the vital structures and the possible anatomical variants is necessary to be a safe and effective surgeon of the first metatarsal.

Neurovascular structures

The first ray complex has a fairly predictable neurovascular arrangement. With the exception of the deep peroneal nerve and the deep plantar artery, the neurovascular structures lie in the subcutaneous layer. This affords an important anatomical landmark during the surgical approach to the osseous tissue. If the surgeon is able to mobilize the skin and subcutaneous layers as a single layer, then the vital structures can be safely preserved and protected during the performance of the procedure. The maintenance of these structures as a single soft tissue envelope also provides for less swelling and allows for a neat and anatomical closure. It also serves to protect the nerves from unnecessary dissection, which can predispose to post-operative scarring around the neural elements.

The saphenous nerve follows the course of the greater saphenous vein and runs just anterior to the medial malleolus at the level of the ankle. The medial marginal vein feeds into the greater saphenous vein at the level of the ankle. The distribution of the saphenous nerve is variable but generally supplies the skin on the proximal dorsomedial portion of the first metatarsal. It can provide cutaneous innervation to an area as far distal to the first metatarsophalangeal joint, but usually ends at the mid-shaft of the metatarsal. Rarely, it will supply the plantar medial aspect of the proximal half of the metatarsal.

The medial dorsal cutaneous nerve, a branch of the superficial peroneal nerve, generally bifurcates from this main trunk at the ankle joint. It then courses medially to bifurcate into a medial and lateral branch. The medial branch courses distally in an oblique fashion and crosses the first ray over the first cuneiform, superficial to the extensor hallucis longus tendon. Once on the medial side of the bone, it proceeds distally to the dorsomedial aspect of the hallux and supplies the anatomy with sensation along its course (**10.1**). The medial dorsal cutaneous nerve must be identified and mobilized in almost any procedure on the first ray. There are two situations where the nerve is especially vulnerable to surgical trauma: during the exposure to the proximal aspect of the metatarsal for a basilar osteotomy or metatarsal cuneiform joint procedure and during most approaches to the first metatarsophalangeal joint. In these two instances, it is critical to maintain the nerve in the subcutaneous envelope.

The deep peroneal nerve, a branch of the common peroneal nerve, courses in the anterior compartment to the level of the ankle and rests on the dorsum of the second cuneiform. At or about this level, the nerve bifurcates into a medial and lateral terminal division. The medial terminal division courses distally to the first web space, where it supplies the dorsal aspect of the space with cutaneous innervation. The lateral terminal division is the motor supply to the extensor hallucis brevis muscle and runs laterally away from the first ray complex.

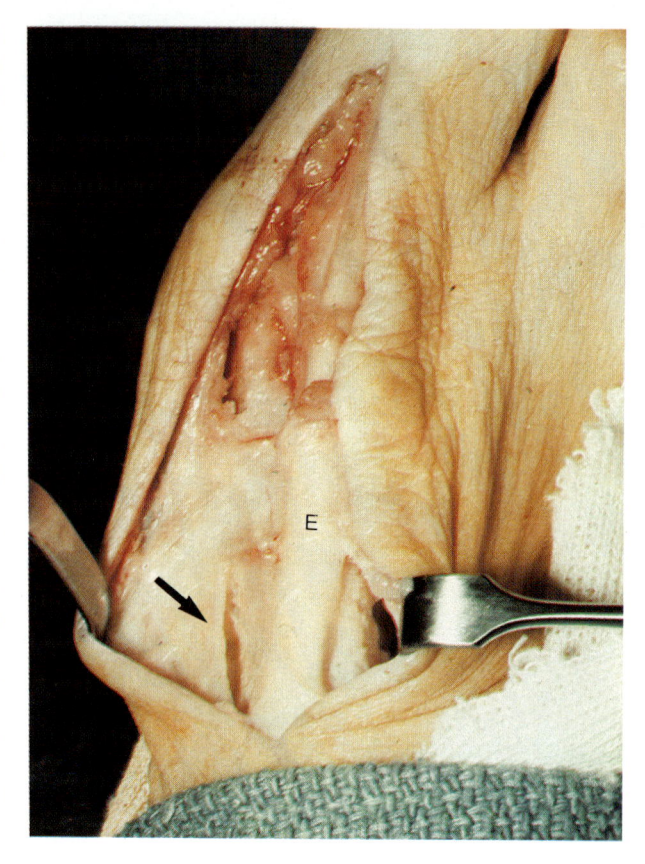

10.1 Intra-operative photograph of the first ray complex. Note the medial dorsal cutaneous nerve in the medial subcutaneous flap (arrow). It follows the course of the bony anatomy. It is always medial to the extensor hallucis longus tendon (E) distal to the first cuneiform.

Muscles

There are four extrinsic muscles and four intrinsic muscles which have distinct attachments and, therefore, direct influence on the first ray function. Understanding the individual and synergistic actions of these muscles on the first ray is paramount to performing logical surgical procedures.

Extrinsic muscles

The peroneus longus muscle inserts into the plantar lateral aspect of the base of the first metatarsal.[1,2] It serves to stabilize and plantarflex the metatarsal. Although it is essentially shielded from the surgeon's view, it must be considered when performing osteotomies of the first metatarsal base or proximal fusion procedures. Inadvertent detachment of the insertion is possible by an ill-directed saw or scalpel blade. The tendon insertion is particularly at risk during fusion procedures because the proximal articulating surface is routinely removed. It is also at risk when closing abductory procedures are performed on the first ray. If a closing abductory procedure is being performed on the first metatarsal cuneiform joint, then the corrective wedging should come from the cuneiform side of the joint so that the peroneus longus tendon does not need to be sacrificed. Loss or attenuation of this muscle's action would further compromise the stabilizing effect on the bone and may defeat the purpose of the operation.

The tibialis anterior muscle inserts into the medial side of the first metatarsal cuneiform joint and serves to stabilize this articulation. This tendon is directly accessible to the operator and thus is less vulnerable to inadvertent trauma. However, it can be detached with overzealous dissection on the medial side of the joint. It is recommended that dissection be performed as close to the osseous structures as possible so that the relatively wide insertional band can have maximal surface area to reattach. If extensive exposure is needed, it is prudent to anchor the insertion with sutures followed by immobilization in the tenuously repaired case.

The extensor hallucis longus tendon essentially runs along the course of the first ray (see **10.1**). It is located in its own sheath, which is attached to the dorsum of the metatarsal. The long extensor inserts into the base of the distal phalanx of the hallux. It is encountered in the overwhelming majority of first ray surgical procedures and, therefore, must usually be mobilized. It is preferred to mobilize the tendon without removing it from its sheath; the gliding function of the tendon is less likely to be disturbed. This is accomplished by mobilization of the sheath by underscoring the entire apparatus just superficial to the periosteum of the first metatarsal. The tendon and its surrounding sheath can be mobilized medially or laterally, according to the demands of the exposure.

The extensor hallucis capsularis is invariably present and emanates from the long extensor tendon in its proximal domain (**10.2**).[2] It courses directly medial to the extensor and inserts along the dorsomedial capsule of the first metatarsophalangeal joint. It serves as an excellent landmark for capsulotomy of the first metatarsophalangeal joint and, because of its tendinous composition, it also serves as a strong anchor point during repair of the capsule.

The flexor hallucis longus tendon runs along the plantar aspect of the first metatarsal to insert into the base of the distal phalanx. At the level of the sesamoid complex, the flexor hallucis tendon is located between the two sesamoids.[3,4] In deformities that involve migration or displacement of the sesamoid apparatus, the flexor longus tendon can usually be located in the same relative position.[5] This is because of the strong ligamentous attachment of the sheath to the sesamoid complex and the investiture of the sheath between the bones.

Intrinsic muscles

The abductor hallucis muscle is located along the medial aspect of the first ray. In the most proximal aspect, the muscle lies plantar and medial to the osseous structure. It then lies directly medial as it courses distally to the medial aspect of the base of the

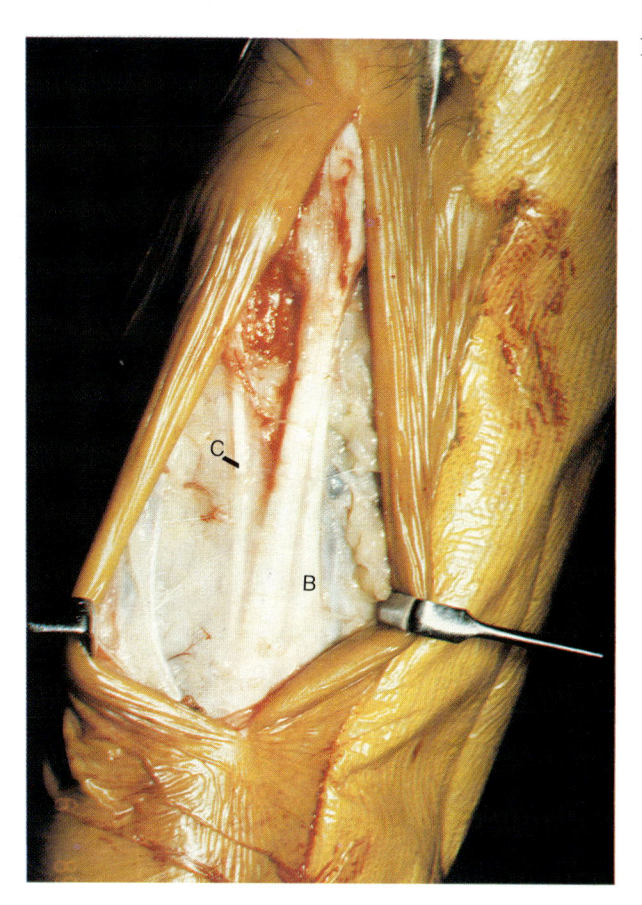

10.2 The extensor hallucis capsularis (C) can usually be found medial to the long extensor to the great toe. It is of variable size and is rarely absent. The extensor hallucis brevis (B) flanks the lateral side of the long extensor. It runs a similar course to the first metatarsophalangeal joint.

proximal phalanx. At the level of the first metatarsophalangeal joint, the muscle is tendinous and lies invested in the medial capsular structures. With a hallux abductovalgus deformity the tendon is located more plantarly, due to the valgus rotation of the hallux. Medial exposure to the first metatarsophalangeal joint can involve partial detachment of the tendinous insertion, but it is rare to encounter a situation where the entire insertion needs to be detached.

The extensor hallucis brevis muscle is actually the medial-most head of the extensor digitorum brevis muscle. As the muscle courses distally from its origin in the sinus tarsi, it approaches the lateral aspect of the first metatarsal. At the base of the bone, it can be found as a tendon between the first and second metatarsal bases. The tendon runs a similar, but more oblique and deeper, course than the long extensor. At the level of the first metatarsophalangeal joint the tendon is contained in the sheath-like structure of the long extensor and then inserts into the base of the proximal phalanx.[2,4]

This muscle can be a deforming force in the pathoanatomy of hallux abductovalgus. It is often advantageous to release the tendon during bunion surgery. It is best performed at the level of the joint, in order to release contiguous attachments that may be contributing to the deformity.

The adductor hallucis is a two-headed structure that is located in the third layer of plantar foot muscles. The oblique and transverse heads unite as the individual heads emanate from their independent insertions. In about 12% of cases, the muscles form one distinct tendon of insertion, which attaches to the lateral condyle of the base of the proximal phalanx. In the remaining instances, the transverse head attaches directly to the epimysium of the oblique head, which itself ends in a distinct tendon of insertion on the phalangeal base. In few cases does the tendon influence or act upon the lateral sesamoid.[6] However, the oblique head and its tendinous insertion are closely adhered to the lateral aspect of the fibular sesamoid. Because the oblique head is almost parallel to the shaft of the metatarsal, there is little lateralizing effect on the sesamoid from contraction of this muscle. The transverse head may serve to alter the angle of pull of the oblique head but has no real effect on sesamoid position, because the insertion is proximal to the point where the oblique head becomes tendinous.[6]

The flexor hallucis brevis is a bipennate muscle with two distinct tendons of insertion. It is located on the plantar aspect of the first metatarsal and inserts directly into the sesamoids. The sesamoids then attach to the plantar aspect of the base of the proximal phalanx through two separate ligaments.[7]

Joints

The hallux interphalangeal joint

The interphalangeal joint, a bicondylar joint controlled by the long hallucial extensor and flexor, is best approached from the dorsum, or the dorsal aspects on either side, depending on the demands of the procedure. Longitudinal linear incisions are generally favoured for procedures on the side of the joint; however, they are not suitable for direct approach to the joint.

When the interphalangeal joint requires fusion, then incisions with a large transverse component are indicated. There are two useful options: (1) two converging transversely oriented semi-elliptical incisions at the level of the joint or (2) an S-shaped incision with the central limb opposed transversely across the joint (**10.3**).

First metatarsophalangeal joint

This major forefoot articulation is quite accessible from the dorsal aspect for virtually any surgical indication. It must be remembered that there are several intrinsic and extrinsic tendons that invest the joint. The long extensor tendon almost always requires mobilization to enter the joint. It is prudent to mobilize the tendon within its synovial sheath, in order to reduce postoperative restriction of motion. Because the capsule is adhered to the tendon sheath, it is usually mobilized by simple reflection of the capsule (**10.4**). On either side of the joint there are collateral ligaments and the sesamoidal metatarsal ligaments. It is best to sever these ligaments as close to bone as possible so as not to thin the structural integrity of the capsule. With this manoeuvre there is no need to differentiate the collateral ligaments from the sesamoid ligaments.

The sesamoid-metatarsal joint

Traditionally, this joint has been overlooked as a source of pathology or arthrosis in this functionally active articulation. The sesamoids glide on the plantar aspect of the metatarsal head as the joint excurses through its range of motion. The crista serves to further guide this excursion.[1] As the crista becomes eroded or adaptively displaced, aberrations in sesamoid tracking are likely to occur. Tracking dysfunctions can be a source for arthrosis and pain. Repositioning of this apparatus must include either repositioning of the metatarsal or release of the ligaments. Arthritic changes in either side of the articulation can be a cause of considerable pain and disability.

First metatarsal cuneiform joint

This articulation is kidney-shaped and is bound by several tendons and ligaments. The deep plantar vessels run directly lateral to the joint between the first and second metatarsal bases. It is quite vulnerable to trauma during procedures on this joint and should be protected carefully. The articulation itself is quite deep, due to the kidney shape of the joint (**10.5**), and can pose a problem with accessibility to the plantarmost aspects of the joint. Long saw blades or osteotomes are often necessary during resection of the articular cartilage. Again, attention must be paid to protection of underlying neurovascular and tendon structures.

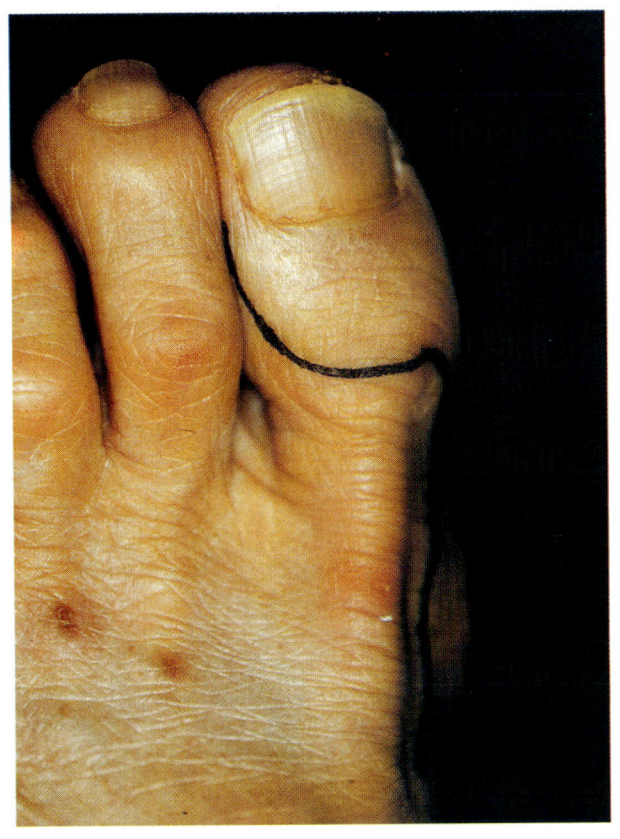

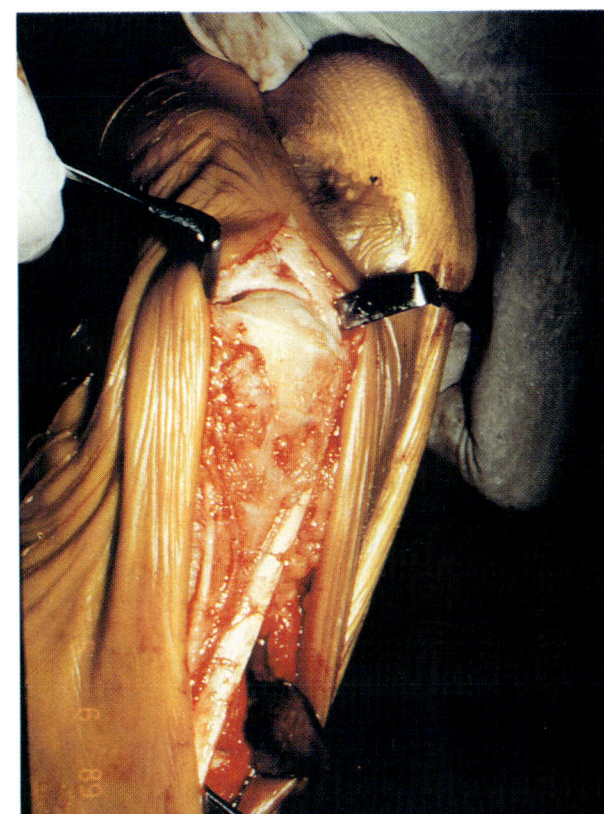

10.3 Approach to the interphalangeal joint of the great toe.

10.4 Intra-operative photograph showing approach to the first metatarsophalangeal joint. Note the extensor hallucis longus tendon is reflected with the capsule to expose the articular surface.

10.5 Photograph of articulated skeleton showing the proximal articular surface of the first metatarsal. It is kidney-shaped, with the convexity facing medially and the concavity laterally.

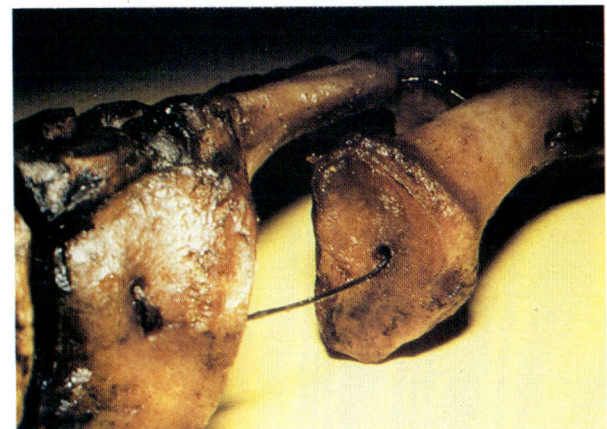

Radiographic assessment

The complete assessment of first ray deformities requires radiographic measurement of basic parameters. Specific angular values are necessary to evaluate the degree of deformity and the need for specific surgical procedures. Radiographic analysis of osseous alignment of areas other than the first ray are also important in evaluating the entire clinical picture and lending insight into the biomechanical profile of the patient. Some of these distant measurements will determine the interdependence of structural and functional relationships and help plan for a more lasting and functional surgical reconstruction.

AP projection

Intermetatarsal (IM) angle

The intermetatarsal angle is the angular relationship between the first and second metatarsal, and is determined by taking the longitudinal bisections of each metatarsal and then measuring the subtended angle. It is normally 0–8° (**10.6**). In the hallux abductovalgus deformity it is almost always accentuated. In the hallux varus deformity it can be normal or even negative, signifying convergence of the first and second metatarsals.[8–10]

Hallux abductus (HA) angle

This angle signifies the degree of deformity at the metatarsophalangeal joint, and is also measured by determining the longitudinal bisections of the first metatarsal and phalanx. It is normally between 10 and 15° (**10.7**). Similar to the intermetatarsal angle, this parameter is increased with the hallux valgus deformity and negative with the hallux varus deformity.

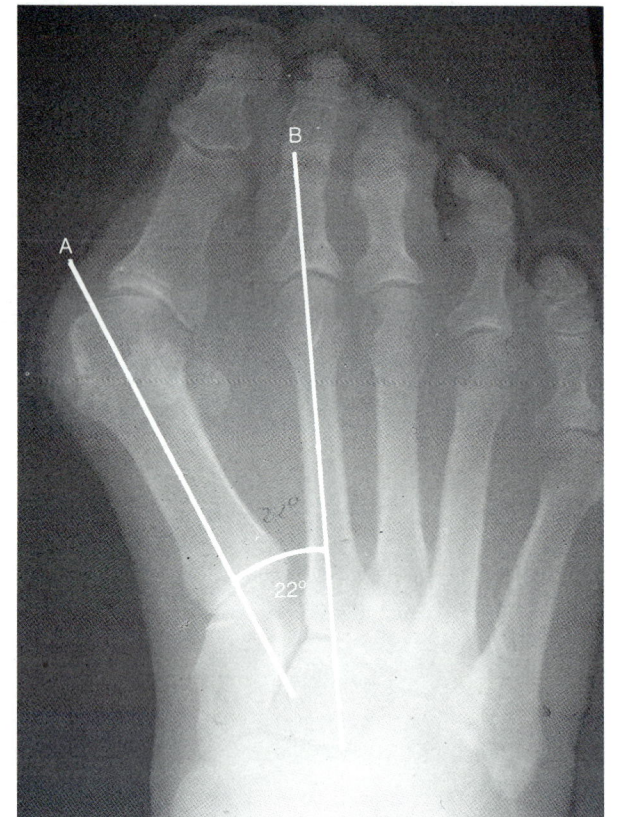

Hallux interphalangeus (HI) angle[11]

This angle quantifies the relationship of the distal and the proximal phalanx. It is normally between 0 and 10°. The distal phalanx is often abducted relative to the proximal phalanx and therefore contributes to the hallux abductovalgus deformity. The angle is formed by the bisections of the proximal and distal phalanges. The distal phalangeal bisection is determined by a line connecting the bisection of the base of the phalanx and a point formed by the intersection of lines drawn as tangents to either side of the phalanx (**10.8**).

Proximal articular set angle (PASA)

This parameter gives the evaluator an approximation of where the distal articular cartilage lies in relationship to the long axis of the bone. It is well known that in the bunion deformity, the articular cartilage may be located in a more lateral position as it functionally adapts to the position of the toe.[12] However, because cartilage is radiographically silent, it is impossible to determine where exactly it lies.[13] It is assessed by first determining the medial and lateral extents of the articular cartil-

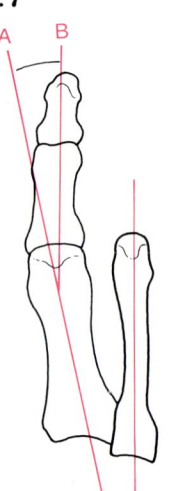

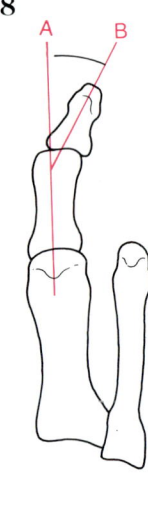

10.6 AP projection of foot. The intermetatarsal (IM) angle is subtended by lines A and B.

10.7 The hallux abductus (HA) angle, subtended by lines A B, measures the degree of lateral deviation of the hallux.

10.8 The hallux interphalangeus (HI) angle is constructed from the intersection of the phalangeal bisections. Note the tangents drawn to the medial and lateral aspects of the distal phalanx.

age. In many cases, the medial aspect of the cartilage is hallmarked by the existence of a prominent sagittal groove. The lateral aspect is often at the most lateral extension of the proximal phalangeal base. However, in the absence of these landmarks, the determinations occur when the distal metatarsal head is completely rounded.

Once the surgeon has determined the approximate extents of the articular cartilage, a line is drawn connecting the two points. A perpendicular line is then constructed which then subtends the proximal articular set angle with the longitudinal bisection of the first metatarsal (**10.9**). It is usually between 7 and 10°.

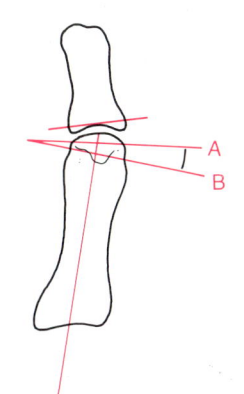

10.9 The proximal articular set angle (PASA) is constructed here by the lines A and B. It represents the approximate position of the articular cartilage relative to the metatarsal shaft.

Distal articular set angle (DASA)

This angle describes the relationship between the articular cartilage of the proximal phalanx and the long axis of the bone. It is normally between 0 and 6°. If accentuated, it signifies deformity within the structure of the phalanx itself. It also can further contribute to the degree of hallux abductus. The angle is determined by finding the extents of the medial and lateral cartilage at the base of the phalanx. It is not nearly as nebulous as that of the first metatarsal head. The perpendicular line constructed to a line connecting the medial and lateral extents forms the angle with the longitudinal bisection of the proximal phalanx (**10.10**).[9,14,15]

Joint congruity

If the PASA and DASA are parallel, the first metatarsophalangeal joint is said to be congruous. If the two lines intersect outside the confines of the lateral extent of the joint cartilage, the joint is said to be deviated. If, however, the lines intersect inside the joint, it is said to be subluxed (**10.11**). The classification is arbitrary, but can serve to guide the surgeon when choosing the surgical procedure. Different philosophies prevail with regard to whether or not to reposition the articular cartilage; therefore, one must use the classification in line with personal preference.[16,17]

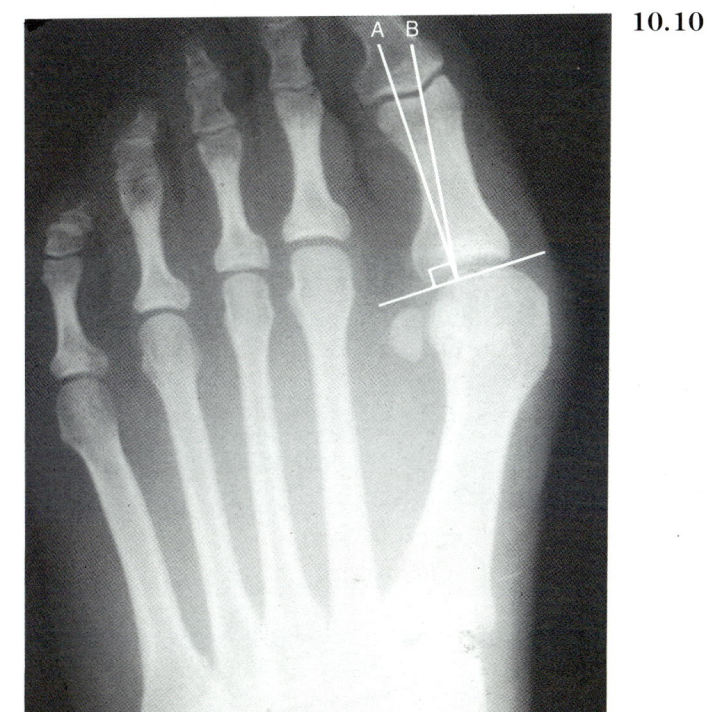

10.10 The distal articular set angle (DASA) is determined by the lines A and B. Both the PASA and the DASA can contribute to the lateral position of the hallux in the transverse plane.

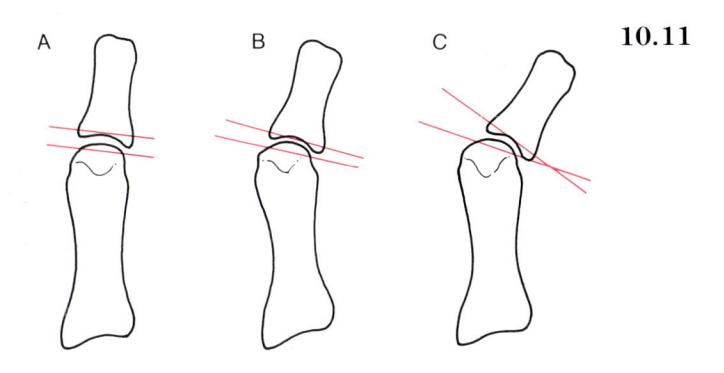

10.11 Determination of first metatarsophalangeal joint position. A, congruous joint; B, deviated joint; C, subluxed joint.

Sesamoid position

The degree of deviation of the sesamoids in the transverse plane is described by the sesamoid position. Normally, the sesamoids occupy the area directly in the centre of the first metatarsal head like two 'eyes on a face'. As the hallux deviates laterally and the first metatarsal medially, it causes the sesamoids to appear displaced relative to their central location. The positional determination is usually based upon the tibial sesamoid position (TSP). Position '1' is the normal sesamoid location. Position '4' is when the tibial sesamoid is centred on the longitudinal bisection of the first metatarsal. Position '7' occurs when the tibial sesamoid is located in the first intermetatarsal space. The remaining positions occupy progressively lateral positions on the continuum (**10.12**).

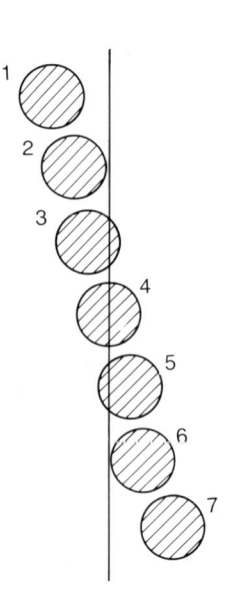

10.12 The right tibial sesamoid position (TSP) is determined by the position of the tibial sesamoid in relation to the bisection of the first metatarsal bone.

Shape of the metatarsal head

The shape of the metatarsal head can be assessed by the AP X-ray. Its significance is nebulous because of the variability of its appearance by the angle of the central ray of the X-ray. As a general guideline, the more round the head, the more likely the patient is to develop transverse plane deviations. The flat or oblique metatarsal head is usually considered to be stable. The patient with a square or irregular-shaped first metatarsal head is more prone to hallux limitus or rigidus type of deformity (**10.13**).[18]

Metatarsal protrusion distance (MPD)

This measurement provides the surgeon with an idea as to the relative length of the first and second metatarsals.[19,20] It is helpful when deciding whether the first metatarsal can withstand a shortening osteotomy or requires a procedure with length preservation. It is determined by extending the longitudinal bisections of the first and second metatarsals until they intersect proximally. A compass is placed at the point of intersection and two arcs are subtended, with radii determined by the distal aspect of each respective bone. The distance between these two arcs is called the metatarsal protrusion distance. Normally, the length of the first metatarsal is one or two millimetres less than the second metatarsal (**10.14**).[21,22]

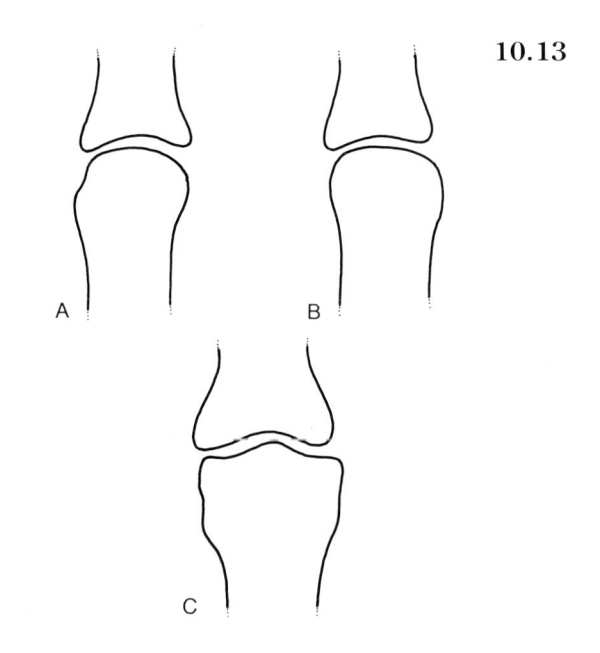

10.13 Metatarsal head shape. (A) Round: may be more prone to hallux abductovalgus and post-operative hallux varus formation. (B) Flat: a relatively stable joint. (C) Square: may be more prone to hallux limitus.

Metatarsus adductus (MA) angle

This measurement indicates the relative adductus of the metatarsus to the midfoot (**10.15**). The importance of this angle is that it prioritizes the significance of the intermetatarsal angle as it contributes to the hallux

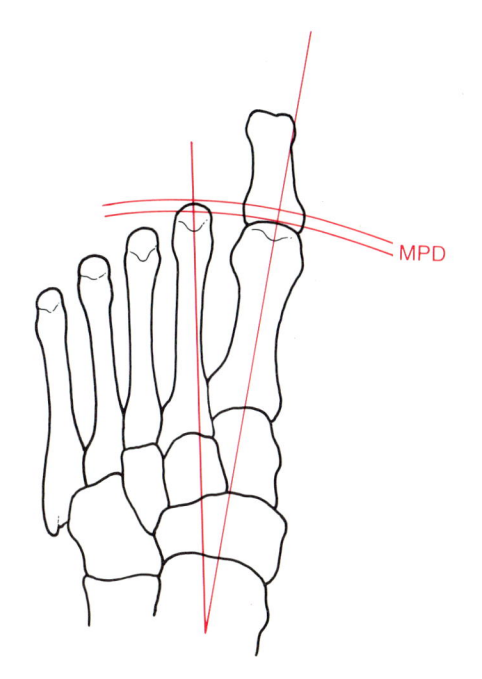

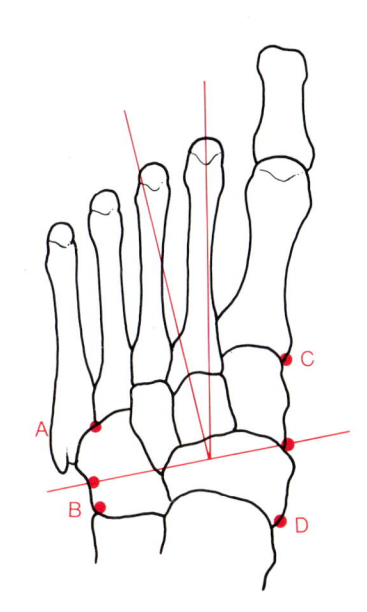

10.14 The metatarsal protrusion distance (MPD) is used to determine the relative lengths of the first and second metatarsal bones. The second metatarsal is usually 1–2 mm longer than the first metatarsal.

10.15 Metatarsus adductus (MA) angle. The bisection of the lesser tarsus is formed by a line connecting the mid-points of lines A–B and C–D. The bisection of the second metatarsal and the perpendicular to the lesser tarsus bisection subtends the metatarsus adductus angle.

abductovalgus deformity. Generally, as the metatarsus adductus angle increases, the more important it is to reduce the intermetatarsal angle on a direct basis. As will be discussed later, proximal osteotomies become more necessary as the metatarsus becomes more adducted.[23]

It is measured by bisecting the lesser tarsus. The medial-most aspect of the first metatarsal cuneiform articulation is located and marked. Then the medial-most aspect of the talonavicular joint is located and marked. A line connecting the two points is constructed, and the mid-point is determined.

A similar procedure is done on the lateral side, using the lateral aspect of the fourth metatarsal cuboid joint and the lateral-most aspect of the calcaneal cuboid joint. The two mid-points are connected and a perpendicular constructed to this line. The longitudinal bisection of the second metatarsal and this perpendicular subtend the metatarsus adductus angle.

Lateral projection

Sagittal intermetatarsal angle[10,12]

This angle depicts the relative parallelism or divergence of the first and second metatarsal on the lateral view. In the normal foot, the first and second metatarsal are relatively parallel. However, in the patient with a hypermobile first ray, the first metatarsal will be more parallel to the supporting surface. In the cavoid foot type, the first metatarsal will be more declinated and the pre-operative absolute value of the angle is not important. It is more important to assess the relative positions of the two metatarsals pre-operatively and determine the amount of change post-operatively (**10.16, 10.17**).

Although it is beyond the scope of this chapter to fully detail procedures, it is important to assure that the

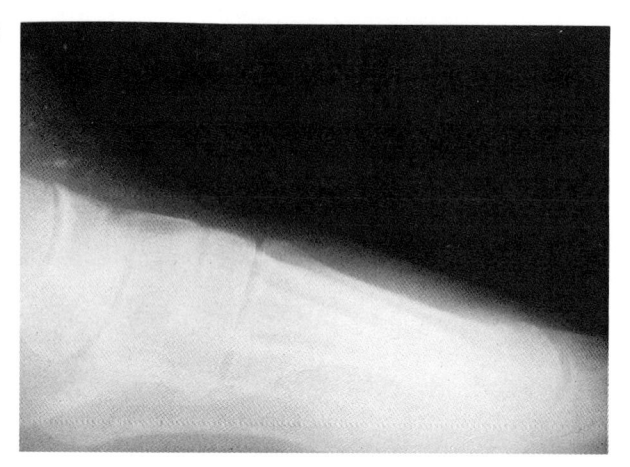

10.16 The sagittal intermetatarsal angle in the pre-operative condition. Note the parallelism of the first and second metatarsals. Here the angle is defined as 0°.

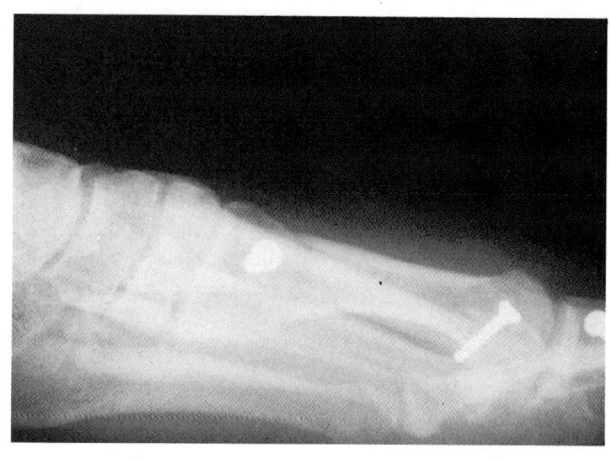

10.17 In this post-operative patient the first metatarsal is elevated, designating a positive angle.

foot is properly positioned for radiographic assessment. Due to the complex arrangements of the facets and articulations, the angles of the skeletal system are highly dependent on the position of the foot and the position of the X-ray tube.

Surgical procedures

This section describes the entire range of first ray surgery, with a special emphasis to the restoration of function. We first discuss the surgical treatment of bunions or hallux abductovalgus, and then cover the other conditions that affect the first metatarsal complex. Some of these procedures can be utilized in both the surgical treatment of bunions and in the other conditions.

soft tissue balancing procedures as pioneered by Hiss,[24] McBride,[25] and Silver.[26] As more correction is required, one must consider the distal metatarsal osteotomies. And finally, the most complicated and advanced deformities often require proximal metatarsal surgery and joint replacement procedures. This section will discuss the entire array of bunionectomies.

Bunionectomies

The term bunion, as it applies to the foot, has a relatively consistent interpretation by the lay public. Most patients can aptly describe a bunion as an enlargement of the great toe joint on the inside of the foot. They are equally as astute to discover that the pain is often relieved by the simple task of removing one's shoes.

However, when the term bunionectomy is interpreted by the public, there is universally a wide variance as to what constitutes this procedure. Descriptions range from the simple shaving of the first metatarsal head to an elaborate and horrifying experience involving reconstruction of the bones of the first ray complex. This variable interpretation as to what is involved in a bunionectomy gives testament to the wide variety of clinical alternatives. There is indeed the relatively simple bunionectomy that involves the elementary task of removing the bump. Intermediate procedures include the

Simple bunionectomy

The simple bunionectomy requires the resection of the medial eminence from the first metatarsal head. It is primarily indicated when there is irritation of the bump from shoe pressure only and there are no functional or radiographic malalignments. There should be no significant abduction of the great toe. It is seldom indicated in the young, active patient. This is because the mere surgical violation of the medial capsule weakens it sufficiently to allow for more lateral deviation of the hallux after the procedure. It is best applied to the elderly patient who has difficulty wearing shoes due to pressure. One does not need to consider bone density in this procedure because there is no dependence on bone healing for the success of the procedure. Although it is usually desirable to resect the medial eminence in such a fashion that the cut surface is flush and parallel with the proximal diaphysis, exceptions can be made on this procedure. In the elderly patient it is acceptable to 'spike the head'. Excessive removal of the bump may provide more comfort to the patient by narrowing the foot even more. The risk of osteoarthritis and an incongruous joint is minimal because of the patient's age and low functional demands.

The capsule may be trimmed of excessive tissue, but it should not be sutured tightly in order not to pull the proximal phalanx over too far and cause either a hallux varus or premature arthrosis as a result of malalignment. In other words, the joint should be maintained exactly as it was in the pre-operative state or corrected only slightly.

Post-operative care entails a wooden-soled shoe for 2–4 weeks and regular loose-fitting shoes when comfort allows.

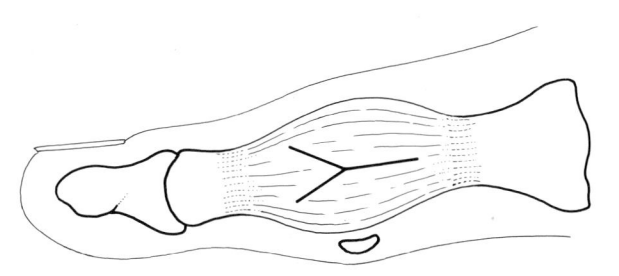

10.18 The Y-capsulotomy of Silver. The fashioning of the flap in this manner allows for capsular correction of the hallux position. The portion that is still attached to the proximal phalanx is pulled proximally and oversewn on the stem portion of the Y.

Silver bunionectomy

The Silver bunionectomy is another simple soft tissue procedure for the patient with a mild deformity.[26] It differs from the simple bunionectomy in that some transverse plane correction of the abducted hallux is obtained. Therefore, it is indicated when there is an offending medial eminence and a positional incongruity of the joint. The age limits are similar to the simple bunionectomy, but this procedure can occasionally be used for the younger patient.

The joint is approached through a dorsomedial incision. The capsulotomy is fashioned in the shape of a Y (**10.18**) and the capsular flaps are elevated.[26,27] The medial eminence is resected, but the head should not be spiked because the capsular correction may cause excessive adduction, leading to hallux varus. If there is tightness of the lateral structures, they can be released (*see* section on lateral release). The capsular flaps are advanced and overlapped. The repair of the capsular plication occurs with the toe held in a slightly overcorrected position. Care should be taken not to overtighten the capsule. It should be just tight enough to maintain the hallux and metatarsal head in a congruous condition. Post-operative management is similar to that for the simple bunionectomy.

McBride bunionectomy

Earl McBride published his benchmark work in 1928.[25] Today, some modification of this procedure is performed in a vast majority of bunionectomies. McBride realized the significance of the lateral structures in maintaining the deformity. He postulated that the lateral sesamoid was the centre of the hub, and the muscles which acted upon it were responsible for pulling the proximal phalanx lateral-ward. This resulted in a secondary increase in the intermetatarsal angle due to retrograde pressure at the joint. McBride felt that by removing the lateral sesamoid and freeing up the structures laterally one could achieve correction of the joint malposition as well as the intermetatarsal angle. The intermetatarsal angle was reduced by transferring the adductor complex directly to the first metatarsal bone. McBride published several subsequent papers on his work which are essentially refinements in the technique and the report of complications from the procedure.[28,29] Even today, the procedure associated with his name has many different descriptions among the surgeons performing it. It has been modified extensively, with variations as plentiful as there are surgeons.

The indications for this procedure alone are quite narrow. This is because the appreciation for correction of structural deformities has permeated our thinking today and the relatively high incidence of hallux varus with this procedure. This procedure is indicated in the patient with a moderate bunion and a positional deformity. The intermetatarsal angle should probably not exceed 15°. It should be flexible and able to be manually reduced. One must inspect the pre-operative X-rays to ensure that the base of the first metatarsal does not articulate with the base of the second metatarsal. Otherwise, the reduction of the IM angle will not be possible with distal metatarsophalangeal joint releases and repositioning. The sesamoid position should be at least 4, or at least the lateral sesamoid should be hanging over the lateral aspect of the metatarsal head. The joint should not be arthritic and there should be minimal deviation of the PASA.

The basic procedure, as it is today, consists of removal of the medial eminence, a lateral sesamoidectomy, and occasional transfer of the adductor hallucis into the medial capsule.[30] This can be accomplished through one or two incisions. The single incisional technique involves a dorsomedial approach with a capsulotomy of choice. The bump is removed in a fashion that will preserve the plantar aspect of the sagittal groove. This is done by taking more bone off the dorsal aspect of the metatarsal head than off the plantar (**10.19**). The tangent to the resection, however, should always be parallel to the long axis of the metatarsal. The precision needed to achieve these objectives is often underestimated and less than optimal bony resections result. The consequence of incorrect medial eminence resection is a high propensity for hallux varus, because there is little to prevent the medial sesamoid from creeping around the over-resected plantar aspect of the metatarsal head (**10.20**). The mechanical advantage that the remaining sesamoid now enjoys will often lead to hallux varus. There is no corresponding lateral sesamoid to counteract the medial structures. One can see it is of the utmost importance to properly resect the medial eminence.

The lateral release

Lateral sesamoid release is an extremely critical component of successful hallux abductovalgus correction. The technique of lateral release is one that can only be mastered by repetition and adherence to basic tenets. It should be stated that the entire sesamoid apparatus and the intrinsic muscles are involved to some degree in the pathoanatomy of the deformity. Although it is commonly misconceived, the sesamoid complex and the associated structures do not actually displace. It is the reciprocal displacement of the first metatarsal relative to a relatively fixed sesamoid apparatus and resultant contracture of the sesamoid ligaments that necessitates the lateral release. With the proper repositioning of the first metatarsal, the sesamoid structures must be mobilized and released from their contracted state to reassume their anatomically correct location.

The first step in performing lateral release is to identify the correct tissue plane. It is best to dissect in the first intermetatarsal space by staying completely superficial to the capsular structures. Dissection is then carried to the level of the superficial transverse metatarsal ligament,[2,29,31] which is severed using a sharp blade or scissors. This allows for additional separation of the first and second metatarsals. Then the oblique head of the adductor hallucis and its tendon are identified. A fresh scalpel blade is then inserted into the interval between the sesamoid and the tendon and the blade is advanced distally in a saw-like motion (**10.21**). This is carried to the level of the proximal phalanx, and the tendon release is completed by turning the blade laterally and thereby transecting the attachment; this furnishes the adductor tendon, with its maximal length, for later transfer if needed (**10.22**).

The second step is to insert the scalpel blade between the sesamoid and the metatarsal head. The knife is advanced distally to transect the entire dorsal attachments of the sesamoid to the metatarsal. Next, the

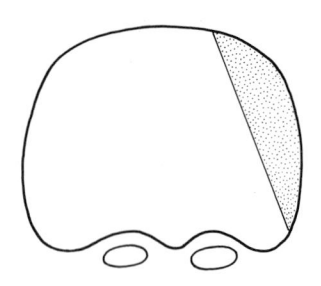

10.19 Cross-section showing the plane of resection of the medial eminence. The plantar aspect of the metatarsal head is only minimally resected, if at all. If one desires a narrower metatarsal head, then more of the plantar aspect can be resected, as long as the sagittal groove is resected.

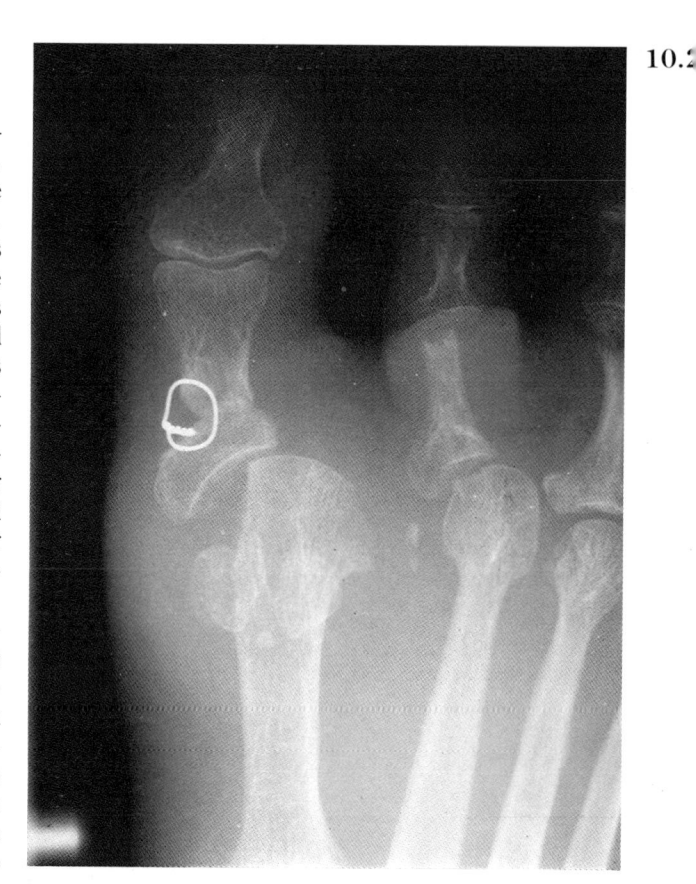

10.20 Post-operative X-rays of a patient who developed hallux varus. This was due to overzealous lateral release and a 'spiked' medial eminence. The sagittal groove was resected, allowing the prominent phalangeal base to hook over the edge.

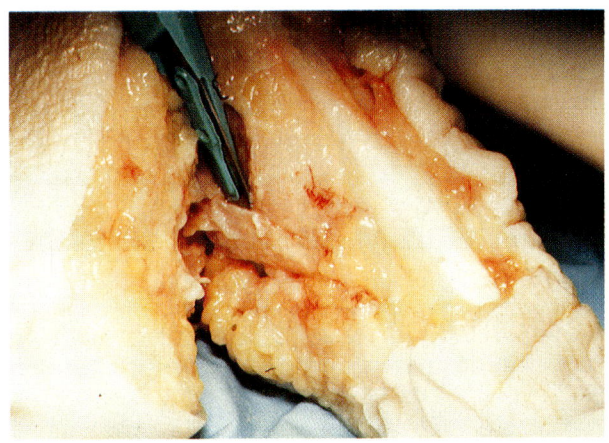

10.21 Cadaveric specimen in which the proper technique for detachment of the oblique head of adductor hallucis is demonstrated. The scalpel blade is inserted between the tendon and sesamoid and then advanced distally to the base of the phalanx.

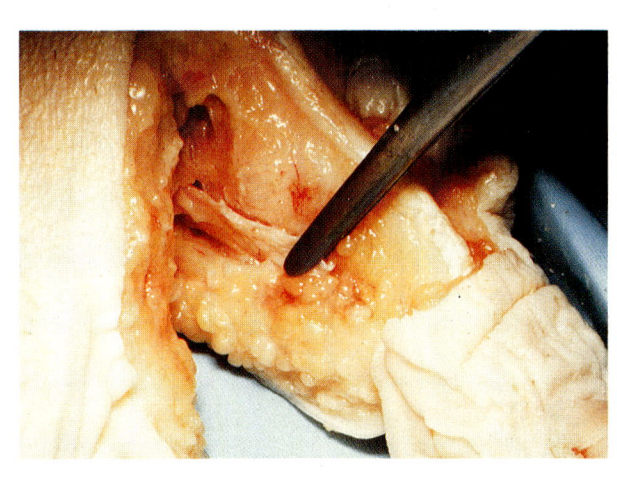

10.22 The same cadaveric specimen as in **10.21**. The entire length of the adductor tendon is retrieved for transfer if desired.

proximal attachment of the lateral head of the flexor hallucis brevis is released, taking care not to injure the long flexor tendon. A vertical lateral capsulotomy is then performed. The extensor hallucis brevis tenotomy is carried out, as mentioned, at the level of the first metatarsophalangeal joint.

Finger palpation is performed to check for any tight structures, and these are released. The hallux should be able to be manipulated into any position if the release has adequately addressed all of the contracted structures.

Approach to the lateral sesamoid from the first intermetatarsal space can lead to iatrogenic injury to the long flexor tendon. Careful control of the scalpel blade is necessary in this area, with excellent mental appreciation for the spatial relationship of the tendon and scalpel blade. If the surgeon wishes to totally extirpate the sesamoid, additional release is required: it can be difficult to remove because it is firmly invested in the sesamoidal ligamentous complex. The sesamoid is often partially sheltered by the lateral aspect of the metatarsal head, especially in those cases where the sesamoid position is 4 or 5. Up to this point, the sesamoid has been freed of all attachments, except for the intersesamoidal ligament and the tendon of the lateral head of the short hallucial flexor, which courses distally from the bone. The tag of tissue that is still attached to the lateral aspect of the sesamoid should be grasped with a multi-toothed forceps and pulled dorsally. Then the distal attachment of the sesamoid is severed sharply with a scalpel, leaving only the intersesamoidal ligament to be severed. This can be carried out by careful manipulation of the sesamoid and, once completed, the bone can be easily removed.

Additional difficulty can arise if the intersesamoidal ligament is calcified or if the two sesamoids are anklylosed. In this case, the connection can usually be broken by using a stout Mayo-type scissors. One must be extremely careful not to damage the long flexor hallucis tendon, which is in close approximation and must be diligently protected. After every sesamoidectomy, the integrity of the long flexor tendon should be examined; if it has been severed, then it should be repaired.

Once the tendon of the oblique head is freed up, it can be transferred into the head of the first metatarsal through the use of nonabsorbable sutures. The IM angle should be manually reduced while the sutures are being tied. The capsule is now repaired by reefing it up on the medial aspect while holding the toe in a corrected or slightly over-corrected position.[32]

Modified McBride bunionectomy

This procedure has many different connotations among podiatric and orthopaedic surgeons. This procedure is described as I employ it. It is almost never used alone, but is an essential component of the bunionectomy. In my hands, this procedure is performed as part of virtually all bunionectomy procedures for hallux abductovalgus.

It involves the McBride procedure, except that the sesamoid is not removed. The reasons for leaving the lateral sesamoid are predicated on stability and the avoidance of hallux varus. When one performs a complete lateral release, the sesamoids can be relocated under the metatarsal head whether one combines the soft tissue procedure with an osseous procedure or not. One must remember that the sesamoids do not actually migrate: it is the first metatarsal that moves away from the intrinsic anatomy. Therefore, the surgeon is merely releasing the long-standing contractures in order for the sesamoids to move independently of the metatarsal.

If one chooses to do an osteotomy, the bone will be moved over the sesamoid complex.[33] If an osteotomy is not chosen, the sesamoid complex can be repositioned through soft tissue plication.

Distal metatarsal osteotomies (DMO)

Distal metatarsal osteotomies are utilized for the reduction of moderately increased intermetatarsal angles.[34] They can also be employed to redirect the orientation of the articular cartilage or reduce the PASA.

The reduction of the IM angle is a relative one, as these procedures merely move the distal aspect of the metatarsal in a lateral direction. Each of these procedures has certain advantages and disadvantages. The procedures are discussed individually and contrasts and similarities made.

Chevron bunionectomy (Austin)

This is probably the most common distal osteotomy performed today for the correction of hallux abductovalgus deformity. It was designed by the late Dr Dale Austin.[35] The osteotomy is truly a chevron-shaped cut in the distal cancellous metaphyseal bone of the first metatarsal. The apex of the cut is pointed distally and the limbs emanate in a proximal direction (**10.23**). The orientation of the osteotomy is the transverse plane;[36] that is, the axis of the apex is on or closest to the

10.23 Diagram depicting the proper orientation of the Austin or chevron bunionectomy. Note that the cut is entirely within the metaphyseal region of the bone and the apex is directed distally.

10.24 Diagram of biplanar chevron bunionectomy. Note that there is more bone removed from the medial aspect of the proximal fragment. The lateral translocation of the head may serve to reduce some of the apparent correction of the proximal articular set angle.

transverse plane. Certain refinements in technique can involve deviations of the axis from the transverse plane, in order to customize the direction of movement of the capital fragment.[37-39]

The basic procedure includes a dorsomedial or medial approach to the metatarsophalangeal joint, with a capsulotomy of choice. The medial eminence is removed but the resection is modified for this procedure. Instead of removing bone in a manner that is flush with the metatarsal shaft, one needs only to make a flat surface on the medial aspect of the head, but removing a much smaller amount of bone. When the metatarsal head is repositioned, it will compensate for the lesser amount of bone. Because only the distal aspect of bone is exposed, it is important to fashion the resected surface as if the metatarsal were a true rectangular volume. The resected surface should parallel the medial side and be exactly perpendicular to the top of the bone. The reason for this is that the surgeon now has an accurate orientation point for the osteotomy. Any lack of precision can cause the axis of the osteotomy to be orientated in a direction that leads to mal-positioning of the capital fragment.[40]

The osteotomy is then made with an oscillating-type saw. It is important first to locate the position of the apex of the cut. It is best positioned in the centre of the metatarsal head on the cut surface. The saw blade should not over-cut the apex. The plantar limb should exit proximal to the sesamoids and the dorsal limb should exit at a similar level on the dorsal cortex. The head is then lateralized and held in the desired location.

Biplanar chevron bunionectomy, which is useful when a reduction of the PASA is necessary as well as a reduction of the IM angle,[41] is accomplished by removing more bone from the medial aspect of the metatarsal shaft fragment (**10.24**). This serves to de-rotate the capital fragment and the articular cartilage when it is impacted or replaced on the metatarsal shaft.

Although the issue of fixation of the osteotomy has never been adequately decided, it is my opinion that all chevron osteotomies deserve some form of fixation. Proponents of leaving the osteotomy unsecured contend that the osteotomy is inherently stable and therefore no fixation is needed.[42] However, the shear forces that are generated in the transverse plane during normal ambulation may overcome the bone-to-bone friction that secures the osteotomy on the transverse plane. It is on this plane that the fracture is not stable.[43] The cost of internal or external fixation is low. One need only experience the post-operative patient where the head of the metatarsal has slipped with a resultant loss of correction or, worse still, the metatarsal head migrates into the interspace, to appreciate the wisdom of fixation.[44] Fixation is generally easy to install and there is a low incidence of complications. The device used is solely dependent on the surgeon's personal preference; devices include K-wires, bone screws, Herbert screws,[45] staples, and monofilament wire. Various modifications have been published to accommodate specific fixation devices. It is my experience, however, that there are low complication rates attributed to the type of fixation alone and, therefore, the issue of fixation is relegated to the issue of whether to use it in the first place. My own preference is a single 2.7 mm cortical bone screw placed from dorsal distal to plantar proximal. The dorsal limb is extended slightly more proximal in order to facilitate screw placement (**10.25**).

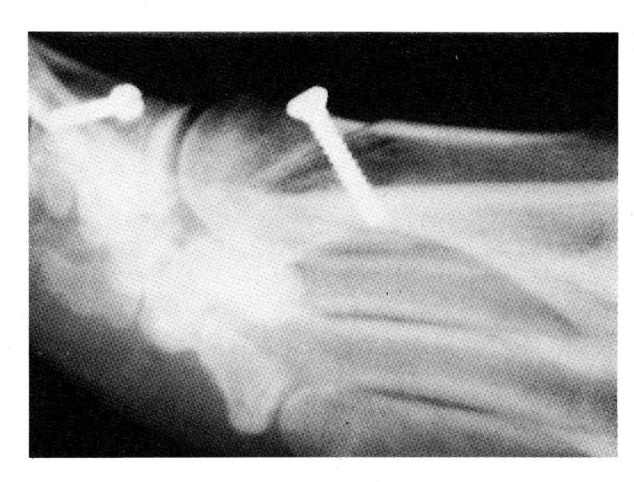

10.25 Post-operative lateral radiograph of Austin bunionectomy fixated with 2.7 mm cortical screw. The proximal dorsal limb of the osteotomy is elongated slightly to facilitate screw placement.

Post-operative care for this procedure generally includes an ambulatory situation in the near post-operative period. This is because the osteotomy is stable, especially when it is fortified with fixation. The inherent nature of the osteotomy does allow for resistance of vertical ground reactive forces. Usually, we give the patient a post-operative wooden shoe and allow full weight-bearing as soon as it is comfortable. This, of course, implies that there were no intra-operative mishaps which render the fracture unstable. External fixation devices can be removed at 4–6 weeks. Radiographs should be checked periodically to ensure good bone apposition and osseous union.

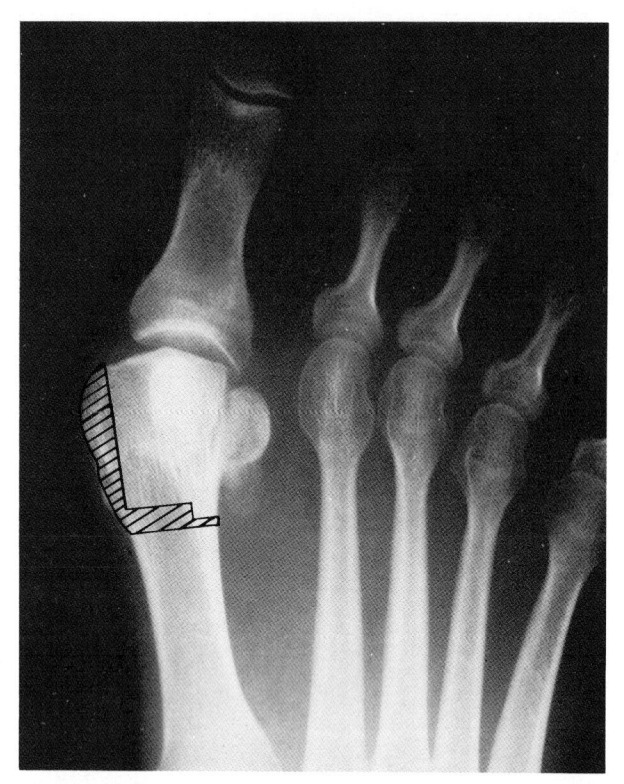

Mitchell bunionectomy

The procedure designed and popularized by Hawkins and Mitchell in 1945[46,47] is slowly becoming an obsolete procedure for the correction of hallux abductovalgus. This is because the procedure has several disadvantages that are avoided by the more commonly utilized chevron osteotomy or its modifications. Nevertheless, satisfactory reports continue to appear.[48] The procedure is described as a double osteotomy in the distal aspect of the metatarsal at the metaphyseal diaphyseal junction (**10.26**). The first cut is made perpendicular to the shaft and is made ⅔–¾ across the bone. The second cut is made parallel to the first at a distance 3–4 mm proximal to the first, but is completely across the bone. The procedure is finished by removing the small rectangle of bone from the metatarsal head fashioned by the incomplete first cut. This leaves the capital fragment with a proximally directed stump of bone. The metatarsal head is now relocated laterally until the stump of bone overhangs the lateral cortex of the shaft (**10.27**). This effectively lateralizes the metatarsal head and shortens the first metatarsal. The shortening of the metatarsal may be necessary in some patients because of a long metatarsal with uncontrolled retrograde forces. In these cases, the Mitchell procedure is indicated if small corrections of the intermetatarsal angle are required.

Fixation of the osteotomy is required. Mitchell first proposed a suture be placed across the osteotomy. Common sense and experience tells us that this is inadequate fixation for several reasons. First, the complete osteotomy is only fixed in one plane. The forces of weight-bearing, or even muscle pull, can serve to rotate the capital fragment in the sagittal plane, thereby destroying the position of the bone. Secondly, Mitchell described the procedure be carried out proximal to the metaphysis in an area that heals poorly. Thirdly, the osteotomy is inherently unstable because of its design and the fact that the metatarsal was shortened. Finally, there is little soft tissue tension available to stabilize the osteotomy.

Therefore, if this procedure is to be used, more stable and useful fixation is required. Crossed K-wires are usually best applied here because the design of the procedure precludes other devices. A recent report of Herbert screw fixation is encouraging, but sagittal plane stabilization may still be suspect.[49]

Post-operative care must be carefully monitored due to the tendency for displacement. The greatest tendency in this regard is in the dorsal direction. Only under the most stable conditions can the patient be allowed to bear weight before complete bony union occurs. If single cortex fixation is utilized, then the patient is best kept off weight-bearing until union occurs.

Complications with this procedure result primarily

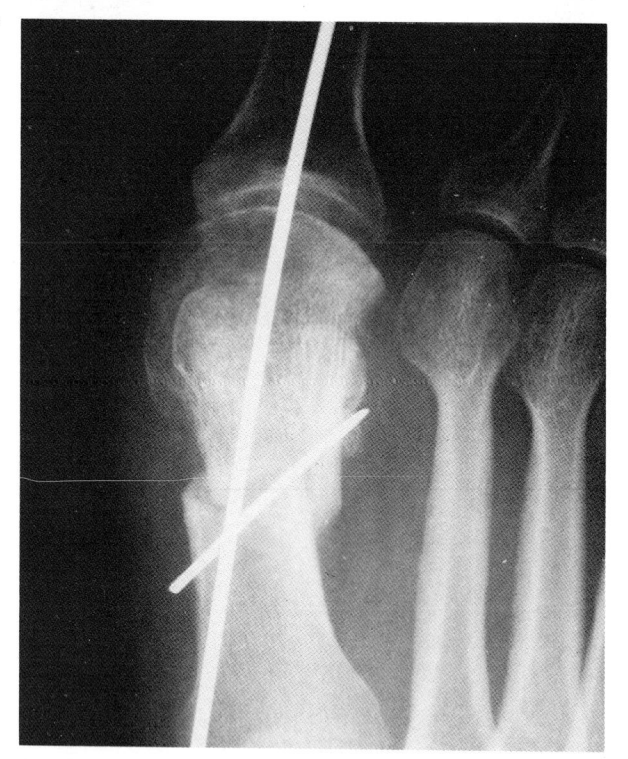

10.26 Mitchell osteotomy prior to the removal of bone. The shaded area represents the amount of bone removed.

10.27 The completed Mitchell osteotomy with the head relocated laterally on the shaft. Fixation is then introduced.

from the dorsal migration of the capital fragment.[48] Transfer lesions to the lesser metatarsals and metatarsalgia are common sequelae and are difficult to manage conservatively in a satisfactory manner to the patient.

Reverdin procedure

This osteotomy is utilized for the realignment of the deviated articular cartilage at the metatarsal head level. A medial closing wedge osteotomy is performed in the distal metaphysis, while leaving an intact lateral hinge (**10.28, 10.29**). The cartilage is thus aligned in a position that is more perpendicular to the shaft of the metatarsal, thereby reducing the PASA. This effectively realigns the first metatarsal joint axis and serves to adduct the hallux. It must be combined with an effective lateral release in order to allow for this correction as well as realignment of the sesamoid complex. This will also utilize the reverse-buckling concept, by virtue of repositioning of the hallux.[32,50]

The indications for this procedure are presence of an abnormal PASA. Other abnormalities in alignment may be present, but they must be corrected with other procedures.

The procedure is carried out by exposing the joint in routine fashion.[51] The head of the first metatarsal is osteotomized using a power saw. The first cut is made approximately 1 cm proximal to the end of the metatarsal and is directed parallel to the articular cartilage. The second cut is made parallel to the long axis of the shaft such that a wedge of bone is fashioned with an intact lateral apex (*see* **10.28, 10.29**). The sesamoids should be protected with a retractor placed under the metatarsal head. The cut is feathered until the capital portion can be closed and aligned on the shaft. Fixation is a matter of personal choice. In some cases, none is required, due to the retrograde pressure of the hallux. Absorbable suture works well if the lateral hinge remains intact: it is simple to implement and provides insurance that the osteotomy will not displace. If the hinge fails, it may be necessary to use K-wire stabilization but joint motion will be compromised.

Post-operative care in the absence of other metatarsal procedures allows early weight-bearing in a wooden or semi-flexible shoe.

Complications of this procedure are common, as a result of the design of the osteotomy. Loss of motion or a stiff first metatarsophalangeal joint is possible because the integrity of the sesamoid articulation with the metatarsal head is disrupted. Also, a modest amount of capsular stripping is necessary for performance of the procedure. The capital fragment may undergo avascular necrosis because of this exposure. We agree with Boberg *et al.*[37] that the lateral aspect of the capsule should be left intact to diminish this possibility. Nevertheless, the Reverdin operation does have some usefulness in a limited patient population.

Reverdin–Green modification

Intrinsic problems of intra-articular violation with the Reverdin procedure led to the Green modification, described in 1977 by Todd.[52] The operation has exactly the same indication as the traditional procedure. The first cut, however, is made in the plantar aspect of the metatarsal head, parallel to the weight-bearing surface, superior to the sesamoids (**10.30, 10.31**). The remaining cuts are the same as the Reverdin osteotomy, except that the cuts end at the confluence of the wedge and the initial plantar cut. This allows for the same degree of correction, but does not violate the plantar aspect of the metatarsal head. This modification is quite stable, due to the plantar shelf, and is even less likely to require fixation, again providing the lateral hinge remains intact. Range of motion exercises are required to prevent post-operative restriction of motion.

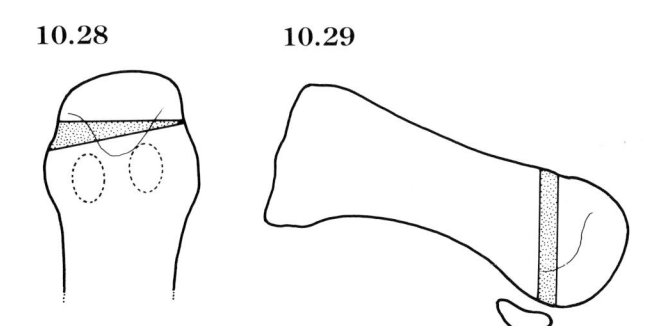

10.28 Dorsal view of the Reverdin osteotomy. The base of the wedge is directed medially and the apex laterally.

10.29 The same osteotomy from the medial aspect. The shaded areas represent the portion of bone to be removed.

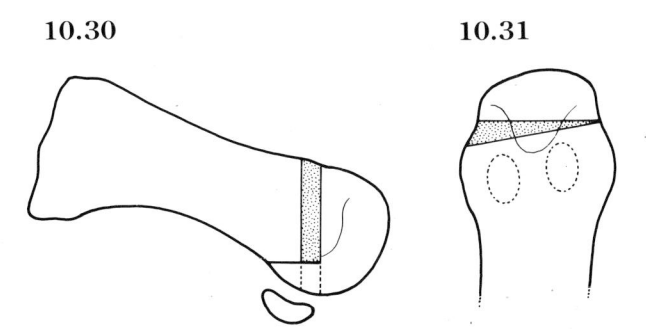

10.30 Medial view of the Reverdin–Green osteotomy. Note that the plantar articular surface for the sesamoids has not been violated by the osteotomy.

10.31 The dorsal view appears exactly the same as **10.28**.

10.32

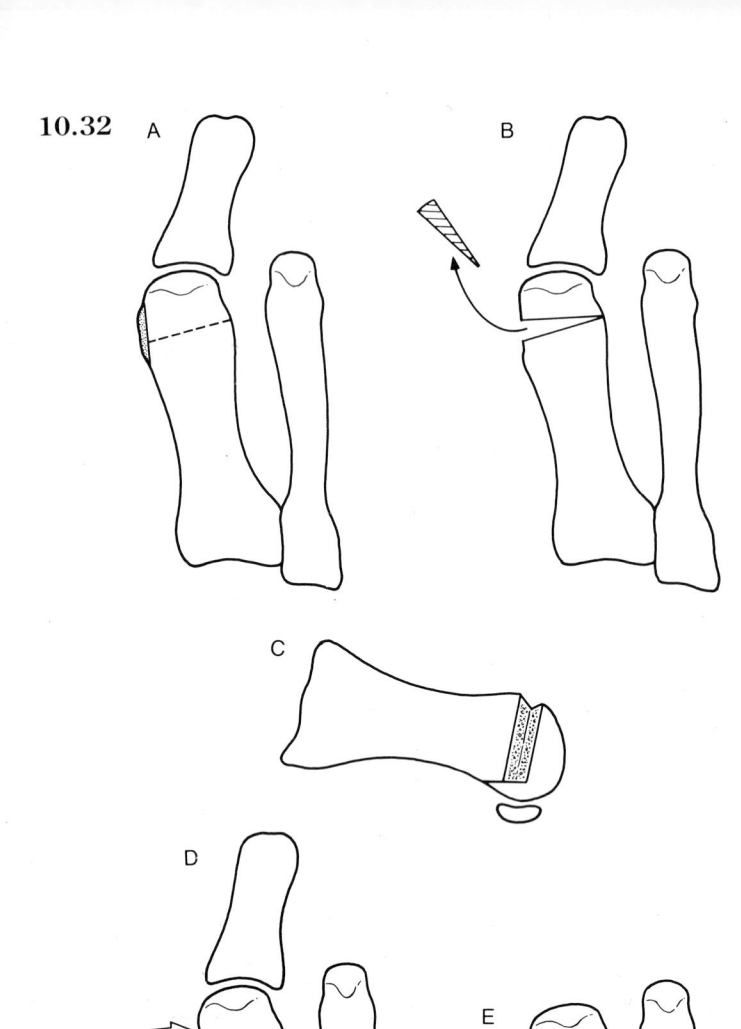

Reverdin–Laird modification[52]

This is yet another modification of the basic Reverdin operation. It is exactly the same as the Reverdin–Green procedure, except that the apex is deliberately cut and the entire distal fragment is transposed laterally (**10.32**). This gives one a relative reduction in the intermetatarsal angle and works similar to the Austin bunionectomy; however, because it is made a bit more distal, the amount of correction attained is somewhat less than in the Austin procedure. The bi-correctional Austin procedure, although more difficult to perform, affords better intrinsic stability and is favoured over the Reverdin–Laird operation when all else is equal. If correction of an abnormal PASA is the first priority over lateralization of the metatarsal head, then the Reverdin–Laird would be the favoured procedure.

10.32 Dorsal view of the Reverdin–Laird osteotomy after transposition of the capital fragment. Some relative reduction of the intermetatarsal angle is realized (E).

Mid-shaft procedures

Z-Bunionectomy

The Z-bunionectomy was designed to overcome some of the inherent difficulties of the first metatarsal elevation with the closing wedge osteotomy. When performed in the traditional fashion, this procedure was predisposed to first metatarsal elevation. The procedure was conceived at the University of Chicago in 1981 and has earned its place in the armamentarium of many foot surgeons.[53] It is utilized for the reduction of the intermetatarsal angle that is moderately increased. One of the advantages of the procedure is that it is extremely stable, as a result of its configuration, and can withstand early weight-bearing without fear of dorsal angulation or displacement.

The osteotomy is fashioned in the shape of the letter Z. The transverse limb of the Z coincides with the longitudinal bisection of the first metatarsal. The dorsal limb is similar to the dorsal leg of the first chevron osteotomy and the plantar limb courses distally towards the first metatarsal head (**10.33**).

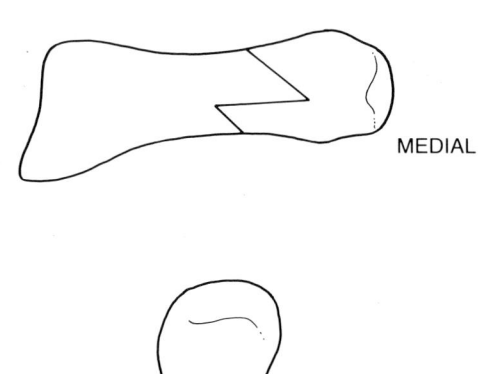

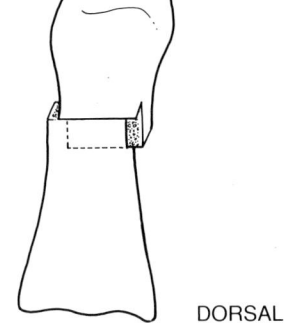

10.33 Z-osteotomy bunionectomy. Sometimes referred to as the scarf procedure, this osteotomy technique is inherently stable but is still usually fixated with screws.

Proximal osteotomies

Proximal osteotomies are valuable procedures in the patient with accentuated IM angles. Reductions of high degrees of metatarsus primus varus deformities are best accomplished at the level of the base of the first metatarsal. The amount of correction that is available is obtained through the application of the simple physical laws of lever arms. As Ruch and Banks[54] point out, the greatest amount of lateral movement of the first metatarsal head occurs with relatively small corrections at the level of the metatarsal base. This is true regardless of the design of the osteotomy.[55]

Closing wedge osteotomies[56,57]

The lateral closing wedge osteotomy is the most commonly utilized proximal metatarsal procedure for the reduction of the intermetatarsal angle, because of its relative ease in performing the procedures and its effectiveness. The indications include an abnormally high IM angle, usually in excess of 15°. However, in some cases where there is significant metatarsus adductus, it can be applied to the IM angle as low as 10°. There should be sufficient length of the metatarsal because some shortening can be expected.[21,22] Adequate bone stock should also be realized although osteoporotic bone does heal as well as dense bone provided it can be stabilized with fixation devices. This procedure is generally reserved for the patient who is under the age of 65. The elderly patient is much less likely to be able to endure the 6-week period of non-weight-bearing in the post-operative period. In addition, the elderly patient is less likely to require the degree of return to function that the closing base wedge osteotomy can provide.

This procedure is almost universally combined with a distal muscle–tendon balancing procedure, such as the modified McBride.[33] In some instances, a distal cartilage repositioning or hallux osteotomy procedure may also be utilized. The distal procedure is performed first, including the lateral release. The basal osteotomy is then performed by either extending the original incision proximally or making a second (or third) approach over the basal metatarsal. I prefer the single incisional approach because it allows for the obligate exposure necessary for repetitive and successful reconstructions.

The favoured approach is a dorsomedial incision that parallels the bony anatomy (**10.34**). The incision is curved slightly lateral as it traverses over the metatarsal base. It ends at the proximal lateral aspect of the metatarsal cuneiform joint. The subcutaneous tissue is swept off the deep fascial structures at the basilar level. This provides complete visualization of the extensor hallucis longus (EHL) and brevis tendons as well as access to the first intermetatarsal space. The deep fascia is then incised several millimetres medial to the EHL tendon but only to the level of the periosteum. I

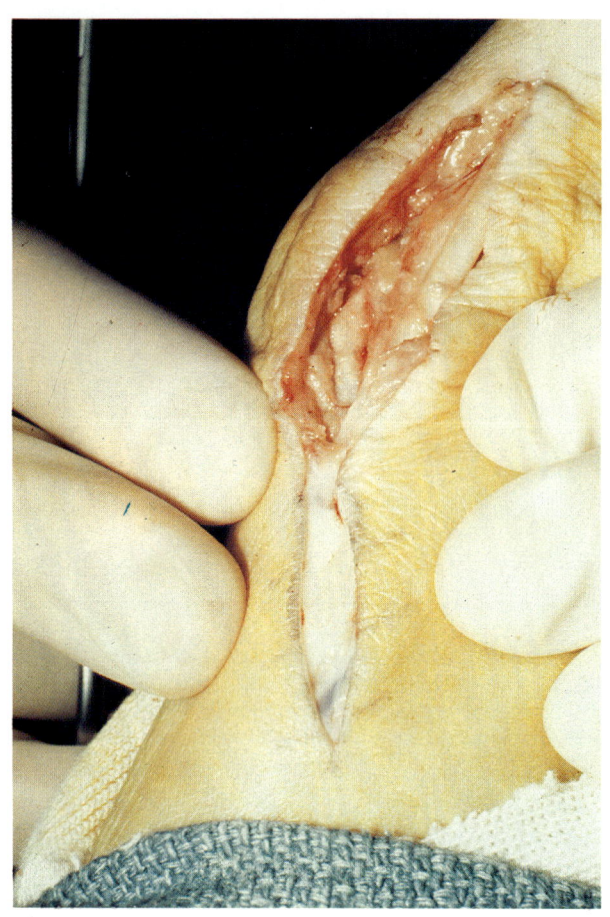

10.34 Incisional approach to the closing wedge osteotomy. The proximal aspect of the incision courses laterally to facilitate visualization of the lateral aspect of the metatarsal base and for adequate retraction of the deep plantar artery and deep peroneal nerve.

believe that there is no need to strip the vascular periosteum from the metatarsal when it may supply up to 25% of the blood supply to the bone. Once this is done, the entire EHL tendon and its sheath can be mobilized laterally, with the tendon completely contained in its sheath. This will prevent post-operative adhesions of the tendon at this level. A Hohmann retractor can then be placed into the interspace, thereby retracting the extensor tendon and protecting the deep plantar artery and the medial terminal division of the deep peroneal nerve. At no time is the periosteum disturbed. Small globules of connective tissue and fat may remain behind attached to the periosteum dorsally, but these are easily removed with a knife and forceps.

We are now ready to perform the osteotomy. The level of the first metatarsal cuneiform joint is marked with either a 25 g needle or a surgical marker. The osteotomy is orientated oblique from an apex; that is, proximal medial to a distal lateral base. The ideal orientation is at an angle of about 45° to the long axis of the bone. The distal cut is made first with a power saw in the direction desired, directly through the periosteum. It is often easier to make the proximal cut first, but care should be taken, regardless of the order of the cuts, to preserve and maintain the integrity of the medial cortical hinge. Loss of the hinge will complicate the fixation and, in all likelihood, the stability. The second cut is made at an angle that will subtend the appropriate amount of bone wedge to obtain the desired amount of correction of the IM angle.[55] The author prefers to strive for an IM angle that approaches 0°; however, in some cases overzealous bony resection leads to a negative IM angle. This can create a propensity towards hallux varus if the distal procedures have been performed improperly. Once the cuts have been completed and the wedge of bone removed, the osteotomy is feathered and readied for fixation. The reader is referred to the excellent detailed description of the technique by Ruch and Banks.[54]

Fixation is best accomplished by a compression screw placed across the osteotomy.[9,21,58,59] The visualization of the lateral aspect of the metatarsal enables accurate placement of the screw. The surgeon should be wary of the situation where the drill or tap migrates within the contents of the first metatarsal base. Each time these instruments are inserted, the exit point on the lateral aspect should be verified by direct visualization.

If there is any degree of failure of the fixation, its stability should be critically evaluated. Supplemental or alternative devices may be necessary to provide stable, but not necessarily rigid, fixation.[21] If the screw threads do not purchase tightly, one may elect to utilize crossed K-wires as an alternative.

Once fixation is achieved, intra-operative X-rays will provide a permanent record of the apposition of the osteotomy site and the degree of bony correction (**10.35**). It is recommended, however, that the surgeon ensures that the osteotomy accomplishes the pre-operative goal before fixation is attempted. It is difficult to undo a fixated osteotomy for adjustments if the X-ray indicates the position is unsatisfactory. An alternative would be to X-ray the patient before fixation devices are placed. However, temporary fixation must be utilized that does not interfere with the intrinsic tensions of the soft tissues. Too often the bone clamp utilized for apposition of the osteotomy will pull or place tension on the long extensor tendon and spuriously influence the degree of correction through the retrograde action of the hallux on the metatarsal. If this approach is chosen, it is better to fixate the osteotomy with a K-wire that does not impinge on significant soft tissue structures.

Closure can begin when there is satisfactory reduction in the deformity. Because the periosteum is not stripped, there is no need to search for a potentially

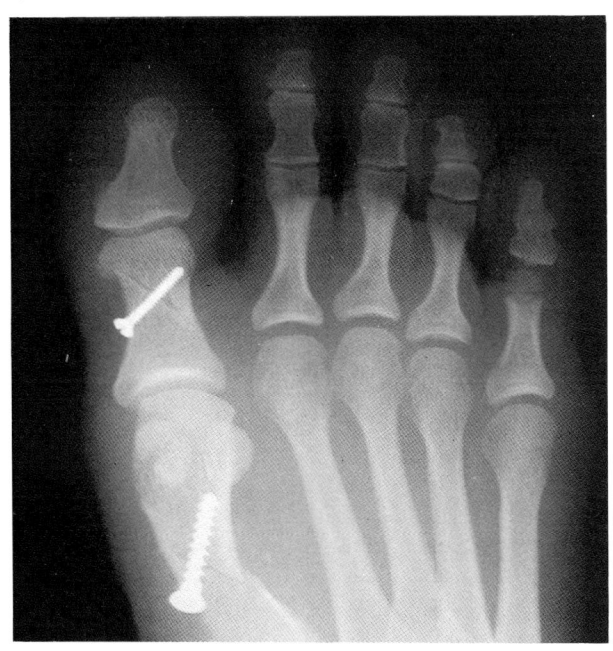

10.35 Intra-operative X-rays of a closing wedge osteotomy that was placed far too distal. In this case, the surgeon chose to fashion the osteotomy with a distal medial apex. Note the apparent over-correction and the intramedullary placement of the screw. The intra-operative discoveries must be addressed.

shredded structure. The extensor hallucis longus sheath can be anchored back into place if desired, although in practice it usually assumes its previous position over the metatarsal. The subcutaneous tissue layer can be re-approximated as well as the skin with the sutures of choice.

Post-operative management consists of non-weight-bearing for a period of 6 weeks or longer. We obtain X-rays at the 10–14 day period, when sutures are removed, and then again at 6 weeks. If adequate bony union has occurred at this time, the patient is allowed to bear weight in a protected fashion. This means a short leg walking cast or a wooden-soled shoe is used for an additional 2 weeks. Only when the surgeon is extremely confident in the stability of the construct can unprotected weight-bearing be allowed at the 6-week time interval.

The conditions during the non-weight-bearing period can vary according to the confidence of the surgeon and the compliance of the patient. If there are ideal conditions of compliance and a stable osteotomy, the patient can be given a removable splint or bivalved cast. Range of motion exercises for the first metatarsophalangeal joint can then be done two or three times a day. If, however, the patient is non-compliant or the rigidity of fixation is suspect, then a short leg cast is in order. This is not to imply that the cast will provide stability with occasional lapses in the non-weight-bearing situation. It only serves as a reminder to the patient and dampens slight amounts of pressure from resting the foot on the ground or in the event of a fall. Repeated loading of the first metatarsal will cause failure of the fixation and post-operative migration. Schuberth et al.[21] demonstrated that 93% of closing wedge osteotomies will show elevation on the sagittal plane if the patient is allowed to bear weight, regardless of the type of fixation and the external immobilization. If there is any delay in bony union, then an additional non-weight-bearing period is indicated.

Opening wedge osteotomy

The opening wedge procedure involves the insertion of a bone graft in the proximal aspect of the metatarsal to close down an abnormally high intermetatarsal angle. The indications are almost identical to those for the closing wedge osteotomy with some exceptions. It should be confined to those patients with a short first metatarsal needing large amounts of correction of the IM angle. It may also be utilized when the risk of shortening may exacerbate a hyperkeratotic lesion under the second metatarsal. Often, however, the lesion may be due to the splay of the first metatarsal and, therefore, the pattern can not be the single aetiological factor. Nevertheless, any patient who has a structural shortening of the first metatarsal and requires IM angle reduction should be considered for this procedure. The pre-operative metatarsal protrusion distance often indicates first metatarsal deficits of 2 mm or more (**10.36**).

Because bone must be inserted into the base on the medial side to reduce the metatarsal angle, the obvious question of where does the bone come from arises. Some authors favour the insertion of the medial eminence from the first metatarsal head into the osteotomy site. I have never found this to be suitable because it is usually not enough bone and cannot be shaped for precise fit and optimal bony apposition. Allograft bone is another choice. It is readily obtainable and can be shaped precisely for good bony apposition. Cortical cancellous samples are ideal for this procedure and are widely available commercially. The biggest disadvantage is the longer incorporation time over that of autogenous bone. The risk of rejection is also real and care should be taken to utilize allograft that is not irradiated as its sole means of sterilization and decreasing antigenicity.

There are several sources of autogenous bone for this procedure. Because a relatively small amount of bone is needed, the distal tibia is an ideal location for graft harvesting. Here a small cortico-cancellous graft can be taken with little risk to the patient. The best place in the tibia is in the distal metaphysis just above

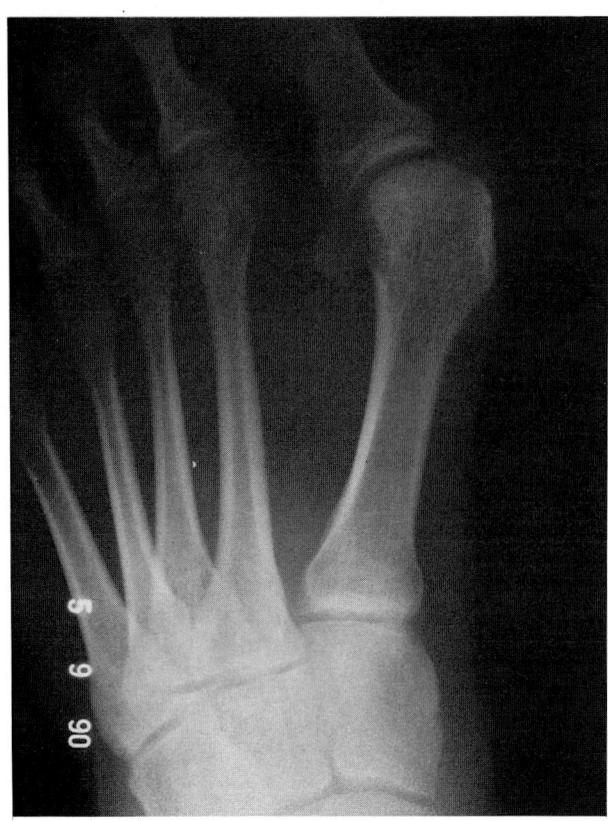

10.36 Pre-operative AP radiograph of a patient with short first metatarsal and large intermetatarsal angle. The metatarsal protrusion distance measures −4 mm. Any osteotomy designed to reduce the IM angle would accentuate the short first ray.

the medial malleolus. Other options include the proximal tibia and the iliac crest.

The approach to the base of the first metatarsal base is the same as for the closing base wedge osteotomy. The periosteum is left intact and a single transverse cut is made in the bone from medial to lateral at a point approximately 1–1.5 cm from the first metatarsal cuneiform joint. The osteotomy stops before it penetrates the lateral cortex. An osteotome is then inserted into the osteotomy site and is used to pry the osteotomy open. The lateral cortex may fracture, but does not always separate into two fragments due to maintenance of the periosteum on this side. The previously harvested graft is then inserted into the site with the apex directed medially.

Fixation of the opening wedge osteotomy is mandatory. Crossed K-wires or Steinmann pins, staples, or even small plates are easily applied. Stability of the construction is dependent on the fixation, due to the tenuous nature of the lateral cortex. This is especially true with iatrogenic violation of the lateral side. In highly unstable cases, external fixation can be used.[60]

If temporary fixation is used, it should be left in place for a long period of time, owing to the use of the bone graft. As the graft incorporates, it may actually demineralize and weaken as osteogenic activity and creeping substitution ensues. Prolonged periods of non-weight-bearing may be necessary. A minimum of 8 weeks is required in almost all cases. Complications include non-union, loss of correction or position, and jamming of the first metatarsophalangeal joint. Elevation of the first ray is not as prevalent as in the closing wedge osteotomy because there is less technical difficulty to the osteotomy.

Crescentic osteotomy

Crescentic osteotomy is designed to overcome the limitations of closing wedge osteotomy with regard to shortening. It is a proximally based osteotomy and is crescentic in nature. By design, the osteotomy is a through-and-through osteotomy that allows for rotation of the distal fragment around the axis fashioned by the osteotomy (**10.37**).

The advantage of this procedure is that it does not significantly shorten the first metatarsal, because there is essentially no bone removed from the metatarsal except that removed by the excursion of the kerf of the saw blade.[22] Large amounts of correction can be obtained by simply rotating the distal portion laterally.[55]

The disadvantages of the procedure are few, but significant. First of all, it is an inherently unstable osteotomy, because there is no intact cortical hinge or periosteal tissue that prevents displacement. Secondly, as more correction is needed, it is obtained at the expense of bone-to-bone contact.[55] Thirdly, this osteotomy is not readily amenable to rigid internal fixation techniques, which may preclude early range of motion exercises.

The approach to the metatarsal can be the same as for the opening or closing wedge osteotomies, or it can be reduced to a separate smaller proximal incision. This is because the osteotomy does not require widespread exposure for technical execution. If this approach is chosen, a single incision over the proximal metatarsal base is made. Again, the deep fascia is incised, as in the closing wedge osteotomy, to the level of the periosteum. Hohmann retractors are placed on either side of the metatarsal to protect the soft tissues. The crescentic-shaped saw blade is placed in an oscillating handpiece and used to cut the bone. The concavity can be positioned either distally or proximally. I feel it is better to place the concave portion distally, because the excursion of the bone is often impeded by the second metatarsal base when the opposite is chosen. The saw should be positioned so that the tangent to the blade is perpendicular to the floor and not to the long axis of the metatarsal. Iatrogenic first metatarsal elevation will be avoided with positioning of the axis of rotation on the pure frontal plane. The osteotomy is made entirely through the bone at a level of about 1 cm distal to the metatarsal cuneiform articulation. Once the metatarsal has been divided into two portions, the distal is rotated in a lateral direction until the desired amount of correction is obtained. Care should be taken to ensure that there is at least 50% apposition of the fragments: optimally, there should be more than that to allow for stable union. One must also ensure that there is not any elevation or plantar displacement of the distal fragment unless pre-operative assessment dictates its necessity. When the desired position is attained, the fixation devices are placed. The simplest method is to use crossed K-wires or small calibre Steinmann pins anchored well into the tarsus. Care should be taken that the pins do not intersect at the osteotomy site, but on one side or the other. This prevents distraction of the site during the resorptive phase of bone healing. Other types of fixation devices are possible, but require some manipulation of the architecture of the osteotomy site for application.

As with most reconstructive procedures, intraoperative X-rays should be taken to ensure satisfactory correction and placement of the hardware. Post-operative care is similar to any of the proximal osteotomies, with absolute non-weight-bearing for a minimum of 6 weeks.

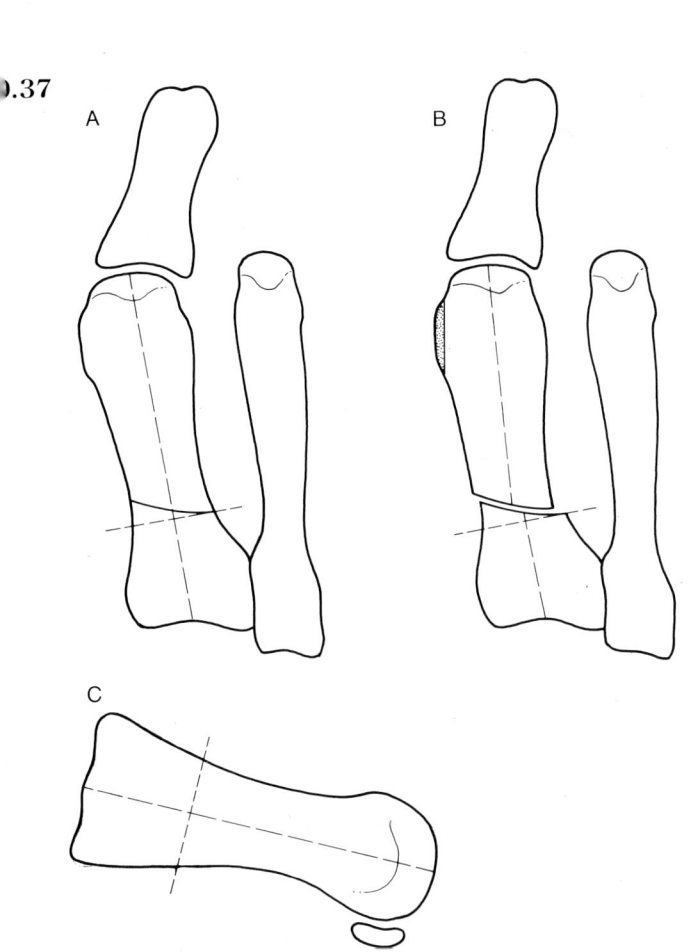

10.37 First metatarsal crescentic osteotomy. The osteotomy is angled so that there is a medial ledge that minimizes the tendency of the fragments to displace.

Fusion procedures

Arthrodesing procedures of the proximal first metatarsal cuneiform joints are valuable in the patient who presents with a hypermobile first ray. The hypermobility may be in the dorsomedial direction or the medial direction. If it is observed in the sagittal plane, in all likelihood, the present symptoms will be a dorsal bunion or hallux limitus rather than the classic hallux abductovalgus deformity. These procedures serve to surgically stabilize the first ray and eliminate the hypermobility that contributes to the splay of the first metatarsal and the overall deformity. These types of procedures are infrequently used but when indicated they allow for post-operative stability of the medial column and provide an excellent long-term result. The use of first metatarsal cuneiform fusions in the juvenile or adolescent bunion patient is increasing. These patients have a high degree of ligamentous laxity and hypermobility.

The aetiology of the hypermobility has been debated for some time in the literature. Whether it is due to the arrangement of the proximal articulation or not leads the controversy.[5,61-63] Certainly, a high percentage of patients that present with hallux abductovalgus and medial metatarsal splay can have some obliquity of the distal first cuneiform facet.[64] However, this medial deviation may actually be more dependent on radiographic positioning than on actual anatomical status. In addition, medial obliquity of the facet does not always correlate with hypermobility, which seems to be more related to ligamentous stability than anything else.[19] The ligamentous complex at the first metatarsal cuneiform articulation may have some inherent weaknesses when compared with the remainder of the tarso–metatarsal junction. This may also contribute to the medial displacement of the metatarsal. Although the exact aetiology is not essential for the selection of the appropriate technique, the surgeon should be aware of both the clinical and radiographic parameters when planning surgical intervention.[65]

The pre-operative clinical examination should note whether the metatarsal splay is reducible or not. If it is not, then the degree of hypermobility, may be difficult to assess. One should look for other signs of hypermobility, such as fifth metacarpal hyperextension, the ability to oppose the thumb to the forearm, and knee hyperextension. If any of these parameters appear exaggerated, then the patient may indeed have hypermobility without obvious pedal signs.

The surgical approach can include a proximal extension of the distal incision, or a separate exposure can be made over the proximal aspect of the metatarsal base. The extensor tendon is again reflected to the lateral side within its sheath and the joint is exposed by a mid-line longitudinal incision directly over the bony structures. The capsule and the periosteum are reflected to give full exposure to the joint without detaching the tibialis anterior insertion. Hohmann retractors are placed on either side of the first metatarsal base in order to protect the deep plantar artery. Dissection should be as extensive as possible to maximize the amount of exposure of the joint. This will facilitate accurate resection of the surfaces as well as removal of the joint surfaces. The first resection should occur on the cuneiform and be relatively perpendicular to the long axis of the bone. This will remove an oblique facet joint, if present, and usually provide adequate correction. The saw blade may need to be changed to a longer one because of the depth of the cuneiform. The saw should be advanced plantarly with caution so as not to sever the flexor hallucis longus tendon or neurovascular structures. Next, the articular surface of the metatarsal base should be removed. The remainder of the correction is obtained with this cut. The degree of resection is limited by the insertion of the peroneus longus tendon on the plantar lateral aspect of the metatarsal. Therefore, if large amounts of abduction are required, it is best to obtain from the cuneiform side of the joint.

Once the cuts are made, the entire joint surfaces are resected together. Two small, flat osteotomes are inserted into each osteotomy site and used as a pry bar to lever the articular surfaces out of the cavity. Once the bone pieces are elevated, they are grasped with a forceps and the remaining plantar soft tissue attachments are severed. The two opposing surfaces are now approximated and the amount of correction is assessed. Refinements can be made if either visual or radiographic inspections are unsatisfactory. Rotational alignment should be checked and, once assured, the fixation is placed.

The technique of fixation is left largely to the surgeon's choice: however, compressive techniques are preferred. The advent of small cannulated screws has simplified the placement of hardware in this area. In the past, the placement of cancellous screws that remain totally within the confines of the first cuneiform was difficult and usually required several intra-operative X-rays.[66] With the cannulated system, the surgeon can introduce the guide pins under fluoroscopic or radiographic control and be assured that the final screw placement will be exactly where the guide pin was placed (**10.38**). Traditional cancellous screws, plates, or even K-wires are also acceptable.

Post-operative care involves a period of non-weight-bearing for no less than 6 weeks. Occasionally, a longer period is required for fusion. After adequate radiographic union, a 2-week stint of a short leg walking cast may be in order.

The disadvantages of this procedure are again related to shortening of the metatarsal. Metatarsalgia is infrequently observed even with significant shortening, due to the stabilizing effect of the fusion on the first ray. The prolonged post-operative immobilization time is also a relative disadvantage. Non-union is rare and can usually be attributed to technique.

If shortening is of significant concern then the same procedure can be carried out, with a bone graft on the medial side, using the same basic principles as the opening wedge osteotomy. Fixation may need to be bolstered on the medial side with a plate, because the graft may not be adequately secured with screws. The tendency is for medial extrusion secondary to the extra tension and the wedge-shaped graft. Placement of a small plate will limit the tendency for extrusion and stabilize the fusion procedure.

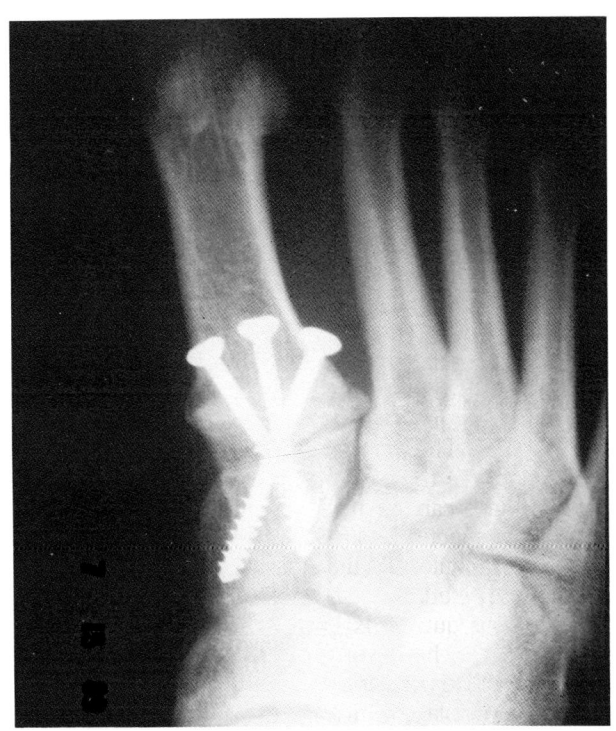

10.38 Post-operative radiograph of the first metatarsal cuneiform fusion. There are three 4.0 mm cannulated screws totally within the confines of the cuneiform and an opening wedge bone graft inserted at the fusion site.

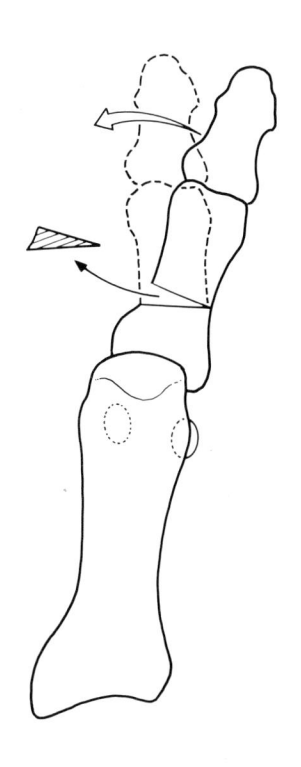

10.39 The Akin osteotomy. The cut should be placed in the metaphysis to enhance healing and maximal correction.

Phalangeal procedures

Even though the proximal osseous segments may be adequately reconstructed, there will be certain patients where there is some deformity at the phalangeal level. The metatarsal may rest in a normal position, but there may be significant abductus of the proximal phalanx. The degree and level of deformity cover a wide range: an abnormal distal articular set angle, a long phalangeal segment, or a deviation of the distal articular surface of the proximal phalanx. These procedures are rarely performed alone: they are most often used to refine the surgical result, either from a cosmetic or functional standpoint.

Akin osteotomy

The basic procedure, developed by O.F. Akin in 1925,[67] is essentially a medial closing wedge osteotomy performed in the proximal metaphysis of the proximal phalanx (**10.39**). Its indication is an abnormal distal articular set angle in the context of a significantly deviated hallux. In general, it should not be performed in the presence of significant degenerative joint disease of the first metatarsophalangeal joint.[68]

Exposure to the proximal phalanx is usually achieved with the standard approach to the first metatarsophalangeal joint. It may be necessary to extend the incision distally for any modifications of the basic technique. It is no less important to also elevate the subcutaneous layer with the skin in this area, which will provide excellent exposure to the bone and tendinous structures as well as protect the neurovascular structures.

The osteotomy is performed by making a transverse cut from the medial side of the bone to the lateral without disrupting the lateral cortex. It is made 7–10 mm distal to the joint and parallel to the proximal articular cartilage. Again, care is taken not to disrupt the long flexor tendon: it should not be pinned inadvertently against the plantar aspect of the phalanx with the retractors but rather left undisturbed. The second cut is made proximal to the first in a direction perpendicular to the longitudinal axis of the phalanx. The wedge is removed and the osteotomy is feathered and closed.

Fixation can be K-wires, monofilament wire,[69,70] or staples (**10.40, 10.41**).[71,72] If monofilament wire is chosen, it should be fashioned so it engages four cortices, especially on the plantar aspect. This will prevent plantar gaping when the forces of weight-bearing are applied. If the lateral cortex fails during perform-

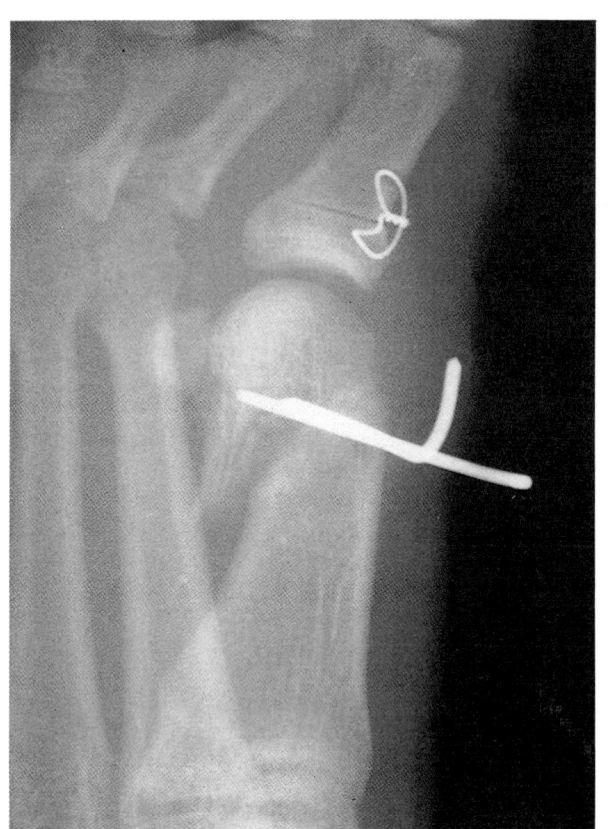

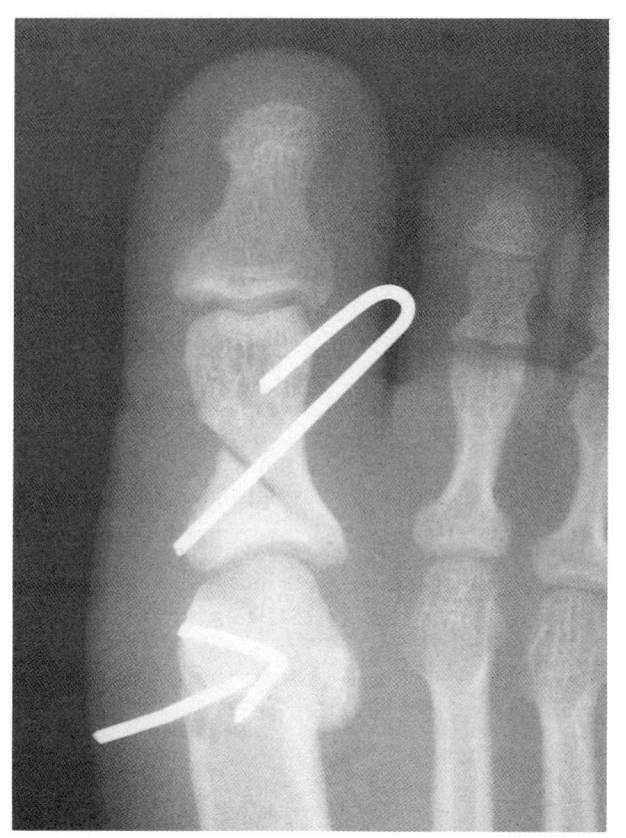

10.40 Radiograph showing Akin osteotomy fixated with 28 gauge monofilament wire.

10.41 Radiograph of Akin osteotomy fixated with single K-wire. This osteotomy was designed for screw fixation but was abandoned due to poor purchase of the screw.

10.42 X-ray of Akin osteotomy fixated with 2.7 mm cortical screw. Note that the apex of the osteotomy is proximal lateral, which maximizes correction.

ance of the procedure, then crossed K-wires should be used.

Modifications of the direction and orientation of the osteotomy can be utilized to facilitate the use of screw fixation.[73,74] It requires more exposure and relies more on cortical rather than cancellous bone healing (**10.42**). Without intra-operative or post-operative fracture, this point is superfluous. However, if there is hinge failure, then the more oblique osteotomy is less likely to heal due to its tendency to displace. Here two screws are indicated.

Valgus de-rotation can often be corrected with some modification of the procedure.[75,76] The procedure involves a manual de-rotation of the hallux prior to the second or distal cut. More extensive feathering may be required to close the osteotomy. This probably necessitates an actual disruption of the lateral cortex since an asymmetric wedge of bone is being fashioned for removal. Purposeful disruption of the cortex may even be in order to facilitate de-rotation. Nevertheless, K-wire fixation is usually required due to the essentially complete osteotomy.

Cylindrical Akin

This procedure was originally designed for the patient with a long proximal phalanx and an increased distal articular set angle: it served to shorten the phalanx while correcting the DASA. This reduces the length of the lever arm of the proximal phalanx, which helps to resist shoe pressure and pronatory forces. With recurrent abduction of the great toe, a recurrence of the deformity could occur. Shortening of a long phalanx also makes shoe-fitting easier.[77]

The procedure can be performed by fashioning the traditional osteotomy as described above. Then the lateral cortex is cut and a cylindrical portion of bone corresponding to the desired amount of shortening is removed. The distal aspect of the phalanx is then fixated to the proximal aspect. Here there is loss of cancellous bone and the shaft of the phalanx may be impacted into the cancellous base of the phalanx. This situation is not only unstable and difficult to fixate, but will require an inordinate amount of time to heal. Therefore, I prefer to use the oblique osteotomy fixated with screws for this modification. The traditional oblique osteotomy is performed with appropriate wedging. The proximal medial cortex is then cut and the phalanx is shortened by sliding the two bone fragments past one another. Small cortical screws or K-wires are used to fixate the osteotomy (**10.43**). Complications again include non-union and plantar gaping, but once more can be attributed to technique in most cases.

Distal Akin

When the patient presents with a structural deformity of the distal articulation of the proximal phalanx, the great toe may impinge on the second toe. Often, this will be associated with a medial pinch callous. The procedure of choice for correction of the transverse plane deviations is the distal Akin, the basics of which parallel the traditional Akin procedure. The closing wedge osteotomy is made in the distal metaphysis of the proximal phalanx. Exposure requires careful protection of the long extensor tendon. The choices for fixation of the osteotomy are the same as for the parent procedure. Similarly, modifications in design can be made to allow for screw fixation, but the hinge must be made distal lateral so as to rotate the distal articular surface into the correct position.

The non-union rate is similarly infrequent, but dorsal displacement is slightly less prevalent due to a shorter lever arm being acted upon by the forces of weight-bearing.

The post-operative management for any of the Akin procedures and their modifications is usually predicated on the accompanying procedures. The Akin itself can withstand immediate weight-bearing in a wooden-soled shoe, provided fixation is adequate.

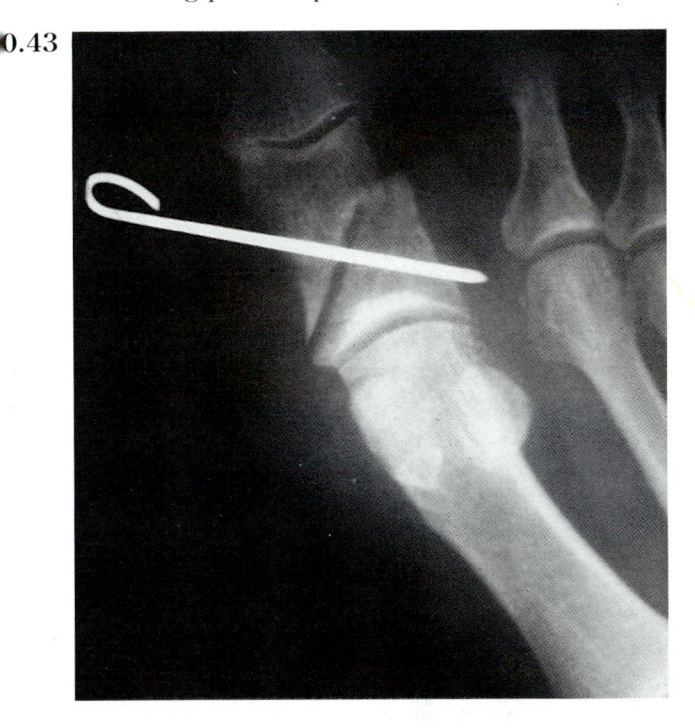

10.43 Radiograph of shortening-type Akin osteotomy. The lateral cortex was severed, allowing the two portions of bone to be transposed past one another. Although in this case only one K-wire provided stability, usually more than one point of fixation is required and is recommended.

Arthroplastic procedures

The problem of hallux abductovalgus is sometimes complicated by the presence of a severe degenerative joint disease of the first metatarsophalangeal joint that precludes the application of standard surgical approaches. The presenting complaint may actually be pain caused by the degenerative diathesis rather than the mechanical irritation of the bunion itself. Astute pre-operative clinical history and examination usually reveal the true source of pain. In conjunction with radiographic examination, this allows the surgeon to perform the appropriate surgical procedure. Joint destructive procedures are indicated when the problem of degenerative arthritis cannot be solved by any other conservative or surgical methods.

Keller procedure

Before the advent of silastic implants, the Keller procedure was the benchmark operation for patients with hallux abductovalgus deformity and significant degenerative disease. The Keller procedure involves the resection of the medial eminence and the proximal aspect of the proximal phalanx, along with some sort of soft tissue interposition. The theory behind the procedure, as it is applied today, is to eliminate the articulation and thereby relieve the symptoms attributed to the arthritic process. When the procedure was conceived, it was designed to provide soft tissue laxity and allow for positioning of the hallux at the end of the metatarsal.[78,79] For a while it was a very popular procedure, because it was easy to do and provided excellent reduction of the deformity.[80] However, it was fraught with long-term complications, especially when applied to the younger patient. The complications were mainly due to the loss of function of the first metatarsophalangeal joint and the lack of toe purchase. Symptoms of lesser metatarsal overload usually were part of the post-operative result. Nevertheless, in an elderly, sedentary patient with severe deviation of the great toe, this procedure still has a place in the foot surgeon's armamentarium.

Another indication is a severe deformity in which an osteotomy of the first metatarsal is contraindicated. Because there is no preservation of the joint, large resections of the medial aspect of the first metatarsal head are well tolerated. It is even acceptable to 'spike the head' in these patients, to reduce the medial prominence and provide even more narrowing of the foot.

Traditionally, the success of this operation was predicated on the surgeon's ability to balance the soft tissue on either side of the first metatarsophalangeal joint. With the increasing trend toward osseous reconstruction and silastic toe prostheses, this art has been largely lost.

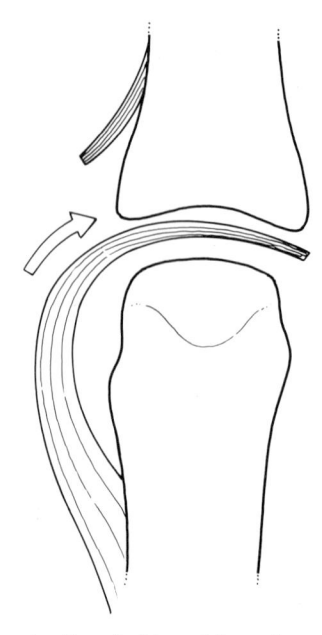

10.44 Capsular flaps fashioned from the medial capsule of the first metatarsophalangeal joint. The capsule can usually be thinned longitudinally and the lateral portion is rotated into the joint.

The Keller procedure involves the standard approach to the joint. A dorsolinear capsulotomy is then made and the entire soft tissue sleeve about the base of the proximal phalanx is sharply detached. Caution should be observed when approaching the plantar aspect of the phalanx because of the close proximity of the flexor hallucis longus tendon. The attachment of the flexor hallucis brevis may be difficult to detach until the bone cut is made. However, it makes for an easier resection of the base of the phalanx if as much soft tissue as possible is deflected off the underlying bone.

When this is completed, the base of the proximal phalanx is osteotomized at the distal aspect of the metaphyseal flare; once again, the long flexor tendon should be unharmed. Attaching a Backhaus towelclamp in the transverse dimension of the phalanx facilitates the side-to-side rotation needed for detachment of all of the soft tissues.[77] The base should now be easily removed from the wound while preserving the soft tissue envelope.

The soft tissue plication necessary for the stabilization of the phalanx on the metatarsal head is the next operation. The technique for this is highly variable and can be as simple as an hourglass-type capsular closure or as elaborate as the fashioning of medial capsular flaps for refined soft tissue balancing (**10.44**).[81,82] If transverse plane correction is required, it will usually lend itself well to a T-capsulotomy by removing a small portion of capsule from the medial side. Re-approximation of the capsular edges will pull the hallux in the medial direction. It may be necessary to reattach the capsule back to the metatarsal neck if it becomes detached or attenuated during exposure. Drill holes into the neck provide an excellent means to anchor the capsule to the bone.[83]

The hourglass manoeuvre is designed to interpose some soft tissue into the dead space and provide a cushion or articular substance for the base of the now resected proximal phalanx.[80] This will minimize shortening of the toe, which may be unacceptable to the patient.

Nonabsorbable sutures are placed into the capsule on the plantar aspect and tied from the plantar side to the dorsal side. The amount of tension placed on the sutures varies according to the amount of tissue interposition desired. It is usually adequate to position the phalanx a distance of 1–1.5 cm from the distal aspect of the metatarsal head. An alternative technique is to place a nonabsorbable stitch around the inside circumference of the capsule and pull the 'purse string' to the desired tautness. Occasionally, K-wire fixation may be necessary to enhance stabilization and promote soft tissue fibrosis. The wire should remain in place for at least 4 weeks, or any long-term stabilizing effect of the K-wire will be lost.

Post-operative care generally allows for early weight-bearing in a wooden shoe. Early motion should not be encouraged because the stability of the final repair is in part dependent on post-operative scarring. Only in those patients where the capsular repair is absolutely stable should the joint be moved early.

Implant arthroplasty

With the advent of silastic implants, the true Keller procedure is seldom used today for correction of hallux abductovalgus. Although there is a long history of the use of various implants, the long-term success rate has been dismal. Once investigators realized that the first metatarsophalangeal joint cannot maintain a luted or constrained prosthesis, results became more favourable. Similarly, the abandonment of rigid materials has added to the success of implants.

The introduction of an implant into the void created by joint resection provides several advantages. The first is the prevention of toe shortening. Although this may seem like a cosmetic advantage, it provides a more functional length for the intrinsic and extrinsic muscles to act upon the hallux. It may also lend stability by the reestablishment of length. This is particularly true in the case of the double-stem implant and when the plantar intrinsics are either preserved or reattached.[84]

The indications for implant arthroplasty parallel those of the Keller operation in the bunion patient.[85]

However, the surgeon must keep in mind that implants should be used conservatively. It should be viewed as a procedure that has no other viable long-term options. Certainly, the heyday of implantation is over with regard to weak indications and injudicious insertion into every patient with even the slightest arthrosis. As one accumulates a group of patients who require implant removal or revision, it becomes evident that they actually fare quite well when the implant is removed. Most patients function no worse than they did prior to implant removal. It is absolutely unreasonable to expect or to lead a patient to believe that the joint will function like a normal one. It is even unreasonable to expect that there will be more mobility at the metatarsophalangeal joint in some cases. Only in the patient with severe restriction of motion pre-operatively can this parameter be expected to improve.

On the other hand, the implant, well inserted into a patient with the proper indications, may provide that patient years of a pain-free and functional joint.[86,87] Certainly as one develops experience with the technique and learns from the honest reporting of others, the results of joint implantation will probably improve. Specifically, the indications for joint implantation are not absolute: they must be tempered with the patient's age, functional limitations and expectations, and the quality of the bone stock. As a rule, implants should not be used on younger patients; it is unrealistic to expect current implants to last 15 or more years. Although it serves no purpose to impose rigid arbitrary limits which preclude implantation, 55 years of age appears to be a reasonable guideline. Other options should be exhausted prior to artificial substitution. Nevertheless, some patients well below this age may be suitable candidates if there are no other reasonable options.

Some degree of degenerative change is required for consideration for implant use. Long-standing hallux valgus, rheumatoid arthritis with hallux valgus, gouty arthritis, or joints with limited and painful ranges of motion are among the possible candidates for implantation.[87,88]

Other considerations include the overall alignment of the osseous segments. If additional procedures are needed, will an implant be compatible? Those patients with a large intermetatarsal angle may not be able to tolerate an implant if the metatarsal is not realigned. Adequate bone stock is a consideration, but weak bone stock does not always preclude implant insertion. If some maintenance of position is expected by the implant, then good bone stock is of more import. If, however, there is no reliance on the implant for positional maintenance and it merely acts as a spacer, then lesser bone stock may still allow for implantation.

Patients with instability or imbalance of the first metatarsophalangeal joint may also be candidates for implantation. Hallux varus is one deformity which may have no other options, especially if the deformity has been long-standing. Patients with recurring bunions or hallux abductus following surgery may also require implantation due to disruption of normal soft tissue arrangements.

Total implant

In the vast majority of cases that are candidates for implantation, the double-stemmed implant is the procedure of choice. Degenerative erosions of cartilage will be seen on both components of the joint in most cases. The double-stemmed implant, if properly placed, has few points of actual contact with the bony structures and therefore the chance of degradation is lessened. In fact, a large percentage of the actual bending and resultant digital motion comes at the expense of the stem–hinge interface and not at the hinge itself. Both the distal and proximal stems are known to piston in and out of the respective medullary canals. Titanium grommets are now available to further reduce the interaction of the hinge–bone interface and thereby prolong the wear.

If peri-operative conditions indicate the use of an implant, then the basic Keller procedure is performed as described above. If one is utilizing the intrinsic muscle preserving total implant by Lawrence, then the angle of resection of the phalangeal side is modified to the demands of the implant.[89,90] The medullary canal of the proximal phalanx is then prepared for acceptance of the stem of the implant. There are several ways to accomplish this, but the overall goal is to be kept in mind. The primary objective is to fashion a square-shaped receptacle so the stem of the implant fits into the medullary canal with rotational stability (**10.45**). This necessitates the milling of the medullary canal and the base of the phalanx. In actuality, only the cross-section of the proximal aspect of the phalanx matters; that is, if the entrance site is square, the implant stem can be accommodated and the shape of the remainder of the medullary canal is inconsequential. The most dense cancellous bone will be at the proximal aspect of the bone and provides the best material for fashioning an appropriate canal. The cortex of the phalanx is often thin and is generally not amenable to customizing. The preferred way of preparing the canal is to begin with a side-cutting power burr and score the confines of the proposed canal. It is easy to lose perspective with regard to rotation of the phalanx, especially in those patients with axial valgus rotation. The loss of orientation is compounded when the base of the phalanx has been resected; therefore, it is best to mill the plantar boundary of the square hole parallel to the plantar aspect of the phalanx. If this is performed accurately, then the rest of the opening will be correctly oriented. Once the boundaries have been transcribed, the canal can be deepened. Either a hand-held broach or a power rasp is best suited for this task.[91] It will provide square corners and smooth the internal aspect of the canal. When using any power instruments, care must be taken not to perforate the plantar cortex of the phalanx as this will allow for migration of the implant long before it can be stabilized by soft tissue ingrowth. Although this milling procedure seems like it is easily accomplished, the plantar aspect of the phalanx takes a precipitous curve dorsally as it courses distally. The canal should not be deepened with the broach or power rasp, only widened. If the canal needs to be deepened, then the side-cutting burr should be used. The depth of the canal is governed primarily by the size of the residual phalanx. It should be deepened as far as the bony confines will allow, without perforating the interphalangeal joint. It should be remembered that some of the distal stem of the implant can be cut off if the canal is not long enough.

If there is weak bone stock, the entire medullary canal can be scooped out with a simple swipe of a freer elevator. Refinement of the canal is difficult and one must be ready to accept a less than perfectly square hole to secure the implant.

The distal aspect of the metatarsal head must be freed of all soft tissue attachments by extending the dissection proximally. The concept of a soft tissue 'envelope' is vital to the success of the procedure. The metatarsal medullary canal is also prepared with the amount of rotation in mind. The plantar sesamoid groove may not be a reliable indicator of the bottom of the metatarsal if there has been some deviation in the course of the development of the deformity. Therefore, careful inspection is required to properly orientate the square canal. It is acceptable to drill the canal. However, it is recommended to resect the cap of cartilage from the metatarsal head. The plane of resection is from dorsal proximal to plantar distal. This will

10.45 Intra-operative photograph of the phalangeal base. Note that the medullary canal has been milled into a square-shaped opening for the distal stem of the implant.

preserve the weight-bearing function of the plantar aspect of the metatarsal head and still alleviate some of the soft tissue tension from the insertion of the implant. The side-cutting burr is used to begin the canal and squared and finished with the hand broach or power rasp. The canal should be fashioned towards the dorsal aspect of the metatarsal head rather than the plantar so there is little chance of bony impingement with dorsiflexion. Additional refinements of the distal aspect of the head may be necessary if one is attempting to insert an implant without reduction of the IM angle; in such a case, the plane of resection should be angled from distal medial to proximal lateral in addition to the dorsoplantar angulation described above.

Once the medullary canal is prepared, the implant is ready for sizing. The sizers are used to determine the appropriate size. Guidelines in this decision are first to utilize an implant that is large enough to overlap the edge of the proximal phalangeal stump: this will inhibit bony hypertrophy and engulfment of the implant. Secondly, an implant should be inserted loosely, both with regard to the longitudinal tension on the entire ray and within the canal itself: the implant should not be so loose that it can rotate within the square canal. Longitudinal tension may be removed by resecting more bone off the phalangeal base. If the implant seats flush against the phalangeal base, the length of the canal is probably too short; this can be remedied by either elongating the canal or trimming off the tip of the implant when it is inserted. It should be remembered that implant sizers are slightly smaller than their silastic counterparts as a result of shrinkage caused by repeated autoclaving.

Once the appropriate size is selected, the real implant is opened aseptically into saline, with or without antibiotic. If any trimming of the stem is required, it can and should be done while the implant is submerged in the saline. Atraumatic forceps can be used to grasp the implant and then 2–4 mm of the stem can be trimmed with a new No. 15 blade. The underwater nature of the manoeuvre prevents contact with surfaces that may impart a static charge to the implant and also prevents the implant from squirting across the operative field if it slips from the surgeon's control. The wound is thoroughly irrigated and the implant is then transferred to the patient's foot and inserted using the no touch technique. It is also preferable to avoid any contact with the skin during insertion to reduce the possibility of infection by *Staphylococcus epidermidis*, which is becoming a common pathogen in cases with implants. Iodine-impregnated adhesive drapes are recommended for implantation as they effectively shield the entire surgical field from contact with the skin. The implant is inserted into the canal with the metatarsal side being seated first. Closure begins immediately. Stay sutures, through drill holes in the phalanx, which are anchored into the medial capsule, may be necessary to prevent migration or drift of the distal segment on the metatarsal head. To give maximal digital purchase, the short flexor can be sutured back to the phalangeal base if there is enough laxity of the soft tissue.[92] Even the long flexor can be tenodesed to the stump at this level to enhance hallux purchase. Any of these modifications should be performed before the implant is inserted or it will need to be removed again. The capsule is closed followed by the subcutaneous layer. It is critical to completely encase the implant in a soft tissue layer to ensure proper encapsulation and prevent infection. Once this is done, the iodine drape can be removed and the skin closed.

Hemi-implant arthroplasty

The single-stem silastic implant is slowly disappearing from the scope of foot surgery, with investigators now recognizing the prevalence of silicone detritus and silicone synovitis secondary to wear of the implant.[90] This wear occurs by abrasion on even the slightest irregularity of the opposing articulating surface. It is highly unlikely to encounter a joint that has degenerative changes isolated solely to the distal aspect. An implant may be indicated if there is significant splay of the first metatarsal and a Keller bunionectomy is considered. However, it may defeat the purpose by eliminating the soft tissue laxity that may be the key to reduction of the deformity. At any rate, the surgeon must be skilled at balancing the soft tissue in order to get the implant to stay perched upon the metatarsal head. The technique for insertion is similar to the phalangeal base preparation of the total implant. Stay sutures should be carefully planned so that tension on either side of the implant is equalized.

Complications of implants generally are more extreme than those seen with the Keller procedure. The problems of rejection, implant failure, and silicone detritus are well covered in other sources.[93–95] Lesser metatarsalgia and lateral overload problems are also somewhat common due to loss of the intrinsic function of the first metatarsophalangeal joint.

Elevating osteotomies

Procedures that are designed to raise the first metatarsal head away from the supporting surface are commonly used to treat painful keratomas under the first metatarsal head. They may also be indicated in the cavovarus-type foot that has a plantar-flexed first ray as a contributor to the deformity. Because the procedure has a simple biomechanical premise of sagittal plane elevation, there are only a few variations of the basic technique. The overall result is a balance of the forefoot, with reduction of reciprocal hindfoot supination.

When evaluating the painful lesion under the first metatarsal head plantar, one must first decide whether it is caused by a functional or a structural imbalance. If it results from a functional imbalance, then a first metatarsal osteotomy is probably not indicated. For example, if a patient presents with a painful first metatarsal head callosity but also has extensor substitution and a hallux hammertoe, the plantar lesion may be due to a reciprocal plantar flexion of the metatarsal head at the first metatarsophalangeal joint. If the biomechanical aberration is short-lived, the plantar flexion of the metatarsal may be reducible. In this case, osseous elevation is not indicated and one must attack the deformity elsewhere. If, however, the deformity has been long-standing, the first metatarsal may be rigidly plantarflexed, necessitating a bony procedure in addition to others.

Secondly, one must also determine if the lesion is caused by hypertrophy of the sesamoids from any cause. If so, the surgeon should direct attention there. One must also rule out the existence of a taut plantar fascia or peroneus longus tendon which may be holding the metatarsal in a depressed position. When all of these other causes for a plantarly positioned first ray have been eliminated and the deformity is rigid, a dorsiflexory osteotomy is indicated.

Because we are dealing with an angular deformity, it must be corrected at the level of deformity. The metatarsal base is the correct location of the osteotomy because it gives one the best lever arm and axis of rotation to achieve correction.[55] Very little bone needs to be removed for marked positional swings in the first metatarsal head location. The osteotomy can be conventionally oriented with the resultant osteotomy perpendicular to the long axis of the bone, or it can be obliquely oriented to facilitate rigid screw fixation. If one chooses the former, it should be realized that screw fixation is not recommended, and other devices such as staples, K-wires, plates, or stainless steel wire must be employed.

The approach is modified to allow for the osteotomy to be made from the side of the bone. This is preferable because one does not have to bury the saw blade in the deep aspect of the metatarsal base in a blind fashion. A lazy S type of incision is made from the dorsoplantar aspect of the metatarsal base proceeding plantar medially. The incision crosses the medial dorsocutaneous nerve, then turns distal along the plantar medial aspect of the metatarsal to approximately the mid-shaft. Again, anatomical dissection is used to peel the subcutaneous layer off the deep fascia. The extensor tendon is mobilized within its sheath by making an incision through the deep fascia along the medial margin of the sheath. It is then reflected laterally and a Hohmann retractor is placed into the first intermetatarsal space. This protects the deep plantar artery. A second Hohmann retractor is placed in the plantar interval between the muscle layer and the metatarsal. The osteotomy is made with a sagittal or oscillating saw from the medial aspect of the bone using the lateral retractor as a stop. The wedge is fashioned and removed. The site is feathered and closed. The three orientations of the osteotomy are seen in **10.46**. The best fixation is achieved if the apex of the osteotomy is plantar proximal and the base dorsal distal. This allows for screw purchase in the dense cortical bone of the metatarsal shaft (**10.47**).

Post-operative care is 6 weeks of non-weight-bearing, followed by progressive amounts of protected and then unprotected weight-bearing as radiographs indicate.

Complications are infrequent as long as one institutes sound fixation. Non-unions are very rare. Nerve entrapment is not as prevalent as expected: in fact, it is extremely unusual.

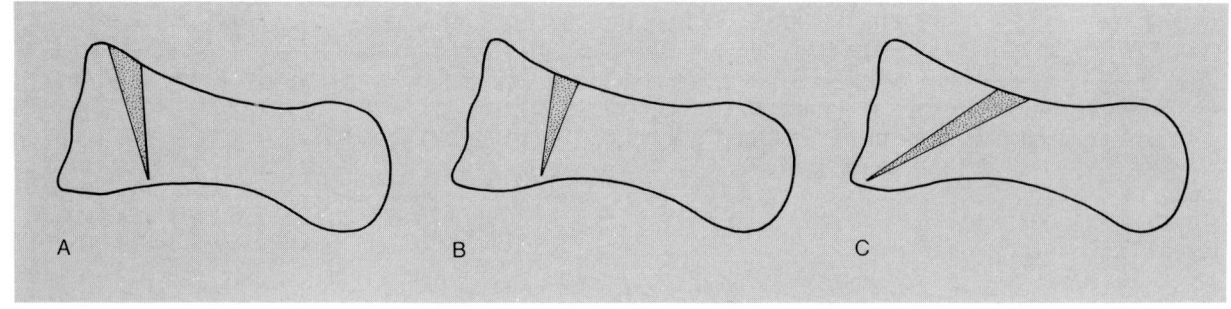

10.46

10.46 The three possible orientations of the dorsiflexory wedge osteotomy at the base of the first metatarsal. A, The apex is plantar distal. B, The apex is centrally located. C, The apex is plantar proximal.

First metatarsal cuneiform exostoses

Exostoses of the first metatarsal cuneiform joint are quite common. Patients usually present complaining of irritation from shoes; rarely are complaints indicative of arthritic change. Conservative treatment is only as useful as the patient's willingness to modify the shoes they wear. The aetiology is uncertain but it is believed to be biomechanically induced. Although there is no consistent pattern of presentation with regard to foot type, the forefoot valgus seems most prevalent. The diagnosis is made almost completely on clinical examination. The local hypertrophy of the metatarsal cuneiform may be quite obvious or may be so minimal that symptomatology seems overstated. Nevertheless, the palpation of firm bony material at the level of the joint gives one the diagnosis. The joint should be put through a range of motion to determine the presence of crepitus. If it is present, then fusion might be considered. One must also make sure the exostosis does not encompass more than one joint. If it does, localized resection is only prone to transfer the pressure laterally.[96] Additionally, symptoms of compression of the medial dorsal cutaneous nerve should not be confused with mechanical irritation of the bone.

Radiographs will seldom assist in the establishment of the diagnosis. The lateral projection may understate the degree of pathology. Even so, the absence of radiographic findings should not deter the surgeon in the patient with legitimate symptoms.

A dorsal approach is made to the joint, directly over the extensor tendon. The medial dorsal cutaneous nerve is consistently in the incision line and should not be pulled out of the subcutaneous tissue, but retracted within the layer. Skin and subcutaneous tissue are reflected as one layer and the tendon sheath is not mobilized separately. An incision directly to bone is made on the medial side of the tendon sheath and the capsular and ligamentous tissue is sharply elevated off the underlying joint. Wide exposure must be obtained. Bony resection is left to an osteotome or power saw. The cuneiform is resected first. A generous portion of bone is resected from proximal to distal. Then the metatarsal base is addressed. It is recommended that the metatarsal be loaded from the plantar in order to simulate weight-bearing. Then, the plane of resection can match the resected surface of the cuneiform, which prevents prominence of the metatarsal base with weight-bearing. A power rotating burr is used to round corners and actually create a dell behind each joint surface, so that the expected bony proliferation will not cause a failure. This is one of several exostectomies of the foot where the amount of bony resection must exceed that which seems adequate. Once accomplished, the deep fascial layer is re-approximated and the skin is closed.

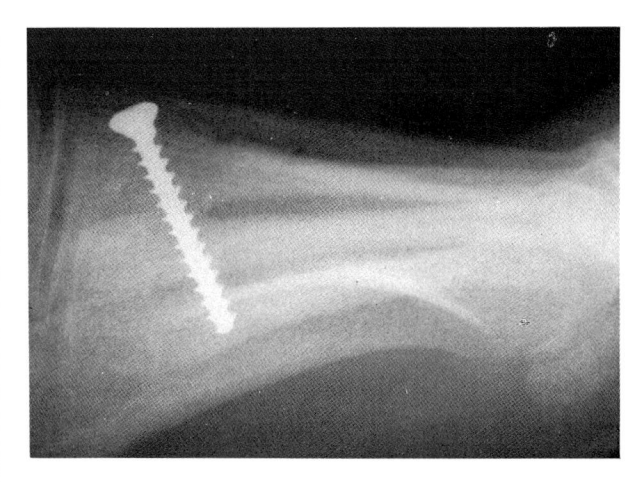

10.47 Radiograph of completed and fixated dorsiflexory osteotomy. The apex is plantar proximal, allowing for purchase of the screw in dense cortical bone.

If the joint appears arthritic, then the chance of failure of the procedure increases. The additional motion is likely to exacerbate an arthritic joint. However, it is surprising that this joint is very forgiving in terms of incongruities and the exostectomy may serve the patient well.

Post-operative care is variable. A short leg walking cast is preferred for comfort, but a wooden-soled shoe may be used instead. The immobilization should be kept in place for 2–4 weeks to allow for some stabilization of the ligamentous structures.

Complications include nerve damage or entrapment and regrowth of the exostosis.

Plantarflexory osteotomies

Procedures that plantarflex the first metatarsal are infrequently required. However, there are certain conditions where their application is absolutely mandatory to the successful surgical result. These conditions include the hypermobile first metatarsal and iatrogenic evaluation of the first metatarsal. Although these problems are distinctly different clinical entities, the approach to a dorsally positioned metatarsal has a fairly consistent solution. The hypermobile first metatarsal has a few more options than a structurally dorsiflexed first metatarsal but will be discussed in the same setting.

The patient who has undergone a prior procedure of the first metatarsal and has been left with a dorsally displaced metatarsal can present with a variety of symptom complexes. The complaints may be distant from the first metatarsal, such as a lesser metatarsalgia, stress fractures, or intractable plantar keratomas. The patient may also complain of first metatarsophalangeal joint pain and dysfunction secondary to jamming of the joint. Either of these two patterns are addressed via the correction of the bony first metatarsal deformity. The metatarsal must be plantarflexed in order to reestablish the normal distribution of weight and allow for normal function of the joint. The peroneus longus will also be able to function effectively if the metatarsal is repositioned.

To choose the most appropriate reconstructive procedure, the surgeon must evaluate not only the presenting complaint but also the radiographic appearance of the foot. If the metatarsal has been excessively shortened as well as elevated, then some consideration should be given to a bone graft in order to restore length. If there is hypermobility of the first ray, fusion procedures should be considered. Fusion of the first metatarsal cuneiform joint is covered later in this chapter in the section on hallux limitus. Three options are available to plantarflex the first metatarsal: closing plantarflexory osteotomy, mid-shaft sliding osteotomy, and opening wedge plantarflexory osteotomy, which is reserved for patients who require lengthening of the first ray. The sliding osteotomy is reserved for those patients where shortening may be detrimental but additional length is not necessary. The closing wedge is the standard procedure, but some shortening is expected. Shortening, however, is not nearly as morbid a condition as dorsal angulation as it relates to the metatarsal head mechanics. If the metatarsal is angulated its usual 20–21°, each millimetre of shortening raises the metatarsal head only 0.33 mm off the ground. This distance is calculated using standard trigonometric ratios.

The closing plantarflexory wedge is performed using the same approach as the dorsiflexory wedge, with the operation best performed from the side for the same reasons (see section on elevating osteotomies). Once the bone is exposed, the same options of osteotomy orientation exist. If fixation other than screws is utilized, then the wedge is best oriented in the plane perpendicular to the long axis. If screw fixation is desired, the apex should be proximal dorsal and the base plantar distal. The proximal-based apex allows for a more anatomical reconstruction, owing to the longer axis of rotation. Post-operative care is similar to any proximal osteotomy of the first metatarsal; that is, 6 weeks of non-weight-bearing. Serial radiographs are taken to ensure adequate bone healing.

If the patient requires a sliding plantarflexory osteotomy, then it is performed in the sagittal plane. Here the approach is dorsomedial. An S-incision can be made to facilitate exposure but is not always necessary. The usual technique of mobilization and extraperiosteal dissection is performed. The cut should be fashioned from proximal medial to distal lateral and should be between the proximal and distal metaphyseal regions (**10.48**). This orientation assures that the deep plantar artery will not be injured. The cut is com-

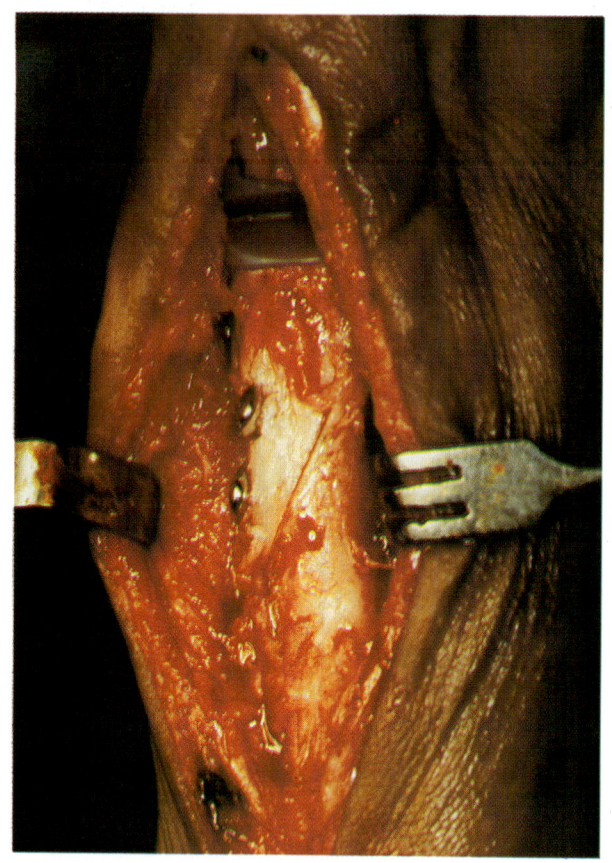

10.48 Intra-operative photograph of right foot, showing recommended technique for the sagittal plane plantarflexory osteotomy. An implant can be seen in the first metatarsophalangeal joint.

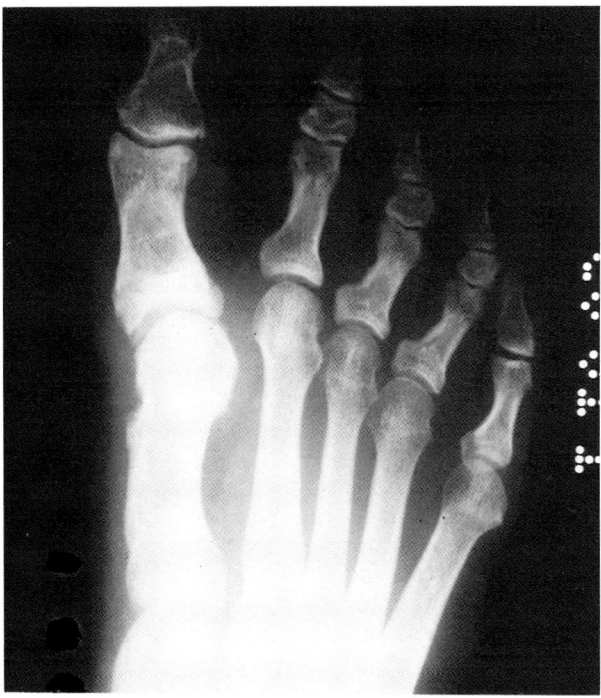

10.49 Pre-operative AP X-ray of a patient who acquired hallux varus deformity and first metatarsal elevation after a base osteotomy and McBride bunionectomy 18 years previously. Note the narrow intermetatarsal angle.

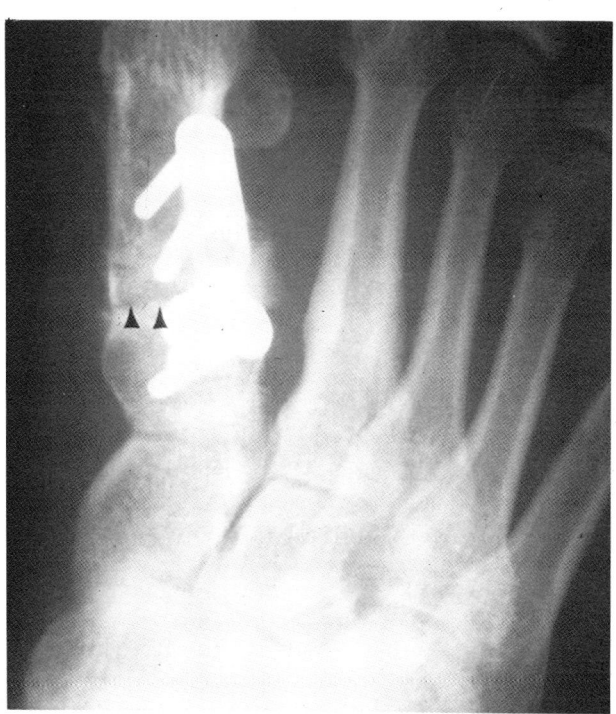

10.50 Post-operative AP X-ray of the same patient as in **10.49** after a plantarflexory opening wedge osteotomy was performed. A small T-plate was used to secure the autogenous bone graft and the osteotomy. The arrows show the proximal extent of the graft.

pletely through the bone, rendering it into a medial and lateral portion. Precise orientation in the sagittal plane is required so as not to spuriously place the metatarsal head in a varus or valgus attitude. The distal portion is then rotated plantarly into the desired position and held in place with a bone clamp. Slight adjustments in length can be made by proximal or distal traction.

Compression is achieved by cortical bone screws placed from medial to lateral: there is no suitable alternative fixation and this is in strictly cortical bone. If total failure of screw fixation occurs intra-operatively, then tenuous fixation may be achieved with K-wires and cerclage wire, but is clearly not recommended, except in this instance.

Post-operative care requires the same period of non-weight-bearing as the other proximal osteotomies, although there may be adequate stability to allow for earlier weight-bearing in the rigidly fixated cases. Nevertheless, failure could occur with premature repetitive loading.

The last option for the dorsiflexed metatarsal is the opening wedge procedure. This requires the use of bone graft, which may be either allograft or autograft. The advantages for each type of graft are discussed in the section on opening abductory wedge osteotomies of the first metatarsal. Either source is useful, but a precise fit is necessary. A wedge of bone deep enough to traverse the entire depth of the first metatarsal is required.

The approach is modified to provide access to the dorsal aspect of the metatarsal to insert the wedge of graft. The position of the osteotomy is at the level of the previous osteotomy, if there was one, or at the proximal metaphysis, if there was not. In other words, it is at the level of the deformity. Again, extraperiosteal dissection is performed and a transverse cut is made in the bone at the appropriate level. If the cut is made in the diaphysis, complete transection of the metatarsal is necessary to attain the required mobility. If the cut is made in the metaphysis, the plantar cortex can be spared and still provide the mobility needed for graft insertion. Once the opening is enlarged, the graft is shaped according to the amount of plantarflexion needed and tamped into place. Temporary K-wires or screws may be used, but a small plate provides the best stability because it forces the wedge-shaped graft to remain in place and uses the soft tissue tension to help compress the graft. A small T-plate is most suitable, although other plates may be utilized. The plate is placed dorsally and secured with cortical screws. Screws through the graft are optional (**10.49, 10.50**).

The post-operative management is similar to the opening abductory wedge procedure. Graft incorporation is likely to take 10–12 weeks and caution should be exercised before allowing unprotected weight-bearing.

Complications are related to union of the osteotomy, particularly in the opening wedge procedure. Delayed or non-unions are possible. Overzealous plantarflexion may also cause intractable sesamoiditis, lateral ankle pain, and fifth ray problems as a result of reciprocal subtalar inversion and lateral overload of the lesser metatarsals.

Hallux limitus

Hallux limitus is a very common condition which the foot surgeon is called upon to treat. Although the deformity can often be managed with conservative means, surgery has a definite place in the scheme of management. This section will focus on early and late hallux limitus because the treatment options and prognosis are dramatically different. Patients who, in the early stages of the deformity, are relatively young should be treated with the philosophy of joint preservation in mind. If the integrity of the joint can be saved, then functional restoration can be achieved. It should be remembered that this problem represents a progression of degenerative change on a well-defined and predictable continuum.[97] Arresting the progression of destruction with early restorative surgery has not yet been fully accepted. As options of the other currently accepted procedures become less favourable, this philosophy will gain more acceptance. The patient's willingness to submit to surgery depends on the functional limitations present. However, the surgeon's presentation of surgery is based on the knowledge of a predictable course of ankylosis and probable discomfort. Only in the older patient are the conventional options of implantation and fusion compatible with a long-term pain-free gait.

Early hallux limitus

The younger patient with hallux limitus may be a candidate for one of several procedures which do not destroy the first metatarsophalangeal joint. The indications depend primarily on the amount of joint destruction and joint space narrowing seen radiographically. If there is still viable articular cartilage throughout most of the joint, then the patient is clearly a candidate. The amount of dorsal proliferative change is immaterial when evaluating these patients because it is almost always removed. The proliferation is only the response to abnormal biomechanical forces acting on the joint. It is incumbent on the surgeon to determine the aetiology of the deformity if possible and address these aetiological factors surgically.[98]

The cheilectomy

Cheilectomy has long been accepted as an approach to hallux limitus. It is based on the premise that removing the offending bone will eliminate the block of motion and restore function to the joint. Although this works empirically on a short-term basis, it does nothing to improve or alter the biomechanical forces of the foot. It is true that functional orthotic control may be used adjunctively to control these pathological forces, but no long-term studies are available. Further investigation is warranted before this procedure can be applied to the young patient with adequate cartilage. The procedure clearly has a place in the treatment of the deformity when reconstructive procedures are done in addition.[99]

The surgical approach is a standard dorsomedial one. Once the subcutaneous layer has been reflected, the hypertrophic joint and capsule are encountered. The capsulotomy is also a dorsomedial one and should be directly to bone. The knife must be placed under the enlarged ridge from the proximal side to enable the reflection of the capsule. The entire capsule is reflected medially and laterally trying to preserve a single envelope of tissue. The hypertrophic bony ridges may make this more difficult than usual. The joint is then remodelled by sequential resection of the dorsal, medial, and lateral sides of the metatarsal head. An osteotome or power saw is used to remodel the dorsum of the head. The redundant bone should be resected at a level that is flush with the shaft. This usually removes all but 2–3 mm of eburnated bone. The medial and lateral side should also be remodelled to the point that it resembles a normal metatarsal head. Corners are rounded with a power rotating burr or rongeur and rasp. Range of motion is checked and if inadequate, the sesamoid complex is checked for adhesions. A McGlamry metatarsal elevator or No. 95 meniscal knife is passed plantarly to free-up any adhesions of the plantar structures to the metatarsal head. This usually provides adequate motion. The use of bone wax on the resected surfaces to prevent bleeding is optional, but has not been necessary in our hands. Eburnated areas about the periphery of the joint or central defects should be drilled with a fine drill or K-wire. The number of holes should be generous as the eburnated bone provides exceptional bony support. The depth of the drill holes should be well into the cancellous bone. The capsule is closed after some of the redundancy is excised. Excessive resection of the capsule will only lead to restriction of motion.

Post-operatively, the joint should be ranged as soon as the patient is comfortable. This should be no later than 48 h after surgery. It is equally important to instruct the patient or physical therapist to perform plantarflexion range of motion exercises as well as dorsally. This will enhance toe purchase and reduce capsulodesis on the dorsum of the metatarsal head. Immediate weight-bearing is permitted if there are no other procedures in which it is contraindicated.

Plantarflexory procedures

In a great majority of patients who present with hallux limitus, there is some degree of first metatarsal elevation. This may be structural and fixed or, more commonly, it may be a hypermobile first metatarsal. This can be determined clinically as well as radiographically. If it is determined that the primary factor in the development of the deformity is indeed hypermobility, the surgical procedure should be directed towards its elimination. Since the hypermobile segment is usually at the first metatarsal cuneiform joint, fusion of this joint is a logical end to the excessive motion. The procedure used can be either an opening or closing wedge, depending on the length pattern of the first metatarsal: if length is deemed to be excessive, then a closing wedge is the procedure of choice; if length is required, then an opening wedge is preferable. Either of these choices is best combined with a cheilectomy. It is surprising that this seemingly logical solution to the problem has not been more widely performed in the past.

Plantarflexory fusion of the first metatarsal cuneiform joint

This procedure is best performed through a dorsomedial approach to the first metatarsal cuneiform joint. If performed with a cheilectomy, a proximal extension of the incision is all that is needed. Care should be taken to protect the tibialis anterior insertion as well as the deep plantar artery. Hohmann retractors are placed on either side of the first metatarsal base after the usual reflection of the long extensor tendon and its sheath. The dorsal, medial, and lateral ligaments are incised and a circumferential release is carried out. The resection of the cartilage should begin from the metatarsal side and should be relatively perpendicular to the long axis of the bone, protecting the attachment of the peroneus longus tendon on the metatarsal base. Next, the corrective resection of the cuneiform articular facet is performed. Once both joint surfaces have been transected, they are extracted from the wound using the two-osteotome technique. A trial fit of the opposing surfaces is done. The amount of plantarflexion is checked radiographically after temporary fixation with a K-wire or guide pin if cannulated screws are used. If the correction is satisfactory, then fixation is applied. If not, then refinements can be made and checked again until adequate correction is obtained. Fixation is similar to the fusion of the first metatarsal cuneiform joint for hallux abductovalgus.

Opening wedge fusions of the first metatarsal cuneiform joint

If the length pattern of the first metatarsal is such that it requires additional length or at least should not be shortened, then an opening wedge is necessary. The approach is exactly the same as for a plantarflexory fusion. The resected surface of the cuneiform is made parallel to the long axis of the bone and a bone graft is inserted (**10.51**). The same principles and procedures for insertion of the bone graft, fixation, and post-operative care are applied as for the plantarflexory opening wedge osteotomy.

We have been using a combination of first metatarsal cuneiform fusion and cheilectomy for the past 4 years. Our series of 21 patients has provided encouraging results over a 2-year follow-up period. Reestablishment of the first metatarsal position enables dorsiflexion of the phalanx on the head. Range of motion has improved considerably and is pain-free.

Complications have been more common in patients receiving bone graft, owing to the longer postoperative course. The incorporation of graft significantly increases post-operative swelling. Overlengthening has also been observed and we now employ the graft only in those cases where length is definitely required. No non-unions have been observed. This procedure, in spite of complications related to our early experience, provides an excellent means of eliminating the morbid forces and reestablishing normal first metatarsophalangeal joint mechanics.

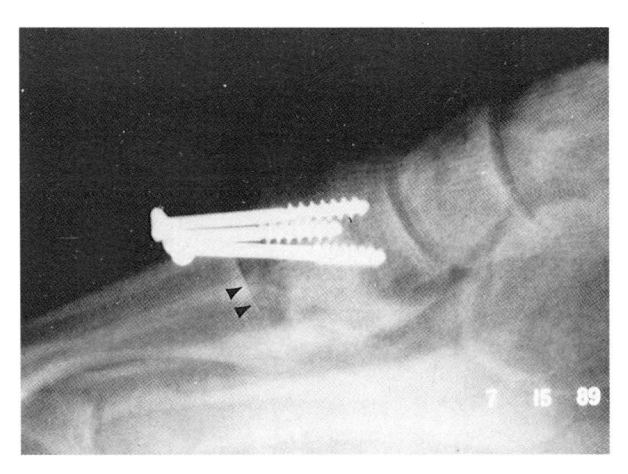

10.51 Post-operative AP X-ray showing insertion of a bone graft into the first metatarsal cuneiform joint.

Late hallux limitus

Patients who present with advanced degenerative destruction of the first metatarsophalangeal joint have limited surgical options. Basically, one can perform a Keller procedure, with or without a total joint prosthesis, or fuse the arthritic joint. Cheilectomy has not proved to be efficacious in patients with severe loss of joint space.[100]

The total joint implant procedure has been described above. It is indicated in the patient over the arbitrary age of 55, but again, may be indicated in the much younger patient who refuses fusion. Long-term wear of the implant can be expected to progress as the activity level of the patient increases and as pathological forces continue to act on the implant. Although it is theoretically sound, repositioning of the first ray is not practical because the implant is still the weak link. Future study may show whether the eradication of hypermobility via osteotomy or first metatarsal fusion will prolong the longevity of the implant. In those patients whose activity level is diminished, longer periods of success will prevail.

First metatarsophalangeal joint fusion

This procedure is becoming less and less popular in the scheme of foot surgery, primarily because it is poorly accepted by patients and is not a functional procedure. It is true that patients can achieve a high level of pain-relief, but the concept of a fused big toe joint is not easily sold. The poor acceptance by patients is a bit surprising because many of the patients have no motion at the joint anyway. Although implants can provide some restoration of motion, it is not their primary purpose. If the patient accepts the risk of implant failure, wear, and the possibility of revision, then it is probably a better alternative to fusion in all but the very young active patient. Conversion to a later fusion is possible in the cases of failed total implant.

Those patients who are arthrodesis candidates must have an adequate interphalangeal joint of the hallux. This is where the vast majority of compensation for loss of the first metatarsophalangeal joint range of motion will occur. In fact, those patients with hallux limitus usually present with some degree of IPJ hyperextension. Therefore, the demands of this joint may not increase substantially.[101-103] If there are seemingly normal IPJ characteristics, then the patient can be expected to develop symptoms in that joint following first metatarsophalangeal joint arthrodesis at some distant point.

The optimal position of fusion is neutral rotation, 20° of abductus, and approximately 15–20° of dorsiflexion.[104] Patients should be cautioned that shoes with heels of more than the average height may be tolerated poorly because of the fixed nature of the hallux. Any strong shoe requirements by the patient should be elicited prior to surgery and accounted for by the position of fusion.[103]

The approach to the first metatarsophalangeal joint is a standard one. Two avenues of technique are available: the peg-and-hole arthrodesis and the direct end-to-end apposition technique; either one is acceptable. The former offers less choices in the type of fixation and the latter is more difficult to adjust position intraoperatively.

Peg-and-hole arthrodesis

The first metatarsal head is denuded of all articular cartilage except for the plantar aspect. It is important to preserve the weight-bearing portion of the bone because there will be no further plantarflexion positioning of the head from reciprocal dorsiflexion of the hallux. The base of the phalanx is burred to accommodate the 'peg-shaped' metatarsal head. Both components must have abundant cancellous bone for optimal contact. The phalanx is positioned in the predetermined attitude and fixated with threaded Steinmann pins. K-wires are probably inadequate, owing to the tremendous muscular and bending forces across this joint.[105]

End-to-end arthrodesis

Here the resection of cartilage is done with a saw and the angle of resection is tailored again to the needs of the fusion. Rotation of the toe may be difficult to control, so careful attention to detail during the procedure is mandatory. Fixation can again be with Steinmann pins, but screw fixation provides for compression and counters the muscular forces better. A single 4.0 mm cancellous screw is often suitable when driven from plantar medial distal to proximal lateral.[106,107] Two screws are preferable.

Weight-bearing is not permitted for 6 weeks or until fusion is evident on radiographs. Complications include IPJ arthrosis, non-union, sesamoiditis, shoe problems secondary to malposition, and lesser metatarsalgia.[101]

Summary

First ray (phalangeal–metatarsal–cuneiform) surgical procedures are multiple and relatively complex in nature. This is due, mostly, to the triplane function and distinct anatomical variables involved in this area. The surgeon needs to have an excellent understanding of not only the anatomy but also the biomechanics of the first ray before embarking upon reconstructive surgical procedures.

References

[1] McCarthy, D.J. The surgical anatomy of the first ray. Part II: the proximal segment. *J. Am. Podiatric Med. Assoc.*, **73**: 244, 1983.

[2] Sarrafian, S.K. *Anatomy of the Foot and Ankle*. Philadelphia, J.B. Lippincott, 1983.

[3] David, R.D., Delagiutte, J.P. and Renard, M.M. Anatomical study of the sesamoid bones of the first metatarsal. *J. Am. Podiatric Med. Assoc.*, **79**: 536, 1989.

[4] McCarthy, D.J. The surgical anatomy of the first ray. Part I: the distal segment. *J. Am. Podiatric Med. Assoc.*, **73**: 111, 1983.

[5] Haines, R.W. and McDougall, A. The anatomy of hallux valgus. *J. Bone Joint Surg.*, **36B**: 272, 1954.

[6] Cralley, J.C. and Schuberth, J.M. The transverse head of adductor hallucis. *Anat. Anz.*, **146**: 400, 1979.

[7] Grode, S.E. and McCarthy, D.J. The anatomical implications of hallux abductovalgus, a cryomicrotomy study. *J. Am. Podiatric Med. Assoc.*, **70**: 539, 1980.

[8] Kashak, T.J. and Laine, W. Surgical Radiology. *Clin. Pod. Med. Surg.*, **5**: 797, 1988.

[9] LaPorta, G., Melillo, T. and Olinsky, D. X-ray evaluation of hallux abductovalgus deformity. *J. Am. Podiatric Med. Assoc.*, **64**: 544, 1974.

[10] Lundberg, B.J. and Sulja, T. Skeletal parameters in the hallux valgus foot. *Acta Orthop. Scandinav.*, **43**: 576, 1972.

[11] Sorto, L.A., Balding, M.G., Weil, L.S. *et al*. Hallux abductus interphalangeus. *J. Am. Podiatric Med. Assoc.*, **66**: 384, 1976.

[12] Armanek, D.L., Mollica, A. and Jacobs, A.M. A statistical analysis on the reliability of the PASA. *J. Foot Surg.*, **25**: 39, 1986.

[13] Palladino, S. PASA changes with unicorrectional Austin bunionectomy. *J. Am. Podiatric Med. Assoc.*, **76**: 636, 1986.

[14] Balding, M.G. and Sorto, L.A. Distal articular set angle. Etiology and X-ray evaluation. *J. Am. Podiatric Med. Assoc.*, **75**: 648, 1985.

[15] Christman, R.A. Radiographic evaluation of DASA. *J. Am. Podiatric. Med. Assoc.*, **78**: 352, 1988.

[16] Frankel, J. Structual or positional hallux abductus. *J. Am. Podiatric Med. Assoc.*, **63**: 647, 1973.

[17] Pressman, M.M., Stano, G.W. and Krantz, M.K. Correction of hallux valgus with positionally increased IM angle. *J. Am. Podiatric Med. Assoc.*, **76**: 611, 1986.

[18] Brahm, S.M. Shape of the first metatarsal head in hallux rigidus and hallux valgus. *J. Am. Podiatric Med. Assoc.*, **78**: 300, 1988.

[19] Hardy, R.H. and Clapham, J.C.R. Observations on hallux valgus. Based on a controlled series. *J. Bone Joint Surg.*, **33B**: 376, 1951.

[20] Morton, D.J. Foot disorders in general practice. *J. Am. Podiatric Med. Assoc.*, **109**: 1112, 1937.

[21] Schuberth, J.M., Reilly, C.H. and Gudas, C.J. The closing wedge osteotomy. A critical analysis of the first metatarsal elevation. *J. Am. Podiatric Med. Assoc.*, **74**: 13, 1984.

[22] Zlotoff, H. Shortening of the first metatarsal following osteotomy and its clinical significance. *J. Am. Podiatric Med. Assoc.*, **67**: 412, 1977.

[23] LaReaux, R.L. and Lee, B.R. Metatarsus adductus and hallux abductovalgus: their correlation. *J. Foot Surg.*, **26**: 304, 1987.

[24] Hiss, J.M. Hallux valgus. Its cause and simplified treatment. *Am. J. Surg.*, **11**: 51, 1931.

[25] McBride, E.D. A conservative operation for bunions. *J. Bone Joint Surg.*, **10**: 735, 1928.

[26] Silver, D. The operative treatment of hallux valgus. *J. Bone Joint Surg.*, **5**: 225, 1923.

[27] Wenig, J.A. Modified V–Y capsulotomy in hallux abductovalgus surgery. *J. Am. Podiatric Med. Assoc.*, **79**: 132, 1989.

[28] McBride, E.D. The McBride bunion hallux valgus operation. Refinements in the successive surgical steps of the operation. *J. Bone Joint Surg.*, **49A**: 1675, 1967.

[29] McGlamry, E.D. and Feldman, M.H. A treatise on the McBride procedure. *J. Am. Podiatric Med. Assoc.*, **61**: 161, 1979.

[30] Kempe, S.A. Modified McBride bunionectomy utilizing the adductor tendon transfer. *J. Foot Surg.*, **24**: 24, 1985.

[31] Valvo, P., Hochman, D. and Reilly, C.H. Anatomic and clinical significance of the first and most medial deep transverse metatarsal ligament. *J. Foot Surg.*, **26**: 194, 1987.

[32] Fenton, C.F. and McGlamry, E.D. Reverse buckling to reduce metatarsus primus varus. *J. Am. Podiatric Med. Assoc.*, **72**: 342, 1982.

[33] Curda, G.A. and Sorto, L.A. The McBride bunionectomy with closing abductory wedge osteotomy. *J. Am. Podiatric Med. Assoc.,* **71**: 349, 1981.
[34] Wilson, J.N. Oblique displacement osteotomy for hallux valgus. *J. Bone Joint Surg.,* **45B**: 552, 1963.
[35] Austin, D.W. and Leventen, E.O. A new osteotomy for hallux valgus. *Clin. Orthop.,* **157**: 25, 1981.
[36] Miller, S. and Croce, W.A. The Austin procedure for surgical correction of hallux abductovalgus deformity. *J. Am. Podiatric Med. Assoc.,* **69**: 110, 1979.
[37] Boberg, J., Ruch, J.A. and Banks, A.S. Distal metaphyseal osteotomies in hallux abductovalgus. *In* McGlamry, E.D. (ed.), *Comprehensive Textbook of Foot Surgery.* Baltimore, Williams & Wilkins, 1987, pp. 173–184.
[38] Duke, H.F. and Kaplan, E.W. A modification of the Austin bunionectomy for shortening and plantar flexion. *J. Am. Podiatric Med. Assoc.,* **74**: 209, 1984.
[39] Youngswick, F. Modifications of the Austin bunionectomy for treatment of metatarsus primus equinus associated with hallux limitus. *J. Foot Surg.,* **21**: 114, 1982.
[40] Gerbert, J. Complications of the Austin type bunionectomy. *J. Foot Surg.,* **17**: 1, 1978.
[41] Gerbert, J., Massard, R., Wilson, F. *et al.* Bicorrectional horizontal osteotomy (Austin type) of the first metatarsal head. *J. Am. Podiatric Med. Assoc.,* **69**: 119, 1979.
[42] Steinbock, G. Austin bunionectomy transpositional V osteotomy of the first metatarsal for hallux valgus. *J. Foot Surg.,* **27**: 211, 1988.
[43] Knecht, J.G. and VanPelt, W.L. Austin bunionectomy with Kirschner wire fixation. *J. Am. Podiatric Med. Assoc.,* **71**: 139, 1981.
[44] Clary, R. A traumatically displaced Austin bunionectomy: a case report. *J. Am. Podiatric Med. Assoc.,* **70**: 247, 1980.
[45] Quinn, M.R., DiStazio, J.J. and Kruljac, S.J. Herbert bone screw fixation of the Austin bunionectomy. *J. Foot Surg.,* **26**: 516, 1987.
[46] Hawkins, F.B., Mitchell, C.L. and Hedrick, D.W. Correction of hallux valgus by metatarsal osteotomy. *J. Bone Joint Surg.,* **27**: 387, 1945.
[47] Mitchell, C.L., Fleming, J.L., Allen, R., *et al.* Osteotomy–bunionectomy for hallux valgus. *J. Bone Joint Surg.,* **40A**: 41, 1958.
[48] Wu, K. Mitchell: An analysis of 430 personal cases plus a review of the literature. *J. Foot Surg.,* **26**: 277, 1987.
[49] Bonner, A.C. Rigid internal fixation of the Mitchell–Hawkins osteotomy/bunionectomy with the Herbert bone screw. *J. Foot Surg.,* **25**: 390, 1986.
[50] Heden, R.I. and Sorto, L.A. The buckle point and the metatarsal protrusion's relationship to hallux valgus. *J. Am. Podiatric Med. Assoc.,* **71**: 200, 1981.
[51] Beck, E.L. Modified Reverdin technique for hallux abductovalgus. *J. Am. Podiatric Med. Assoc.,* **64**: 657, 1974.
[52] Todd, W.F. Osteotomies of the first metatarsal head. Reverdin, Reverdin modifications, Peabody, Mitchell, and Drato. *In* Gerbert, J. (ed.), *Textbook of Bunion Surgery.* Mt. Kisco, New York, Futura, 1981.
[53] Zygmunt, K.H., Gudas, C.J. and Laros, G.S. Z-bunionectomy with internal screw fixation. *J. Am. Podiatric Med. Assoc.,* **79**: 322, 1989.
[54] Ruch, J.A. and Banks, A.S. Proximal osteotomies of the first metatarsal in correction of hallux abductovalgus. *In* McGlamry, E.D. (ed.), *Comprehensive Textbook of Foot Surgery.* Baltimore, Williams and Wilkins, 1987.
[55] Doll, P.J. and Esposito, F.J. Angular analysis of wedge type osteotomies. *J. Am. Podiatric Med. Assoc.,* **74**: 587, 1984.
[56] Balacescu, J. Un caz de hallux valgus simetric. *Rev. Chir.,* **7**: 128, 1903.
[57] Loison, M. Note sur la traitement chirurgicale de hallux valgus d'apres l'étude radiographique de la deformation. *Bull. Mem. Soc. Chir.,* **27**: 528, 1901.
[58] Gudas, C.J. Compression screw fixation in proximal first metatarsal osteotomies for metatarsus primus varus. Initial observations. *J. Foot Surg.,* **18**: 10, 1979.
[59] Kirchwein, W. Cross screw compression fixation technique in proximal osteotomies of the first metatarsal for hallux abductovalgus. *J. Foot Surg.,* **27**: 412, 1988.
[60] Armaneck, D.L., Juda, E.J. and Oloff, L.M. Opening base wedge osteotomy of the first metatarsal utilizing rigid external fixation. *J. Foot Surg.,* **25**: 321, 1986.
[61] LaPorta, G.A., Richter, K.P. and Jolley, G.P. Pressure osteosynthesis for internal fixation of metatarsal angulational osteotomies. *J. Am. Podiatric Med. Assoc.,* **66**: 173, 1976.
[62] McCrea, J.D. and Lichty, T.K. The first metatarsocuneiform articulation and its relationship to metatarsus primus adductus. *J. Am. Podiatric Med. Assoc.,* **69**: 700, 1979.
[63] McNerney, J.E. and Johnson, W.B. Generalized ligamentous laxity, hallux abductovalgus, and the first metatarsocuneiform joint. *J. Am. Podiatric Med. Assoc.,* **69**: 69, 1979.
[64] Lapidus, P.W. Operative correction metatarsus primus varus in hallux valgus. *Surg. Gynecol. Obstet.,* **58**: 183, 1934.
[65] Bacardi, B.E. and Boysen, T.J. Considerations for the Lapidus operation. *J. Foot Surg.,* **25**: 133, 1986.
[66] Sangeorzan, B.J. Modified Lapidus procedure for hallux valgus. *Foot Ankle,* **9**: 262, 1989.
[67] Akin, O.F. The treatment of hallux valgus—a new operative procedure and its results. *Med. Sentinal,* **33**: 678, 1925.
[68] Gerbert, J., Spector, E. and Clark, J. Osteotomy procedures on the proximal phalanx for correction of a hallux deformity. *J. Am. Podiatric Med. Assoc.,* **64**: 617, 1974.
[69] Gerbert, J. and Melillo, T. A modified Akin procedure for the correction of hallux valgus. *J. Am. Podiatric Med. Assoc.,* **66**: 384, 1976.

[70] Murphy, J.S., Mozena, J.D. and Walker, R.E. K-wire technique for fixation of the Akin osteotomy. *J. Am. Podiatric Med. Assoc.*, **79**: 291, 1989.

[71] CollCra, B. and Weitz, E.M. Proximal phalangeal osteotomy in hallux valgus. *Clin. Orthop.*, **54**: 105, 1967.

[72] Lauf, E. Akin osteotomy of the proximal phalanx utilizing Richards mini-staple fixation. *J. Foot Surg.*, **26**: 178, 1987.

[73] Langford, J.H. ASIF Akin osteotomy. A new method of fixation. *J. Am. Podiatric Med. Assoc.*, **71**: 390, 1981.

[74] Levitsky, D.R., DiGilio, J. and Kander, R. Rigid compression screw fixation of the first proximal phalanx osteotomy for hallux abductovalgus. *J. Foot Surg.*, **21**: 65, 1982.

[75] Schwartz, N.H., Lannuzzi, P.P. and Thurber, N.B. Derotational Akin osteotomy. *J. Foot Surg.*, **25**: 479, 1986.

[76] Schwartz, N. and Hurley, J.P. Derotational Akin osteotomy: further modification. *J. Foot Surg.*, **26**: 419, 1987.

[77] McGlamry, E.D., Kitting, R.M. and Butlin, W.E. Hallux valgus repair with correction of coexisting long hallux. *J. Am. Podiatric Med. Assoc.*, **60**: 86, 1970.

[78] Keller, W.L. Surgical treatment of bunions and hallux valgus. *New York Med. J.*, **80**: 741, 1904.

[79] Keller, W.L. Further observations on the surgical treatment of hallux valgus or bunions. *New York Med. J.*, **95**: 696, 1912.

[80] Kaplan, E.G. and Kaplan, G.S. The Keller procedure. *J. Am. Podiatric Med. Assoc.*, **64**: 603, 1974.

[81] Fuson, S.M. Modification of the Keller operation for increased functional capacity. *J. Foot Surg.*, **21**: 292, 1982.

[82] Ganley, J.V., Lynch, F.R. and Darrigan, R.D. Keller bunionectomy with fascia and tendon graft. *J. Am. Podiatric Med. Assoc.*, **76**: 7302, 1986.

[83] McGlamry, E.D., Kitting, R.W. and Butlin, W.E. Keller bunionectomy and hallux valgus correction—further modifications. *J. Am. Podiatric Med. Assoc.*, **63**: 237, 1973.

[84] Kravette, M.A. and Baker, G.I. The Swanson arthroplasty of the great toe: a prospective study. *J. Foot Surg.*, **17**: 155, 1978.

[85] Swanson, A.B. Implant arthroplasty of the great toe. *Clin. Orthop.*, **85**: 75, 1972.

[86] Cracchiolo III, A., Swanson, A.B., DeGroot, X. and Swanson, G. The arthritic great toe metatarsophalangeal joint. *Clin. Orthop.*, **157**: 64, 1981.

[87] Weil, L.S., Pollak, R.A. and Goller, W.L. Total first joint replacement in hallux valgus and hallux rigidus. *Clin. Podiatry,*, **1**: 103, 1984.

[88] Fenton, C.F., Gilman, R.D., and Yu, G.V. Criteria for joint replacement surgery in the foot. *J. Am. Podiatric Med. Assoc.*, **72**: 535, 1982.

[89] Jarvis, B.D., Moats, D.B., Burns, A. and Gerbert, J. Lawrence design first metatarsophalangeal joint prosthesis. *J. Am. Podiatric Med. Assoc.*, **76**: 617, 1986.

[90] Lawrence, B.R. and Papier, M.J. Implant arthroplasty of the lesser metatarsophalangeal joint—a modified technique. *J. Foot Surg.*, **19**: 16, 1980.

[91] Nuzzo, J. Intramedullary power broaching. *J. Am. Podiatric Med. Assoc.*, **76**: 84, 1986.

[92] McGlamry, E.D., Kitting, R.M. and Butlin, W.E. Keller bunionectomy and hallux valgus correction. An appraisal and current modifications sixty-six years later. *J. Am. Podiatric Med. Assoc.*, **60**: 161, 1970.

[93] Vanore, J.V., O'Keefe, R.G. and Pikscher, I. Silastic implant arthroplasty: complications and their classification. *J. Am. Podiatric Med. Assoc.*, **74**: 423, 1984.

[94] Verhaar, J., Balstra, S. and Walenkamp, G. Silicone arthroplasty for hallux rigidus. Implant wear and osteolysis. *Acta Orthop. Scand.*, **60**: 30, 1989.

[95] Worsing, R.A., Engber, W.D. and Lange, T.A. Reactive synovitis from particulate silastic. *J. Bone Joint Surg.*, **62B**: 551, 1982.

[96] Smith, T.F. Resection of common pedal prominences. *J. Am. Podiatric Med. Assoc.*, **73**: 93, 1983.

[97] Drago, J.J., Oloff, L. and Jacobs, A.M. A comprehensive review of hallux limitus. *J. Foot Surg.*, **23**: 213, 1984.

[98] Gould, N. Hallux rigidus: cheilectomy or implant? *Foot Ankle*, **1**: 315, 1981.

[99] Hattrup, S.J. and Johnson, K.A. Subjective results of hallux rigidus following treatment with cheilectomy. *Clin. Orthop.*, **226**: 182, 1988.

[100] Pontell, D. and Gudas, C.J. Retrospective analysis of surgical treatment of hallux limitus/rigidus: clinical and radiographic follow up of hinged, silastic implant arthroplasty and cheilectomy. *J. Foot Surg.*, **27**: 503, 1988.

[101] Fitzgerald, J.A.W. A review of long term results of arthrodesis of the first metatarsophalangeal joint. *J. Bone Surg.*, **51B**: 488, 1969.

[102] Harrison, H.M. and Harvey, F.J. Arthrodesis of the first metatarsophalangeal joint for hallux valgus and rigidus. *J. Bone Joint Surg.*, **45A**: 471, 1963.

[103] Thompson, F.R. and McElvenny, R.T. Arthrodesis of the first metatarsophalangeal joint. *J. Bone Joint Surg.*, **22**: 555, 1940.

[104] Lipscomb, P.R. Arthrodesis of the first metatarsophalangeal joint for severe bunions and hallux rigidus. *Clin. Orth. Rel. Res.*, **142**: 48, 1979.

[105] Schlefman, B.S., Fenton, C.F. and McGlamry, E.D. Peg-in-hole arthrodesis. *J. Am. Podiatric Med. Assoc.*, **73**: 187, 1983.

[106] KcKeever, D.C. Arthrodesis of the first metatarsophalangeal joint, hallux rigidus, and metatarsophalangeal varus. *J. Bone Joint Surg.*, **34A**: 129, 1952.

[107] Raymakers, R. and Waugh, W. The treatment of metatarsalgia with hallux valgus. *J. Bone Joint Surg.*, **53B**: 684, 1971.

11 Surgical complications of the forefoot

JEFFREY C. CHRISTENSEN

A surgical complication is an unexpected set of circumstances which occurs during the peri-operative setting that directly or indirectly prolongs the patient's functional recovery period. This prolonged recovery period varies according to the severity, as well as the speed of diagnosis and treatment of the complication. Therefore, there are temporary as well as permanent types of surgical complications. If appropriately anticipated, some complications are preventable, while the effect of other complications can be minimized with early diagnosis.

Surgical complications, unfortunately, are inherent to all types of surgical procedures, and forefoot surgery is no exception. Complications can be broken down into two basic categories: preventable and non-preventable. The most preventable complication involves the surgeon's judgement pre-operatively. First, the surgeon must carefully consider if the patient is a good surgical candidate for the proposed surgery; secondly, the surgeon must make an accurate diagnosis; and thirdly, the procedural selection must clearly address the pathological condition. If there is an error in the pre-operative surgical judgement, then there is an increased risk for post-operative complications. Other forms of preventable complications are proper patient education as to risks of potential complications and informing the patient that certain measures must be followed to prevent potential problems.

This chapter discusses the most commonly encountered complications associated with forefoot surgery. It is the intent of the author to heighten the awareness of these complications and underscore some of the common pitfalls in forefoot surgery and to assist the surgeon or trainee in preventing potential surgical complications.

Since the foot is a primary weight-bearing structure and is mechanically complex, it is to be expected that the majority of surgical complications involving the foot are mechanically related. The general surgical standards of wound management and osteosynthesis need to be observed by the foot surgeon; however, because of excessive mechanical stresses placed on the foot, compliance of strict structural and mechanical principles must be adhered to in order to assure a successful functional result.

A thorough understanding of all surgical principles pertaining to foot surgery is needed to produce consistent and uncomplicated results. It is recommended that no surgical procedure should be attempted by a surgeon unless that surgeon is sufficiently prepared to diagnose and manage the potential subsequent complications.

Delayed wound healing

Delayed wound healing is one of the most common complications associated with forefoot surgery. The aetiology of delayed wound healing is varied (**Table 11.1**). In most cases, delayed wound healing is self-limiting and does not lead to surgical failure unless significant infection or reduced blood supply is present.

Table 11.1 Aetiology of delayed wound healing

Infection
Suture reaction
Wound margin strangulation
Excessive prolonged wound retraction
Foreign body reaction
Haematoma formation
Vascular compromise
Excessive joint movement

Simple wound delay

Most cases of delayed wound healing involve little or no tissue loss. In minor cases of delayed healing, simple postponement in suture removal usually facilitates adequate healing of the incision, unless the delayed healing is due to a suture reaction. Suture reaction is usually seen with absorbable types of suture; however, nylon and dacron are also commonly involved. If suture reaction is suspected, then the sutures should be removed, and the wound can then be stabilized with adhesive strip closures. In cases of true suture reaction, the wound rapidly proceeds into normal healing once the sutures have been removed. Application of topical antiseptics will also assist in the wound-healing process during the simple cases without tissue loss.

Skin slough

The causes of skin slough are outlined in **Table 11.2**. Skin slough involves necrosis of the skin, with tissue loss. In forefoot surgery, this most commonly occurs with bunion surgery. Historically, semi-lunar incisions for bunionectomy involved significant undermining of skin that led to frequent skin slough.[1] Currently, most approaches for bunion correction utilize longer linear or near-linear approaches requiring less undermining of skin.

The use of tourniquet haemostatic control during reconstructive foot surgery increases the chances of haematoma and skin slough. There is too much reliance on pressure bandages after tourniquet use to control post-operative bleeding. If a tourniquet is to be used, it is good practice to release it after the reconstructive work is completed to allow for ligation or cauterization of any bleeders. The presence of haematoma can lead to delayed wound healing and skin slough, as well as to infection. If untreated, further tissue loss and progression of the complication is possible.

The most preventable cause of skin slough is overzealous dissection techniques or retraction of tissues. This is a situation where too much or too little dissection can lead to wound margin injury and the same complication. To prevent tissue slough, a thorough knowledge of vascular supply and all aspects of incision placement, length, and dissection techniques must be considered relative to tissue planes. Extensive subcutaneous dissection will interrupt the essential perforator blood supply that comes from underlying muscle (**11.1**).[2]

Table 11.2 Aetiology of skin slough

Infection
Excessive skin undermining
Subincisional haematoma
Overzealous skin retraction
Wound margin strangulation
Stretching of vascular elements
Blood flow interruption
Lack of venous outflow
Excessive compression from dressings

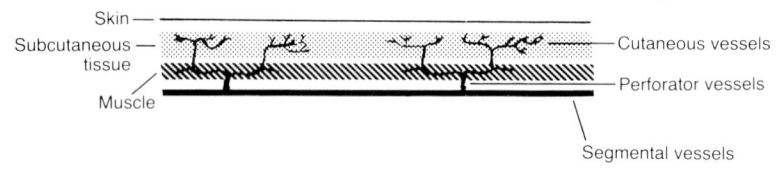

11.1 Schematic drawing of blood supply to skin, subcutaneous tissues, and underlying musculature. (From Christensen and Dockery[2].)

Cutaneous complications

In recent years, foot surgeons are utilizing retained metallic hardware more frequently. Erythema, swelling, dermatitis, and other manifestations present themselves as a direct response to the underlying metal in those patients who have metal allergies: this is especially true in hardware that contains nickel alloys. Surgical stainless steel is the most common metal used in hardware for bone surgery. In patients who show allergies to stainless steel, other metals such as titanium and vitallium may be used. If internal hardware is being planned as part of the surgical procedure, it is important to obtain a good history of metal allergies from the patient. Asking about allergies to jewellery, such as the metal post of earrings, may be a clue to metal allergy. If metal allergy is suspected following placement of deep-buried hardware, then simple removal of the metal may be in order and the tissue reaction is usually reversible.

Excessive scar formation

This post-surgical condition includes hypertrophic and keloid-type scars. A keloid is an exaggerated fibroblastic reparative response to skin injury. Clinically, the keloid presents as a red, raised, and thickened lesion that may be pruritic.[3] The tendency to form keloid scars is believed to be genetic.[4] Hypertrophic scars are widened raised scars which differ histologically from keloids. Clinically, the hypertrophic scar is encountered relatively frequently and stays within the boundary of the wound site (**11.2**), whereas the keloid is relatively rare and has a markedly raised and malignant-like growth which can encompass normal adjacent tissue and may become pedunculated or pendulous (**11.3**).[4] It is important for the surgeon to determine if a patient undergoing elective surgery has any history of scar-forming problems and to determine if they are keloid formers. It is recommended that elective surgery in documented keloid formers should be avoided if possible.

Hypertrophic scars are generally caused by the same aetiological mechanisms as delayed wound healing (see **Table 11.1**). Excessive motion, at incision sites that cross joints, early in the wound-healing process also leads to a propensity for development of scar hypertrophy. Therefore, it is advisable, in a clinical setting of delayed wound healing, to limit activity, which would otherwise further complicate the situation.

11.2 Photograph of a hypertrophic scar following proximal phalanx osteotomy. (Courtesy of Dr G. Dockery, Seattle, USA.)

Neurovascular complications

Haemorrhagic complications

It is not within the scope of this chapter to discuss primary haematological defects that affect the clotting mechanism. Bleeding problems, if elicited, should be appropriately investigated and elective foot surgery should be carefully assessed in the patient with a blood factor or clotting deficit. This section, however, discusses several haemorrhagic complications that are commonly associated with forefoot surgery.

In patients with a normal platelet count and intact clotting mechanism having forefoot surgery, the presence of severe haemorrhagic complications is low. The foot seems to respond reasonably well to compression dressings after most surgical procedures. As long as good surgical technique with adequate haemostasis is accomplished, combined with care and concern while operating around vascular bundles, then severe haemorrhagic complications will rarely be encountered.

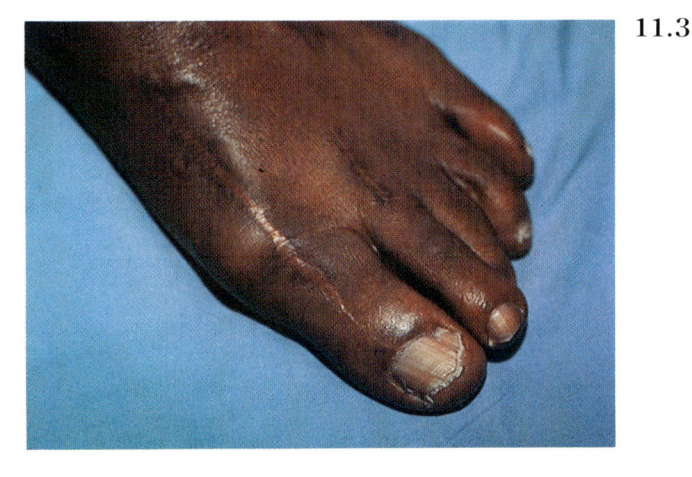

11.3 Photograph of moderate keloid formation following bunion surgery. (Courtesy of Dr G. Dockery, Seattle, USA.)

Haematoma

The most frequently encountered complication in forefoot surgery is probably the simple haematoma. As discussed in the delayed wound healing section, the presence of haematoma relates to the use of tourniquet control and the lack of deflation prior to wound closure to ensure complete haemostasis. In surgical situations where haemostasis is difficult, such as extensive surgical dissection, and medullary or cancellous bone bleeding, a closed suction drainage system is frequently beneficial in preventing haematoma.

When bleeding is significant from involved reconstructive procedures, dead space from extensive dissection, or generalized cancellous bone haemorrhage, the potential for development of haematoma increases. The wound should then be adequately drained to prevent any potential complications associated with haematoma. In this surgical setting, it is recommended that a form of closed suction drainage be utilized as a preventative measure to avoid haematoma formation.[5] Since haematoma or seroma increases the potential for wound infection, antibiotic prophylaxis is recommended in surgical procedures that are prone to haematoma formation: this permits incorporation of antibiotics within the haematoma. If a haematoma is diagnosed early, then it may be prudent to attempt to aspirate the haematoma and re-evaluate a few hours later. If haematoma development or excessive bleeding into dressing persists, then the wound should be opened and examined to determine the source of the haemorrhage (**11.4**).

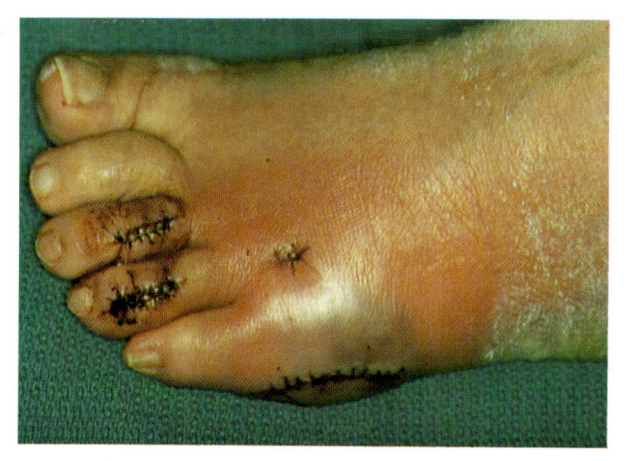

11.4 Photograph of secondary infection from haematoma formation after hammertoe surgery and correction of tailor's bunion. Proper haemostasis was not maintained and a drain was not utilized.

Drug-induced haematologic disorders

The potential for haematoma development increases with platelet inhibition induced by aspirin (acetylsalicylic acid) and non-steroidal anti-inflammatory products. Platelets are permanently inhibited by aspirin intake and a patient should be taken off aspirin products before elective surgical procedures. Non-steroidal anti-inflammatory medications cause a reversible platelet inhibition; therefore, they may be discontinued 3–4 days before surgery to get adequate platelet-binding activity.

Reflex sympathetic dystrophy

Reflex sympathetic dystrophy (RSD) is a syndrome of burning pain, hyperaesthesia, swelling, hyperhidrosis, and trophic changes of the skin and bone of the affected extremity. It is well known that it starts almost invariably at some time following an injury. A major or minor trauma may be associated with the development of RSD. The disease was first described by Mitchell under the term causalgia during the American civil war. Over the past 100 years it has been determined that RSD involves an over-activity of the sympathetic nervous system.

This disease entity is described in stages, whereby a series of symptoms and signs occur at rather non-specific intervals after onset of the disease. For the most part, each case of RSD is expressed differently. Classically, after the initial injury, there is a pattern of progressive discomfort, followed by a period of 2 weeks to 2 months post-injury where there develops evidence of vasoconstriction. This causes ischaemic pain—the pain of inadequate blood supply which, consistently, is extremely painful in all documented cases of RSD. In addition to vasoconstriction, over-activity of the sympathetic nervous system also seems to amplify the pain.

In most cases, as the disease evolves, the pain is intense and is severely aggravated by any movement or pressure, such as weight-bearing. Commonly, even wearing a slipper or sock is painful. Physical examination frequently reveals a shiny skin and diffuse swelling to the injured part. Skin temperature of the affected area becomes strikingly lower than the unaffected extremity.

With continued sympathetic activity, RSD progresses, with an inflammatory response occurring in the bone. This inflammation is caused by poor blood supply and disuse of the body part due to the extreme pain. The effect on bone can be measured with positive bone scan findings and eventual radiographic changes in bone appearance with the hallmark of patchy osteoporosis, which is termed Sudeck's atrophy.

Treatment of reflex sympathetic dystrophy

Treatment of RSD depends in part on the status of the disease at the time a definitive diagnosis is made. If treatment is initiated before osteoporosis develops and while there is still good motion in the extremity, the prognosis is improved somewhat. The treatment of the cases that have radiographic evidence of patchy osteoporosis is usually far less successful.

Reflex sympathetic dystrophy is known to respond to various kinds of therapy, including physical therapy, pain control, sympathetic blocks with local anaesthetic, chemical sympathetic blockade, steroid therapy, and surgical sympathectomy.

Interruption of sympathetic overflow to the affected limb is a well-documented treatment. Serial lumbar sympathetic blocks and use of drugs that induce chemical sympathectomy, such as guanethidine, reserpine, and bretylium—injected into the affected extremity via a modified Bier technique—can provide significant relief of sympathetic over-activity from hours' to months' duration, depending on the severity of the condition. These periods of resolution then permit vigorous physical therapy.

Surgical removal of a portion of the sympathetic ganglia, which is attributed to some of the sympathetic overflow, may permanently reduce the sympathetic overflow and usually relieve all or some of the pain associated with RSD (**11.5**). For chronic intractable cases where other treatments have failed, there have been encouraging results with epidural morphine pumps.

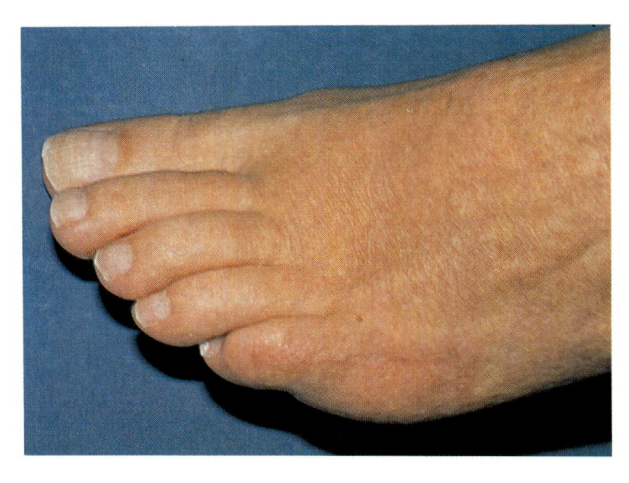

11.5 Photograph of segmental reflex sympathetic dystrophy (RSD) after fifth metatarsophalangeal joint arthroplasty. Note loss of skin tone, hair loss, and colour changes.

Symptomatic incisional neuromas

Peri-incisional sensory nerve neuromas are a common complication of forefoot surgery. The incidence of occurrence is not known; however, the clinical presentation of peri-incisional anaesthesia, dysaesthesia or paraesthesia is well documented.[6] Neuromas develop when a nerve is accidentally sutured, traumatically retracted, transected (bulb neuroma), or entrapped in scar tissue. According to Sunderland's classification, a spindle neuroma is a neuroma where the perineurium is intact, a lateral neuroma is where the perineurium has been breached, and bulb neuromas form on the ends of transected or severed nerves.[7] A symptomatic sensory neuroma can be extremely painful and totally disabling. The clinical presentation associated with the diagnosis of peri-incisional sensory neuroma is a history of paraesthesias, anaesthesias or dysaesthesias over the incision site. Positive physical findings include a Tinel's sign over the incision and an area of decreased or altered sensation distal to the entrapment site. Treatment options include neurolysis, proximal nerve resection, nerve capping, and nerve grafting.

The use of the dorsal medial incision for bunion correction, placed over the dorsal proper digital nerve, is frequently associated with nerve entrapment or injury. A longer, more dorsally placed, incision for bunionectomy is recommended, with incisional placement just medial to the extensor hallucis longus tendon.

It is best to understand the aetiology of peri-incisional neuromas and take precautions to prevent this condition. Good incisional placement, meticulous dissection, gentle retraction, and control of haemostasis are all factors that will help in preventing incisional neuromas.

Osseous-related complications

Thermal necrosis

With the general acceptance of power instrumentation in the performance of forefoot surgery, there is an increased risk of surgical complication as a direct result of improper use or technique, causing thermal necrosis of bone. Thermal injury from pin insertion has been documented and is related to the configuration of the pin tip.[8] The trochar tip generates the most heat, whereas the drill tip pin the least. Excessive heat generated from pin placement can cause cylindrical heat necrosis and lead to pin-tract infections.

During the creation of an osteotomy with the use of pneumatic saws, a high temperature can be reached, imparting a significant adjacent zone of osseous thermal necrosis that can affect the rate or ability to adequately heal the osteotomy site. There is a spectrum of thermal injury that can cause damage to bone, ranging from slight delay in bone union to an overt fibrous non-union. It is imperative that the surgeon utilizes sharp saw blades and properly irrigates the surgical wound during osteotomy placement to prevent thermal necrotic injury and eventual delayed healing or non-union.

Micromotion

The purpose of internal fixation is to achieve accurate reduction of the fracture or osteotomy and provide rigid maintenance of the bone fragments to permit immediate mobilization of the articulations. Motionless rigid fixation and accurate reduction are the primary prerequisites for the efficient use of internal fixation. Interfragmentary micromotion, consisting of movement in excess of 1 µm, can cause significant pressure necrosis and resorption at the fracture or osteotomy site, which can significantly delay or disable bone healing. It is therefore necessary to achieve rigid internal fixation with interfragmentary compression at the osteotomy or fracture site to prevent interfragmentary motion and strain.[9] In a transverse osteotomy, resorption of one to two cell layers in thickness will abolish the compression present at the osteotomy.[10]

Delayed union and non-union

All osteotomy, arthrodesis, and fracture sites that are going to heal will have healed or showed signs of healing within 4 months. The differentiation between delayed union and non-union is defined as sites not healed at 4 months and sites not healed at 9 months, respectively: this is an arbitrary classification, but one that is widely accepted. There are several major causes of delayed unions and non-union (**Table 11.3**) and control of these factors may prevent their occurrence. Delayed unions or non-unions in the forefoot are at times very problematic because of difficulty in preventing relative motion at the fracture or osteotomy site with cast immobilization only. Therefore careful attention to internal fixation is especially important in forefoot surgery to decrease the incidence of delayed union or non-union.

Non-unions are divided into two categories: (1) hypertrophic (elephant foot) type, and (2) atrophic. Hypertrophic forms are caused by excessive motion occurring between the bone fragments, whereas atrophic non-unions are caused by inadequate vascularity or infection at the non-union site (**11.6**).[11]

Osteomyelitis

Post-surgical osteomyelitis is a direct infection of bone from an exogenous source (**11.7, 11.8**). A significant cause for delayed or non-healing of bone is osteomyelitis. Bacteriological breakdown of bone matrix in an environment of relatively diminished blood perfusion creates a clinical situation which is difficult to manage.[12]

It is important for the forefoot surgeon to be aware of antibiotic prophylactic methods and have a high index of suspicion for osteomyelitis when delayed bone healing is discovered. Early discovery and prompt aggressive treatment is imperative to limit the potential destructive nature of this condition.

Generally, treatment is indicated in acute osteomyelitis in the foot, especially if there is evidence of abscess formation or poor response to antibiotics. In chronic osteomyelitis, surgery is necessary to remove all septic and dysvascular tissue (sequestra). Historically, osteomyelitic bone was considered a barrier to antibiotic treatment, however, recent investigations have shown that antibiotic penetration is not impaired by osteomyelitic bone.[13] Therefore, surgical treatment for osteomyelitis needs only to resect devitalized bone whereby residual infected living bone can be treated via antibiotic therapy. It is prudent to obtain a medical consultation or request assistance from an infectious disease specialist for this complication.

Table 11.3 Aetiology of delayed union and non-union

Inadequate rigid internal fixation
Distraction between fragments
Gaping between fragments
Interposed tissue between fragments
Malposition of fragments
Infection
Various systemic conditions/disorders

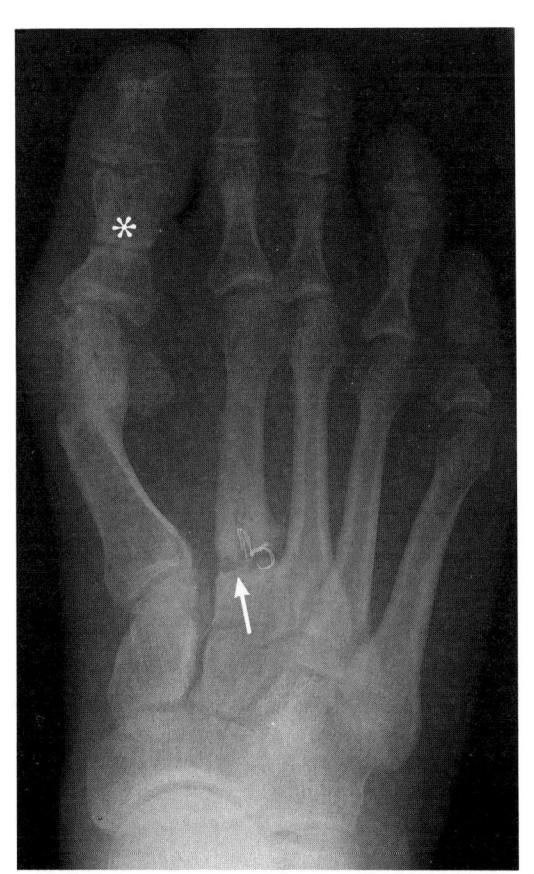

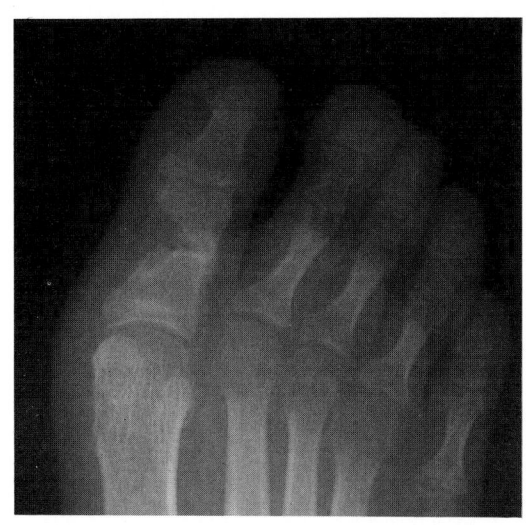

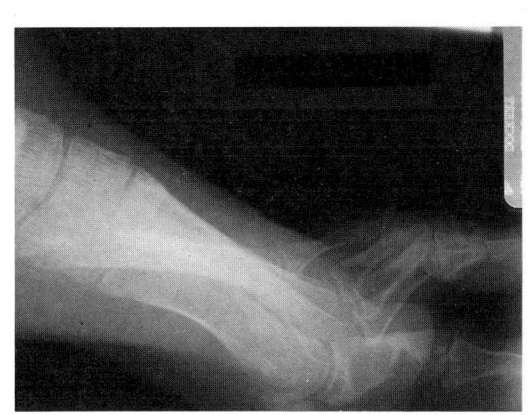

11.6 Radiograph of a symptomatic hypertrophic non-union at the base of the second metatarsal (arrow head) and an asymptomatic atrophic non-union of the proximal phalanx of the hallux (asterisk). The hallux non-union was caused from a screw supporting a gaped osteotomy site (note the sclerotic margins). The second metatarsal base osteotomy was inadequately fixated with monofilament wire.

11.7, 11.8 Radiographs of a chronic osteomyelitis of an osteotomy site from a proximal phalanx osteotomy of the hallux.

Technical osteotomy complications

The technical aspects of osteotomy placement at times can be very challenging and may lead to surgical complications. A very difficult to manage complication is osteotomy misplacement. This usually occurs when the surgical site is under-dissected, or from surgical inexperience. Spacial interrelationships can be misinterpreted and the osteotomy location wrongly placed. This can be very dangerous if localized near joint structures or diaphyseal bone, if the osteotomy is designed to be located in metaphyseal bone.

Other technical complications of osteotomies include errors in osteotomy configuration/design (**11.9**). This is especially true in forefoot surgery where the osteotomies are very complex as in bicorrectional types of osteotomies. If the saw cut is slightly off, it can be very difficult to close, as well as to fixate. An example of this is an Austin chevron osteotomy of the first metatarsal head that has cut surfaces that diverge from medial to lateral. This would prevent transposition of the distal fragment. Conversely, Austin chevron osteotomy cuts that converge from medial to lateral will lose significant bone surface congruity, which may lead to delayed union or non-union.

Complications in osteotomy fixation are encountered in forefoot surgery especially when the surface area of the osteotomy is limited or the configuration of the cut forces the surgeon to utilize a less than optimal fixation approach. Other types of fixation errors occur when improper technique is utilized (**11.10**).

Bone stock complications

There are instances of intra-operative complications that are related to the quality of bone stock. This is usually not a problem in younger patients; however, there are times where benign lesions may interfere with osteotomy placement or fixation methods. More frequently, the foot surgeon is faced with a situation of trying to fixate osteoporotic bone that can be most challenging and may lead to potential fixation failure complications.

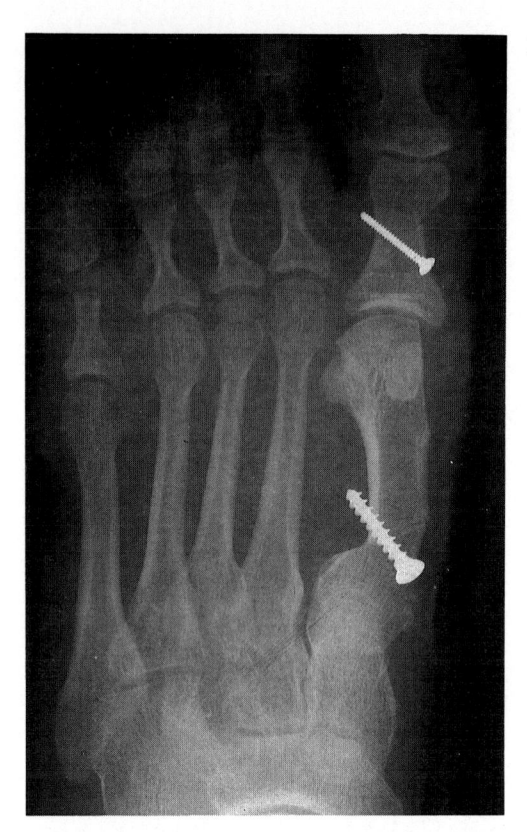

11.9 Radiograph of a misplaced (mid-shaft) first metatarsal osteotomy. Note the overcorrection of the distal fragment.

Soft tissue surgery of the forefoot

Complications of Morton's neuroma

A common complication following Morton's neuroma surgery is the development of a haematoma (see section on Haematoma complications).[14] Other complications include stump neuroma, infection, and transection of lumbrical tendon with associated digital diversion.

Skin flap failure

Flap failure continues to be a common clinical complication with plastic surgical procedures of the forefoot. Currently, the aetiology of flap failure is attributed to intrinsic or extrinsic factors. The only intrinsic factor

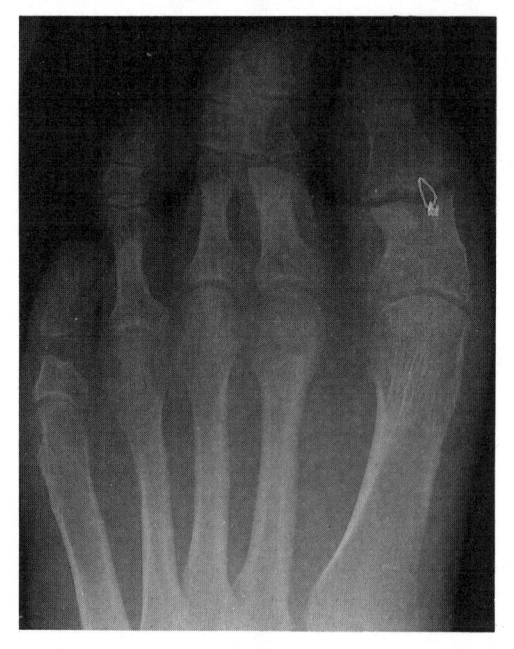

11.10 Radiograph depicting a failed hallux interphalangeal joint arthrodesis site due to an error in fixation technique. A single loop of monofilament wire creates a situation of one-point fixation, which is unstable at any arthrodesis site.

known to cause flap failure is a lack of nutrient blood flow. Whether flap survival relative to blood flow is due to venous or arterial insufficiency has not been clearly delineated. Some investigators conclude that venous insufficiency is the primary cause of necrosis in pedicle flap tissue, even if there appears to be adequate arterial inflow.[15] Other authors base flap necrosis primarily on inadequate arterial blood flow.[16] Extrinsic factors that lead to flap failure include infection, arteriosclerosis, hypotension, and diabetes mellitus. Local factors are excessive skin traction, haematoma, anastomotic thrombosis, excessive compression, and kinking of the pedicle flap.

A pedicle flap that is surviving on marginal blood flow is very susceptible to infection. Once infection has set in, it is necessary to debride the necrotic tissue; otherwise, the necrotic tissue may further thrombosis and possibly threaten the viability of the remainder of the flap.[2] Flap survival variables are different for each type of flap and for each anatomical location. One must have sound knowledge of tissue survivability for all types of flaps, or a high rate of failure may be experienced. A thorough knowledge of blood flow patterns of the foot and leg are paramount as well as an insight into the fundamental concepts of flap mechanics, including the delay phenomenon, designing flaps, length-to-width ratios and evaluation of flap vascularity. Inappropriate or poorly performed flap procedures may create situations that are more difficult to manage than the original problem; therefore, judicial use of these procedures is recommended.

First ray surgical complications

Hallux varus

Acquired hallux varus is a dynamic abducted deformity of the hallux which has been known to be a postoperative complication of hallux abductovalgus surgery (especially the McBride procedure). Treatment frequently centres around tissue balancing in acute cases or joint implant replacement in more chronic conditions.

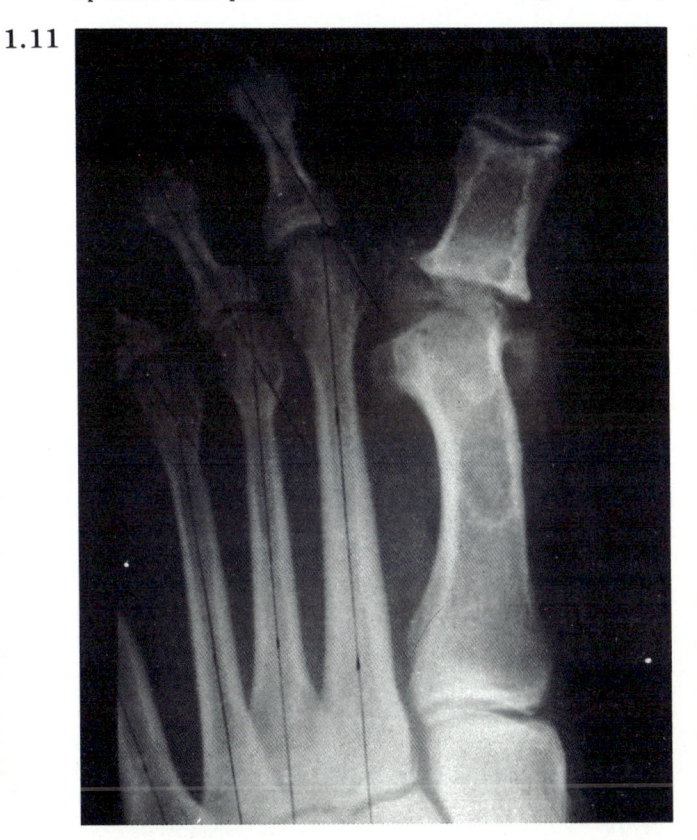

11.11 Radiograph of a hallux varus condition secondary to failure of a total silicone elastomer joint implant.

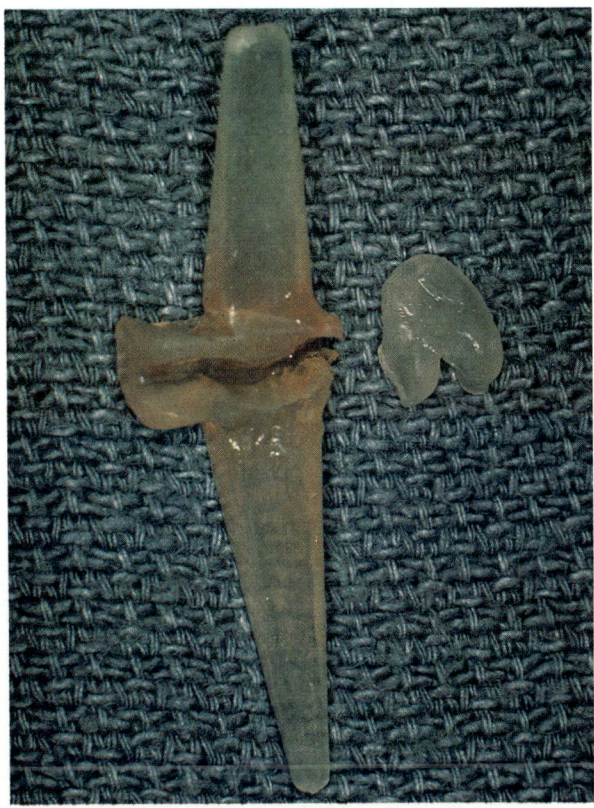

11.12 Photograph of the failed total joint implant.

However, hallux varus may even occur when the first metatarsophalangeal joint has been replaced with a total hinged implant that has failed (**11.11, 11.12**). When the severity of the hallux abductovalgus deformity is underestimated, a futile attempt by the surgeon is sometimes made to over-reef the medial joint capsule and release the lateral joint structures. This may unbalance the periarticular structures and lead to a hallux varus condition. **Table 11.4** reviews other possible aetiologies for developing a hallux varus complication. Isolated fibular sesamoidectomy or bunionectomy combined with sesamoidectomy and its relationship towards a hallux varus condition must be emphasized. Once a diagnosis of hallux varus is made, then it should be aggressively treated with an attempt to rebalance the periarticular structures; otherwise, progression of the deformity may occur with increased severity, hammering of the hallux and adductus migration of the second digit (**11.13**).

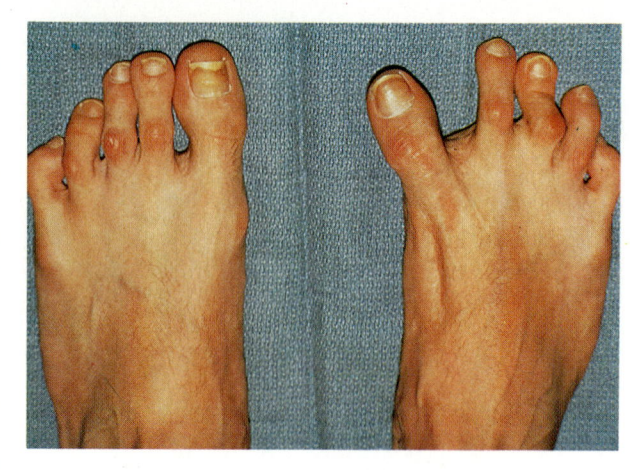

11.13 Photograph of severe hallux varus condition with second and third digital hammering.

Table 11.4 Aetiology of hallux varus

Over-reefing of medial joint structures
Staking or excessive medial resection of first metatarsal head
Over-correction of intermetatarsal angle
Fibular sesamoidectomy
Excessive release of lateral joint structures

Adhesive capsulitis

Adhesive capsulitis following simple bunionectomy procedures is a common occurrence and rarely leads to any long-term sequelae. Usually near normal range-of-motion returns to the first metatarsophalangeal joint within a couple of months, unless overzealous capsulorrhaphy or extensive capsular release was accomplished.

Bunionectomy without osteotomy

The prototype procedure of this group is the McBride procedure. This method is generally utilized for mild symptomatic bunion conditions.

Undercorrection/error in procedure selection

A surgical error in performing a bunionectomy without osteotomy is attempting soft tissue correction in situations that require osseous correction (**11.14**). There

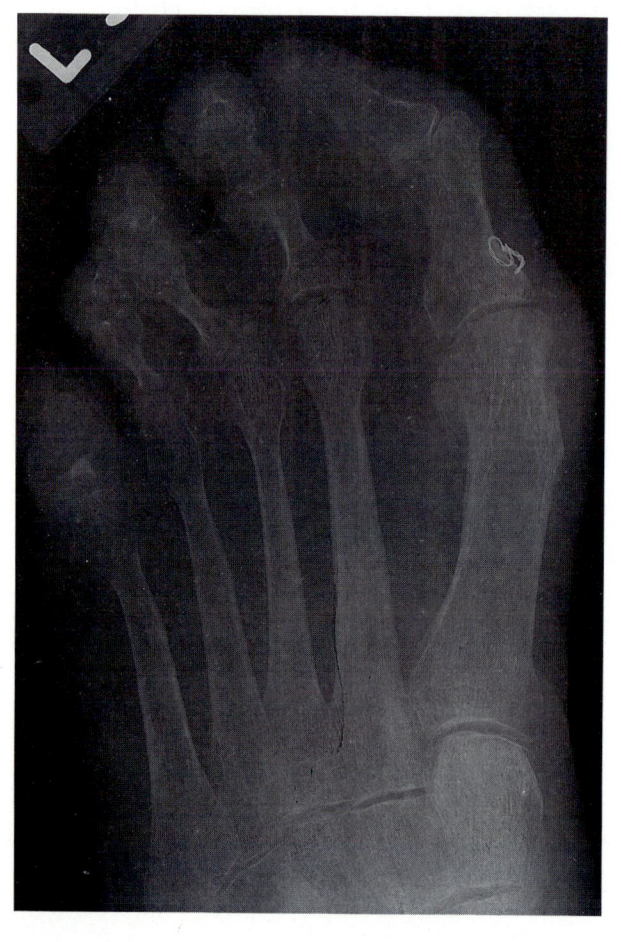

11.14 Radiograph of a recurrent hallux abductovalgus deformity following a modified McBride-type bunionectomy with osteotomy of the proximal phalanx of the hallux.

are instances where osseous correction is the only mechanism to achieve adequate correction of the deformity. To get consistent results with bunion surgery, a thorough knowledge of the limitations of the various techniques is necessary to prevent errors in procedure selection. In this clinical situation, the performance of a soft tissue correction procedure will lead to an undercorrection of the deformity or a rapid recurrence of the deformity.

First metatarsal neck osteotomy

Bunionectomy with metatarsal neck osteotomy is usually reserved for mild-to-moderate bunion deformities with a metatarsal primus varus of less than 15°. There are numerous complications associated with first metatarsal neck osteotomies (**Table 11.5**). The most common complication is the frequently described limited joint range-of-motion. Other notable complications include avascular necrosis, first metatarsal shortening, and metatarsal head displacement.[17–19] These may be under-reported complications and can be very disabling and lead to surgical failure. Inadequate, failure, or lack of internal fixation may lead to metatarsal head displacement or dislocation. Avascular necrosis of the first metatarsal head has been reported to be associated with first metatarsal neck osteotomies; however, the incidence is very low and its occurrence seems to be related to over-aggressive first metatarsophalangeal joint dissection combined with first metatarsal neck osteotomy.

Under-correction of a bunion condition can result from attempting to correct a large metatarsus primus varus position. Other complications may occur with errors in surgical technique, especially with complicated osteotomy cuts. Pitfalls may not only involve the osteotomy but the fixation techniques as well.

Incidence of delayed union and non-union of the first metatarsal after osteotomy is low, with or without weight-bearing. Weight-bearing will compress most neck osteotomy configurations and with the osteotomy located in metaphyseal bone this allows for rapid healing in most instances.

In cases of fixation failure and loss of correction, if alignment is unacceptable, the surgeon must re-operate. If the alignment is acceptable, then it is recommended to place the patient in a non-weight-bearing status (**11.15**).

In a series of 33 Mitchell osteotomies a 9% incidence of second metatarsalgia was demonstrated as the most common complication. Two cases of second metatarsal stress fracture were also noted. These complications are probably related to first metatarsal shortening.[18]

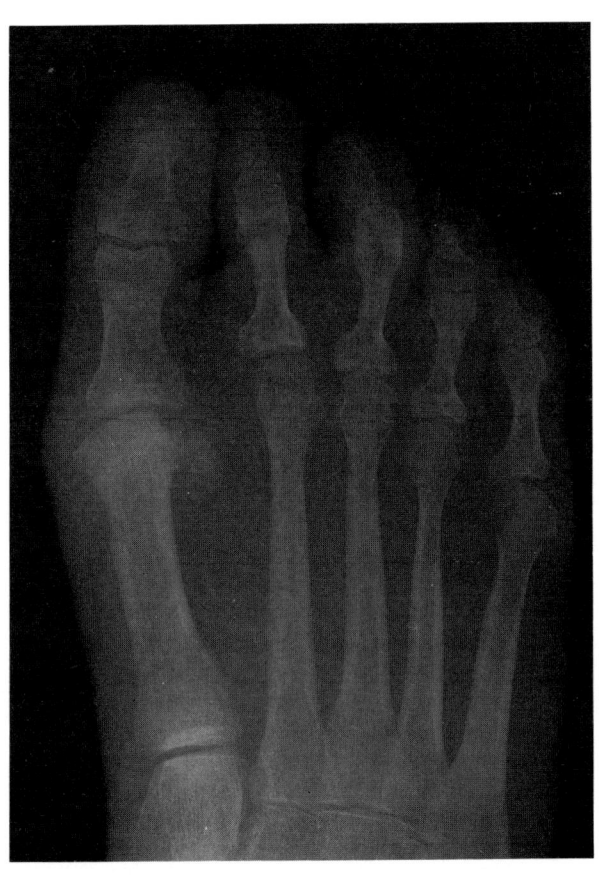

11.15 Radiograph of a medially displaced first metatarsal neck osteotomy that healed uneventfully with non-weight-bearing.

Table 11.5 First metatarsal neck osteotomy complications

Delayed/non-union
Malunion
Avascular necrosis of first metatarsal head
Hallux varus
Metatarsal head displacement/dislocation
Fixation failure
Technical osteotomy complications
Adhesive capsulitis

First metatarsal base or shaft osteotomy

The base or shaft osteotomy of the first metatarsal is very useful in reducing the metatarsus primus adductus component of hallux abductovalgus deformity. The majority of the complications associated with this class of surgical procedure are associated with fixation failure and osteotomy displacement (**11.16**). This can lead to a complete loss of correction and elevation deformity of the first metatarsal (metatarsus primus elevatus) due to the effect of ground reactive forces. Other complications include osteotomy placement errors which result in malalignment of the distal metatarsal fragment (**Table 11.6**). Osteotomy misplacement can lead to over- or under-correction of the intermetatarsal angle. A more severe complication is improper osteotomy configuration, where the distal metatarsal fragment is elevated from the weight-bearing plane (**11.17**). An elevated first metatarsal usually is associated with lesser metatarsalgia, transfer lesions, lesser metatarsal stress fractures, and first metatarsophalangeal joint stiffness. Curda and Sorto in their series of closing base wedge osteotomies with wire fixation discussed complications including residual hallux abductovalgus, hallux varus, first metatarsal elevation, and other joint complaints.[20]

The location of a first metatarsal osteotomy to a more proximal position poses an increased risk for mechanically induced displacement from premature weight-bearing. Schuberth et al.[21] noted in a retrospective study of 159 feet with closing first metatarsal base wedge osteotomy that 93.7% had post-operative elevation and the average elevation was 6.7° on the sagittal plane. This study suggests that unilateral surgery, screw fixation, and post-operative immobilization with non-weight-bearing cause less distal metatarsal elevation.

Ground reactive forces on the first metatarsal with a basal osteotomy impart a greater force on the osteotomy site than an osteotomy localized to the metatarsal neck. Sagittal plane displacement can occur with a weight-bearing cast. Therefore, to prevent dorsal displacement of the proximal metatarsal osteotomy, it is imperative that the patient maintain a non-weight-bearing status for 4–6 weeks.

Table 11.6 Complications of metatarsal base wedge osteotomy

Distal segment elevation
Delayed/non-union
First metatarsal shortening
Over-reduction of intermetatarsal angle
Technical osteotomy complications
Fixation failure/early weight-bearing

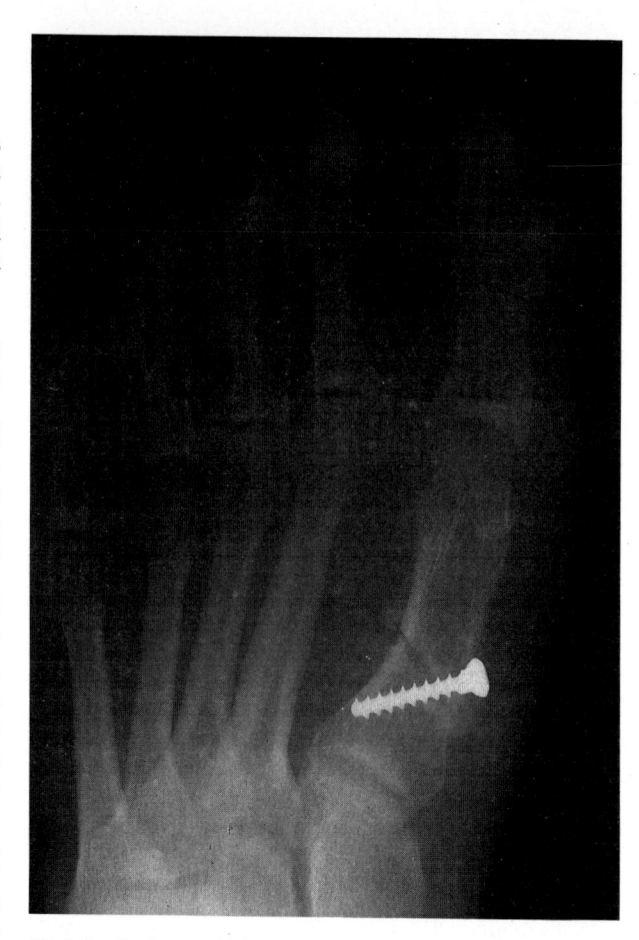

11.16 Radiograph demonstrates fixation failure of a first metatarsal closing base wedge osteotomy with bone callous formation around the osteotomy site as a result of intrafragmentary micromotion.

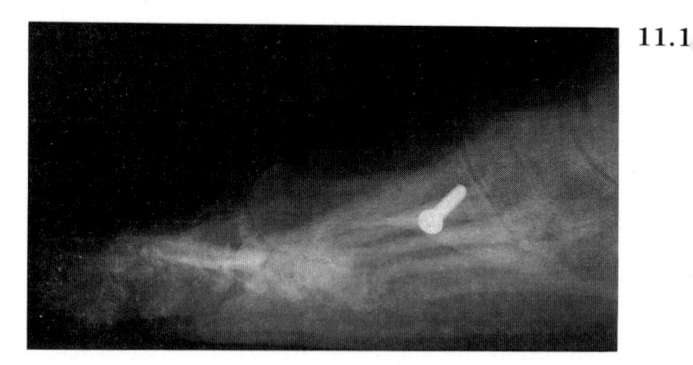

11.17 Radiograph depicts a healed oblique first metatarsal osteotomy with marked elevation of the distal segment within the sagittal plane (metatarsus primus elevatus). This is caused from wedging the metatarsal perpendicular to the shaft rather than perpendicular to the weight-bearing plane.

First metatarsal cuneiform joint arthrodesis

Frequently described as the Lapidus procedure,[22] this procedure effectively decreases first ray movement and will correct the deformity of metatarsal primus varus. A side effect associated with this procedure is the elimination of first ray movement. In some instances this will lead to an eventual long-term complication of hallux limitus and potential degeneration of the first metatarsophalangeal joint. It is also associated with a high non-union rate (reports of up to 30%). First ray position and length complications have also been reported.

Restriction of first-ray movement

Performing a first metatarsal cuneiform joint arthrodesis effectively reduces first ray hypermobility and there is usually residual but limited first ray movement. If the arthrodesis is extended to include the base of the second metatarsal, then complete first-ray motion will be eliminated. This effectively causes a functional hallux limitus and eventual first metatarsophalangeal joint breakdown (**11.18**).

First metatarsophalangeal joint arthrodesis (Table 11.7)

Malposition

Malposition-related complications are very common types of complaints noted with this procedure. Malposition usually occurs in the transverse and sagittal planes: most of the problems are found in female patients, as a result of the additional biomechanical demands associated with female shoe styles. There is evidence of a long-term complication of hallux interphalangeal joint degeneration with this procedure, which seems to be more of a problem if there is little or no valgus position of the toe at the time of fusion.[23]

Non-union/fixation failure

Technically this is not a difficult joint to fuse unless there have been prior procedures that could potentially complicate the healing capacity of the bone. In the event of non-union, re-operation is generally indicated due to pain at the arthrodesis site.

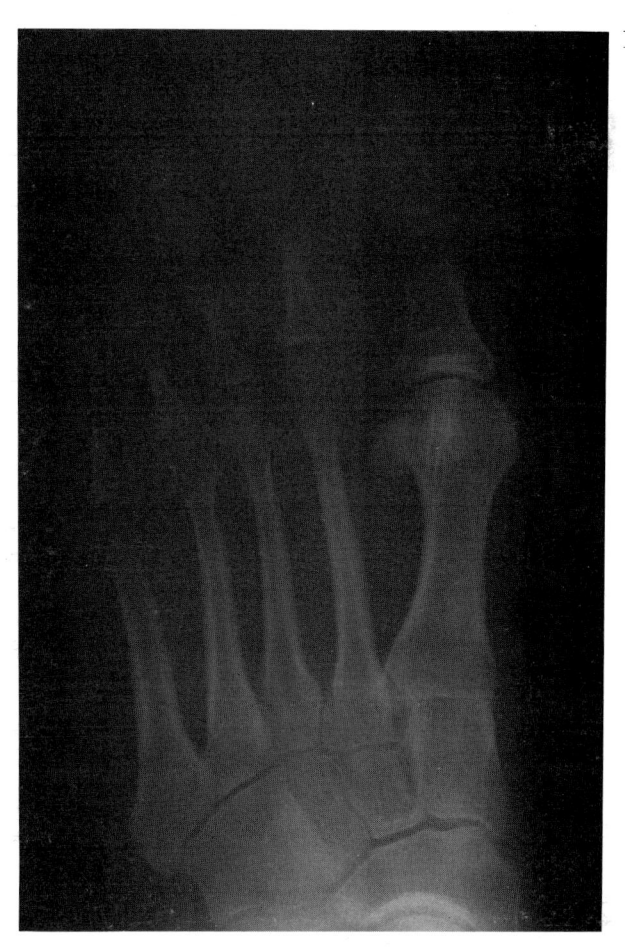

11.18 Radiograph of a modified Lapidus base arthrodesis 6 years post-operatively. This surgery fused the first metatarsal cuneiform joint and the first and second metatarsal bases.

Table 11.7 Complications of first MPJ fusion

Metatarsalgia
Interphalangeal joint arthritis
Hallux malposition
Non-union
Alterations in gait
Difficulty in wearing certain shoe styles

First metatarsophalangeal arthroplasty

The Keller procedure is the eponym associated with the resection of the base of the proximal phalanx for treatment of hallux valgus condition. This is the most commonly accepted of first metatarsophalangeal joint destructive procedures. Because of the severely high functional complication rate with isolated metatarsal head procedures they should only be performed under extreme and necessary circumstances. The Keller procedure has been reported to relieve the pain and disability of the hallux valgus condition, but it does so at the expense of hallux function. Therefore as Lapidus[22] described: 'The big toe becomes a short dangling appendage, held above the ground' and the loss of propulsive properties of the hallux as a result of the Keller operation by Joplin is a consistent side effect of the Keller and should not be considered a complication of the procedure *per se*.[24]

First metatarsophalangeal joint replacement (Table 11.8)

Implant failure

Implant failure is generally caused by technical errors in placement or excessive demands on the implant (*see* **11.11, 11.12**). Not removing sufficient bone at the joint level causes excessive pressure and demands on the implant. This type of surgical error is responsible for implant particulate matter formation and breakage of the implant itself.

Lack of toe purchase

A common occurrence with this procedure, lack of toe purchase is not considered a complication but merely a mechanical side effect of the procedure. This problem can sometimes be controlled by the reattachment of the short flexor tendon to the base of the proximal phalanx prior to implantation.[25–27]

Technical errors in placement

The most devastating problem associated with implant surgery is placement of the prosthesis with too little bone removed, which causes avascular necrosis and breakdown on all osseous interfaces. Telescoping deformities with the implant being swallowed by the adjacent bone have been attributed to excessive tightness of fit and placement of too small an implant.[26]

Procedure selection errors

Alignment of the osseous structure is necessary prior to completing implantation of a joint (**11.19**).
Complete sesamoidectomy with implantation will cause a lack of purchase of the first metatarsophalangeal joint, which may lead to some balance problems and potentially chronic lesser metatarsalgia and stress fracture of adjacent metatarsals.

Table 11.8 Errors in flexible joint implant placement

Too little bone removed
Uncorrected joint alignment
Implant too small
Sharp bone margins at hinge–stem interface
Breach of cortex within stem holes
Improper positioning of stem holes
Improper handling of implant

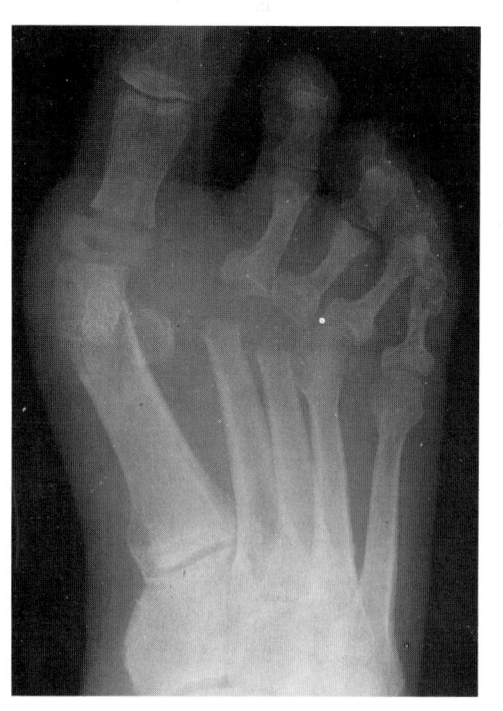

11.19 Radiograph of an implant arthroplasty improperly placed due to failure to correct the alignment at the joint level. Note the improper placement of the implant stems.

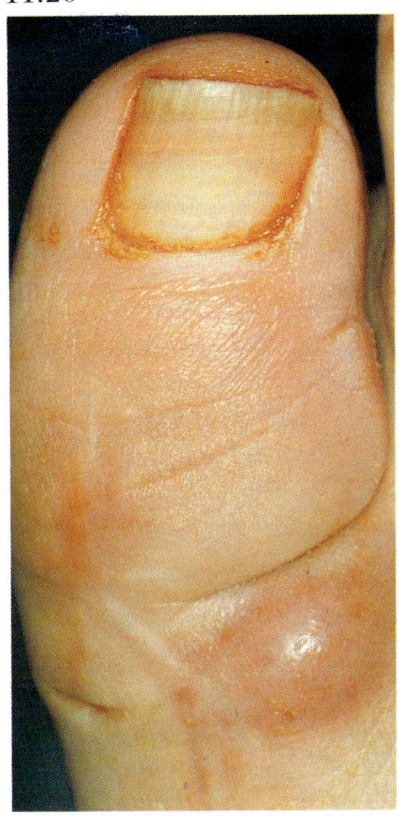

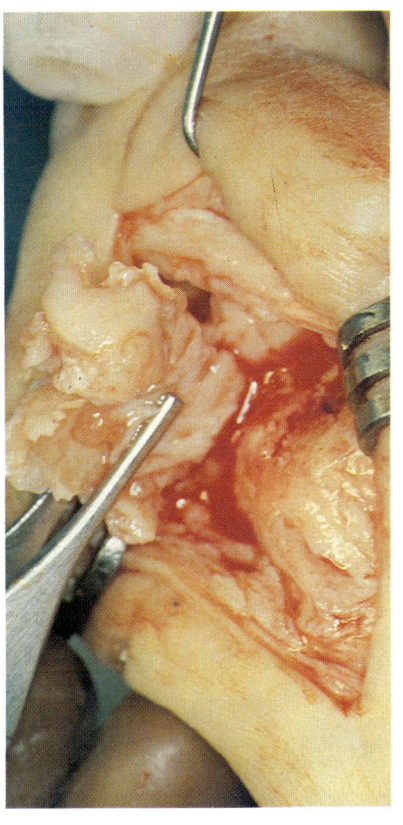

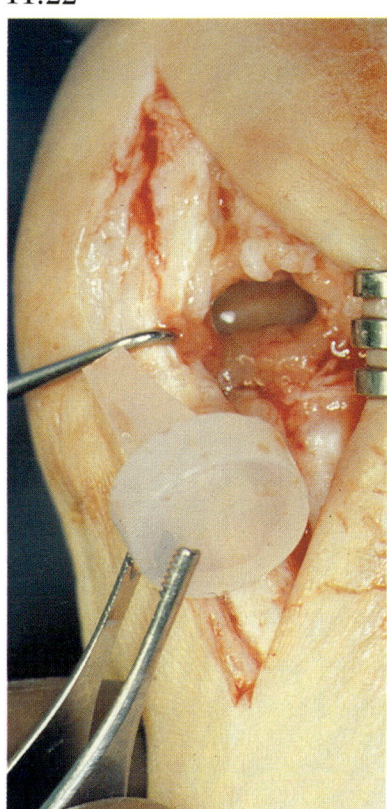

11.20 Cutaneous erythema caused from a fulminant implant foreign body reaction.

11.21 Intra-operative photograph of reactive synovitis and foreign body reaction secondary to the implant.

11.22 A rejected silicone great toe hemi-implant during implant removal.

Detritic synovitis with histological evidence of giant cell formation and synovial shards have been described in numerous cases.[25–27] This condition is attributed to the exposed bone-wearing and abrading of the smooth surface of the implant. Flexible implants are designed to piston and move within the medullary canal to increase the available motion at the implant site. This leads to a low grade foreign body reaction to these particles. In situations of excessive wear due to inappropriate fit or excessive demands on the implant, the particulate matter can be seen with a clinically significant foreign body reaction and possible implant failure (**11.20–11.22**). The development of medullary grommets has helped decrease the potential abrasion at the hinge–bone interface, where wear and failure are most significant.

Lesser metatarsal surgery

The same complications with osteotomy and joint implantation of the first metatarsal occur with the lesser metatarsals (**Table 11.9**). When a simple fifth metatarsal head procedure is being performed for the correction of tailor's bunionette or prominent condyle, the same considerations for removal of bone from the head are present as when the procedure is on the first metatarsal. When too much bone is removed from the lat-

Table 11.9 Complications in implant arthroplasty

Hallux extensus
Recurrence of hallux abductovalgus
Short hallux
Transfer lesions
Implant failure
Hallux varus
Lesser metatarsal stress fracture
Implant dislocation
Metatarsalgia sub second
Infection

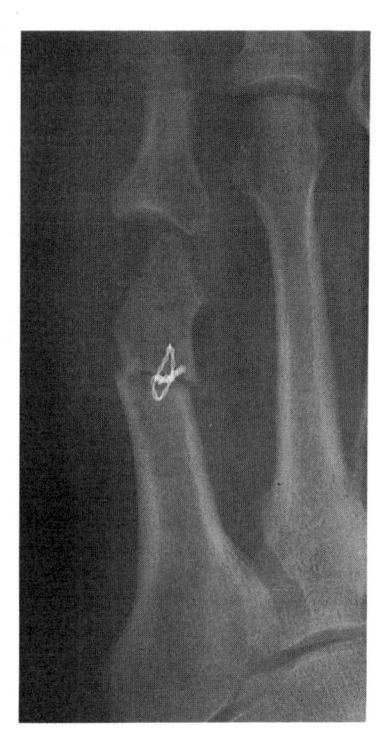

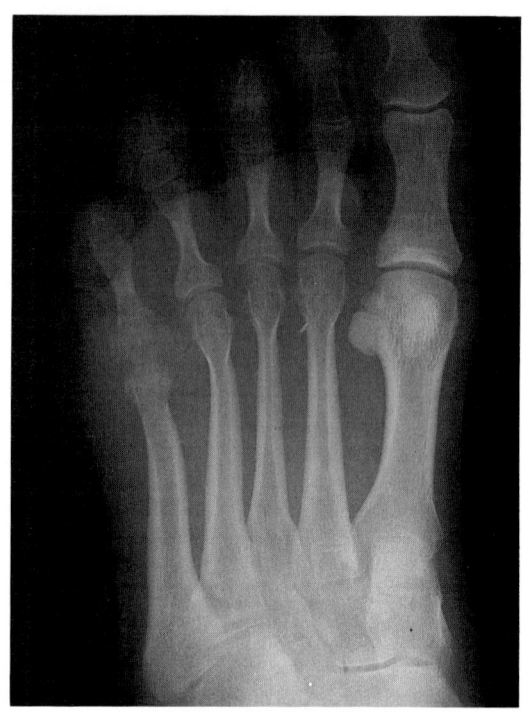

11.23 Radiograph of a 'staked' fifth metatarsal head causing severe joint pain postoperatively, with a poorly fixated transverse osteotomy which eventually resulted in a delayed union.

11.24 Radiograph of an improperly placed fifth metatarsophalangeal joint total implant which is too large for the digital and metatarsal bone stock.

eral head-condyle area of the fifth metatarsal, the joint will frequently become unstable and joint stiffness with pain may result (**11.23**).

Additionally, joint replacement in the fifth metatarsophalangeal joint is under similar demands as the first. Using too large or improperly placed implant may result in a complication of stiffness, swelling, pain or failure of the implant (**11.24**).

Hallux surgery complications

Interphalangeal arthrodesis

Historically, this is a very difficult joint to fuse. Recent advances utilizing screw fixation have dramatically diminished the frequency of non-union. However, even in the event of non-union, it is rarely a significant complication because there is usually an adequate fibrous union that is acceptable and rarely produces a disabling result.

Akin (proximal hallux phalanx osteotomy) complications

Contrary to hallux interphalangeal arthrodesis, the Akin osteotomy has a very low non-union rate, even with weight-bearing. Most of the complications result from separation of the osteotomy site with fixation failure. Rarely does fixation failure and separation of the osteotomy site cause a need to re-operate unless the cortical hinge also breaks, rendering a totally unstable osteotomy. Usually splintage or percutaneous pinning, combined with weight-bearing reduction techniques, will suffice in getting the osteotomy healed. Complications involving infection could certainly cause non-union and osteomyelitis as seen in **11.7, 11.8**.

Fixation errors

The type of fixation used does not seem to play an important role in the Akin osteotomy. Most of the fixation errors occur when the hinge of the osteotomy is broken. If the surgeon does not take into account the lack of stability of the osteotomy when fixation takes place, the hinge side of the osteotomy can be displaced. This situation can lead to dorsal displacement of the distal phalanx segment. When the osteotomy fails, a large osteotomy gap can result and the fixation device may provide a distractive force, which further complicates the situation.

Over-correction errors

The Akin osteotomy is frequently utilized to help correct mild hallux abductus or hallux interphalangeus deformities. If too much wedge is removed, a hallux varus can occur (**11.25**). If the deformity is not within the proximal phalanx, a bayonet deformity may occur.

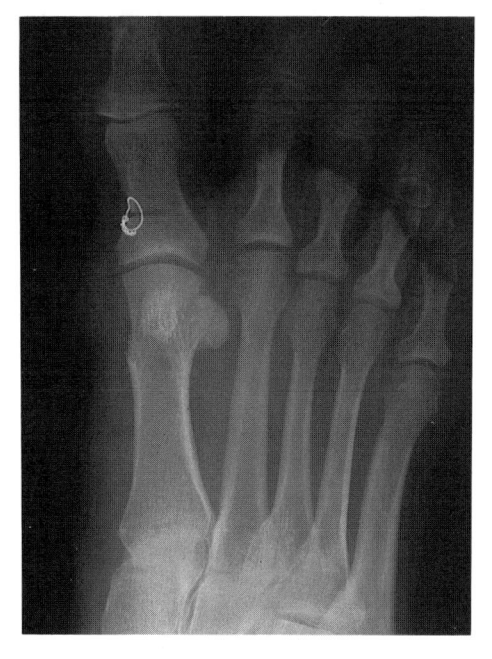

11.25 Radiograph of a hallux varus caused by an excessive bone wedge taken from a proximal phalanx osteotomy of the hallux.

Lesser digital surgery complications

As in other types of surgery, complications like infection, swelling, and skin slough can occur in lesser digits. However, managing these digital complications can be difficult and situations that are out of control or undertreated may result in digital amputation. Therefore, early diagnosis and aggressive treatment is necessary and may be the critical factor in ultimately saving the digit.

Mechanical dysfunction is probably the most common of all digital complications. The lesser digits of the foot are frequently the most unpredictable and problematic structures of the foot. Many foot surgeons relate that digital surgery is the most frustrating aspect of their practice. In the treatment of digital deformities, it is important to assess the exact nature of the deformity. Is the deformity flexible or fixed? How does weight-bearing affect the toe position? It is not uncommon to see a sagittal plane contracture of a digit, with normal alignment in the transverse plane off weight-bearing, which will deviate in the transverse plane with weight-bearing. Accurate assessment with improved procedure selection will make the final surgical outcome much more predicable.

Infection

Digital infections may be seen after minor toenail procedures or after major reconstructive surgery (**11.26**). At the earliest signs of infection, the patient should be assessed and appropriate diagnostic and therapeutic measures taken. Frequently, patients are treated much too conservatively during the early stages of infection and the complications appear to be greater in these cases. Cultures and antibiotic disc sensitivities should be performed as soon as there is drainage or material for testing. Placing the patient on suitable topical or oral antibiotic agents as soon as possible will be very important.

Digital osteomyelitis

Digital soft tissue infections that are undiagnosed or treated inappropriately may result in deep infections with secondary osteomyelitis (**11.27**). When radiographic evidence of osteomyelitis is present, surgical intervention may be necessary to achieve the best results.

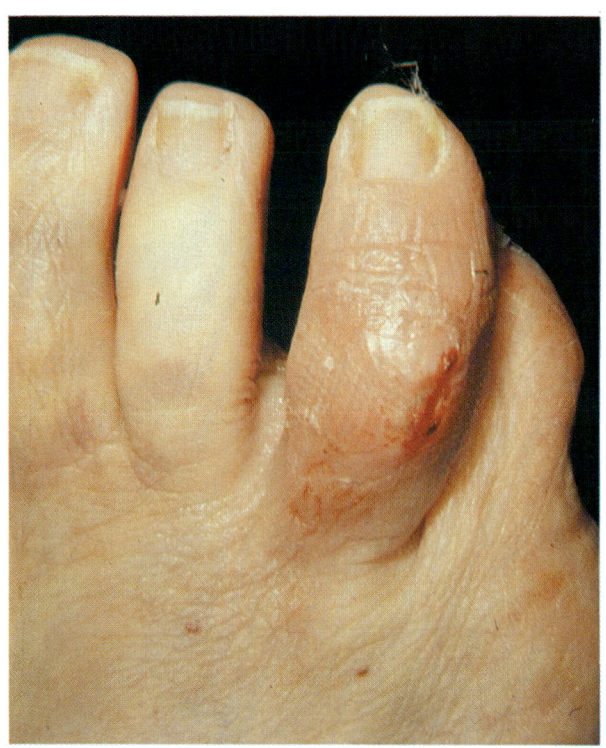

11.26 Infected fourth digit following simple bursa removal. (Courtesy of Dr G. Dockery, Seattle, USA.)

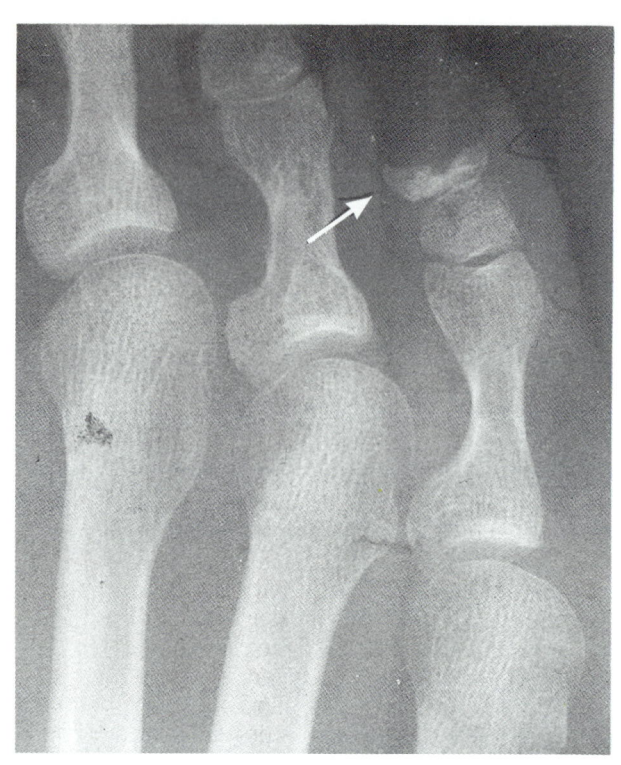

11.27 Osteomyelitis of the distal phalanx fifth digit following toenail surgery. (Courtesy of Dr G. Dockery, Seattle, USA.)

Skin slough

The skin edges may pull apart early after wound closure. This wound dehiscence may be followed by sloughing of the skin in and around the surgical site (**11.28**). The primary conditions that result in sloughing of the skin following surgery include suture reaction, stitch abscess, superficial wound infection, poor blood flow, oedema, haematoma, increased pressure, and increased motion at the incision site. For most cases of skin slough the treatment consists of proper wound care, antibiotics, debridement, and protection of the healing edges. Drying foot soaks may speed up healing and in some cases of massive skin slough, secondary covering with skin grafts may be necessary.

Swollen toe

Swelling of the digit may occur following minor surgery, injury or infection (**11.29**). There are numerous causes for swelling following surgery to digits. The primary causes include seroma, haematoma, tissue injury, inflammation, infection, and damage to the lymphatic drainage system. Most of the known causes respond to some form of therapy and with a little

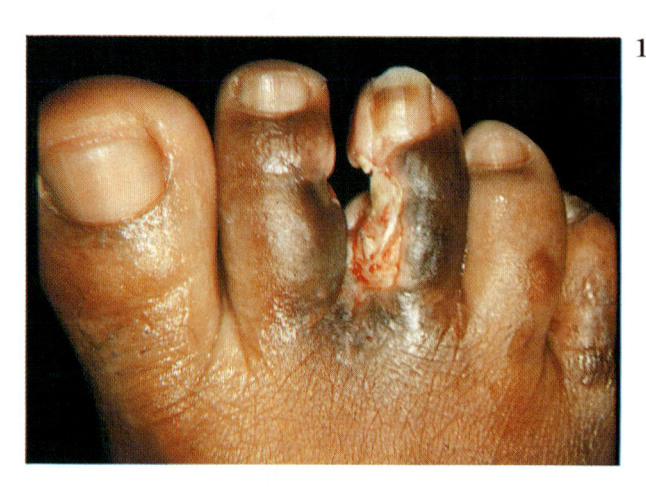

11.28 Skin slough of digits following attempted desyndatylism procedure. (Courtesy of Dr G. Dockery, Seattle, USA.)

patience, and a lot of persistence, the oedema may be reduced. In general, the swelling should be minimalized by massage, manipulation, and compression. With appropriate antibiotics or anti-inflammatory drugs, the conservative treatment programme is usually successful.

Sausage toe

This is a descriptive condition of a severely swollen digit that can occur in situations of infection, haematoma, or severe inflammation (**11.30**). The sausage toe may be seen in non-surgical cases of gouty arthritis and seronegative spondyloarthropathies. Surgically related sausage toe is also a common complication. Usually a post-operative sausage toe is self-limiting but must be carefully evaluated to ensure that it is not infected. Treatment is similar to that for a swollen toe. One additional treatment that is very popular for the true sausage toe is intra-digital steroid injections. In most cases, a single injection of 0.25 ml of triamcinolone acetonide injected throughout the digit will cause a significant reduction in the chronic swelling. Following injection, the toe should be massaged and wrapped in a compressive (but not constrictive) wrap. Additional injections may be performed with the caution to discontinue this form of treatment when the toe approaches normal appearance, or any side effects appear.[28]

Interphalangeal arthroplasty

This is the most common lesser digital procedure performed. Complications with this procedure are usually associated with the amount of bone resected. If too little bone is resected, there may be complications with bone regeneration, stiffness, and bone impingement. Bone impingement may also occur if the cut portion of bone is not resected in a smooth or complete manner. The success of this procedure is based on an appropriate amount of bone being resected with interposed scar tissue to occupy the space of the resected bone. If too much bone is resected then a flail or floppy toe (**11.31**) or over-shortened toe (**11.32**) may develop.

Transverse plane instability is a complication with interphalangeal arthroplasty. This is seen in the second digit, especially with a concomitant deformity of hallux valgus. The second digit will yield to the hallux deformity and the resultant deformity increases with time. This complication may be avoided by addressing the hallux condition and performing an arthrodesis procedure on the digit in order to provide more transverse stability.

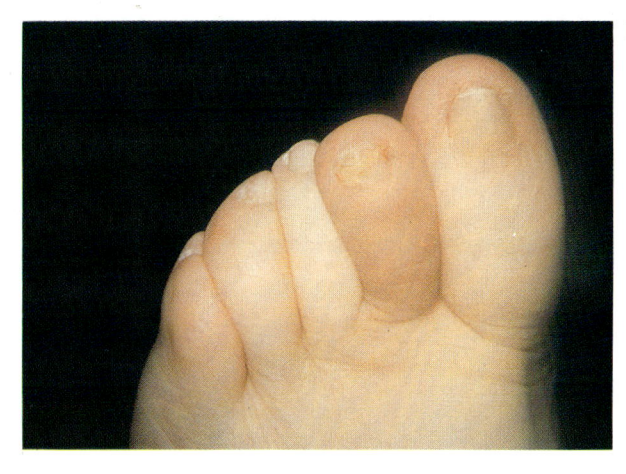

11.29 Swollen second digit following simple toenail surgery. (Courtesy of Dr G. Dockery, Seattle, USA.)

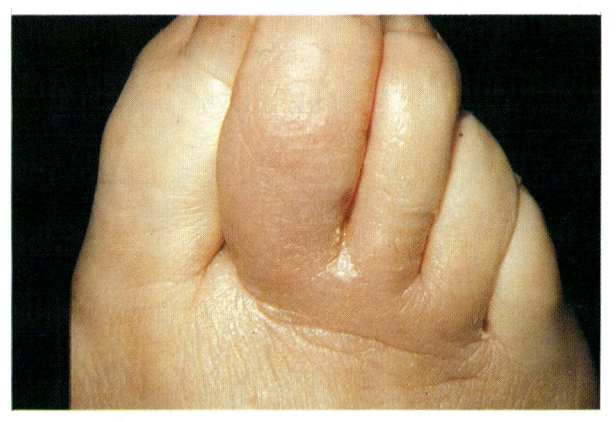

11.30 An example of a sausage toe. Usually a result of disruption to the digital lymphatic drainage system. This condition produces more induration than general swelling. (Courtesy of Dr G. Dockery, Seattle, USA.)

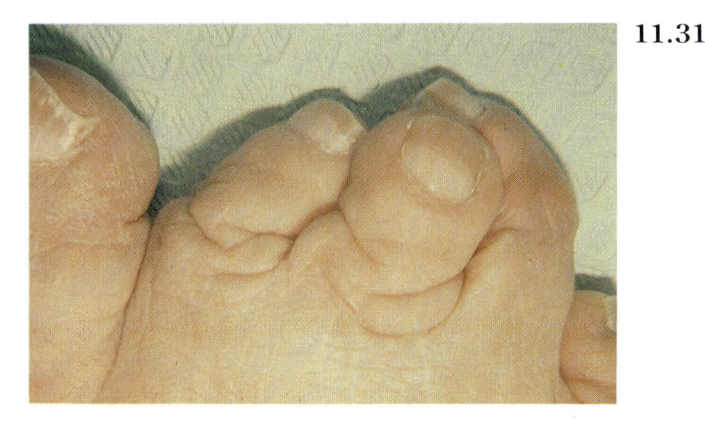

11.31 Severe floppy toes. In this case, excessive bone was removed from the digits during attempted hammertoe correction. (Courtesy of Dr G. Dockery, Seattle, USA.)

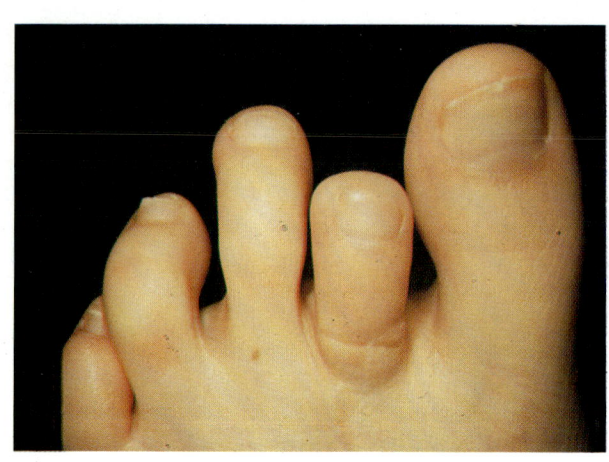

11.32 Over-shortened second toe, from removal of the proximal phalanx base. (Courtesy of Dr G. Dockery, Seattle, USA.)

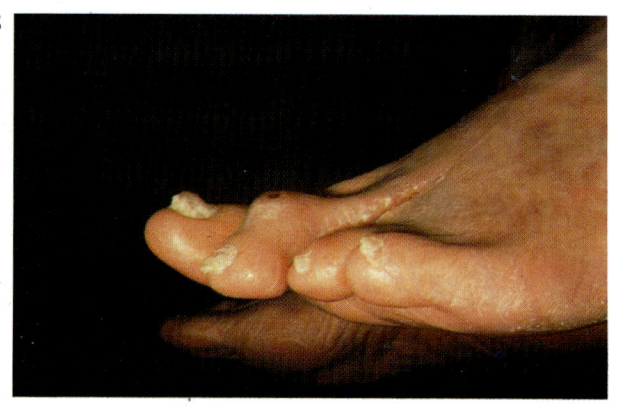

11.33 Mallet toe condition following arthrodesis of the proximal interphalangeal joint secondary to flexor tendon contracture. (Courtesy of Dr G. Dockery, Seattle, USA.)

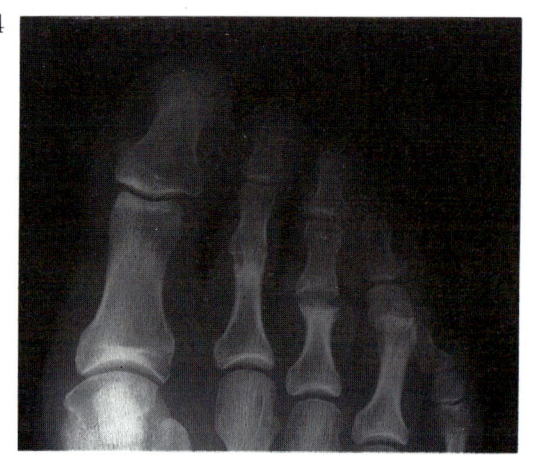

11.34 Pseudoarthrosis of attempted third digit arthrodesis. Note successful arthrodesis of second digit.

Interphalangeal arthrodesis

Arthrodesis is a commonly performed procedure aimed at correcting digital contractures and providing stability of the digit post-operatively. Digital stiffness is not considered a complication but rather a side effect of the procedure. The most common complication with this procedure is a floating toe. This condition may be difficult to prevent and frequently requires a flexor tendon transfer to help with toe purchase, especially if there is dorsal contracture at the metatarsophalangeal joint level.[29]

A complication specific to an arthrodesis of the proximal interphalangeal joint is a subsequent mallet toe deformity (**11.33**). This is especially true in cavus feet. Fusion of both of the interphalangeal joints or flexor transfer would be effective in preventing this problem. Non-union is also a relatively common complication; however, in most cases, they become asymptomatic and function as a fibrous union (pseudoarthrosis), similar to that seen with the digital arthroplasty (**11.34**).

Digital implants

Several designs of lesser digital implants are available for the proximal interphalangeal joint (see Chapter 7). These implants are made of silicone elastomer and suffer the same complications as other silicone implants. Sausage toe may occur if the implant is abraded by the adjacent bone and leads to detritic synovitis from silicone shards and foreign body giant cell reaction. Long-term studies for this type of implant have not been performed; therefore it is difficult to determine if the procedure has more benefit than the time-tested arthroplasty and arthrodesis procedures that are more commonly performed. However, it is well known that improper placement of digital implants will lead to rapid degeneration of the implant and early implant rejection. In some cases, digital implants are used inappropriately to try to straighten hammered toes (**11.35**).

Flexor tendon transfers

These effective procedures to help maintain toe purchase are usually used in conjunction with digital arthroplasties and arthrodesis procedures. The most common complication of this procedure is failure due to the tendon attachment tearing or the tendon being sutured too loosely. This will result in a floating or sometimes floppy toe deformity. Flexor transfers may take on a sausage toe appearance because of the increased bulk of tendon around the proximal phalanx. It is also not unusual to see some erosive changes at the phalangeal attachment site of the tendon, which tend to be asymptomatic.

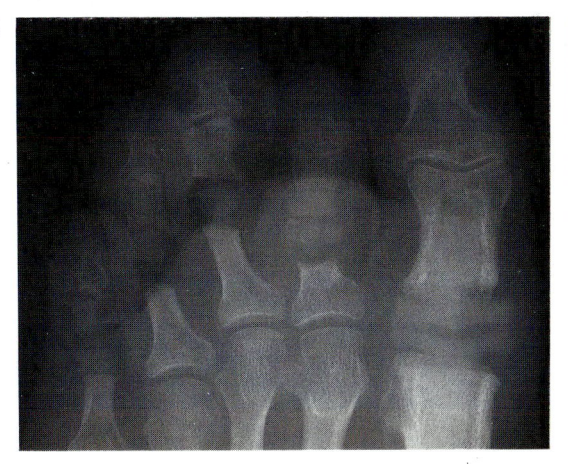

11.35 Improper selection, use, and criteria for digital implants. Note improper size, position, and displacement of implants in each digit.

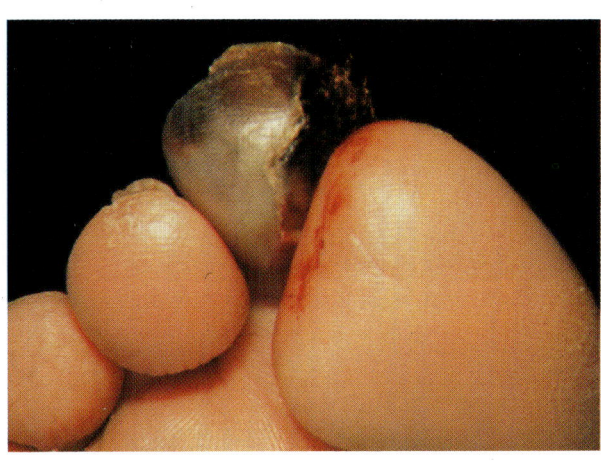

11.36 Vascular compromise to the toe, causing tissue damage or gangrene, may occur after any surgical procedure that damages the digital blood vessels. (Courtesy of Dr G. Dockery, Seattle, USA.)

Other digital complications

A less common, but certainly severe, complication of digital surgery is vascular impairment of the digit. This can occur whenever extensive surgery is performed at or adjacent to multiple vascular bundles to the toe. Adjacent intermetatarsal neuroma surgery can put a digit at risk of vascular compromise. Pan metatarsal head resection may also result in vascular compromise as a result of inadvertent sectioning of the neurovascular bundle (**11.36**).

Underlying conditions of diabetes, arterial sclerosis, scleroderma, or Raynaud's disease are relative contraindications for digital surgery and must be properly worked-up and the patient well informed before surgery is undertaken.

Summary

The accomplished forefoot surgeon is one who is not only familiar with the various surgical and medical treatment options available but also with the potential complications that may arise before, during, and after treatment. The surgeon should be able to anticipate and take steps towards preventing or at least reducing the potential end results.

Once a surgeon is aware of the various forms of complications inherent to forefoot surgery, then an index of suspicion must be exercised to make an accurate and timely diagnosis in order to initiate proper treatment. All surgeons have complications of varying degrees; however, it is the exceptional surgeon who can recognize and rapidly implement a treatment programme to reduce the morbidity that can be associated with various complications. The fact that complications occur with certain techniques does not interdict their proper use. It is essential for the forefoot surgeon to constantly evaluate and critique his or her own work. The ultimate lesson a foot surgeon can learn to prevent surgical complications is that healing must be cultivated and not imposed.

References

[1] Kelikian, H. *Hallux Valgus, Allied Deformities of the Forefoot and Metatarsalgia.* Philadelphia, W.B. Saunders, 1965.

[2] Christensen, J.C. and Dockery, G.L. Flap classification and survival factors: current concepts. *Clin. Podiatric Med. Surg.,* **3**: 579, 1986.

[3] Murray, J.C., Pollack, S.V. and Pinnell, S.R. Keloids and hypertrophic scars. *Clin. Dermatol.,* **2**: 121, 1984.

[4] Kwiecinski, M.G. and Reinherz, R.P. Keloids and hypertrophic scars in the foot. *J. Foot Surg.,* **26**: 293, 1987.

[5] Miller, S.J. Surgical wound drainage system using silicone tubing. *J. Am. Podiatry Assoc.,* **71**: 287, 1981.

[6] Kenzora, J.E. Sensory nerve neuromas—leading to failed foot surgery. *Foot Ankle,* **7**: 110, 1986.

[7] Sunderland, S. *Nerves and Nerve Injuries,* 2nd edn. New York, Churchill Livingstone, 1978.

[8] Matthews, L.S., Green, C.A. and Goldstein, S.A. The thermal effects of skeletal fixation-pin insertion in bone. *J. Bone Joint Surg.,* **66A**: 1077, 1984.

[9] Perren, S.M. Physical and biological aspects of fracture healing with special reference to internal fixation. *Clin. Orthop. Rel. Res.,* **138**: 175, 1979.

[10] Huntzschenreuter, P., Steinemann, S., Perren, S.M., Geret, V. and Klebl, M. Some effects of rigidity of internal fixation on the healing pattern of osteotomies. *Injury,* **1**: 77, 1969.

[11] Muller, M.E., Allgower, M., Scheider, R. and Willenegger, H. (eds). *Manual of Internal Fixation. Techniques Recommended by the AO Group,* 2nd edn. Berlin, York, Springer-Verlag, 1979.

[12] Waldvogel, F.A., Medoff, G. and Swartz, M.N. Osteomyelitis: A review of clinical features, therapeutic considerations and unusual aspects. *New Engl. J. Med.,* **282**: (5) 260, 1970.

[13] Fitzgerald, R.H., Jr. Antibiotic distribution in normal and osteomyelitic bone. *Orthop. Clin. N. Am.,* **15**: 537, 1984.

[14] Miller, S.J. Surgical technique for resection of Morton's neuroma. *J. Amer. Podiatry Assoc.,* **71**: 181, 1981.

[15] Reinisch, J.F. The pathophysiology of skin flap circulation. *Plast. Reconstr. Surg.,* **54**: 585, 1974.

[16] Kerrigan, C.L. Skin flap failure: pathophysiology. *Plast. Reconstr. Surg.,* **72**: 766, 1983.

[17] Meisenhelder, D.A., Harkless, L.B. and Patterson, J.W. Avascular necrosis after first metatarsal head osteotomies. *J. Foot Surg.,* **23**: 429, 1984.

[18] Donovan, J.C. Results of bunion correction using Mitchell osteotomy. *J. Foot Surg.,* **21**: 181, 1982.

[19] Gerbert, J. Complications of the Austin-type bunionectomy. *J. Foot Surg.,* **17**: 1, 1978.

[20] Curda, G.A. and Sorto, L.A. The McBride bunionectomy with closing wedge abductory wedge osteotomy. *J. Am. Podiatric Med. Assoc.,* **71**: 349, 1981.

[21] Scuberth, J.M., Reilly, C.H. and Gudas, C.J. The closing wedge osteotomy: a critical analysis of first metatarsal elevation. *J. Am. Podiatry Assoc.,* **74**: 13, 1984.

[22] Lapidus, P.W. The author's bunion operation from 1931 to 1959. *Clin. Orthop.,* **42**: 119, 1962.

[23] Fitzgerald, J.A.W. A review of long-term results of arthrodesis of the first metatarso-phalangeal joint. *J. Bone Joint Surg.,* **51B**: 488, 1969.

[24] Cleveland, M. and Winant, E.M. An end result study of the Keller operation. *J. Bone Joint Surg.,* **32A**: 163, 1950.

[25] Kravette, M.A. The Swanson arthroplasty of the great toe: a prospective study. *J. Foot Surg.,* **17**: 155, 1978.

[26] Mondul, M., Jacobs, P.M., Caneva, R.G. *et al.* Implant arthroplasty of the first metatarsophalangeal joint: a 12-year retrospective study. *J. Foot Surg.,* **24**: 275, 1985.

[27] Swanson, A.B., Lumsden, II, R.M. and Swanson, G.D. Silicone implant arthroplasty of the great toe. *Clin. Orthop. Rel. Res.,* **142**: 30, 1979.

[28] Dockery, G.L. and Nilson, R.Z. Intralesional injections. *Clin. Podiatric Med. Surg.,* **3**: 473–485, 1986.

[29] Kuwada, G.T. and Dockery, G.L. Modification of the flexor tendon transfer procedure for the correction of flexible hammertoes. *J. Foot Surg.,* **19**: 38–40, 1980.

Index

References in light type are to page numbers, those in **bold** type are to illustrations.

Abductor digiti quinti 163
Abductor hallucis 197
Abnormal dip phenomenon 169
Adductor hallucis 198
Adductovarus contracture 125
Adrenaline 21, 37–8
Advancement flaps 23, **1.35**, **1.38**
AIDS 189
Akin osteotomy 219–21, 252–3, **10.39–10.43**, **11.25**
Allergies
    foreign body reaction 251, **11.20–11.22**
    metal 238
Alvarado incisions 31, **1.62**
Angiofibrolipoma 186
Angioleiomyomas 188
Angiomyolipoma 188
Anterior tarsal tunnel syndrome 176
AO bone screw fixation 147, **7.15**
Arteries, perforating 112
Arthrodesis
    first metatarsal cuneiform joint 232, 249–50
    first ray 217–32
    interphalangeal 252, 256
    lesser digits 147–9
    peg-in-hole 148, 232, **7.16**
    proximal interphalangeal joint 148–9
Arthroplastic procedures 222–30
    Freiberg's infraction 123, **6.27**
    hammertoe 145–7, **7.13**
    interphalangeal 255
Atrophic non-union 242
Austin bunionectomy 208–9, **10.23–10.25**
Avulsion fractures 121, **6.18**
Axial pattern flap 22, **1.34**
Axon sprouts 173–4, **8.27**
Axons 164

Bandages
    Esmarch 68, **3.8–3.11**
    flaps 32
    grafts 18, 32
Basal osteotomy 213
Benign hypermobile joint syndrome 126
Bevelled incisions 11, **1.10–1.11**
Biopsies 183
Blades 10, **1.8–1.9**
Boll's technique 68
Bone
    allografts 215
    complications of surgery 242–4
Bow tie incision 31, **1.62**
Brachymetatarsia 122, **6.24–6.25**
Bunion 204
    tailor's, *see* Tailor's bunion
Bunionectomies 204–12
    without osteotomy 246–7, **11.14**

Bürow's wedges (triangles) 23, **1.36**
Bursitis 183, 190, **9.12–9.13**

Capsulitis, adhesive 246
Capsulotomy 104, 147, **5.9–5.10**
    Silver's 205, **10.18**
    vertical lateral 207
Carbolic acid 138
Cauterization 73–7, 138
Cheilectomy 230–1
Chevron (Austin) bunionectomy 208–9, **10.23–10.25**
Circular defects 24–5
Clayton's procedure 130
Closing wedge osteotomies 213–15, **10.34–10.35**
Cocaine 25, **2.1**
Combined-V incision 31, **1.62**
Common peroneal nerve 43, **2.6–2.7**
    nerve block 52, **2.13–2.14**
Compression syndromes 159, 174–9
Computerized axial tomography (CAT) 118, 183
Convoluted nail plate 66, **3.5**
Creep 7
Crepitus 227
Crescentic osteotomy 216–17, **10.37**
Crista 198
Crush injuries 121
Curvilinear incisions 10, 183–4, **1.7**
Cyanosis 172–3
Cysts, fluid-filled 183, 184, **9.1–9.2**

DASA, *see* Distal articular set angle
Deep peroneal nerve 159, 196, **2.12**, **8.29**
    compression neuropathy 176
    nerve block 58, **2.26–2.28**
Deep transverse intermetatarsal ligament 166, 171–2, **8.12–8.13**
Dehiscence 184, 254
Dermatofibroma 183, 185, **9.3**
Dermatofibrosarcomas 185
Dermatomes
    nerve fibres 162–4, **8.3–8.6**
    skin grafts 20, **1.31**
Diabetes mellitus 159, 186
Diaphysectomies 155
Digits
    arthrodesis 147–9
    blocks (total ring blocks) 61–2, **2.30–2.33**
    exostoses 85–91, **4.1–4.3**
    implants 256, **11.35**
    innervation 43–5
    joint prosthesis 151–3
    mechanical dysfunction 253
    osteomyelitis 253, **11.27**
    plethysmography 137
    surgery 137–58, 253–7, **11.26–11.27**
    surgical anatomy 111–14
Distal articular set angle (DASA) 201, 221, **10.10**
Distal metatarsal osteotomies (DMO) 208–12
Distal transverse plane osteotomy 129, **6.39**

Dog-ear deformities 12, 23, **1.12**
Donor sites 19, 21
Dorsal digital nerves 43, **2.11**
Double osteotomy 210
Double-chevron osteotomy 124, **6.28**
Double-S incision 31, **1.62**
Double-stemmed implant 224
Double-Z rhomboid flap 30–1, **1.60–1.61**
Dressing grafts 19
Dufourmentel rhomboid flap 30, **1.58**
Dupuytren's contracture 185

Electrodesiccation 76
Elevating osteotomies 225–6, **10.46–10.47**
Elongated toes 123–4, 155, **7.21**
EMLA 51
End-to-end arthrodesis 232
Endoneural oedema 167
Endoprostheses 151–3, **7.18**
Entrapments 159, 165, 174–9
Epinephrine (adrenaline) 21, 37–8
Epineurium 164
Eponychium 138
Equinus 125
Erythromelalgia 159
Esmarch bandage 68, **3.8–3.11**
Eucraine 25, **2.1**
Exostoses, digital 85–91, **4.1–4.3**
Exsanguination of the toe 68, **3.8–3.11**
Extensor hallucis brevis 197
　tenotomy 207
Extensor hallucis capsularis 197
Extensor hallucis longus (EHL) 213
　tendon 197
Extensor hood 113, 138, **6.7, 7.2**
Extensor sling 113
Extensor substitution 125

Fascicles 164, **8.9**
Fasciotomy, percutaneous 171–2
Felypressin (Octapressin) 38
Femoral nerve 162
Fibrinoid necrosis 190
Fibrosarcomas 185
Fibular sesamoidectomy 102–5, 107, 176, 246
Field blocks 61
Fifth metatarsal
　fractures 119
　internal fixation **6.22**
　range of motion, evaluation of **6.34**
　staked 252, **11.23**
First digital interspace 43–5, **2.12**
First metatarsal
　hypermobile 228
　iatrogenic elevation 217
　osteotomy 247–8, **11.16–11.17**
　sesamoids 95–8, **5.2–5.7**
　short 215, **10.36**
First metatarsal cuneiform joint 198, **10.5**
　arthrodesis 249, **7.12, 11.18**
　exostoses 227
　fusion 218, **6.33, 10.38**
　opening wedge fusion 231, **10.51**
First metatarsophalangeal joint 95–8, 198, **5.3–5.6, 10.4**
　arthrodesis 232, 249–50
　entrapment neuropathy 175–6
　implant 246, 250–1, **11.11–11.12**
First ray
　arthrodesis 217–32
　hypermobile 217–18
　muscles 196–8, **10.2**
　neurovascular structures 195–6, **10.1**
　plantar-flexed 225
　procedures 195–235, 245–51
Flail (floppy) toe 255, **11.31**
Flaps, *see* Skin flaps
Flexor digitorum brevis 163
　sling 167
Flexor hallucis brevis 198
Flexor hallucis longus tendon 197
Flexor stabilization 125
Flexor substitution 125
Flexor tendon transfers 149–51, 256
Floating toe 122, 155–7, 256, **6.24, 7.22–7.23**
Floppy toe 255, **11.31**
Foreign body reaction 251, **11.20–11.22**
Fractures
　avulsion 121, **6.18**
　Jones 119, 122, **6.17, 6.23**
　lesser metatarsal 119–22
　sesamoids 101
　styloid process 122
Free flap axial pattern 22, **1.34**
Freiberg's infraction 123, **6.26–6.27**
　implants 132, **6.47**
Frost procedure 80–2, **3.32–3.46, 7.7**
　subungual exostectomy 90, **4.5**
Full-thickness skin grafts (FTSGs) 19
Fusiform closure 21, **1.32**
Fusiform incision 145
Fusiform neuroma 171
Fusion, *see* Arthrodesis

Ganglia 183, 184, **9.1–9.2**
Gangrene 37–8, 173
Giannestras step down osteotomy 117
Giant cell tumours (pigmented villonodular synovitis) 186–7, **9.6**
Girdlestone procedure 149
Glomus tumours 190
Grafts
　allograft bone 215
　cortico-cancellous 215
　skin 18, 19–21, 32
Granuloma pyogenicum (pyogenic granuloma) 189–90, **9.10–9.11**

Haematoma 16, 238, 240, **11.4**
　neuroma surgery 172
Haemorrhage 239
Hallux abductus (HA) angle 200, **10.7**
Hallux abductus deformity 99–100, 197, 245–6
Hallux interphalangeal joint 198, **10.3**

Hallux interphalangeus (HI) angle 200, **10.8**
Hallux limitus 217, 202, 230–2
Hallux varus 205–6, **10.20**
    acquired 245–6, **11.13**
    implant arthroplasty 223–4
Hammertoe 125, 126, 145–9
Heloma dura 145–6
Heloma molle 145–6, 153
Herbert screw 210
Hibbs' tensosuspension procedure 125, **6.32**
Histiocytoma, cutaneous fibrous (dermatofibroma) 183, 185, **9.3**
Hoffman's procedure 130
Hourglass manoeuvre 222–3
Hypercholesterolaemia 186
Hypermobility
    first metatarsal 228
    first ray 217–18
Hypertrophic non-union 242, **11.6**
Hypertrophic scars 239, **11.2**
Hyponychium 65, 138

Implants
    arthroplasty 132, 223–5, **6.47**
    digital 256, **11.35**
    failure 225, 245–6, 250, **11.11–11.12, 11.19**
    lesser metatarsal 132, **6.47**
    prosthetic joint 151–3, **7.18**
Incisional nail procedures 78–83
Incisional neuromas 241
Incisions 9–15
    Alvarado 31, **1.62**
    hammertoe 145
    Morton's neuroma 170–1, **8.19–8.21**
    sesamoidectomy 102–5
    soft tissue masses 183–4
Infection
    implants 225
    lesser digital surgery 253, **11.26–11.27**
    non-incisional nail procedures 78
Innervation 43–50, 159–64
    digits 43–5
    first ray 195–6, **10.1**
    metatarsals 112–13
    see also Nerves; Peripheral nerves
Instruments 8, 20–1, **1.3–1.4, 1.31**
Intermediate dorsal cutaneous nerve 159
Intermetatarsal (IM) angle 200, **10.6**
    increased 126, 213–14, 215
Intermetatarsal neuroma (Morton's neuroma) 165, 166–74, **8.10–8.27**
Intermetatarsal plantar neuromas 175
Internal fixation
    complications 242
    digital arthrodesis 147–9
    errors 253
    fifth metatarsal **6.22**
    isolated midshaft fractures 122, **6.22**
    midshaft fractures 121, **6.21**
Interosseous muscles 111–12, 159, **6.5**
Intersesamoidal ligament 207
Interstitial disorders 165

Intoed gait 124
Inverted spoon (embedded) nail 67, **3.7**
Inverted-V capsulotomy 104, **5.9**
Involuted nail plate 66, **3.4**
Iontophoresis 183
Ischaemia 159, 240
Island axial pattern 22, **1.34**
Isoxuprine (Vasodilan) 172

Jacoby V-osteotomy 117, **6.12**
Jimenez double oblique osteotomy 117
Joint congruity 201, **10.11**
Joint implants 151–3, **7.18**
Jones fractures 119, 122, **6.17, 6.23**
Jones-type splint 148–9
Joplin's neuroma 175, **8.28**

K-wire fixation
    digital arthrodesis 147–9, **7.14**
    elongated toes 155, **7.21**
    floating toe syndrome 155–7
    mid-shaft fractures 121, **6.21**
Kaposi's sarcoma 189
Keller procedure 222–3, 250, **10.44**
Keloid scar formation 239, **11.3**
Keratomas 225, 228
Kernan's tumours 185
Koehler's second disease 123
Kuwada modified CAP procedure 118
Kuwada technique **7.11**
Kuwada–Dockery flexor tendon transfer 149, **7.17**

Lapidus technique 249, **6.33, 7.12, 11.18**
Laser matrixectomy 139, 143–4
Lateral bowing 127, **6.36–6.37**
Lateral sesamoid 198
    release 206–7, **10.21–10.22**
Lateral squeeze test 168, **8.15**
Lawrence implant 224
Leiomyomas 188
Lepird procedure 124, **6.31**
Lesser digits, *see* Digits
Lesser metatarsals, *see* Metatarsals
Lignocaine 35, **2.2**
Limberg rhomboid flap 29–31, **1.57**
Lines of maximum extensibility (LME) 21, **1.32**
Lipomas 186
Lisfranc fracture–dislocation 111, 119, **6.16**
Lo–Dye strapping 169, **8.17**
Local anaesthetics 35–63
Lumbricals 112, **6.6**
    tendon 172
Lunula 138

McBride bunionectomy 205–6, 207–8, 213, **10.19–10.20**
Magnetic resonance imaging (MRI) 118, 175, 183, **6.13**
Mallet toe deformity 256, **11.33**
Master Knot of Henry 163
Matrix 65, 138–9
    partial removal 68–76, **3.8–3.22**
    total removal (matrixectomy) 138–44, **7.4–7.28**

Mayo block 62
Mechanical entrapment neuropathy 166
Medial dorsal cutaneous nerve 159, 196
Medial pinch callous 221
Mercado's 'fish mouth' incisional approach 89, **4.4**
Metal allergy 238
Metatarsalgia 125
Metatarsals
   base fractures 119
   deformities 119–32
   elongated 123–4
   equinus (plantarflexed lesser metatarsus) 125–6, **6.32**
   fifth, *see* Fifth metatarsal
   first, *see* First metatarsal
   head
      resection, rheumatoid foot 130, **6.44–6.46**
      shape 202, **10.13**
   implants 132, **6.47**
   length formula 111
   neck fractures 119, 121, **6.14, 6.19**
   osteotomies 117, **6.11**
   pads 169, **8.16**
   protrusion distance (MPD) 202, **10.14**
   shape and position 111, **6.1–6.4**
   splay 218
   surgery 111–135
      complications 251–2, **11.23–11.24**
   traumatic deformities 119–22
   tumours 129–30, **6.41**
Metatarsophalangeal joint apparatus 113, **6.8**
Metatarsus adductus 124, **6.29–6.31**
Metatarsus adductus (MA) angle 202–3, **10.15**
Metatarsus primus varus deformities 213
Midshaft fractures 119, **6.15**
   isolated 122
   wire fixation 121, **6.21**
Mitchell osteotomy 210–11, **10.27–10.28**
Morton's neuroma 165, 166–74, **8.10–8.27**
Morton's syndrome 122
Mucocutaneous cysts (digital mucous cysts) 184
Mulder's sign 168
Muscles
   first ray complex 196–8, **10.2**
   interosseus 111–12, 159
   plantar 162–3
Myelin 164

Nail
   anatomy 138–9, **7.3**
   avulsion **7.4–7.8**
   bed 65, 137, **7.1**
   curvature 66, **3.3**
   matrix, *see* Matrix
   pathology 67–83
   plate 65–6, 137, 138, **3.3–3.5, 7.1**
   surgery 65–83
   unit, normal anatomy 65–6, **3.1–3.2**
Needles 40–1, **2.3–2.4**
Negative galvanism 75–6, 139
Nerves
   blocks 51–62
   capping 241
   entrapments 159, 165, 174–9
   fibres 164, **8.7**
   first ray complex 195–6, **10.1**
   grafting 241
   injuries 174–7
   pain 175
   sheath tumours 165
   see also Innervation; Peripheral nerves
Neurilemmoma (schwannomas) 187, **9.7–9.8**
Neurodermatomes 162–4, **8.3–8.6**
Neurofibroma (von Recklinghausen's disease) 188, **9.9**
Neuromas 165, 187, 241
   adjacent intermetatarsal space 172
   intermetatarsal plantar 175
   Joplin's 175, **8.28**
   Morton's 165, 166–74, **8.10–8.27**
   recurrent (stump) 173, **8.24–8.26**
   sensory 176–7
Neuromatous zone (N-zone) 176–7, **8.30**
Neuropathies 159, 165–6
Neurovascular complications of surgery 239–41
Non-incisional nail procedures 67–78
Non-union 242

Onychauxis 67, 138
Onychocryptosis (ingrown toenails) 138
Onychodystrophy 184
Onychogryphosis (onychodystrophic toenails) 67, 138
Onycholysis (separated toenail) 138
Onychomycosis (fungal nails) 67, 138
Opening wedge osteotomy 215, 228, 229, **10.49–10.50**
Os trigonum syndrome 177
Osteochondrosis 123, 125, **6.26–6.27**
Osteomyelitis 242, **11.7–11.8**
Osteotomies
   Akin, *see* Akin osteotomy
   basal 213
   closing plantarflexory 228
   crescentic 216–17, **10.37**
   distal metatarsal (DMO) 208–12
   distal transverse plane 129, **6.39**
   double 210
   double-chevron 124, **6.28**
   elevating 225–6, **10.46–10.47**
   Giannestras 117
   Jacoby V 117, **6.12**
   Jimenez 117
   lesser metatarsal 117, **6.11**
   Mitchell 210–11, **10.27–10.28**
   plantarflexory 228–30, **10.48–10.50**
   proximal 213
   technical complications 243–4, **11.9–11.10**
   wedge, *see* Wedge osteotomies
Over-shortened toe 255, **11.32**

Pacinian corpuscles 166
Panner's disease 123
Pantographic expansion 23, **1.37**
Paraesthesias 159, 174
Parenchymatous disorders 165
Partite sesamoids 95, 101, **5.2**

PASA, *see* Proximal articular set angle
Pedicle flaps 245
Peg-in-hole arthrodesis 148, 232, **7.16**
Peninsular axial pattern 22, **1.34**
Perineural fibroma (Morton's neuroma) 165, 166–74, **8.10–8.27**
Peripheral nerves
    anatomy 164, **8.7–8.9**
    leg 159–64, **8.1–8.2**
Periungual exostectomy 85–91
Periungual fibromas 185
Peroneus longus muscle 196
Peroneus longus tendon 218
Peyronie's disease 185
Phalangeal procedures 219–21
Phenol matrixectomy 139
Phenolization 73–4, **3.23–3.24**
Phentolamine (Regitine) 172
Phonophoresis 183
Pigmented villonodular synovitis 186–7, **9.6**
Pinch grafts 20, **1.30**
Plantar compartments 114, **6.10**
Plantar condylectomy 117
Plantar digital nerves 43, **2.9**
Plantar fibromas 185, **9.4–9.5**
Plantar incisions 170–1, 184, **8.19–8.20**
    sesamoidectomy 102
Plantar muscles 113–14, **6.9**
Plantar nerves 162–3
Plantarflexed lesser metatarsus (metatarsus equinus) 125–6, **6.32**
Plantarflexory osteotomies 228–30, **10.48–10.50**
Pleomorphism 185
Porta pedis 162
Posterior tibial nerve 159, 162, **8.31–8.32**
    entrapment 177–8
Procaine 35, **2.2**
Proliferative synovitis 130
Pronation 114–15
Propulsive gait 126
Proximal articular set angle (PASA) 200–1, 208, 209, 211–12, **10.9**
Proximal interphalangeal joint arthrodesis 148–9
Proximal osteotomies 213
Pseudoarthrosis 256, **11.34**
Pyogenic granuloma 189–90, **9.10–9.11**

Quadratus plantae 163

Radiculopathy 159
Random pattern flaps 22, **1.33**
Ray resection 117
Recurrent neuroma 173, **8.24–8.26**
Reflex sympathetic dystrophy (RSD) 240–1, **11.5**
Regrowth
    exostectomy 90
    non–incisional nail procedures 78
Relaxed skin tension lines (RSTL) 7, **1.1–1.2**
Retinacular release 176
Reverdin procedure 211, **10.28–10.31**
Reverdin–Green modification 211
Reverdin–Laird modification 212, **10.32**

Rheumatoid arthritis 126, 130, **6.42–6.46**
Rheumatoid nodules 183, 190
Rhomboidal (rhombic) flaps 29–31, **1.57–1.60**
Rotation flaps 24–7, **1.39–1.55**

S-shaped incisions 10, 15, **1.7**
Sagittal groove 201, 205
Sagittal intermetatarsal angle 203–4, **10.16–10.17**
Saphenous nerve 43, 159, 162, 195–6, **2.5–2.6**
    nerve block 52–3, **2.15–2.18**
Sausage toe 255, **11.30**
Scar formation 147, 239, **11.2–11.3**
Scarf procedure 213, **10.33**
Schink Metatarsal Spreader 171, **8.22**
Schrudde slide-swing plasty 25, **1.45–1.55**
Schwann cell 164, 188, **8.8**
Schwannomas 187, **9.7–9.8**
Sciatic nerve 43, **2.7**
Scived incisions 11. **1.10–1.11**
Sensory neuromas 176–7
Serial casting 124, **6.30**
Sesamoid bones 93–110
    distribution and morphology 93–4, **5.1**
    pain, non-invasive treatment 102
    position 202
    replacement 108
Sesamoid complex
    bunionectomy 208
    flexor longus tendon 197
    intersesamoidal ligament 207
Sesamoid-metatarsal joint 198
Sesamoidectomy 93–110
Sesamoiditis 102
Sgarlato's technique 117, 149
Silicone caps 173, **8.26**
Silicone synovitis 225
Silver bunionectomy 205, **10.18**
Simple transposition flaps 28, **1.56**
Skin 7
    complications of surgery 238
    extensibility 7
    flaps 21–32
        failure 244–5
    grafts 19–21
    lesser digits 137–8
    marker lines 9, **1.5–1.6**
    retractors 8, **1.3–1.4**
    slough 238, 254, **11.28**
    tension 7
Sliding plantarflexory osteotomy 228–9, **10.48**
Soft tissue damage, lesser metatarsal fractures 121, **6.20**
Soft tissue tumours 183–93
Solitary benign bone tumour 129, **6.41**
Splay foot 126
Split-thickness skin grafts (STSGs) 19–20
Sponsel procedure 127, **6.38**
Stent dressing 18
Steri-strip tape sutures 16
Steroid flare 170
Stress relaxation 7
Stump neuroma (recurrent neuroma) 173, **8.24–8.26**

Styloid process fractures 122
Subtalar joint pronation, abnormal 126
Subungual (periungual) exostectomy 85–91
Sudeck's atrophy 240
Superficial peroneal nerve 43, 196, **2.6, 2.10**
    nerve block 59, **2.29**
Suppan cartilaginous articulation preservation (CAP) procedure 117
Suppan nail technique 140, **7.8, 7.10**
Sural nerve 43, 159, **2.6–2.7, 2.10**
    entrapment 176
    nerve block 57, **2.25**
Surgical ablation 139, 140
Sutures
    reaction 238
    removal 32
    techniques 16–17, **1.24–1.29**
Swelling 254–5, **11.29**
    hammertoe arthroplasty 146–7
    non-incisional nail procedures 78
Sympathectomy 241
Syndactylism 153–4, **7.19**
Synovitis
    detritic 251
    pigmented villonodular 186–7, **9.6**
    proliferative 130
    silicone 225

T-capsulotomy 222
Tailor's bunion 126–9, **6.35**
    associated neuromas 175
Tarsal tunnel syndrome 177–8
Teardrop incision 154
Tendon lengthening 149–51
Tendon transfers 149–51
Tent nail 67, **3.6**
Thermal necrosis 242
Tibial nerve 43, **2.7–2.8**
    nerve block 54–6, **2.19–2.24**
Tibial sesamoid 100
    position (TSP) 202, **10.12**
    removal 102–5, 106–7
Tibialis anterior muscle 196
Tinel's sign 177, 241
Titanium grommets 224
Toe crest pads 169
Total ring (digital) block 61–2, **2.30–2.33**

Tourniquets 238
Trap-door deformity 29
Triangular defects 24
Trochar tip 242
Tropocaine 35, **2.1**
Tuberous sclerosis 185
Tumours
    fibrous 185
    glomus 190
    Kernan's 185
    metatarsal 129–30, **6.41**
    nerve sheath 165
    soft tissue 183–93
    solitary benign bone 129, **6.41**
Turk's test 177

Ultrasound 183
Union, delayed 242

V-blocks 59
V–Y-plasty procedure 14, 154, **1.21–1.22**
Valleix phenomenon 177
Varus toe 154, **7.20**
Vascular impairment
    digital surgery 257, **11.36**
    neuroma surgery 172–3
Vasoconstriction 37–9, 240
Von Recklinghausen's disease 188, **9.9**

Washington monument capsulotomy 104, **5.10**
Web-splitting 170, **8.19**
Webster 30° transposition flap 30, 1.59
Wedge osteotomies 102
    closing 213–15, **10.34–10.35**
    oblique base 129, **6.40**
    opening 215, 228, 229, **10.49–10.50**
Winograd procedure 79, **3.25–3.31, 7.6**
    modified for subungual exostectomy 90
Wound healing, delayed 237–8

Xanthomas 186

Y-capsulotomy of Silver 205, **10.18**

Z-bunionectomy (scarf procedure) 213, **10.33**
Z-plasty procedure 12, **1.14–1.20**
Zadik's procedure 68, 80, 140, **7.9**